A Textbook of Regional Anatomy

A Textbook of Regional Anatomy

J. Joseph, MD, DSc, FRCOG

Professor of Anatomy, Guy's Hospital Medical School, London

First published 1982 by
THE MACMILLAN PRESS LTD
London and Basingstoke
Companies and representatives
throughout the world

Typeset in 10/12pt Press Roman by
ILLUSTRATED ARTS
Sutton, Surrey

Printed in Hong Kong

ISBN 0 333 28911 0 (hard cover)
      0 333 28912 9 (paper cover)

To my wife Carol
and our twins Nicholas and Andrew

Contents

Preface

One must assume that some justification is required for another textbook on human anatomy. Two main reasons can be put forward. Because of the very large changes in the preclinical curriculum there have also been changes in the teaching of anatomy both quantitatively and qualitatively. The introduction of new subjects in many of the medical curricula (psychology and sociology for medical students, genetics and statistics) has resulted in the time spent on anatomy being reduced. Within anatomy itself the amount of time spent on dissection has been curtailed and other aspects of anatomy have claimed an increased proportion of the time spent on the subject. In spite of this it may be said that although other aspects of anatomy have increased in importance, for example cellular biology, experimental and comparative embryology, neuroanatomy, a corpus of knowledge about the topography of the human body together with ways of studying living gross anatomy remains an essential part of the basic knowledge of anyone studying medicine, or any other subject involving the examination and treatment of a human being. After all the changes, gross anatomy, together with some knowledge of osteology and surface and radiological anatomy, can be regarded as one limb of the many appendages which belong to the subject. Hence the first reason for writing another textbook — to give a medical student or doctor, in a fairly brief compass and within the limits of the time available, sufficient information to enable him or her to learn and understand the basic gross structure of the different regions of the body.

The second reason for writing this book was the encouragement by several people to put on record the experience of teaching the subject for more than 35 years. It is possible to make much of anatomy interesting, some of it easy to understand and remember, and a small part even amusing. It is regrettable that one cannot make the whole of anatomy all of these. However, it has been suggested that putting good teaching into written and pictorial form is *nearly* as important as publishing research. The author himself cannot say that his teaching is good. He must leave that to his students, and it is appreciated that good oral teaching does not necessarily make a good textbook. The reverse of what was said about Oliver Goldsmith may be true:

> 'Here lies Nolly Goldsmith, for shortness called Noll
> He wrote like an angel and talk'd like poor Poll'
> (David Garrick, impromptu epitaph)

Modern educationalists say that examinations should be an extension of teaching. They seldom approve of the corollary that teaching should be based on examinations. In fact it is often claimed that teaching should have no relationship to examinations, but since examinations are there, students are inevitably interested in them. Broadly speaking this book, except for some of the clinical applications, contains much of what most examiners expect students to learn during a course in topographical anatomy, and hence what they require for their examinations, written or oral. They are, however, not expected to know everything in this book. It must be added that it is assumed that courses in cellular biology (histology, microscopic anatomy), embryology and neuro-anatomy, together with some lectures on general topics, form other parts of the anatomical curriculum. Reference to these aspects of anatomy are therefore incidental to the main description of the regional anatomy of the body.

It is hoped that the different subdivisions of anatomy are integrated so that students are learning the gross anatomy of a part of the body at the same time as they are learning its microscopic structure and development. Integration between the different preclinical departments, and with clinical medicine is also a feature of some medical schools. Whatever the organization of the curriculum, a knowledge of gross anatomy is a basic essential of medical education. Its importance in the past may have been overestimated but attempts to eliminate it have resulted in its being quickly restored as one of the pillars of a sound medical curriculum.

Acknowledgements

Very few books are the result of one person's efforts. It gives me great pleasure to thank Frank Price (thorax), Paul Darton (abdomen and pelvis), Bridget Hough (head and neck) and Anne Barrett (limbs) for their drawings. I am very grateful to Kevin Fitzpatrick (photography), Department of Anatomy, and Jerry Rytina (reproductions of X-rays), Department of Medical Illustration, both of Guy's Hospital Medical School, for their substantial contribution to the illustrations. The publishers and editors of *Hamilton's Textbook of Human Anatomy* have very kindly given permission for the reproduction of a number of illustrations from that book, and I would like to thank Dr John Keishishian for permission to reproduce figure 148.

I owe a great debt to Margaret Collins for her typing, and retyping, the text and to Elizabeth Horne and The Macmillan Press for their encouragement and co-operation. Thanks are due to them, to Drs Sue Standring and Michael Hutchinson of the Department of Anatomy, Guy's Hospital Medical School, for their reading the manuscript and making many corrections and helpful suggestions and to Dr Nigel Bickerton for reading the page proofs and noticing all the errors which I overlooked.

London, 1981   J.J.

Anatomical Terminology

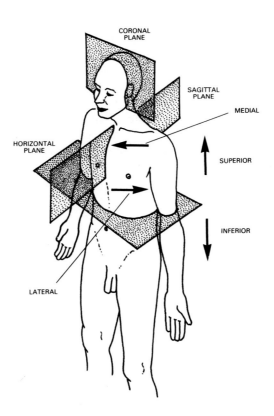

Figure 1   The anatomical position and some common anatomical terms.

In order to facilitate the description of parts of the body and to relate accurately one part to another, a standard position of the body is used. This is the *anatomical position* (figure 1) in which the body is erect with the head facing forwards, the upper limbs are at the sides of the trunk with the thumb pointing outwards, and the lower limbs are together and parallel to each other with the feet pointing forwards. In all relations between structures, the body is assumed to be in the erect position.

The three cardinal planes which are used are the *sagittal* (*sagitta* = *arrow*, Latin), a vertical plane in the midline running anteroposteriorly, the *coronal* (*frontal*) (*corona* = *crown*, Latin), a vertical plane at right angles to the sagittal and the *horizontal* (*transverse*) running at right angles to the other two. The sagittal plane is often called the *median* and *parasagittal planes* are parallel to the sagittal. All vertical planes at right angles to the sagittal are called coronal.

The front surface of the body is *anterior* (*ventral*) and the back surface is *posterior* (*dorsal*). (In biology the term *anterior* means nearer the head.) These terms are also used to describe relative positions of parts of the body to one another, as are the terms *medial* and *lateral* which refer to the midline. The former is nearer the midline; the latter is further away from the midline. For example, in the anatomical position the index finger is medial to the thumb and the thumb is lateral to the index finger. Vertical relationships are indicated by the terms *superior* and *inferior*. For example, the head is superior to the neck. *Cephalad* (nearer the head; *cephale* = *head*, Greek), *cranial* and *rostral* (nearer the beak; *rostrum* = *beak*, Latin) are synonyms for superior, and *caudal* (nearer the tail; *cauda* = *tail*, Latin) is synonymous with inferior. The terms *superficial* (nearer the surface) and *deep* (nearer the inside) refer to the surface of the body on any of its aspects. *External* and *internal* have similar meanings but refer especially to cavities or hollow organs. In the limbs a *proximal* structure is nearer the trunk and a *distal* structure is nearer the fingers or toes.

There are some common terms used for movements. *Flexion* is a forward movement about a transverse axis in the sagittal plane and *extension* is a backward movement about the same axis. *Abduction* is a movement about an anteroposterior axis in the coronal plane away from the midline of the body, and *adduction* is a movement towards the midline about the same axis. Many special terms are used to describe movements at various joints, such as *pronation* and *supination* of the forearm.

In general the terms used in this book are the accepted English translations of or the most recently revised version of the Nomina Anatomica. Frequently terms are translated or explained and common alternative terms, even if eponymous, are given, together with the dates, country and speciality of the individual after which a structure has been named. If it is thought that the first reference to a structure requires further explanation, more information is given, for example a spinal nerve or the term *anastomosis*.

Part 1

The Thorax

1

The Thoracic Skeleton and Walls

The thorax is the upper part of the trunk and contains the heart and lungs and the structures associated with them — the large blood vessels, the trachea and bronchi. The oesophagus also passes through the thorax in or near the midline from the neck to the abdominal cavity, as do two autonomic structures, the vagus nerve and the sympathetic trunk on each side. The phrenic nerves pass from the neck through the thorax to the diaphragm. The thoracic walls, moved by muscles, expand and contract during respiration. The diaphragm, lying between the thoracic and abdominal cavities, makes a large contribution to the changes in volume of the thoracic cavity during this activity. The conical shape of the thorax can only be appreciated after removal of the pectoral girdle, formed by the scapula and clavicle, and the muscles which attach the upper limb to the trunk.

The Thoracic Skeleton

The bony skeleton of the thorax consists of the twelve *thoracic vertebrae* posteriorly, the *sternum* anteriorly and the *ribs* and *costal cartilages* at the back, sides and front. The cartilages join the upper seven ribs to the sternum (figures 2, 3). The upper opening of the thorax is called the *inlet* and the lower, the *outlet*. The *inlet* is formed by the upper anterior border of the body of the first thoracic vertebra posteriorly, the medial border of the first rib laterally and the upper border of the sternum anteriorly (figure 4). The inlet is about 6 cm antero-

posteriorly and 10 cm from side to side, and slopes downwards from behind. This slope is important because it results in some structures in the thorax, such as the apex of the lung, extending upwards into the neck behind the anterior end of the first rib. Posteriorly they reach the first rib.

The *outlet* of the thorax is bounded posteriorly by the twelfth thoracic vertebra and twelfth and eleventh ribs and anteriorly by the tenth, ninth, eighth and seventh costal cartilages where they join and form a continuous border called the *costal arch* (*margin*). The right and left edges of the costal margin form the *infrasternal angle*. The outlet slopes upwards from behind because the sternum is much shorter than the thoracic part of the vertebral column. The transverse diameter of the thorax is greater than the anteroposterior. This is a human characteristic.

The thoracic vertebrae

One may regard a description of a typical thoracic vertebra (figure 5) as an illustration of the basic structure of all vertebrae. It has an anterior cylindrical *body* and a posterior *vertebral arch* which consists on each side of a rounded *pedicle* (*pes = foot*, Latin) passing backwards and laterally from the upper part of the body and a flat *lamina* passing medially to complete the arch (*lamina = flat plate*, Latin). The back of the body and the vertebral arch enclose the *vertebral foramen* (*foramen = hole*, Latin) in which lie several structures, the most

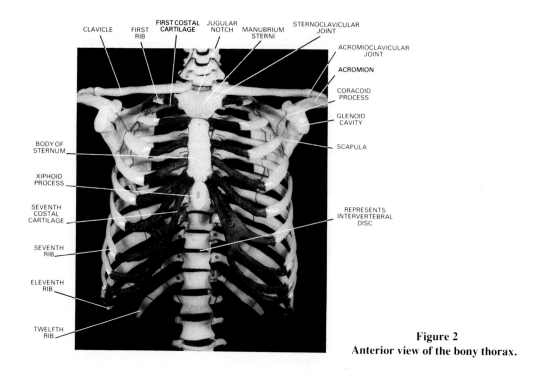

Figure 2
Anterior view of the bony thorax.

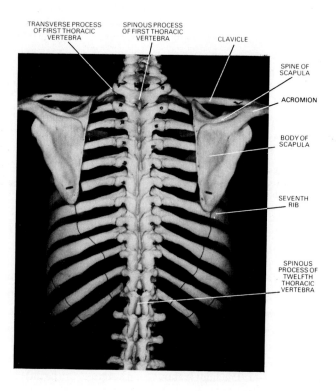

Figure 3
Posterior view of the bony thorax.

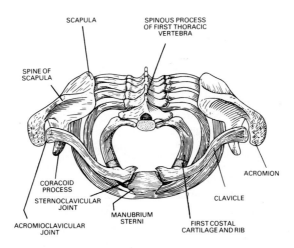

Figure 4   Superior view of the bony thorax and its inlet.

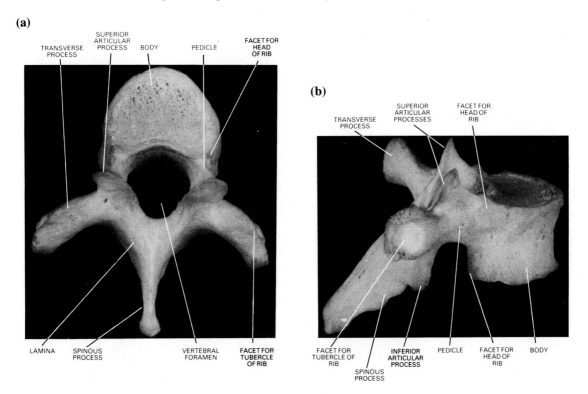

Figure 5   A typical thoracic vertebra: (a) superior view; (b) lateral view.

important being the spinal cord and its membranes. Projecting downwards and backwards from the back of the arch is the *spinous process (spine)* and projecting laterally and backwards on each side from the junction of the pedicle and lamina is a *transverse process*. The *articular processes*, two *superior* and two *inferior*, project upwards and downwards respectively from the vertebral arch. All thoracic vertebrae have one or two facets on the body for articulation with the head of a rib.

This is the feature which distinguishes a thoracic from other types of vertebra. Only the upper ten thoracic vertebrae have an articular facet on the front of the transverse process for the tubercle of a rib. The eleventh and twelfth do not have this facet. Consequently, although a facet on the transverse process distinguishes the thoracic vertebrae, it is the facet on the body which makes it possible to identify all of them.

The body of the first thoracic vertebra has features which resemble that of a cervical vertebra. The lowest three or four thoracic vertebrae resemble the lumbar vertebrae below them, especially in relation to the spinous process (figure 6). They also have only one facet on the body for the rib, unlike the upper eight or nine which have two facets. The bodies increase in size from above downwards. This reflects the weight-bearing function of the vertebral column.

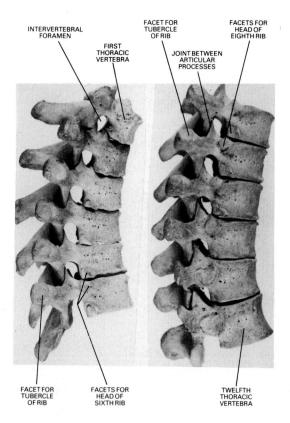

INTERVERTEBRAL FORAMEN
FIRST THORACIC VERTEBRA
FACET FOR TUBERCLE OF RIB
JOINT BETWEEN ARTICULAR PROCESSES
FACETS FOR HEAD OF EIGHTH RIB
FACET FOR TUBERCLE OF RIB
FACETS FOR HEAD OF SIXTH RIB
TWELFTH THORACIC VERTEBRA

Figure 6   Right lateral view of the 12 thoracic vertebrae.

The *ossification* of a thoracic vertebra can be regarded as typical of that of all vertebrae. They ossify in cartilage and there are three primary centres, one for the body and one for each half of the vertebral arch. These appear at about the eighth week of fetal life. The adult body of a vertebra is derived from the ossifying centre of the body (the *centrum*) and also from the adjacent part of the vertebral arch.

At birth a vertebra is in three parts. The halves of an arch unite posteriorly during the first year and the arch unites with the body after the third year. There are five secondary centres, one for each transverse process, one for the spinous process and one on the upper and lower surfaces of the body. They all appear at about 15 years and fuse by about 25 years. The epiphyses of the body are annular in structure. Failure of fusion of the halves of the arches posteriorly results in a condition known as *spina bifida*. This almost invariably occurs in the lowest part of the vertebral column.

Two further features of the thoracic vertebrae, common to all the vertebrae except the sacrum, should be noted. On the posterior surface of the body there is a foramen from which emerges a large vein. This is related to the blood-forming properties of the marrow inside the body. Secondly, if two adjacent vertebrae are articulated, an *intervertebral foramen* is formed, bounded above and below by the two pedicles (figure 6). A spinal nerve emerges from the foramen, the first thoracic spinal nerve between the first and second thoracic vertebrae, and the twelfth nerve between the twelfth thoracic and first lumbar vertebrae. This foramen is related anteriorly to the joint between the articular processes. Disease of these joints is common and can result in pressure on the spinal nerve, although it should be pointed out that this is more likely to occur in the cervical and lumbar regions. Pressure on a spinal nerve results in sensory and motor disturbances along the distribution of the nerve.

Thoracic vertebrae articulate with each other by means of a secondary cartilaginous joint between the bodies, and a plane or gliding synovial joint on each side between the superior and inferior articular processes.

A *secondary cartilaginous joint* is one in which the ends of the bones forming the joint are covered by hyaline cartilage and there is a disc of fibrocartilage uniting the two bones. A *synovial joint* has four basic features: (1) the bone ends are separate; (2) the bones are held together by a fibrous capsule; (3) the fibrous capsule is lined by synovial membrane; (4) the bone ends are covered by articular cartilage which is usually similar to hyaline but may be fibrous. The synovial membrane ends where it meets the articular cartilage. Synovial joints are classified according to the shape of their joint surfaces and/or the type of movement which occurs at the joint. A plane or gliding synovial joint has more or less flat surfaces and only gliding movements can occur. Tilting can also take place but movements are usually very limited.

The disc of fibrocartilage between the bodies is called the *intervertebral disc*. This is the structure referred to in the terms *slipped*, *torn* or *prolapsed disc*. The disc has an outer circular fibrous part called the *anulus fibrosus* and an inner softer part called the *nucleus pulposus*. (The correct spelling of the word *anulus* = ring, Latin, may be with one *n*, there is some doubt about this, but the English word *annular* is always spelt with two *n*s.) If the anulus is torn, and it most frequently tears posterolaterally, the nucleus may bulge out and press on the spinal nerve. Actually this occurs most commonly in the lower lumbar region. Pressure on the nerve

can also occur due to degeneration of the disc so that the bodies of the vertebrae come closer together and the intervertebral foramen is narrowed. It should be emphasised that considerable narrowing can occur without pressure on the nerve.

The structure of the joints between the vertebrae is such that only limited movement between adjacent vertebrae is permitted. However, even a small amount of movement will summate so that the change in position between, for example, the first and twelfth thoracic vertebrae becomes quite large. A bending forwards, flexion, of only 3° between each vertebrae will give a total of 33° between the upper and lower ends of the thoracic part of the vertebral column. Movement in all directions is also limited by the presence of the ribs, and backward movement (extension) is limited by the long spinous processes. The coronal plane of the gliding joints between the articular processes also limits movements but permits a certain amount of rotary movement.

The ribs

There are twelve pairs of ribs (figures 2, 3). All the ribs articulate posteriorly with the bodies of one or two thoracic vertebrae. Anteriorly each rib is attached to a *costal cartilage*. The first seven cartilages articulate with the sternum (*true ribs*) and the eighth, ninth and tenth (*false ribs*) articulate

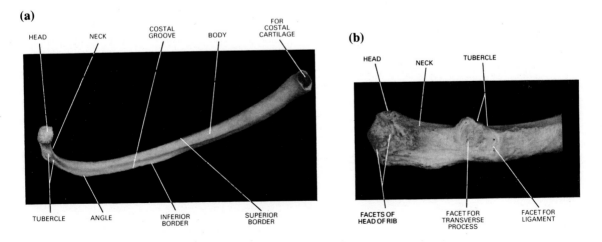

(a)

HEAD   NECK   COSTAL GROOVE   BODY   FOR COSTAL CARTILAGE

TUBERCLE   ANGLE   INFERIOR BORDER   SUPERIOR BORDER

(b)

HEAD   NECK   TUBERCLE

FACETS OF HEAD OF RIB   FACET FOR TRANSVERSE PROCESS   FACET FOR LIGAMENT

Figure 7   (a) The internal surface of a typical left rib. (b) Details of the posterior end.

with each other and form the costal margin of the thoracic outlet (figure 2). The eleventh and twelfth cartilages end in the abdominal wall (*floating ribs*).

A typical rib (figure 7) has a *head* posteriorly which articulates with the bodies of two adjacent vertebrae and the intervertebral disc. Next to the head is the *neck*, about 2 cm long, and lateral to the neck there is a *tubercle* posteriorly. The tubercle has a smooth medial part for articulation with the transverse process and a rough lateral part for the attachment of a ligament. (This is characteristic of the surface of bones — the attachment of ligaments and tendons is usually indicated by a rough area.) The posterior end of the rib continues into the *shaft* (*body*) which after a short distance bends forwards at the *angle*. The shaft continues forwards and downwards and then medially and becomes attached to its costal cartilage. The *costal groove* is on the inner side of the shaft posteriorly near its lower border.

The ribs increase in length and obliquity down to the seventh or eighth rib (figures 2, 3). These are the ribs which are most likely to be fractured as a result of pressure on the chest wall. The site of the fracture is frequently where the rib bends at the angle. The first rib, which is the shortest, also differs from the rest of the ribs in so far as it has upper and lower surfaces, and lateral and medial borders instead of lateral and medial surfaces, and upper and lower borders (figure 4). The second rib is intermediate in shape between the first and lower ribs. The first rib has a number of important structures related to its upper surface. These are described in a later section (p. 231).

The ribs *ossify* in cartilage from one primary centre which appears in the shaft at about the eighth week of fetal life, and from secondary centres in the tubercle and head which appear at about 15 years and fuse at about 25 years.

The costal cartilages undergo calcification and ossification after the age of about 55 years. These changes reduce the resilience of the rib cage and produce shadows on an X-ray.

The sternum (breast bone)

This is a flat bone in the midline of the thorax

anteriorly. It consists of three parts, an upper *manubrium* (*manubrium = handle*, Latin), a middle body and an inferior *xiphoid process* (*xiphos = sword*, Greek) (figure 2). The manubrium, about 4–5 cm wide and long, is roughly square with a marked *jugular* (*suprasternal*) *notch* (*jugulum = throat*, Latin) on the upper border. This is at the level of the second thoracic vertebra. On the upper lateral angle of the manubrium there is a notch for articulation with the medial end of the clavicle. Below this notch there is another depression to which the first costal cartilage is attached. There is a secondary cartilaginous joint between the lower border of the manubrium and the upper border of the body. The anterior edges of this joint project and form the *sternal angle*, or *angle of Louis* (P. Louis, 1787–1872, French physician). This is an important, easily palpable landmark. It indicates the level of the second costal cartilage, which articulates laterally with the sternum at the manubriosternal joint, and corresponds with the level of the fourth or fifth thoracic vertebra. Bony union (*synostosis*) often occurs after the age of 40 years between the body and manubrium.

The body is about 8–9 cm long. It has the second to the seventh costal cartilages articulating with its lateral border; the areas for the sixth and seventh are adjacent to each other at the inferolateral angle. The xiphoid process articulates with the lower border of the body and projects downwards into the anterior abdominal wall. It indicates the level of the ninth or tenth thoracic vertebra.

The sternum consists of cancellous bone covered by a thin layer of compact bone. Samples of the red bone marrow in the cancellous bone of the sternum are taken because it is subcutaneous. This procedure is known as *sternal puncture*.

The sternum *ossifies* in cartilage from about six centres, one in the manubrium and the rest in the body. They appear during the last 3 months of fetal life. The xiphoid process ossifies after birth (at about 3 years). The centres of the body unite with each other after puberty.

The radiology of the thoracic vertebrae

An anteroposterior X-ray of the thoracic vertebrae

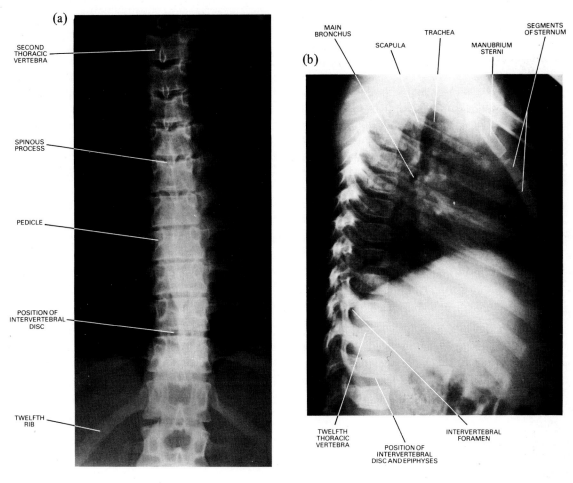

Figure 8   **(a) Anteroposterior X-ray of the thoracic vertebrae. (b) Lateral X-ray of the thoracic vertebrae in a child aged 8 years.**

is shown in figure 8(a), and the individual parts which can be identified are indicated. Figure 8(b) is a lateral view in a child aged 8 years. That the vertebral bodies are growing is indicated by the relatively large spaces between the bodies. This is due to the translucent intervertebral discs and the cartilaginous epiphyses on the upper and lower surfaces of the bodies. The individual segments of the sternum can also be seen.

The Thoracic Walls

The skeletal surface markings

One can palpate the jugular (suprasternal) notch *in the midline at the upper end of the sternum, the* sternoclavicular joint, *where the clavicle projects above the manubrium, the whole length of the* clavicle *and the* acromioclavicular joint *(figure 2). The anterior surface of the* sternum *is subcutaneous and a finger moving downwards from the jugular notch can feel a transverse ridge about 4 cm below the notch. This is the* sternal angle *and indicates the level of the second costal cartilage by means of which one can count intercostal spaces, costal cartilages and ribs. At the lower end of the sternum the* xiphoid process *can be felt. The vertebral levels of the jugular notch, sternal angle and xiphoid process are the second, fourth, and ninth thoracic vertebrae respectively.*

The costal margin *can be palpated as it passes downwards and outwards. Its lowest part is formed by the tenth rib which is at the level of the second or third lumbar vertebra and is only about 5–6 cm above the highest point of the iliac crest of the pelvis. Posteriorly the* spinous processes *of the* seventh cervical vertebra *and* first *and* second thoracic vertebrae *can be seen or felt if the head is bent forwards. The most prominent may be that of the seventh cervical vertebra (*vertebra prominens*) but is frequently that of the first thoracic. The* spine of the scapula *at its medial end is about the level of spinous process of the third thoracic vertebra. The* superior angle of the scapula *is opposite the spinous process of the second and its* inferior angle *is opposite that of the seventh thoracic vertebra.*

The skin

The skin covering the thoracic wall is on the whole typical skin with a variable amount of hair. The amount depends on age, sex and race. Within the male sex there is very marked individual variation which appears to be genetically determined. In addition there is in men an inverse relationship between the amount of hair on the head and the amount on the chest. This explains the advertisements for transplanting small areas of skin of the chest to the head as a treatment for baldness.

The skin of the thorax is innervated mainly by the cutaneous branches of the ventral rami of the *thoracic spinal nerves* in sequence from the second at the level of the clavicle to the sixth at the level of the xiphoid process (figure 9). The *ventral rami* (*ramus = branch*, Latin) of the thoracic spinal nerves become the intercostal nerves. The skin immediately above the clavicle is supplied by the ventral ramus of the fourth cervical spinal nerve. The ventral rami of the spinal nerves between the fourth cervical and second thoracic innervate the skin of the upper limb. It should be added that the skin of the back on either side of the midline for about 5 cm is supplied by the *dorsal rami* of the thoracic spinal nerves, although there appears to be some doubt as to how many spinal segments are

(a)
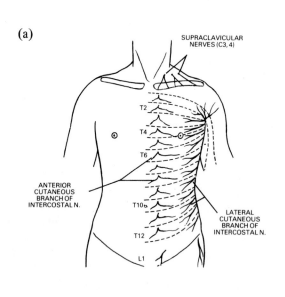

(b)
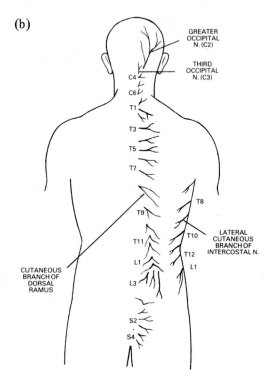

Figure 9   The segmental innervation of the skin of the trunk: (a) anterior; (b) posterior.

missing, that is whether the skin near the midline of the upper part of the back is innervated in such a way that the seventh cervical spinal nerve segment of skin is adjacent to the first thoracic, as indicated in figure 9(b). The area of skin supplied by one spinal nerve is called a *dermatome*.

Spinal and *cranial nerves* form the *peripheral nervous system*, and the brain and spinal cord form the *central nervous system*. The spinal nerves arise by rootlets from the spinal cord and the cranial nerves arise within the skull. There are 31 pairs of spinal nerves — eight cervical, 12 thoracic, five lumbar, five sacral and one coccygeal, and they all are formed and divide in the same way (figure 10). A spinal nerve is formed by the union of a *dorsal root*, which is sensory, and a *ventral root*, which is motor. (Actually a number of dorsal rootlets form a dorsal root and a number of ventral rootlets form a ventral root (figure 10).) On the dorsal root there is the *dorsal root ganglion*, in which are the cell bodies of the sensory neurons. The spinal nerve, which is both sensory and motor, is short and lies in the intervertebral foramen. Just outside the

foramen the nerve divides into a small *dorsal ramus*, and a large *ventral ramus*. These rami are both sensory and motor. The upper cervical ventral rami form the *cervical plexus* and the lower cervical and most of the first thoracic ventral rami form

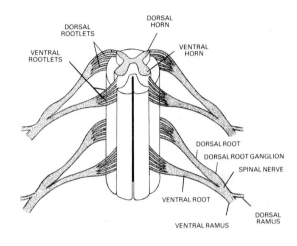

Figure 10   The formation of a typical spinal nerve.

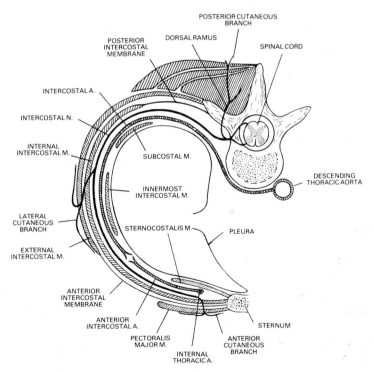

Figure 11   The distribution of an intercostal nerve in the thorax (the lower intercostal nerves end in the anterior abdominal wall).

the *brachial plexus*. The second to the eleventh thoracic ventral rami continue as the *intercostal nerves* and the twelfth thoracic ventral ramus as the *subcostal nerve*. The lumbar and sacral ventral rami form the *lumbosacral plexus*.

In general, the dorsal rami supply the vertebral muscles on either side of the midline of the back, and the skin of the back on either side of the midline for about 5 cm, from the posterior part of the scalp to the lowest part of the vertebral column, the coccyx. As a rule there is no cutaneous branch of the dorsal ramus of the first cervical nerve.

The intercostal nerves from the second to the eleventh give off a *lateral* and *anterior cutaneous branch* (figure 11). The lateral branch divides into two, one of which passes backwards and one forwards. The anterior branch supplies the skin near the midline. In this way the skin of the whole trunk receives a sensory nerve supply because the lower intercostal and subcostal nerves pass into the abdominal wall. Cutaneous nerves contain, in addition to sensory fibres from the skin, postganglionic sympathetic fibres which supply the blood vessels, sweat glands and smooth muscle in the skin.

Clinically, a knowledge of the segmental innervation of the skin enables one to determine the level of an injury to the spinal cord. In addition, a lesion (impairment of function) of a spinal nerve manifests itself as a motor and/or sensory disturbance along its distribution. However, it was emphasised many years ago (Sir H. Head, 1861–1940, British neurologist) that no area of the skin of the trunk is supplied by only one spinal nerve. There is an overlap in the distribution of the spinal nerves to the skin.

The mammary gland (breast)

The breast remains rudimentary in the adult male although it may undergo some temporary changes at puberty. In the female it varies in size and shape in different individuals, and with age and its functional state. On the surface of the skin over the breast, about at its middle, there are the projecting conical *nipple* and the surrounding pigmented skin called the *areola*. The nipple contains circular smooth muscle which on contraction causes it to

become erect. This occurs due to superficial stimulation such as suckling. The nipple has a rich sensory innervation. A nipple may be retracted but this is frequently only an apparent state since surface stimulation causes the nipple to become erect. If permanent, retracted nipples will obviously cause difficulty in suckling. The ducts of the mammary lobes, about 15, open individually on to the nipple.

The areola (*areola = space, area*, Latin) is pink in the nulliparous woman but becomes darker during pregnancy. It contains a number of sebaceous glands which enlarge during pregnancy (*Mongomery's tubercles*; W. Montgomery, 1797–1859, Irish gynaecologist). Their oily secretion assists in keeping the nipple supple during lactation.

The breast itself lies in the superficial fascia outside the deep fascia on the front of the chest. Typically its deep surface extends vertically from the second to the sixth rib and horizontally from the edge of the sternum to the midaxillary line, a vertical line through the middle of the armpit (axilla). The deep surface lies mainly on the pectoralis major but extends laterally on to the serratus anterior and downwards on to the sheath covering the rectus abdominis. The breast extends upwards and laterally into the axilla, the *axillary tail*, which may pierce the deep fascia.

The Structure of the Breast. The breast of a nulliparous woman consists mainly of fat. This varies in quantity and the size of a breast does not indicate its secretory potential. The glandular tissue is in the form of about 15 radially arranged lobes embedded in the fat (figure 12). For this reason a breast abscess should be incised radially. The duct of each lobe is enlarged to form the *lactiferous sinus* before narrowing and opening on to the nipple. Before pregnancy the glandular tissue consists largely of ducts with a small number of non-secreting alveoli. During the first half of pregnancy the duct tissue increases and in the second half the secretory tissue proliferates. Following the birth of the child the secretory tissue produces milk. The breast thus enlarges considerably during pregnancy and lactation. Following the cessation of lactation the breast decreases in size but does not return to its nulli-

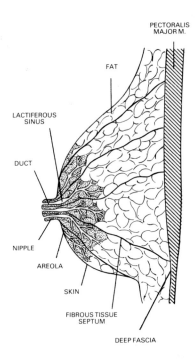

Figure 12   A longitudinal section through the breast of an adult nulliparous woman.

parous structure. After the menopause the breast usually becomes much reduced in size due to the reduction in glandular and connective tissue. Sometimes the breast enlarges due to deposition of fat.

The glandular tissue and fat are embedded in a connective tissue framework. Distinct septa of fibrous tissue pass through the gland from the fascia over the pectoralis major to the overlying skin and the nipple. These are called the *suspensory ligaments* (*of Cooper*; Sir A. Cooper, 1768–1841, British surgeon). If infiltrated by cancer cells these ligaments become contracted and cause pitting and retraction of the skin and nipple.

The Blood Supply and Lymphatic Drainage of the Breast. The breast receives its arterial blood supply from the thoracic branches of the axillary artery on the lateral side and the mammary branches of the internal thoracic (mammary) artery on the medial side. The internal thoracic artery is a branch of the subclavian artery, arises in the neck and runs down-

wards on the inside of the thoracic wall about 1 cm lateral to the sternal edge. Its mammary branches perforate the structures in the anterior ends of the intercostal spaces to reach the breast.

Cancer of the breast is common (more than 10 000 women die each year as a result of this disease). The lymphatic drainage of the breast determines to a large extent the dissemination of the disease and also its treatment, although secondary cancer can also be spread by the blood vessels. The lymphatic vessels of the breast drain mainly to the lymph nodes in the axilla. These nodes, which also receive the lymphatic vessels of the upper limb and the wall of the trunk as far as the umbilicus, are arranged in five groups. The three primary groups, that is the nodes to which most of the vessels drain, are *lateral* along the axillary vein, *posterior* (*subscapular*) on the back wall of the axilla and *medial* (*pectoral*) along the lower border of the pectoralis major on the chest wall (figure 13). All these groups drain into a *central group* lying in the fat of the axilla and these in turn drain into an *apical group* at the apex of the axilla where the armpit communicates with the lowest part of the neck. From the apical lymph nodes the *subclavian*

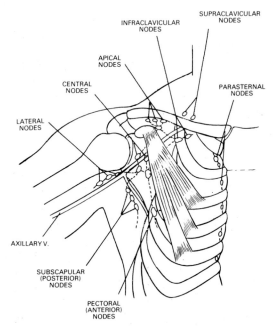

Figure 13   The arrangement of the main lymph nodes draining the breast.

lymphatic trunk drains the lymph into one of the larger veins in the upper part of the thorax.

The tissues of the medial part of the breast drain into the nodes at the anterior end of the intercostal spaces along the internal thoracic vessels.

Within the breast there is a plexus of vessels under the areola, the *subareolar plexus (of Sappey)* (Marie Sappey, 1810–96, French anatomist), to which the vessels of the breast itself go and which drains into the axillary nodes. It is now suggested that vessels also go directly from the breast to the nodes and not necessarily via the subareolar plexus. There is also a plexus of lymphatic vessels on the deep surface of the gland. This plexus was thought to drain into the subareolar plexus. It is said that this deep plexus does not function unless the sub-areolar plexus is blocked.

Other possible lymphatic connections from the breast are (1) with the opposite breast and axilla, (2) with nodes below the clavicle, (3) with nodes above the clavicle, (4) with the peritoneum lining the abdominal cavity through the rectus sheath, (5) with the pleura lining the thoracic wall.

The muscles on the outside of the chest wall

These muscles should be regarded as either upper limb muscles or muscles of the anterior abdominal wall. Anteriorly the large *pectoralis major* is attached medially to the clavicle, sternum and costal cartilages and passes laterally, converging to its attachment to the humerus. Deep to this muscle the *pectoralis minor* is attached below to the third, fourth and fifth ribs and above to the coracoid process of the scapula (figure 14(a)).

The *rectus abdominis* is attached anteriorly to the lower costal cartilages lateral to the midline, the *internal oblique* is attached to the lower ribs more laterally and the *external oblique* to the sides of the lowest eight ribs. All these muscles can be followed downwards into the anterior abdominal wall. The *serratus anterior* is attached laterally to the upper eight ribs, passes backwards round the chest wall anterior to the scapula and is attached to the vertebral border of that bone (figure 14 (a), (b)). Posteriorly the *trapezius* has a midline attachment extending from the skull down to the twelfth

thoracic vertebra (figure 14(b), (c)). Its fibres pass laterally and converge on to the clavicle and scapula. At a lower level and partly deep to the inferior part of the trapezius, the *latissimus dorsi* also has a midline origin, passes upwards round the lower part of the thoracic wall and is attached to the humerus. It is also attached to the lower four ribs.

The muscles are described in more detail with the upper limb (p. 347) and the anterior abdominal wall (p. 69).

The intercostal spaces

The *intercostal muscles* fill the intercostal spaces and pass from the lower border of the rib above to the upper border of the rib below. These muscles are in three layers (figures 11, 15). The outer layer forms the *external intercostal muscle* and passes obliquely between the ribs. The *internal intercostal muscle* is the second layer and runs at right angles to the external muscle. The third layer is called the *innermost intercostal* and runs in the same direction as the internal muscle. The external muscle is membranous anteriorly and the internal is membranous posteriorly. The innermost intercostal muscles are often missing in some parts of the thorax and are regarded as part of a third layer of muscle which includes the *sternocostalis*, attached to the inner aspect of the sternum and costal cartilages, and the *subcostal muscles*, seen between the inner surfaces of adjacent ribs posteriorly. Since this third layer is regarded as similar to the third layer of muscle in the anterior abdominal wall, it is often called the *transversus thoracis*.

All these muscles are supplied by intercostal nerves. Their functions are discussed later (p. 20).

Lying between the internal and innermost intercostal muscles in the upper part of the intercostal space in or near the costal groove is a *neurovascular bundle* consisting of an *intercostal vein, posterior intercostal artery* and *intercostal nerve* from above downwards (figure 15). The intercostal veins drain backwards to the longitudinally running *azygos vein* on the right, and to the *hemiazygos veins* on the left (*azygos = not one of a pair*, Greek). The hemiazygos veins cross to the right to join the azygos vein, which drains into the superior vena

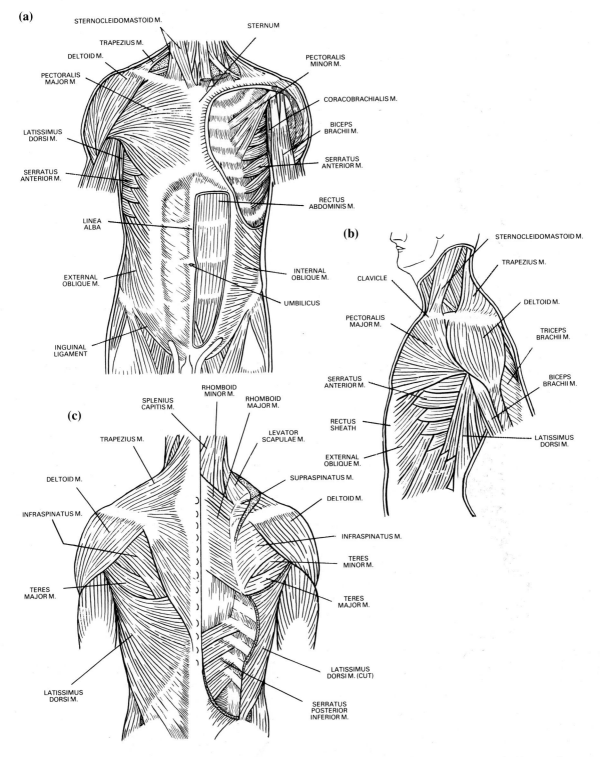

Figure 14 **The muscles attached to the external surface of the thoracic wall: (a) anterior; (b) lateral; (c) posterior.**

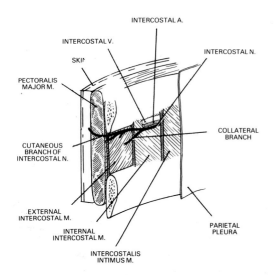

Figure 15   A section of the posterolateral part of the chest wall to show the arrangement of the muscles and the neurovascular bundle.

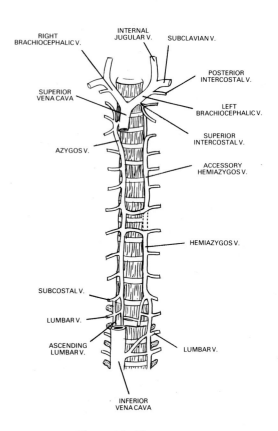

Figure 16   The azygos veins.

cava (figure 16). Since the azygos vein usually begins inferior to the diaphragm and receives blood from the posterior abdominal wall, it provides a possible alternative route for the return of blood from the abdomen and lower limbs if the inferior vena cava is blocked. The veins in the upper three intercostal spaces usually join the large veins in the upper part of the thorax.

The *posterior intercostal arteries* come from the descending thoracic aorta, except for the upper two which come from a branch of the subclavian artery. Passing backwards from the *internal thoracic artery* are *anterior intercostal arteries*. In one type of congenital condition called *coarctation of the aorta*, the aorta is narrowed beyond the origin of the left subclavian artery. Blood can pass from the subclavian artery on each side into its branches, one of which is the internal thoracic artery. Its branches, the anterior intercostal arteries, become enlarged and link up with the posterior intercostal arteries. In this way blood is conveyed to the descending thoracic aorta beyond the narrowing.

The *intercostal nerves* are the ventral rami of the thoracic spinal nerves. (The ventral ramus of the twelfth thoracic spinal nerve is called the *subcostal nerve* and most of the ventral ramus of the

first thoracic nerve passes into the brachial plexus which supplies the upper limb.) The lower five intercostal nerves pass into the abdominal wall so that, for example, the tenth nerve reaches the level of the umbilicus. The intercostal nerves give off *lateral and anterior cutaneous branches* to the skin of the trunk (figure 12). They also supply the intercostal and anterior abdominal muscles. The parietal pleura and peritoneum are supplied by the intercostal nerves.

Reference to the *internal thoracic (mammary) artery*, its mammary branches and the lymph nodes related to it has already been made (p. 13). The artery runs vertically downwards about 1 cm lateral to the lateral border of the sternum and gives off the *anterior intercostal arteries* which run laterally in the intercostal spaces. When it reaches the sixth intercostal space the artery divides into the *musculophrenic* and *superior epigastric arteries*. The former runs laterally and downwards between the diaphragm and the rib cage and gives off branches to the lower intercostal spaces and diaphragm, as well as the pericardium and pleura. The superior epigastric artery passes through the diaphragm near the xiphoid process and enters the abdominal wall where it runs in the rectus sheath.

The *internal thoracic vein* accompanies the artery and receives tributaries corresponding to the branches of the artery. The vein ends in the brachiocephalic (innominate) vein.

The safest and easiest site for the insertion of a needle into the pleural cavity is the third or fourth intercostal space in the midaxillary line. There are no overlying muscles nor underlying organs which could be involved, although care has to be taken not to penetrate the lung. This was the site used for inducing an artificial pneumothorax (air in the pleural cavity) in the treatment of pulmonary tuberculosis. If there is a small amount of fluid in the pleural cavity (p. 23), the sixth or seventh intercostal space posteriorly is used, but entering a lower space than the seventh involves the danger of perforating the diaphragm. In order to avoid the intercostal vessels and nerve the needle should be nearer the lower border of the space than the upper.

If it is necessary to insert a needle into the heart the best site is the fifth left intercostal space 2 cm from the edge of the sternum. This avoids the internal thoracic vessels and the pleura and lung (p.30).

The Diaphragm

The *diaphragm* is a dome-shaped musculotendinous sheet separating the thoracic from the abdominal cavity (figure 17). The muscular part is peripheral and the tendinous part central. The muscle is attached to the xiphoid process (*sternal part*), to the inside of the lower costal cartilages and ribs by digitations (*costal part*) and to the vertebral column (*vertebral part*). The vertebral part requires a fuller description. On either side of the midline the right and left *crura* are attached to the bodies of the lumbar vertebrae (*crus = leg* or *elongated structure like a leg*, Latin), the *right crus* to the upper three and the *left* to the upper two (figure 17). The crura pass upwards and at the level of the twelfth thoracic vertebra cross and pass forwards into the diaphragm. At the side of each crus the muscle fibres arise from the *medial* and *lateral arcuate ligaments*,

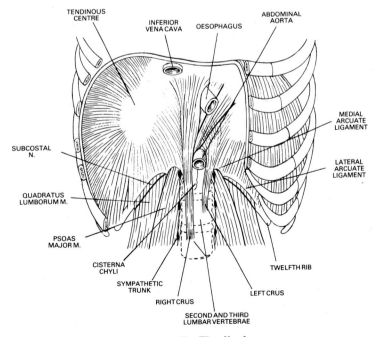

Figure 17   The diaphragm.

thickened fascia over the upper part of two muscles on the posterior abdominal wall, medially the *psoas* and laterally the *quadratus lumborum*. These muscle fibres arch forwards into the tendinous part of the diaphragm. It is important to appreciate that the posterior part of the diaphragm is much lower than the anterior part.

The upper surface of the diaphragm is related to the lungs and pleurae laterally and to the heart and pericardium between the lungs. The fibrous pericardium is attached to the tendinous part and moves with it. The right half of the diaphragm is somewhat higher than the left. Inferiorly on the right is the right lobe of the liver and on the left are the left lobe of the liver and the fundus of the stomach. The kidneys and suprarenal glands are adjacent to the crura and the spleen on the left lies on the posterolateral part of the diaphragm. The inferior surface of the diaphragm is covered by peritoneum except where it is in direct contact with what is referred to as the bare area of the liver.

The Diaphragmatic Openings. There are three main openings in the diaphragm (figure 17). The *aortic opening* transmits the descending thoracic aorta from the thorax to the abdomen where it becomes the abdominal aorta. This opening actually lies *behind* the diaphragm in the midline at the level of the twelfth thoracic vertebra. The thoracic duct and the beginning of the azygos vein on the right of the aorta pass upwards through this opening. The *oesophageal opening* is about 2 cm to the left of and anterior to the aortic opening. Because it is more anterior, this opening is at the level of the tenth thoracic vertebra. The anterior and posterior gastric nerves pass through the oesophageal opening. The *opening for the inferior vena cava* is about 3 cm to the right of the midline and is more anterior than the other two so that it lies at the level of the eighth thoracic vertebra and passes through the tendinous area of the diaphragm. The right phrenic nerve passes through this opening to the inferior surface of the diaphragm.

Additional structures passing through the diaphragm posteriorly are the subcostal nerve behind the lateral arcuate ligament, the sympathetic nerve trunk behind the medial arcuate ligament and the greater and lesser splanchnic nerves through the crus. Anteriorly the superior epigastric artery passes between the sternal and costal parts of the diaphragm.

The Nerve Supply of the Diaphragm. The diaphragm is supplied by the *right* and *left phrenic nerves* which arise in the neck from the ventral rami of the third, fourth and fifth cervical nerves, especially the fourth. The diaphragm develops mainly from a structure in the neck and is pushed downwards by the developing heart and lungs. It takes its nerve supply with it. The phrenic nerve passes downwards in the neck, enters the thorax behind the subclavian vein and passes downwards anterior to the hilum of the lung to the diaphragm. Each phrenic nerve supplies its own half of the diaphragm. About one-third of the fibres of the phrenic nerve are sensory and supply the parietal pleura, pericardium and peritoneum on the inferior surface of the diaphragm. The last mentioned is particularly important clinically, because irritation of this part of the peritoneum produces pain at the tip of the shoulder over the acromioclavicular joint, an area which is supplied by the same spinal nerve as the diaphragm. (This is an example of *referred pain*.) The peripheral part of the diaphragm receives a sensory nerve supply from the lower intercostal nerves.

The Functions of the Diaphragm. The diaphragm is the main muscle of respiration. When it contracts it moves downwards and increases the vertical diameter of the thorax. In respiration it works reciprocally with the muscles of the anterior abdominal wall. When the diaphragm descends, the abdominal muscles are pushed forwards. When the diaphragm ascends the abdominal muscles move backwards. These movements are considered in more detail later (p. 19).

The diaphragm is also involved in activities in which increased abdominal pressure occurs due to contraction of the anterior abdominal muscles. If the activity is associated with emptying a hollow viscus downwards, for example defaecation, the pelvic diaphragm is relaxed and the thoracic diaphragm is fixed. The reverse can also occur, for example in vomiting, in which the thoracic diaphragm is relaxed and the pelvic diaphragm is contracted.

Diaphragmatic Hernia. Although the diaphragm develops from a number of structures, failure of fusion of these structures is not common. If there is a failure of fusion a herniation of one or more of the viscera of the abdomen into the thorax is possible. More commonly, herniation occurs as an acquired condition through the oesophageal opening. This takes two forms. In one, the lower end of the oesophagus and upper part of the stomach herniate into the thorax through the oesophageal opening. In this type (*sliding*) there is interference with the sphincter mechanism at the junction of the oesophagus with the stomach. In the second type (*para-oesophageal*) only a part of the stomach passes upwards in front of the oesophagus and the sphincter mechanism is not affected.

The Movements of Respiration

These movements involve muscles (the diaphragm, anterior abdominal muscles, intercostals and accessory muscles of respiration), bones (the ribs, sternum and thoracic vertebrae) and joints (the costovertebral, costotransverse, chondrosternal and manubriosternal).

The costovertebral and costotransverse joints are synovial and are between the head of a rib and bodies of two adjacent vertebrae, and the tubercle of a rib and the transverse process of a vertebra respectively (figure 18(a), (b)). In the first, tenth, eleventh and twelfth costovertebral joints the head articulates with only one body, and the eleventh and twelfth costotransverse joints are fibrous joints, that is the bones are united by fibrous tissue. The chondrosternal joints are synovial and are between the second to the seventh costal cartilages and the sternum. The joint between the first rib and the sternum is a *primary cartilaginous joint*, that is the bones are united by hyaline cartilage. The manubriosternal joint is a secondary cartilaginous joint (p. 8). During respiration the capacity of the thorax is increased in inspiration when the lungs

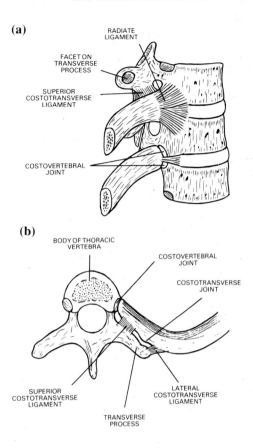

Figure 18   (a) The costovertebral joints. (b) A costotransverse joint.

expand and decreased in expiration when the lungs contract. These changes are due to movements of the diaphragm and ribs. Respiration can conveniently be considered as *quiet*, *deep* and *forced*. Quiet respiration takes place when an adult subject is at rest in reasonably warm surroundings, deep respiration normally occurs during and following exercise, and forced respiration when there is an obstruction to breathing.

In *quiet respiration* the diaphragm has a total excursion of about 1–2 cm (figure 19). It moves downwards in inspiration and displaces the abdominal viscera downwards. The anterior abdominal wall moves forwards to accommodate the viscera. In expiration the diaphragm is relaxed and moves upwards due to the elastic recoil of the lungs, the abdominal viscera move upwards and the abdominal wall moves backwards. In some subjects the muscles

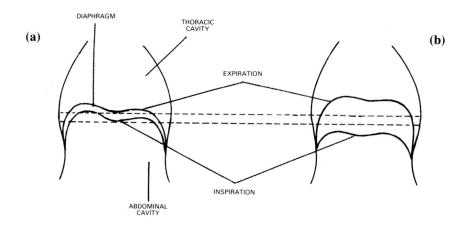

Figure 19 The extent of the movement of the diaphragm: (a) in quiet respiration; (b) in deep respiration. (The dotted lines indicate the excursion of the diaphragm in quiet respiration.)

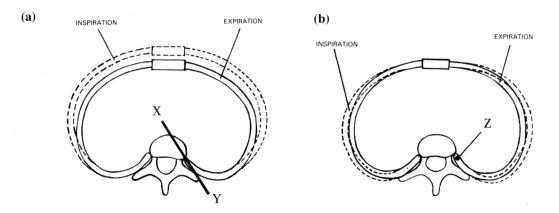

Figure 20 The way in which the ribs move: (a) the upper ribs move about the axis XY (pump handle movement); (b) the lower ribs move about a vertical axis through Z (caliper movement).

of the abdominal wall contract at the end of quiet respiration. Shallow breathing occurs following abdominal surgery because of the pain caused by moving the wounded abdominal wall. This shallow breathing can have deleterious effects on the circulation through the lungs. The diaphragm moves more when the subject is lying down, less when standing up and least when sitting and leaning forwards. If the subject lies on one side the inferior part of the diaphragm moves more than the superior.

In inspiration the upper ribs move in such a way that the transverse and anteroposterior diameters are increased. When the lower ribs move, only the transverse diameter is increased. The upper ribs move about an axis through the head and tubercle (the *pump handle movement* in which the anterior end of the rib is raised and lowered) and the lower ribs about a vertical axis through the neck (the *caliper movement* in which the anterior end of the rib moves outwards) (figure 20). The difference in movement between the upper and lower ribs is related to the shape and position of the costotransverse joints. The upper have curved surfaces and are on the front of the transverse process and the lower are flat and nearer the upper surface of the transverse process (figure 6). The first and second ribs move less than the others because of the slight angulation which occurs at the manubrio-sternal joint in inspiration.

There is considerable controversy as to which muscles move the ribs. The intercostals may be responsible, but many workers using electromyography found no evidence of their contraction. The diaphragm may move the lower ribs which, through their indirect attachment to the lower end of the sternum, can move the whole rib cage. In some subjects the scalene muscles, attached above to the cervical vertebrae and below to the first and second ribs, contract and lift the rib cage from above.

The movement of the diaphragm is responsible for about two-thirds of the increase in the capacity of the chest when standing and about three-quarters when lying down.

In *deep breathing* the total excursion of the diaphragm is about 10 cm (figure 19). There is an increase in movement in both inspiration and expiration. The downward movement of the diaphragm is associated with a marked bulging forwards of the abdominal wall. The upward movement in expiration is assisted by a strong contraction of the lateral muscles of the abdominal wall. This contraction pushes the diaphragm upwards. There is also a marked increase in the circumference in the chest of about 4–5 cm as compared with the 1 cm of quiet respiration. There is a strong contraction of the intercostal muscles in both inspiration and expiration. It has been suggested that the main function of this contraction is to prevent the rib spaces from being sucked in during inspiration and pushed out during expiration. The scalene muscles in the neck are contracted in deep inspiration and this may be the main factor in the increased movement of the chest wall.

In *forced inspiration* it is said that every muscle which can enlarge the capacity of the chest is brought into play. These accessory muscles of respiration, the pectoralis major and minor and the serratus anterior, acting on a fixed upper limb and pectoral girdle, pull on the ribs and attempt to increase the thoracic volume. Experimental work has questioned this. There is no doubt that the scalene muscles of the neck and the sternocleidomastoid muscles, attached above to the skull and below to the clavicle and sternum, contract very strongly and lift up the rib cage. In forced expiration the lateral abdominal muscles contract strongly as does the latissimus dorsi. This is seen in normal activities involving forced expiration such as coughing and sneezing.

Important factors in respiratory movements are the subatmospheric pressure in the pleural cavity and the elasticity of the lungs. If the pressure in the pleural cavity is greater than that of the atmosphere, full expansion of the lungs is impossible. This may be seen in *spontaneous* and *artificial pneumothorax* (air in the pleural cavity). Quiet expiration is largely a passive act and is due to elastic recoil of the lungs. In some diseases of the lungs their elasticity is lost and the result is that deep breathing is impossible because the lungs cannot be stretched and compressed sufficiently in deep inspiration and expiration.

The terms *thoraco-abdominal* and *abdomino-thoracic* were used to describe two types of respiration. In the former the chest wall moved more than the abdominal wall, that is the diaphragm, and in the latter the reverse occurred. Women were assumed to use the thoraco-abdominal type of breathing, as compared with men who used the abdominothoracic type. There is, however, little justification for continuing to use these terms, although by means of training, the relative contributions made by the movement of the diaphragm and the movement of the chest wall to the increase of the capacity of the chest in inspiration can be altered.

2

The Contents of the Thorax
I. The Lungs and Heart

The Arrangement of the Contents (figure 21)

On either side there is a *lung* covered by its serous membrane, the *pleura*. The lungs occupy most of the space within the thorax. The region between the *pleural sacs* is called the *mediastinum* (*mediastinum = the part in the middle*, Latin) in which lie the *heart* in its *pericardium*, the large blood vessels (mostly above the heart), the *trachea* and the *oesophagus*. There are also three longitudinally running nerves on each side, the *vagus*, the *phrenic* and *sympathetic nerves*. The main lymph vessel, the *thoracic duct*, passes upwards through the thorax.

The mediastinum is divided into *superior* and *inferior* parts by a horizontal plane passing through the manubriosternal joint and the intervertebral disc between the fourth and fifth thoracic vertebrae.

The Pleura

The *pleura* is one of the three *serous membranes* in the body, the others being the *serous pericardium* and the *peritoneum*. They are all derived from the lining of the coelomic cavity which becomes separated into the pleural, the pericardial and peritoneal cavities. All the organs of the thorax and abdomen

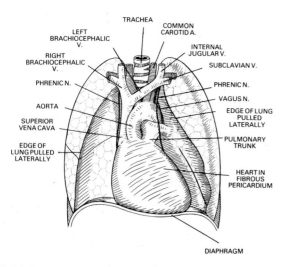

Figure 21   The general arrangement of the main structures in the thorax.

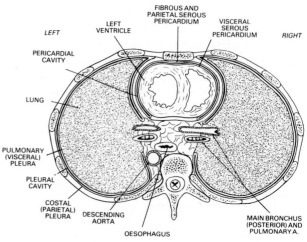

Figure 22   A transverse section through the thorax at the level of the hilum of the lungs to show the arrangement of the pleurae.

are outside the serous membranes and may invaginate them. A serous membrane, as the name implies, is a sheet of connective tissue which produces a small amount of serous fluid.

Each lung is covered by its own pleural sac which has two layers (figure 22). One covers the lung (the *visceral* or *pulmonary layer*) and the other lines its own half of the thoracic cavity (the *parietal layer*; *paries = wall*, Latin). The layers are continuous with each other at the hilum of the lung. The visceral layer is adherent to the surface of the lung and extends into the depth of its fissures. The parietal layer lines the ribs, costal cartilages, sternum and vertebrae (the *costal pleura*), covers the upper surface of the diaphragm (the *diaphragmatic pleura*), and covers the lateral wall of the mediastinum (the *mediastinal pleura*). The apex of the lung is covered by pleura which is called the *dome of the pleura* or *cervical pleura*. Posteriorly this reaches the neck of the first rib but anteriorly, because of the sloping inlet of the thorax, it extends above the anterior end of the rib (and the medial third of the clavicle) into the neck for about 3 cm. The cervical pleura is covered by a fairly dense layer of connective tissue called the *suprapleural membrane* (*Sibson's fascia*; F. Sibson, 1814–76, English physician) which is attached above to the transverse process of the seventh cervical vertebra and inferiorly to the medial border of the first rib.

The mediastinal pleura covers the right and left walls of the mediastinum (figures 23, 24). On the right side it is related to the right atrium of the heart in its pericardium. Entering the right atrium from above is the superior vena cava and more superiorly are the right brachiocephalic vein and, arching forwards, the vena azygos which joins the superior vena cava. The trachea, oesophagus and vertebral column are above the vena azygos. On the right mediastinal wall the vagus nerve is lateral to the trachea and the phrenic nerve is lateral to the superior vena cava and heart. On the left mediastinal wall the arch of the aorta passes upwards and backwards from the left ventricle and is crossed by the phrenic and vagus nerves. The former is anterior to the latter. The phrenic nerve continues

downwards on the pericardium. The left common carotid and subclavian arteries, as they pass upwards from the aortic arch, are covered by the pleura, as is the oesophagus where it lies in front of the vertebrae.

Inferior to the hilum of the lung the mediastinal pleura becomes continuous with the visceral pleura some distance below the structures entering and leaving the hilum. The result is a sickle-shaped fold of pleura passing from the region of the oesophagus to the lung (figures 23, 24). This is called the *pulmonary ligament*.

The costal pleura is continuous with the diaphragmatic pleura along the outer margin of the diaphragm and this marks the lowest limit of the parietal pleura. Since the corresponding border of the lung (between its costal and diaphragmatic surfaces), does not extend as far downwards as the parietal pleura, there is a potential space between the costal and diaphragmatic parietal pleura, the *costodiaphragmatic recess*. The lung in quiet respiration does not fill this recess and is about 4 cm above it. In deep respiration the lower border of the lung moves down much more and enters the recess. There is a similar recess between the costal and mediastinal parietal pleurae anteriorly behind the costal cartilages and sternum, the *costomediastinal recess*.

Normally during respiration the adjacent surfaces of the pleura slide smoothly on each other but due to their being slightly moist they do not separate. When the chest walls move and enlarge the thoracic cavity, the lungs expand with them. There is a potential cavity between the pulmonary and parietal pleurae, the *pleural cavity*, in which in pathological conditions fluid and/or air can accumulate. This interferes with the expansion of the lung during respiration. In the upright position free fluid in the pleural cavity gravitates into the costodiaphragmatic recess.

The loose connective tissue of the pleura contains blood and lymphatic vessels and nerves. The parietal pleura receives branches from the intercostal and internal thoracic arteries. Its veins drain into corresponding veins and its lymphatics pass to nodes on the inner aspect of the thoracic walls. Its

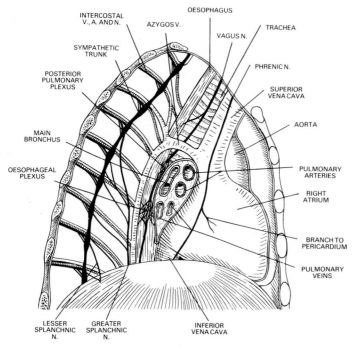

Figure 23   **The right wall of the mediastinum.**

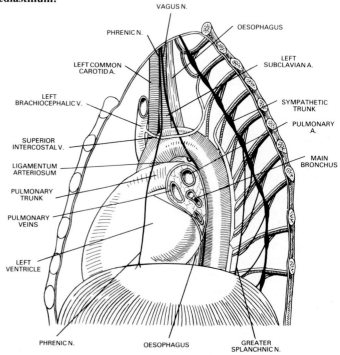

Figure 24   **The left wall of the mediastinum.**

nerve supply is derived from somatic nerves, the intercostal and phrenic. Pain due to irritation of the lower part of the costal pleura can be referred along the distribution of the nerves supplying it, that is to the abdominal wall. The visceral pleura on the other hand receives its arteries from the vessels of the lung, has a lymphatic drainage which goes with that of the lung to nodes at the hilum and is innervated by sensory autonomic nerves.

The Lungs

The two *lungs* are the organs within which gaseous exchange takes place between the air-containing respiratory passages and the blood. The lungs occupy most of the space in the thoracic cavity and are separated from each other by the structures in the mediastinum, mainly the heart and large blood vessels (figure 21). Each lung lies within its own pleural sac within which it is free to expand and contract. Its most fixed part is the hilum, where the structures which enter and leave the lung form the *root of the lung*.

The External Features of the Lungs. The living lung is mottled deep to its smooth surface formed by the visceral pleura (figure 25). On close examination the mottling is seen to consist of lines marking small polyhedral areas, within which are finer lines subdividing these areas. The lines are due to the deposition of fine particles of carbon which have been inhaled and deposited in the areolar tissue near the surface of the lung. In a newly born child the lines are very faint and the whole of the lung is pink. In people who have lived in the country the mottling is much less marked than in those who have lived in industrial areas. Due to its elasticity the lung shrinks when the chest is opened but it does not expel all the air contained in it. The result is that a lung *post mortem* remains crepitant to the touch, produces frothy fluid if the cut surface is squeezed, and floats in water. In an infant who has never breathed, the lung is firm to the touch, does not produce frothy fluid from its cut surface and sinks in water. This is of some forensic importance in determining whether a dead infant has breathed after birth. In the embalmed cadaver the lungs are much firmer to the touch, relatively pale and do

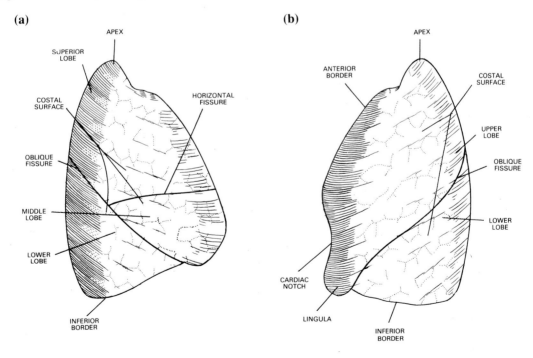

(a)

(b)

Figure 25   The costal surface of (a) the right lung, (b) the left lung.

not shrink from the chest wall. Antemortem adhesions between the visceral and parietal pleurae may also prevent shrinkage of the lungs.

Each lung is cone-shaped with its *apex* superior (figure 25); inferiorly the surface in contact with the diaphragm is called the *base* and is concave. The convex surface in contact with the ribs and costal cartilages is called the *costal surface*. The medial surface is mainly flat and is related anteriorly to the mediastinum and posteriorly to the vertebral column. The edges between the base and costal surface, between the base and medial surface and anteriorly between the costal and medial surfaces, are sharp. This is in contrast to the rounded edge posteriorly between the costal and medial surfaces where a large mass of the lung lies in a deep hollow formed by the sides of the vertebrae and the backwardly projecting posterior ends of the ribs.

The Main Structures Related to the Lungs. The apex projects into the neck due to the obliquity of the inlet of the thorax. It is covered by the dome of the pleura which fits closely over it. The dome is closely invested by the suprapleural membrane.

Posteriorly the apex of the lung reaches as high as the first rib but anteriorly it projects about 3 cm above the medial third of the clavicle. A knowledge of the arrangement of the structures at the inlet of the thorax and in the superior mediastinum (figure 26) makes it much easier to remember the structures related to the apex. The apex is grooved anteriorly by the subclavian artery and vein, and posteriorly, from medial to lateral, are the first thoracic ganglion of the sympathetic trunk, the superior intercostal artery and the ventral ramus of the first thoracic spinal nerve. Medially are structures passing into and out of the thorax. In the midline are the trachea and oesophagus. Medial to the right apex are the brachiocephalic artery and right brachiocephalic vein and medial to the left apex are the left subclavian vein and the left brachiocephalic vein.

The diaphragm separates the base of the right lung from the right lobe of the liver and the base of the left lung from the left lobe of the liver, the spleen and stomach.

The structures related to the medial surface of the lungs are more easily remembered if they are considered in a certain sequence. The heart pro-

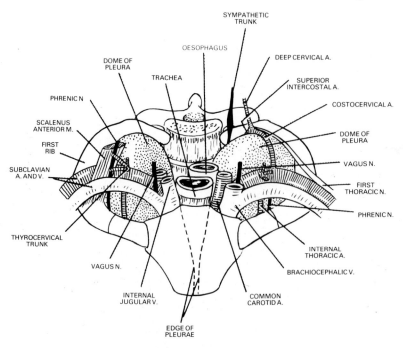

Figure 26   The structures related to the apex of the lung.

(a)

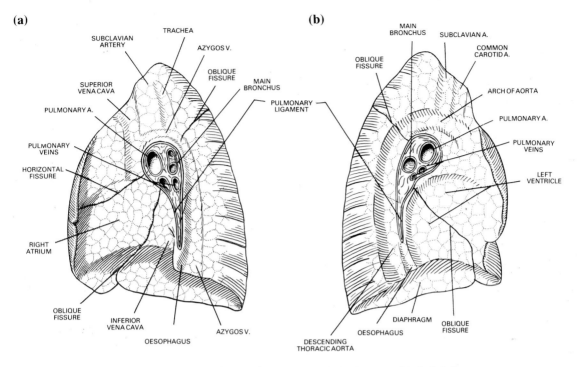

(b)

Figure 27   The mediastinal surface of (a) the right lung, (b) the left lung.

duces a concavity deeper on the left side than on the right. Above and behind this hollow area is the *hilum* where the structures of the root of the lung enter and leave the organ. On the right lung (figure 27(a)) the cardiac area is related mainly to the right atrium and auricle. Vertical grooves above and below the cardiac area indicate the position of the superior and inferior venae cavae respectively. The superior groove is in front of the hilum and a groove arching forwards above the hilum marks the position of the azygos vein. The oesophagus lies behind the hilum and the trachea and vagus nerve are above the groove for the azygos vein.

The cardiac area of the left lung is related mainly to the left ventricle (figure 27(b)). There is a wide groove above and behind the hilum extending to the lower border of the lung. The arch of the aorta and then the descending thoracic aorta lie in this groove. Passing upwards from the groove for the arch are the grooves for the left common carotid and left subclavian arteries. The oesophagus is related to the left lung anterior to the thoracic aorta just above the lower border of the lung.

The hilum is the site of entry and exit of vessels and other structures into and out of the lung. Broadly speaking the arrangement of the largest structures is the same for both lungs, the main bronchus is posterior, the pulmonary artery is anterior to the bronchus, and one pulmonary vein is in front of the artery and one inferior to the bronchus and artery. These relations appear to be altered if the structures are cut nearer to or further away from the lung surface. Nearer the lung the subdivisions of the structures referred to are seen. In addition the main bronchus on the right gives off its upper lobe bronchus earlier than is the case with the left main bronchus and its upper lobe branch. The upper lobe bronchus on the right passes above the pulmonary artery and is consequently often called the *eparterial bronchus*. The bronchus and pulmonary artery and veins are the largest structures forming the root of the lung. At the hilum there are also bronchial arteries and veins which are posterior to the main bronchus, an autonomic plexus of nerves and lymph nodes. The root of the lung is surrounded by the pleura which extends downwards as the pulmonary ligament. Anterior to the root of the lung are the phrenic nerve with an accompanying artery and vein and the anterior pulmonary autonomic plexus of nerves, and posterior are the vagus nerve and the posterior pulmonary nerve plexus.

The Lobes and Fissures of the Lungs. The right lung has three lobes and the left lung has two. Each lung is divided by an *oblique fissure* (figures 25, 27). This begins at the upper, posterior part of the hilum and passes upwards and backwards to the posterior border at a point about 6 cm below the apex. It then extends round the costal surface downwards and forwards to the lower border near its anterior junction with the medial surface and finally passes upwards and backwards on the medial surface of the lower border of the hilum. The left lung consists of two lobes divided by the oblique fissure. The *upper (superior) lobe* includes the apex and parts of the costal and medial surfaces and the *lower (inferior) lobe* includes the remainder of the costal and medial surfaces, most of the base and a large part of the rounded posterior border which lies at the side of the vertebrae. What is more important is that a large part of the lower lobe lies behind the upper lobe. In the right lung there is, in addition to the oblique fissure, a *horizontal fissure* which passes forwards from the anterior edge of the hilum to the anterior border and across the costal surface to meet the oblique fissure in the midaxillary line. The upper lobe is thus divided into a *middle lobe* and an *upper lobe*. The middle lobe is wedge-shaped.

There is one further difference between the right and left lungs. The anterior border of the left lung deviates to the left for about 4 cm at what corresponds with the fourth left costal cartilage and then turns downwards to the lower border which it meets at the level of the sixth costal cartilage. This is called the *cardiac notch* (figure 25). The pleura does not deviate to the left to the same extent so that the heart and its pericardium at this site are covered by only two layers of pleura.

There are thus three important differences between the two lungs — the relations of the medial surfaces, the cardiac notch and the number of lobes. The last mentioned, however, may be more apparent than real since the *lingula* is the name

given to a small projection at the lower part of the cardiac notch and the subdivisions of the main bronchi suggest that basically there are three lobes in the left lung. There are other minor differences between the lungs. The right lung is somewhat larger than the left and the right may have an additional lobe due to a fissure separating off the medial part of the apex in which lies the azygos vein (*azygos lobe*). The base of the right lung is more concave than that of the left.

The Lobar and Segmental Bronchi (Bronchopulmonary Segments)

The lung is divided into lobes and each lobe into segments called *bronchopulmonary segments* which may be defined as subdivisions of a lobe each supplied by a segmental bronchus and all its branches. In terms of its air passages the segments can be regarded as independent structural units. Although each segment has an almost independent blood supply from a branch of the pulmonary artery, the pulmonary veins of adjacent segments are not so markedly separate nor are the lymphatics which form connections between segments. Each *main (principal* or *primary) bronchus* is thus divided into *lobar (secondary) bronchi* and each lobar bronchus is divided into *segmental (tertiary) bronchi*. The right main bronchus gives off the upper lobe bronchus, continues downwards and laterally, gives off the middle lobe bronchus and continues as the lower lobe bronchus. The upper lobe bronchus divides into three segmental bronchi, the middle lobe bronchus into two segmental bronchi and the lower lobe bronchus into five segmental bronchi. Each segmental bronchus has a name and supplies a bronchopulmonary segment (figure 28). The arrangement is different on the left. The left main bronchus gives off the upper lobe bronchus and continues downwards and laterally as the lower lobe bronchus. The upper lobe bronchus divides into two. One is similar to the upper lobe bronchus on the right side in that it divides into three segmental bronchi and the other goes to the lingula (*lingular bronchus*) and like the middle lobe bronchus of the right side divides into two segmental bronchi. The left lower lobe bronchus

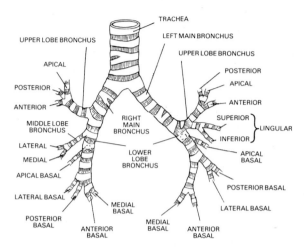

Figure 28 **The main lobar and segmental bronchi.**

divides into five segmental bronchi.

The segmental subdivisions of the lobes of the lung are important because disease may be limited to one segment before spreading to another. This is not the case with disease which spreads via lymphatic vessels, for example cancer of the lung. Interpretation of bronchograms, in which the air passages are made radio-opaque, and what is seen in bronchoscopy require a knowledge of the normal arrangement of the segments. Physiotherapists, who wish to drain one of the segments by different postures (*postural drainage*), need to know the direction of the different segmental bronchi which may pass superiorly, inferiorly, medially, laterally, anteriorly or posteriorly. Surgeons may also remove one or more diseased segments of a lobe.

A segmental bronchus divides and subdivides within its own segment becoming smaller in diameter with each subdivision. The term *bronchus* may be applied to about ten generations of subdivisions and when the diameter of a subdivision is about 1 mm, the term *bronchiole* may be used.

The Blood Vessels and Nerves of the Lungs

The *pulmonary artery* enters the hilum of the lung and divides into lobar branches and then segmental branches. Further subdivisions correspond with the subdivisions of the bronchi and finally a capillary network is formed in relation to the alveoli. The capillary plexus forms venules which in turn form *pulmonary veins*. These do not run with the branches of the pulmonary artery and the bronchioles and bronchi until they become relatively large. Finally two pulmonary veins emerge from the hilum of each lung and go to the left atrium.

The small *bronchial arteries*, usually one right and two left, come from the thoracic aorta or the upper posterior intercostal arteries. They enter the lung at the hilum and accompany the bronchi and their subdivisions to the level of the respiratory bronchioles. They supply oxygenated blood to the walls of the air passages, as well as the walls of the large branches of the pulmonary artery and veins. Some of the blood in the bronchial arteries returns by way of the pulmonary veins. The rest of the blood draining into the bronchial veins comes mainly from the main bronchi, a plexus deep to the visceral pleura and the hilar lymph nodes. The veins end in the azygos system of veins.

There are anastomotic channels (the term *anastomosis* is discussed on p. 37 and illustrated in figure 40) between the bronchial and pulmonary arteries near the smaller bronchi and these may form arteriovenous connections with the pulmonary veins. There may also be arteriovenous shunts between pulmonary arteries and veins.

The lungs are innervated by parasympathetic nerves from the vagus and sympathetic nerves from the ganglionated trunk in the thorax. Both types of autonomic nerve fibres supply the large *posterior pulmonary plexus* and the smaller *anterior pulmonary plexus*. The nerves enter the lung at the hilum and run in the walls of the bronchi and round the blood vessels. The fibres supply the smooth muscle, glands and epithelium of the bronchi and the walls of the vessels. The vagus causes contraction and the sympathetic relaxation of the muscle of the bronchi down to the alveolar ducts and the sympathetic causes vasoconstriction. The vagus is secretomotor to the glands and supplies sensory fibres to the visceral pleura, the connective tissue of the septa and the epithelium of the air passages. Very few of the sensory fibres are sympathetic. The *lymphatic drainage* of the lungs is described on p. 54.

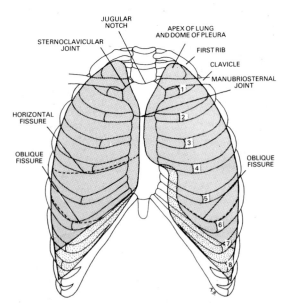

Figure 29   The surface markings of the pleurae, lungs and fissures (dark stipple, lungs; light stipple, pleura).

The Surface Markings of the Pleurae, Lungs and Fissures (figure 29)

The apex of the lung *and* dome of the pleura *can be indicated on both sides by a curved line convex upwards, reaching 3 cm above the medial third of the clavicle. The* anterior borders of the right lung and pleura *pass downwards from the sternoclavicular joint to the sternal angle near the midline and then to the sixth costal cartilages. The* lower border of the right lung *can be followed round the chest along the sixth costal cartilage and rib to the midclavicular line, then to the eighth rib in the midaxillary line and then to the tenth rib about 5 cm from the midline. The* edge of the pleura *is at a lower level and reaches the eighth rib at the midclavicular line, the tenth rib at the midaxillary line and the twelfth rib 5 cm from the midline. The upper pole of the kidney especially on the left lies behind the lower border of the pleura in the region of the eleventh and twelfth ribs. The* posterior borders of the lung and pleura *continue upwards parallel to and 5 cm from the midline of the back.*

The anterior borders of the left lung and pleura *pass downwards from the sternal angle to the*
fourth costal cartilage and then deviate to the left for about 3 cm and pass downwards to the sixth costal cartilage. The margin of the pleura does not deviate to the left as much as that of the lung. From the sixth costal cartilage, the* lower and posterior borders of the left lung and pleura *have the same surface markings as those of the right.*

The oblique fissure of both lungs *begins posteriorly at about the spinous process of the third thoracic vertebra (at the level of the spine of the scapula) and follows the sixth rib round the chest wall to the costal margin. The* transverse fissure of the right lung *is indicated by a horizontal line corresponding with the fourth right costal cartilage and rib from the sternum to where it meets the oblique fissure, usually about the midaxillary line.*

X-rays relevant to the lungs are described at the end of the section on the heart.

The Heart

The pericardium

The heart is surrounded by a double fold of serous membrane, the *serous pericardium*, which is inside a dense connective tissue sac, the *fibrous pericardium*. The fibrous pericardium can be compared with a bag in which the heart lies. The mouth of the bag is superior and fuses with the walls of the large vessels emerging from and entering the upper part of the heart (figure 21). The fibrous pericardium is attached below to the central tendon of the diaphragm, anteriorly to the sternum, and above to the pretracheal fascia.

The outer layer of the serous pericardium is called the *parietal*, and is firmly adherent to the inner surface of the fibrous pericardium (figure 22). The inner layer, the *visceral pericardium*, is adherent to the heart wall and is also called the *epicardium*. The two layers of serous pericardium are continuous with each other where the visceral layer is reflected off the heart wall round the blood vessels. If the fibrous together with the parietal serous pericardium is opened it is possible to pass a hand below and behind the heart. This space within the serous pericardium is called the *oblique sinus* and is limited to the right by the inferior vena cava and above by the pulmonary veins (figure 30).

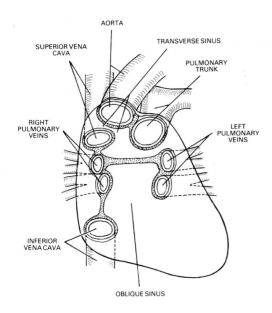

Figure 30 **The reflection of the serous pericardium. The heart has been removed and the large blood vessels cut at their entry into or exit from the heart.**

(*Sinus = cavity* or *space*, Latin, has no specific meaning in anatomy. Often the word is qualified in terms of its contents, for example an *air* sinus or a *venous* sinus.)

One would expect a similar reflection of the visceral serous pericardium behind the aorta and pulmonary trunk but the intervening pericardium breaks down and it is possible to pass one's fingers behind the aorta and pulmonary trunk from one side to the other in front of the superior vena cava and above the left atrium (figure 30). This is called the *transverse sinus*.

The main relations of the pericardium are as follows. The lungs and pleura are lateral, posterior and anterior but due to the left deflection of the lower part of the anterior border of the left pleura and lung, the pericardium comes in contact with the fourth and fifth left costal cartilages. The phrenic nerves, one on each side, lie lateral, and the oesophagus with its plexus of nerves and the descending thoracic aorta are posterior to the pericardium.

The fibrous and parietal serous pericardium are innervated by the phrenic, a somatic nerve, and the visceral by the vagus and sympathetic, autonomic nerves. This arrangement of innervation is common to all the serous membranes. The parietal layer of all serous membranes has a somatic innervation and the visceral an autonomic innervation.

The pericardium moves downwards with the diaphragm on inspiration. The arrangement of the pericardium permits the heart to expand and contract. Its overdistension may be prevented by the strong fibrous pericardium. Fluid in the pericardium or thickening of the adjacent surfaces of the serous pericardium limit the expansion and contraction of the heart and thus limit its functions.

The position and external appearance of the heart

Although the heart changes its position with respiration and posture, one should be able to place the heart approximately in the thorax. *One-third of the heart lies to the right of the midline and its right border extends from the third right costal cartilage 1 cm to the right of the sternal border to the sixth right costal cartilage 1 cm to the right of the sternal border (figure 31). The left border slopes downwards and to the left from the second*

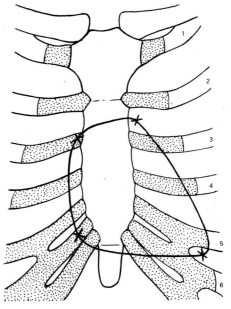

Figure 31 **The surface marking of the outline of the heart.**

left costal cartilage 1 cm to the left of the lateral border of the sternum to the fifth left intercostal space 8 cm from the midline. The last surface marking indicates the position of the apex *of the heart. The* apex beat *can usually be felt here, and is defined as the place where the heart beat can be most easily palpated furthest downwards and to the left. It may not be in the fifth left interspace nor 8 cm from the midline.* The size of the heart varies directly with body size and its shape to some extent with body type. The heart in a child is relatively larger, higher and more transversely placed as compared with that in an adult. In inspiration the heart is lower, narrower and longer than in expiration (figure 42). In the recumbent position the heart is about 2 cm higher than when standing and the apex may move 2–3 cm from its usual position as a result of lying on one side.

The heart is approximately cone-shaped with the apex of the cone below and to the left and the base posterior and to the right. It is about 9 cm wide, 12 cm high and 6 cm anteroposteriorly and weighs about 300 g in the male and 250 g in the female.

The heart has four surfaces, a *right*, a *diaphragmatic* (inferiorly), a *sternocostal* (anteriorly) and a *left* which is also superior. The posterior surface is called the *base*. This is a confusing term and is best understood as that part of the heart opposite the apex, as in a cone, the apex being to the left, anteriorly and inferiorly (figure 32).

There are four chambers in the heart, right and left ventricles (*venter = stomach*, Latin; the word is used for an organ with a cavity) and *right* and *left atria* (*atrium = the main chamber in a Roman house*, Latin). With the heart in its normal position the right atrium is to the right, the left ventricle is to the left and the right ventricle lies between these two chambers (figure 32). The right ventricle forms most of the anterior surface of the heart and extends inferiorly. The right atrium forms the right border, between the anterior and right surfaces, and the whole of the right side. The left ventricle forms the left border, a small part of the anterior surface and the apex but most of it is on the inferior surface. It also forms a small part of the posterior surface. There are two grooves on the anterior surface, the *coronary sulcus* (*atrioventricular groove*) between the right atrium and right ventricle, and the *anterior interventricular sulcus* between the ventricles. The right coronary artery lies in the coronary sulcus and the anterior interventricular artery in the anterior interventricular sulcus.

The *pulmonary trunk* passes upwards from the right ventricle. To its right and behind it the *ascending aorta* passes upwards and slightly to the right. The notched *right auricle* (*auris = ear*, Latin) pro-

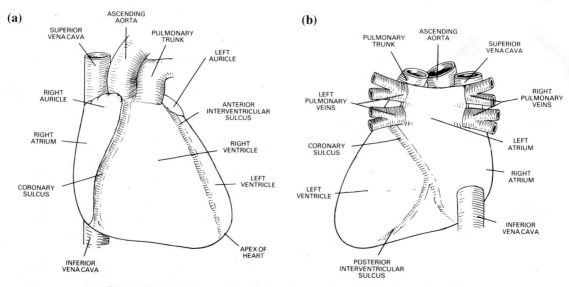

Figure 32   (a) The anterior surface and (b) the posterior surface of the heart.

jects forwards from the right atrium to the right of the aorta and pulmonary artery, and the left auricle projects from the left atrium to the left of the pulmonary artery. (In human anatomy the main part of the chamber is called the *atrium* and the projecting part referred to is called the *auricular appendage* or *auricle*.) The *superior vena cava* passes downwards to the right atrium to the right of the aorta. The *inferior vena cava* is inferior and posterior on the right and enters the right atrium.

When the heart is viewed from behind (figure 32), the *left atrium* is seen to lie entirely on the posterior aspect of the heart. The four *pulmonary veins*, two on each side, enter the left atrium more or less horizontally. Part of the left ventricle lies to the left of the left atrium and part of the right atrium lies to the right of the left atrium. The coronary sulcus separates the atria from the ventricles. The right coronary and circumflex arteries and coronary sinus lie in this sulcus. The circumflex artery is a continuation of the left coronary artery (p. 37).

On the inferior surface of the heart the right and left ventricles are separated by the *posterior interventricular sulcus* in which lies the posterior interventricular artery.

The relations of the heart are similar to those of the pericardium.

The interior of the chambers of the heart

The heart is divided into right and left halves by a septum and each side is divided into an upper atrium and a lower ventricle. The *interatrial septum* between the right and left atria is almost in the coronal plane so that the right atrium is anterior as well as to the right of the left atrium.

The Right Atrium. Its interior (figure 33) has a number of features which are best considered in the following order. The right atrium is divided into a smooth posterior part, the *sinus venarum*, into which the venae cavae open, and a ridged anterior part. The ridges radiate from a vertical line, the *crista terminalis*, which corresponds with the *sulcus terminalis* on the outside, anterior to the venae cavae, on the right surface of the atrium.

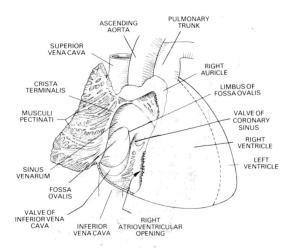

Figure 33   The interior of the right atrium.

The ridges extend into the auricle, contain muscle and are called *musculi pectinati* (*pecten* = *comb*, Latin). The *valve of the inferior vena cava* is a fold anterior to the opening of the inferior vena cava. Its concave free margin passes upwards to the left and is continuous with a fold on the interatrial septum called the *limbus* (*anulus*) *of the fossa ovalis*. The *fossa ovalis* is a depression on the interatrial septum which marks the site of the *foramen ovale*, an opening in the septum of the fetal heart between the right and left atria. The valve of the inferior vena cava in the fetus directs the blood from the inferior vena cava into the left atrium through the foramen ovale. The sinus venarum develops from the sinus venosus and the rest of the atrium and auricle from the atrium of the fetal heart.

On the posterior wall of the right atrium there is a small projection, the *intervenous tubercle*, which lies inferior to the opening of the superior vena cava. In the fetus it may help to direct the blood from this vessel into the right ventricle. The *right atrioventricular opening*, 3 cm in diameter, is below and to the left. Between this opening and the fossa ovalis to the right there is the *opening of the coronary sinus* which returns most of the blood from the heart wall to the right atrium. The *valve of the coronary sinus* is a semilunar fold which lies inferiorly, covers the opening and prevents blood being forced into the coronary sinus during atrial systole.

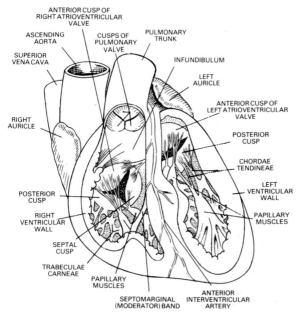

Figure 34   The interior of the right and left ventricles.

The Right Ventricle. This chamber forms most of the sternocostal (anterior) surface of the heart. The *interventricular septum* is oblique so that it forms a posterior left wall of the right ventricle. The septum bulges into the right and is as thick as the rest of the left ventricular wall. The uppermost part of the septum is membranous and not muscular. If followed upwards, the interior of the right ventricle leads into the *infundibulum* (*conus arteriosus*) which is cone-shaped and gives origin to the pulmonary trunk. The ventricular wall is markedly ridged due to the muscle forming columns called *trabeculae carneae* (figure 34) (*trabs = beam, carneae = fleshy*, Latin). Some of these muscles are attached to the ventricular wall along their whole length, some only at their ends and others only at one end. Those attached only at one end pass into the cavity of the ventricle and become attached to the chordae tendineae of the cusps of the atrioventricular valve (*papillary muscles*). The wall of the infundibulum is smooth and is separated from the ridged part by the *crista supraventricularis* which lies between the right atrioventricular opening and the pulmonary opening.

The right atrioventricular opening is on the right side of the cavity of the ventricle and is guarded by the *right atrioventricular (tricuspid) valve.* It con-

sists of three triangular *cusps — anterior, posterior* and *septal*. The septal cusp is next to the interventricular septum and the anterior cusp is between the right atrioventricular opening and the infundibulum (figure 34). The bases of the cusps are attached to a fibrous ring surrounding the opening and are joined to each other. The apices of the cusps project into the ventricular cavity. Fibrous cords attached to the apices and edges of the cusps are called the *chordae tendineae*. The *papillary muscles, anterior* and *posterior*, are attached to the chordae tendineae. The anterior papillary muscle is attached to the anterior and posterior cusps and the posterior muscle to the posterior and septal cusps. The *moderator band* or *septomarginal trabecula* is a muscular band which passes from the interventricular septum to the base of the anterior papillary muscle (figure 34). It contains part of the conducting tissue of the heart. In addition it is thought to play a part in preventing over-distension of the ventricle.

The cusps consist of a small amount of fibrous tissue covered on both sides by a layer of endothelium, the lining of the heart. Except for the part next to the atrium, the cusps are almost avascular. The anterior cusp is the largest. When the valve is closed during ventricular systole the cusps overlap each other and are prevented from being pushed into the atrium by the chordae tendineae and the contraction of the papillary muscles.

The *pulmonary opening* leading into the pulmonary trunk is about 3 cm in diameter and lies at the upper end of the infundibulum. It is above and to the left of the atrioventricular opening. During ventricular diastole it is closed by the *pulmonary valve* which consists of three *semilunar cusps* (also called *valvulae*). Each cusp is attached to the wall of the pulmonary trunk and has a free border projecting upwards into the lumen of the vessel. In the adult heart there are two anterior (right and left) and one posterior cusps. In the fetus there are two posterior (right and left) and one anterior. An anticlockwise rotation of the pulmonary trunk at its origin from the heart produces this change. The beginning of the aorta shows a similar rotation but its cusps change from being two anterior (right and left) and one posterior, to one anterior and two posterior (figure 35). In the middle of the free

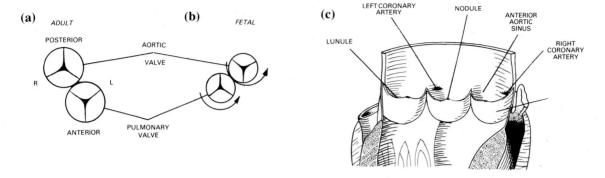

Figure 35   The position of the cusps of the aortic and pulmonary valves (a) in the adult, (b) in the fetus. (c) The cusps of the aortic valve. (The beginning of the aorta has been opened and laid flat.)

border of the cusps there is a thickened *nodule* which assists in closing the central areas of the edges of the cusps. Each cusp consists of a double layer of endothelium containing a small amount of fibrous tissue. The *pulmonary sinuses* are the slight dilatations of the trunk opposite each cusp.

The Left Atrium. This chamber is rectangular in shape with its long axis horizontal. It lies behind the inferior part of the pulmonary trunk and aorta and the right atrium, and extends forwards as the *left auricle* to the left of the pulmonary trunk (figures 34, 38). Two pulmonary veins on each side open into the left atrium. Internally the lining of the wall is smooth except for that of its auricle which is ridged. Almost the whole of the left atrium develops from pulmonary veins. Only the auricle develops from the atrium of the fetus. The four openings of the pulmonary veins, which have no valves, are posterosuperior and the *left atrioventricular opening* lies below and to the left. It is about 2 cm in diameter. The interatrial septum is on the right anteriorly.

The Left Ventricle. This forms the apex of the heart, a small part of the sternocostal surface on the left, and more than half of the diaphragmatic surface. In cross-section, the cavity of the ventricle is circular in shape and its wall is about 1 cm thick, three times the thickness of the right ventricular wall. In other respects the interior of the left ven-

tricle is similar to that of the right ventricle. There are *trabeculae carneae* of the same three types, but they are more numerous and form a denser network. The two *papillary muscles* are thicker. The anterior is attached to the sternocostal wall of the heart and the posterior to the diaphragmatic wall. The left atrioventricular opening, about 2 cm in diameter, is guarded by the *left atrioventricular* (*bicuspid* or *mitral*) *valve* (figure 34). It has two triangular *cusps*, an *anterior*, between the atrioventricular and aortic openings, and a *posterior*, which is smaller and lies behind and to the left of the atrioventricular opening. The bases of the cusps are attached to a fibrous ring round the left atrioventricular opening and their free edges are attached to *chordae tendineae* which in turn are attached to the papillary muscles.

The *aortic opening*, about 3 cm in diameter, lies anterior and to the right of the atrioventricular opening. It is guarded by the *aortic valve* (figure 35(c)). The aortic valve has three *semilunar cusps* with *nodules* and there are marked *sinuses* at the beginning of the aorta opposite the cusps which are anterior, and right and left posterior in position. The part of the ventricle immediately below the aortic opening is called the *aortic vestibule* and has a fibrous wall.

Congenital abnormalities of the heart are fairly common. The foramen ovale in the interatrial septum may remain patent (it remains patent in more than 10 per cent of subjects but usually produces no clinical disturbance) or there may be a larger septal defect. The result is that some of the blood is shunted from the right to the left side of the heart without going through the lungs. Similarly there may be an interventricular septal defect which occurs most commonly in the upper membranous part.

The surface markings of the valves and the propagation of the heart sounds which are related to the closure of the valves are shown in figure 36. The sites where the sounds related to the individual valves can best be heard are as follows: (1) for the tricuspid valve, *the lower end of the sternum to the right; (2) for the* mitral valve, *the apex of the heart; (3) for the* pulmonary valve, *the medial end of the second left intercostal space; (4) for the* aortic valve, *the medial end of the second right intercostal space.*

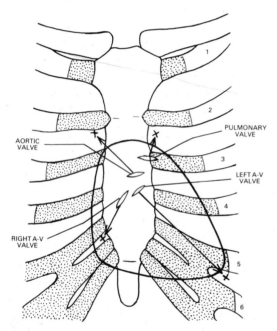

Figure 36   The surface markings of the valves of the heart, the propagation of the heart sounds and the best sites (×) for hearing the sounds associated with the individual valves.

Disease of the valves of the heart is common and can be either congenital or acquired. The mitral valve is the most commonly affected and defects are almost invariably acquired. If affected the valves may be narrowed (stenosis) or incompetent

or both. The normal heart sounds, which are caused mainly by the closure of the valves, are altered. It is therefore important to know the best site for listening to the sounds produced by the individual valves.

The structure of the heart wall

The heart wall consists of an inner layer, the *endocardium*, which is endothelium similar to that lining the blood vessels, a middle layer of cardiac muscle, the *myocardium*, and an outer layer, the *epicardium*, which is the visceral serous pericardium. A *skeleton of fibrous tissue* surrounds the aortic and pulmonary openings and the atrioventricular openings (figure 37). This fibrous tissue is in the form of rings. The ring round the pulmonary opening is the most anterior and is joined posteriorly by fibrous tissue to the fibrous ring round

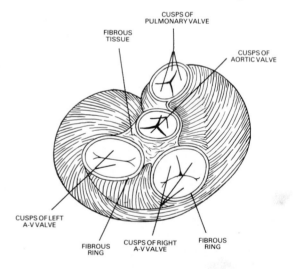

Figure 37   The fibrous framework of the heart.

the aortic opening. The rings round the atrioventricular openings form a figure eight and are joined by fibrous tissue to the ring round the aortic opening which lies anterior to and between them (figure 37). The cusps of all the valves and the cardiac muscle are attached to the fibrous rings. The atrial and ventricular muscle fibres are completely separate. The arrangement of the atrial fibres is relatively simple. The superficial layers encircle the two atria but the deeper muscle fibres surround each atrium separately. Some of the deeper circular fibres extend into the venae cavae. The arrangement of the ventricular muscle fibres is much more complex. Most of the fibres pass in a series of spiralling layers round both ventricles.

The blood supply and venous drainage of the heart

The heart is supplied by two *coronary arteries* from the ascending aorta just above its origin from the heart. They arise from the upper part of the sinuses or even above the level of the free edge of the cusps. The *right coronary artery* arises from the anterior aortic sinus and passes forwards and to the right between the pulmonary trunk and the right auricle (figure 38). It then turns downwards in the coronary sulcus between the right atrium and right ventricle to the lower border of the heart where it passes on to the back of the heart. It continues to the left as far as the posterior interventricular groove where it anastomoses with the left coronary artery. The right coronary artery supplies the right atrium and gives off a *marginal branch* which passes along the inferior border of the heart.

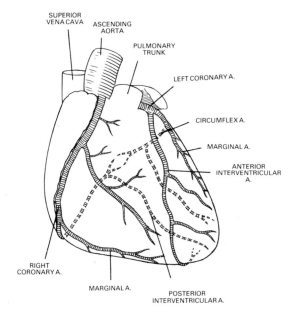

Figure 38 The main arteries supplying the heart.

This branch runs to the left towards the apex of the heart and supplies both ventricles. At its termination the right coronary artery gives off the *posterior interventricular artery* which passes inferiorly in the posterior interventricular groove towards the apex and supplies both ventricles and the posterior part of the interventricular septum. A branch of the right coronary artery near its origin forms a plexus round the beginning of the superior vena cava. From this plexus, in about 60 per cent of hearts, a branch is given to the sinu-atrial node.

The *left coronary artery* arises from the left posterior aortic sinus and passes forwards between the pulmonary trunk and the left auricle. It turns to the left in the coronary sulcus and winds round the left border of the heart on to its posterior surface where it passes to the right and anastomoses with the right coronary artery. The left coronary artery supplies the left atrium and as it turns to the left in the coronary sulcus it gives off the large *anterior interventricular artery* which passes downwards in the anterior interventricular groove towards the apex of the heart and supplies both ventricles and the interventricular septum. The left coronary artery also gives off a *marginal branch* which runs along the left border of the heart. In about 40 per cent of hearts the sinu-atrial node is supplied by an early branch of the left coronary artery.

It can be seen that the left coronary artery follows a course similar to that of the right. The new terminology has changed this. The left coronary artery is now described as having a short course (as far as the anterior interventricular groove) and then dividing into an anterior interventricular branch and a *circumflex branch* which continues in the coronary sulcus and winds round to the back of the heart.

The coronary arteries and their large branches are functional *end-arteries*. An end-artery is one which does not have a precapillary anastomosis large enough to provide an alternative blood supply to a part if the main artery is blocked. An *arterial anastomosis* is a communicating channel or channels between two arteries, before the artery breaks up into capillaries (*anastomein = to provide with a mouth*, Greek; *ana* is a prefix not a negative). There are other types of anastomosis (figure 40).

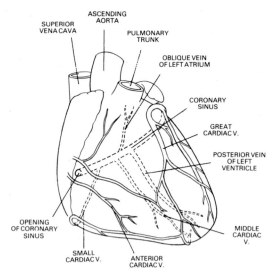

Figure 39   The main veins draining the heart.

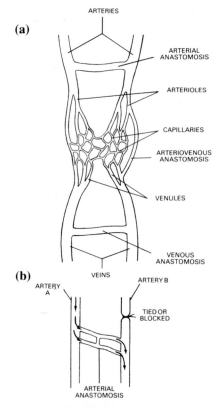

Figure 40   (a) Diagram to illustrate the different types of anastomoses. (b) If artery B is blocked the anastomotic channels from artery A can maintain the supply of blood through artery B beyond the block.

A blood vessel may join a small artery to a small vein, thus bypassing the capillaries. This forms an *arteriovenous anastomosis*. There is also a *venous anastomosis* in which a vein provides a cross-channel communication between two veins. Sudden blockage of a coronary artery or one of its large branches almost invariably causes death. The blockage of a smaller artery causes what is known as a heart attack. There is, however, postmortem evidence that anastomotic channels can open up in the heart if the blockage of an artery takes place very slowly, for example over a number of years. Narrowing of the lumen of the coronary arteries or their branches results in reduction of the blood supply (*ischaemia*) to the muscle of the heart and causes a condition called *angina pectoris* in which the patient complains of retrosternal pain often radiating down the left upper limb. This pain is brought on by muscular effort which requires the heart to increase the blood supply to the rest of the body. The heart is unable to respond to this demand because the coronary arteries or its branches are narrowed. The anoxia of the heart muscle results in an accumulation of metabolites which stimulate the sensory nerve endings in the heart.

Most of the veins draining the heart wall end in the *coronary sinus* which lies in the posterior part of the coronary sulcus between the left atrium and left ventricle (figure 39). It is about 3 cm long and its opening with its valve into the right atrium has already been described. Unfortunately the veins draining into the coronary sinus are named differently as compared with the names of the arteries.

The *great cardiac vein* begins at the apex of the heart and passes upwards in the anterior interventricular groove. At the coronary sulcus it turns to the left and on to the back of the heart where it enters the coronary sinus. It receives a large tributary which runs along the left border of the heart and also receives veins from the ventricles and left atrium.

The *small cardiac vein* lies in the coronary sulcus to the right of the coronary sinus and enters the sinus close to its termination. It receives blood from the right atrium and ventricle. The *middle cardiac vein* begins at the apex of the heart, lies in the posterior interventricular groove and passes backwards to end in the coronary sinus. A large vein called the *posterior vein of the left ventricle* runs on the diaphragmatic surface of the heart to the left of the middle cardiac vein and enters the beginning of the coronary sinus. The *oblique vein of the left atrium*, a small vein on the back of the left atrium, ends in the coronary sinus. It is a remnant of the left common cardinal vein of the fetus.

Some veins to not end in the coronary sinus. The *anterior cardiac veins* on the front of the right ventricle and atrium open directly into the right atrium. The *venae cordis minimae* (the *very small veins of the heart*) consist of a number of small veins opening into the cavities of all the chambers, especially the right atrium.

The conducting system of the heart

This refers to specialised cardiac muscle fibres in the form of aggregations of cells (nodes) and bundles of fibres which are found in certain regions of the heart (figure 41). They are responsible for the rhythmic initiation and propagation of the impulse associated with the heart beat and also coordinate the contraction of the atria and ventricles. The parts of the conducting system are (1) the *sinuatrial node*, (2) the *atrioventricular node*, (3) the

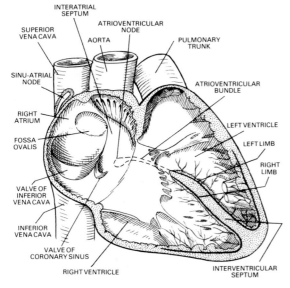

Figure 41   The nodal and conducting tissues of the heart.

atrioventricular bundle with its two *divisions*, (4) the *Purkinje fibres* which form subendocardial plexuses in the ventricles. Purkinje fibres have on the whole a larger diameter than the rest of the myocardial fibres and have extensive contact with one another. They are not found in the atria (J.E. von Purkinje, 1787–1869, German anatomist and physiologist).

The *sinu-atrial node* is about 10 mm long and 4 mm wide and is situated on the right side of the junction between the superior vena cava and right atrium, in the upper part of the crista terminalis. It occupies the whole thickness of the wall. The cells, smaller than those of cardiac muscle, are arranged in a network. This node is called the *pacemaker of the heart* because it controls the frequency of the heart beat. Although there are many nonmyelinated fibres in the node, nerve cells are found adjacent to the node and not in it. Since there is no conducting tissue in the wall of the atrium the impulse from the node is conveyed to the atrioventricular node by the atrial myocardial fibres with which the nodal fibres are in close contact. The sinu-atrial node receives both a sympathetic and parasympathetic nerve supply. Impulses from the former make the heart beat faster. The parasympathetic makes the heart beat more slowly.

The *atrioventricular node* is about 5 mm long and 3 mm wide and is situated in the lower part of the interatrial septum. The node is continuous with the *atrioventricular bundle* (*of His*) which passes towards the interventricular septum in which after a short course it divides into the *right* and *left limbs* of the bundle (W. His, Jr, 1863–1934, German physician). These pass downwards in the subendocardial tissue of the septum towards the apex of the heart. The right limb enters the moderator band of the right ventricle and reaches the anterior papillary muscle where it becomes continuous with a plexus of Purkinje fibres. These fibres are found deep to the endocardium of the whole of the right ventricle and establish close contact with its muscle fibres. The left limb breaks up into several branches as it passes towards the apex of the heart. The cells of the atrioventricular node and bundle and first part of the limbs are similar to those of the sinu-atrial node. Gradually they change into the larger Purkinje cells which are found throughout both ventricles deep to the endocardium. An obvious differentiation of the conducting tissue from the surrounding heart muscle and the histological differences between the cardiac muscle cells and the Purkinje cells are much less marked in man than in large mammals, such as the horse and cow, in which there is a distinct connective tissue covering.

The atrioventricular node has a large number of non-myelinated nerve fibres and a number of nerve cells closely related to it. The fibres are both sympathetic and parasympathetic. It appears that an impulse reaches this node from the atrial muscle and is then conveyed to the ventricular muscle by the atrioventricular bundle. In normal circumstances nerve impulses are not responsible for the propagation of the impulse beyond the sinu-atrial node. If the atrioventricular bundle is interrupted, for example if its blood supply is cut off due to a vascular lesion, a condition known as *total heart block* results and the ventricles beat slowly and rhythmically at their own rate independently of the atria which beat at a rate determined by the pacemaker of the heart. The right coronary artery supplies the atrioventricular node and bundle and its right limb. The sinu-atrial node and the left limb are supplied by either the right or left coronary artery. They are seldom supplied by both.

The nerve supply of the heart

The nerve supply of the heart is derived from both the sympathetic and parasympathetic parts of the autonomic nervous system. The fibres come from the *cardiac plexuses* of nerves, a small *superficial* plexus (inferior to the arch of the aorta) and a large *deep* plexus (behind the arch on the bifurcation of the trachea).

The superficial plexus receives branches from the left sympathetic trunk and vagus nerve (these branches arise in the neck and descend into the thorax) and gives branches to the deep plexus and the right coronary artery. The deep plexus receives branches from the right and left sympathetic trunks and vagus nerves which are given off both in the neck and in the thorax. Most of the branches of the deep plexus reach the heart as plexuses round the coronary arteries but there are some direct branches to the atria.

The preganglionic parasympathetic efferent fibres have their cell bodies in the dorsal nucleus of the vagus in the hindbrain and synapse in the cardiac plexuses, mainly the deep. Some fibres synapse with ganglion cells in the walls of the atria near the nodes of conducting tissue. The preganglionic sympathetic efferent fibres have their cell bodies in the first to the fifth thoracic spinal nerve segments and synapse in the upper five thoracic sympathetic ganglia and the cervical ganglia. Their postganglionic fibres go to the cardiac plexuses and to the heart without synapsing.

There are also sensory sympathetic and parasympathetic fibres from the heart. The sympathetic fibres from the first four or five thoracic spinal nerves are associated with the painful sensations experienced in the condition called angina pectoris (p. 38). Pain is felt deep to the sternum and may be referred to the left shoulder and upper limb areas related to the distribution of the appropriate thoracic spinal nerve segments. It is more difficult to explain pain referred to the left side of the head and neck and to the abdomen. The afferent parasympathetic fibres are associated with cardiac reflexes.

The activity of the sinu-atrial node is regulated by autonomic nerves. In this way these nerves influence the rate and rhythmicity of the heart beat. Nerve fibres without specialised nerve endings are found in close relation to the cardiac muscle fibres, but the function of these nerve fibres in the ordinary activity of the heart is not known.

The radiology of the heart and lungs

A standard X-ray of the chest (figure 42(a)) is obtained with the subject standing 2 m from the X-ray tube with his back to the tube so that the beam passes postero-anteriorly through the chest. The subject is asked to bring his shoulders forwards so that the heart and lungs are obscured as little as possible by the scapulae. The X-ray is taken with the subject holding his breath in deep inspiration.

The structures are examined systematically. One can see the clavicle along most of its length

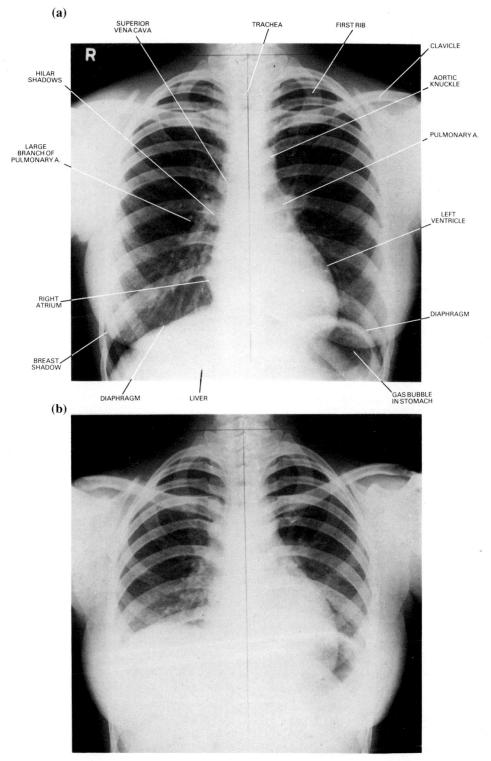

(a)

SUPERIOR
VENA CAVA

TRACHEA

FIRST RIB

CLAVICLE

AORTIC
KNUCKLE

HILAR
SHADOWS

R

PULMONARY A.

LARGE
BRANCH OF
PULMONARY A.

LEFT
VENTRICLE

RIGHT
ATRIUM

DIAPHRAGM

BREAST
SHADOW

DIAPHRAGM

LIVER

GAS BUBBLE
IN STOMACH

(b)

Figure 42   X-rays of the chest: (a) on deep inspiration; (b) on deep expiration.

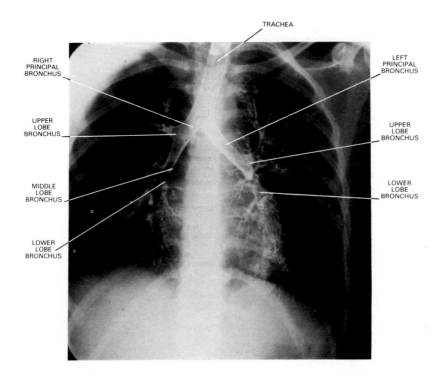

TRACHEA

RIGHT
PRINCIPAL
BRONCHUS

LEFT
PRINCIPAL
BRONCHUS

UPPER
LOBE
BRONCHUS

UPPER
LOBE
BRONCHUS

LOWER
LOBE
BRONCHUS

MIDDLE
LOBE
BRONCHUS

LOWER
LOBE
BRONCHUS

Figure 43   Bronchogram showing the principal bronchi.

and also the upper 10 ribs. The anterior ends of the ribs are much lower than their posterior ends, for example the level of the anterior end of the fifth rib corresponds with the level of the ninth posteriorly. The costal cartilages are not visible in figure 42. They may be seen if they are calcified or ossified. The details of the scapula are not seen and the vertebrae are invisible or only vaguely seen in the upper midline region.

The shadow of the heart is clearly seen. Its right border is formed by the right atrium and the left border by the left ventricle. The size of the heart can be estimated. The upper narrow part of the heart shadow bulges to the left and forms the *aortic knuckle* which is formed by the arch of the aorta. Inferior to this there is often another bulge to the left due to the pulmonary artery. The right border of the narrow part is formed by the superior vena cava.

The translucent lungs are on each side of the heart. The large pulmonary vessels near the hilum of the lung (*hilar shadows*) can be seen radiating

outwards and especially downwards. The periphery of the lungs where the vessels are small show only faint shadows. Circular dots near the hilum are due to large pulmonary vessels seen end on.

In the standard X-ray one can also see (1) the position of the diaphragm – on the right it is the upper border of the inferior opaque area caused by the underlying liver; on the left it is the upper border of the clear area; (2) the gas bubble in the fundus of the stomach; (3) the right and left breast shadows; (4) a vertical clear area in the midline superiorly due to the air in the trachea.

Some of the differences due to deep inspiration and deep expiration can be seen by comparing figure 42(a) with figure 42(b). Vertical and horizontal axes have been drawn to enable measurements to be made. In figure 42(b) the heart is higher, shorter and broader, the diaphragm is higher and the lungs are less translucent. It is more difficult to see that the ribs in figure 42(b) are lower than the ribs in figure 42(a) (compare the seventh rib in the two figures).

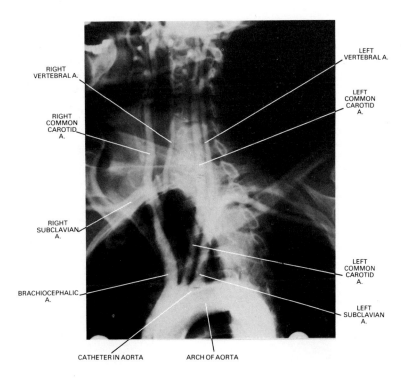

RIGHT VERTEBRAL A.

RIGHT COMMON CAROTID A.

RIGHT SUBCLAVIAN A.

BRACHIOCEPHALIC A.

LEFT VERTEBRAL A.

LEFT COMMON CAROTID A.

LEFT COMMON CAROTID A.

LEFT SUBCLAVIAN A.

CATHETER IN AORTA   ARCH OF AORTA

Figure 44   Aortic arteriogram showing the arch of the aorta and its main branches.

Lateral and oblique views are also used to obtain further information about the organs in the thorax. A right oblique view is taken with the subject standing at about 45° to the film with his back to the tube and right shoulder nearer the plate. In a left oblique view the left shoulder is nearer the plate. On anatomical grounds one can appreciate that, for example, a right oblique view presents the right ventricle as the left border of the heart and a left oblique presents the arch of the aorta as passing from right to left instead of mainly backwards (figure 44).

Special techniques are used to show individual organs or various parts of their structure. These involve the introduction, directly or indirectly, of a contrast medium which may be radio-opaque or translucent. By means of a rubber tube introduced into the nose or a plastic tube into the larynx, a radio-opaque fluid can be introduced into the bronchi and their subdivisions. The fluid coats their lining and makes them visible (figure 43).

This is called a *bronchogram*. Oblique views help to distinguish the different segmental bronchi. The aorta and its branches can also be made opaque by the introduction of radio-opaque material into the aorta through a catheter passed upwards through the femoral artery in the groin. In figure 44 the aorta and its three large branches can be clearly seen (*aortic arteriogram*) and the catheter in the aorta is indicated. The continuation into the neck of those large arteries are visible. An oblique view is required to show the arch of the aorta passing from right to left.

By passing a catheter into the right cephalic vein on the outer side of the upper limb and pushing it upwards until it eventually lies in the right atrium, radio-opaque material can be introduced into the right atrium and ventricle and is seen to enter the pulmonary artery and its branches. Figure 45(a), (b) shows these vessels 3 and 4 s, respectively, after injection of this material.

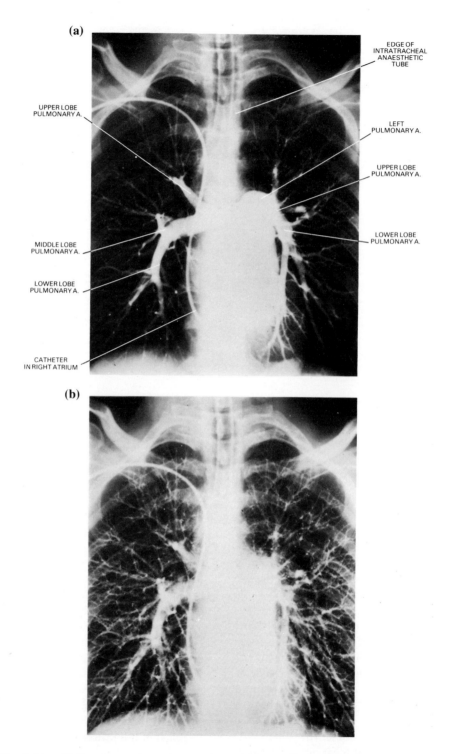

(a)

EDGE OF
INTRATRACHEAL
ANAESTHETIC
TUBE

UPPER LOBE
PULMONARY A.

LEFT
PULMONARY A.

UPPER LOBE
PULMONARY A.

LOWER LOBE
PULMONARY A.

MIDDLE LOBE
PULMONARY A.

LOWER LOBE
PULMONARY A.

CATHETER
IN RIGHT ATRIUM

(b)

Figure 45   The right and left pulmonary arteries are shown following the introduction of radio-opaque material into the right ventricle.

3

The Contents of the Thorax
II. The Remainder of the Mediastinum

The General Arrangement of the Structures (figures 46, 49)

The superior mediastinum lies above the plane through the sternal angle and the fourth thoracic vertebra. In it are the major part of the aortic arch, with the beginning of its large branches, the veins forming the superior vena cava, the vagus and phrenic nerves and sympathetic trunk as they descend into the thorax, the trachea and the oesophagus with the thoracic duct behind it. The general arrangement of these structures is as follows:

(1) The oesophagus is in the midline in front of the vertebral column.

(2) The thoracic duct lies behind the left border of the oesophagus.

(3) The trachea lies in front of the oesophagus as far as the fourth or fifth thoracic vertebra where it divides to the right of the midline into the right and left bronchi.

(4) The left recurrent laryngeal nerve lies between the oesophagus and trachea.

(5) The arch of the aorta is in front of the division of the trachea and the remains of the thymus separate the aortic arch from the sternum.

(6) The brachiocephalic artery passes upwards in front of and then to the right of the trachea and the left common carotid artery lies to the left of the trachea with the left subclavian artery more laterally.

(7) The left brachiocephalic vein runs downwards and to the right along the upper surface of the aortic arch in front of the large arteries and joins the right brachiocephalic vein to the right of the aorta. They form the superior vena cava which runs downwards to the right atrium on the right of the ascending aorta. The azygos vein arches over the hilum of the right lung and joins the superior vena cava.

(8) The right vagus nerve lies to the right of the trachea and the right phrenic nerve to the right of the right brachiocephalic vein and superior vena cava. The left vagus nerve is between the left common carotid and left subclavian arteries and the left phrenic nerve is behind the left brachiocephalic vein lateral to the left subclavian artery. The left vagus and the left phrenic nerves pass to the left of the arch of the aorta with the phrenic nerve anterior to the vagus nerve. The sympathetic trunk lies on the heads of the ribs lateral to the bodies of the vertebrae.

The pulmonary trunk

The *pulmonary trunk (artery)* passes upwards from the right ventricle, lies at first to the left and in front of the aorta and then to its left and is about 5 cm long and 2.5 cm wide (figure 46). *It begins at the sternal end of the second left intercostal space.* It divides into the *right* and *left pulmonary arteries* inferior to the arch of the aorta. The fibrous layer of the pericardium fuses with the tunica adventitia of the pulmonary trunk. The right pulmonary artery passes to the right lung behind the ascending aorta, superior vena cava and upper right pulmonary vein and in front of the oesophagus

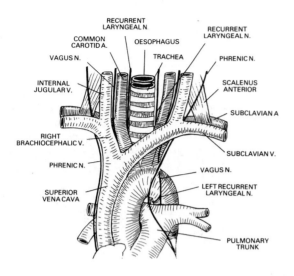

Figure 46   The arrangement of the main structures in the superior mediastinum.

and right main bronchus. The left pulmonary artery goes to the left lung in front of the descending aorta and left main bronchus.

The *ligamentum arteriosum*, the fibrous remnant of the ductus arteriosus of the fetus, is attached to the upper border of the left pulmonary artery and the concave inferior surface of the arch of the aorta (figures 24, 46). The left recurrent laryngeal nerve, a branch of the vagus, lies to the left of the ligamentum. In the fetus the blood from the superior vena cava bypasses the lungs by means of the *ductus arteriosus*. The ductus usually closes at birth due to the smooth muscle in its wall and subsequently becomes fibrous. If it remains patent, aortic blood, because its pressure is higher, enters the pulmonary artery.

Another congenital defect involving the pulmonary trunk is stenosis (narrowing). This may also affect the valve. The right side of the heart undergoes hypertrophy in order to overcome the obstruction. Pulmonary stenosis forms one feature of what is known as *Fallot's tetralogy*, a congenital condition in which there is also a septal defect and an overriding aorta (an aorta whose opening overlies the septal defect with the result that blood from both ventricles enters the aorta). The fourth feature is the hypertrophied right ventricle already referred to (E.L. Fallot, 1850–1911, French physician).

The aorta

The aorta extends from its origin from the left ventricle to its division on the posterior abdominal wall at the level of the fourth lumbar vertebra. At its beginning it passes upwards to the right and is called the *ascending aorta*. It then arches backwards to the left (the *arch of the aorta*), and on the left of the fourth thoracic vertebra continues downwards as the *descending thoracic aorta* to the diaphragm behind which it passes and becomes the *abdominal aorta*.

The *ascending aorta* is about 3 cm wide and 5 cm long (figure 46). *It begins at the level of the third left costal cartilage behind the left side of the sternum and, since it passes to the right, extends upwards behind the lower part of the manubrium sterni nearer the midline.* The main structures related to the ascending aorta have already been indicated – the pulmonary artery is at first to the left and anterior, and then to the left, the superior vena cava is to the right and posterior, the right lung and pleura and remains of the thymus are in front and the right pulmonary artery and main bronchus are posterior. Other features of the beginning of the ascending aorta have already been mentioned – the fibrous pericardium, the aortic valve, the aortic sinuses and the origins of the coronary arteries.

The *arch of the aorta* begins behind the manubrium at the level of the lower border of the first intercostal space and ends at the level of the second left costal cartilage at the edge of the sternum. Its upper border is about the level of the middle of the manubrium.

Because the arch of the aorta passes backwards as well as to the left the structures on the right are also posterior. The left side is crossed by the phrenic and vagus nerves with cardiac autonomic nerves from the neck to the superficial cardiac plexus. The left recurrent laryngeal nerve, a branch of the vagus nerve, hooks round the aortic arch to the left of the ligamentum arteriosum and passes upwards behind the arch. The left superior intercostal vein passes from left to right between the phrenic and vagus nerves. To the right of the arch are the trachea and oesophagus with the left recurrent laryngeal nerve between them and behind the

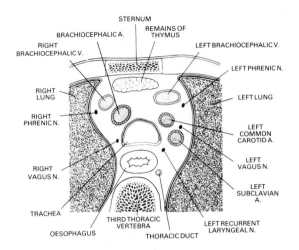

Figure 47 Transverse section of the thorax at the level of the third thoracic vertebrae to show the relations of the main structures (the upper section looked at from below).

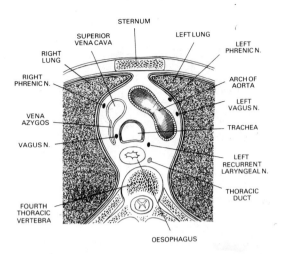

Figure 48 Transverse section of the thorax at the level of the fourth thoracic vertebra (the upper section looked at from below).

oesophagus are the thoracic duct and the vertebral column (figure 48).

The left brachiocephalic vein passes from left to right on the upper surface of the aortic arch. Inferior to the arch are the bifurcation of the pulmonary trunk and the left main bronchus.

The large branches of the aortic arch are the *brachiocephalic (innominate)*, *left common carotid* and *left subclavian arteries* (figure 46). The *bronchial arteries* to the lungs and the *thyroidea ima artery* to the thyroid gland usually arise from the aortic arch.

The *brachiocephalic artery* runs upwards, backwards and to the right. At the level of the right sternoclavicular joint it divides into the right subclavian and right common carotid arteries. At its beginning the left brachiocephalic vein lies in front of the artery, which is anterior and then lateral to the trachea (figure 46). The vagus nerve is on the right of the upper part of the brachiocephalic artery. The right brachiocephalic vein is on the right of the artery and the left common carotid artery is on its left (figure 47).

The *left common carotid artery* has a short course in the thorax before reaching the level of the left sternoclavicular joint and passing into the neck. In the thorax the artery lies in front of and

then to the left of the trachea (figure 46). The left brachiocephalic vein is anterior and left vagus and phrenic nerves are to the left of the artery.

The *left subclavian artery* also has a short thoracic course before entering the neck. The left brachiocephalic vein is anterior to the artery, and sandwiched between the artery and vein are the left vagus and phrenic nerves. As the artery passes upwards it grooves the mediastinal surface of the lung which is lateral to it. The trachea and oesophagus with the left recurrent laryngeal nerve between them are medial to the artery.

The *descending thoracic aorta* begins on the left of the fourth thoracic vertebra and passes downwards and somewhat medially until it reaches the diaphragm in the midline (figure 49). It lies behind the root of the left lung and then behind the left atrium. Superiorly the oesophagus is on its right but inferiorly the oesophagus passes anterior to the thoracic aorta and lies on its left. The azygos vein is on the right of the thoracic aorta and the hemiazygos veins are on its left.

The thoracic aorta gives off branches to the viscera of the thorax — *bronchial*, *oesophageal* and *pericardial arteries*. The branches to the oesophagus supply its middle part and anastomose with branches from the inferior thyroid artery at its

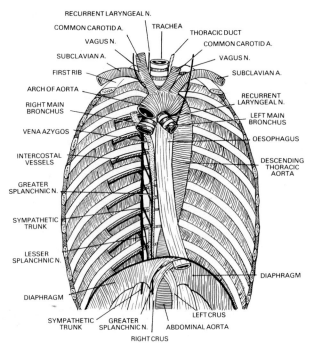

Figure 49   The structures in the posterior part of the thorax.

upper end and branches from the left phrenic and left gastric arteries at its lower end.

Its largest branches are the nine pairs of *posterior intercostal arteries* which go to the lower nine intercostal spaces (figure 49). The right cross the vertebral column and pass behind the oesophagus, thoracic duct and vena azygos to reach their appropriate space. The left pass behind the hemiazygos veins. Both the right and left arteries are posterior to the ganglionated sympathetic trunk and splanchnic nerves. The posterior intercostal artery enters its space lateral to the head of the rib and passes slightly upwards to reach the costal groove in which it runs with an intercostal nerve, and an intercostal vein (p. 14). Anteriorly the artery anastomoses with an anterior intercostal artery a branch of the internal thoracic or musculophrenic artery.

Each posterior intercostal artery gives off a *dorsal branch* which arises at the posterior end of the space, and runs with the dorsal ramus of a spinal nerve and supplies the muscles and skin of the back. The dorsal branch also supplies a *spinal branch* to the spinal cord. The posterior intercostal arteries supply the intercostal muscles and the skin

of the chest wall. The lower intercostal arteries also supply the anterior abdominal wall.

The *subcostal artery* is in series with the posterior intercostal and runs laterally, inferior to the twelfth rib on the posterior abdominal wall after passing below the lateral arcuate ligament. The subcostal artery then enters the abdominal wall.

The veins

The sternoclavicular joint is an important landmark because it indicates the entry and exit of the large arteries and veins from the thorax to the neck (figure 50). The brachiocephalic veins are formed by the union of the subclavian and internal jugular veins behind the sternoclavicular joint. The *right brachiocephalic vein descends perpendicularly for about 2.5 cm to the level of the first right intercostal space at the edge of the sternum where it is joined by the left brachiocephalic vein to form the superior vena cava* (figure 50). The *left brachiocephalic vein* as it passes downwards to the right lies on the upper surface of the arch of the aorta and crosses anterior to the large branches of the arch. The remains of the thymus separate it from the sternum. The right phrenic nerve is posterolateral to the right brachiocephalic vein and the left phrenic and vagus nerves run downwards behind the left vein. On both sides the internal thoracic

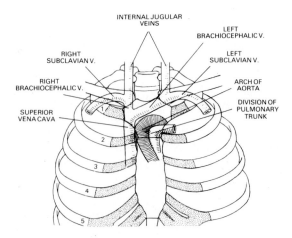

Figure 50   The surface markings of the pulmonary trunk, ascending aorta, arch of the aorta, brachiocephalic veins and superior vena cava.

artery is posterior to the beginning of the veins.

Each vein receives the vertebral and internal thoracic veins. Both inferior thyroid veins usually end in the left brachiocephalic vein. Some of the veins in the upper intercostal spaces go to the brachiocephalic veins. The thoracic duct on the left and the right lymph duct on the right end at the commencement of the respective brachiocephalic veins.

The *superior vena cava* is about 7 cm long and descends vertically *from the first right intercostal space next to the sternum, to the third right intercostal space*, at which level it enters the upper posterior part of the right atrium (figures 46, 50). The superior vena cava is overlapped anteriorly by the right lung and pleura which separate it from the internal thoracic artery and costal cartilages. The right phrenic nerve is to its right and the ascending aorta to its left. The root of the lung is behind the superior vena cava. It is joined by the azygos vein which arches forwards above the root of the lung.

The *azygos vein*, which passes upwards on the right of the front of the thoracic vertebral bodies, has already been described (p. 14). There is considerable variation in the way it begins above or below the diaphragm but its communications with the lumbar veins and the inferior vena cava are important. The thoracic duct and the descending thoracic aorta lie to the left of the azygos vein, and where it arches over the root of the lung, the oesophagus, trachea and right vagus nerve lie to its left. The right posterior intercostal arteries pass behind the vein. The azygos vein receives the hemiazygos veins from the left and also all the right posterior intercostal veins directly or indirectly. (The first may go to the right brachiocephalic vein.) It also receives bronchial, oesophageal and mediastinal veins.

The *hemiazygos* and *accessory hemiazygos veins* are on the left of the front of the thoracic vertebral bodies. The latter receives the veins from the fourth to the eighth left intercostal spaces and the former the veins from the lower intercostal spaces. (The veins from the upper three intercostal spaces go to the left brachiocephalic vein.) Both hemiazygos veins cross to the right behind the oesophagus and join the azygos vein. The hemiazygos veins

also connect the veins of the abdomen with the superior vena cava (figure 16).

The nerves and nerve plexuses

The *right phrenic nerve* enters the thorax between the subclavian artery and vein, passes medial to the internal thoracic artery and descends lateral to the right brachiocephalic vein, the superior vena cava and the right atrium (figure 46). As it does so it lies in front of the root of the lung. The nerve passes through the vena caval opening in the diaphragm and supplies the muscle of the diaphragm. Many of the fibres in the phrenic nerve are sensory and are distributed to the fibrous pericardium, parietal pleura and peritoneum on the inferior surface of the diaphragm. The latter branches are important because pain due to inflammation of the peritoneum on the inferior surface of the diaphragm can be referred to the tip of the shoulder. The phrenic nerve is formed by branches of the ventral rami of the third, fourth and fifth cervical nerves and the skin over the tip of the shoulder is supplied by cutaneous branches of the fourth cervical nerve.

The *left phrenic nerve* enters the thorax between the left subclavian and left common carotid arteries and is crossed anteriorly by the left brachiocephalic vein (figure 46). The nerve then runs forwards in front of the vagus nerve and runs downwards to the left of the arch of the aorta. It passes in front of the root of the lung and lateral to the left ventricle to reach the diaphragm. The distribution of the left phrenic nerve is similar to that of the right. Each phrenic nerve supplies its own half of the diaphragm. If one phrenic nerve is interrupted (crushing the phrenic nerve used to be a fairly common operation in the treatment of pulmonary tuberculosis) only the corresponding half of the diaphragm is paralysed.

The *right vagus nerve* enters the thorax in front of the subclavian artery and behind the subclavian vein (figure 46). It becomes deeper in position and passes medially to run downwards along the right surface of the trachea behind the superior vena cava. The nerve goes behind the right bronchus to the posterior pulmonary plexus where it breaks up. It continues as two or three branches and passes downwards to the posterior part of the oesophageal plexus. From this plexus the nerve re-forms and enters the abdomen through the oesophageal opening as the *posterior gastric nerve*.

The *left vagus nerve* enters the thorax between the left common carotid and left subclavian arteries (figure 46). It passes downwards behind the left brachiocephalic vein and then to the left of the aortic arch behind the phrenic nerve. At the lower border of the arch, the vagus nerve gives off the left *recurrent laryngeal nerve* which passes backwards lateral to the ligamentum arteriosum and runs upwards behind the arch. The left recurrent laryngeal nerve has a different origin from that of the right for embryological reasons. Both nerves arise distal to the sixth arch artery and pass upwards behind it. On the right almost the whole of the sixth arch artery disappears. On both sides the fifth arch artery does not develop. The result is that on the right the recurrent laryngeal nerve hooks round the fourth arch which becomes the subclavian artery. On the left the sixth arch artery persists as part of the left pulmonary artery and the ligamentum arteriosum which joins it to the aortic arch. The result is that the left recurrent laryngeal nerve hooks round the arch of the aorta lateral to the ligamentum arteriosum.

The main trunk of the vagus nerve passes behind the root of the lung to the posterior pulmonary plexus from which branches pass to the anterior part of the oesophageal plexus. The nerve re-forms and passes through the oesophageal opening of the diaphragm anterior to the oesophagus as the *anterior gastric nerve*.

Each vagus nerve gives branches to the posterior and anterior pulmonary plexuses of its own side. Both nerves give branches to the deep cardiac plexus and the oesophageal plexus. The left recurrent laryngeal nerve gives branches to the deep cardiac plexus, trachea and oesophagus. The vagal fibres are mainly motor parasympathetic and produce contraction of the smooth muscle of the trachea, oesophagus and lung and slow the rate of contraction of the heart. The vagus nerves are also secretomotor to the glands of the trachea, bronchi, lungs and oesophagus and supply sensory fibres to these organs.

The *thoracic part* of the *sympathetic nerve trunk* (figure 49) on each side is continuous above with the cervical sympathetic trunk and below with the lumbar part, as the nerve trunk passes downwards behind the medial arcuate ligament which is attached to the body and transverse process of the first lumbar vertebra. The thoracic part of the trunk consists of a series of *ganglia*, 11 or 12 in number, joined by vertically running fibres. The upper ganglia lie on the heads of the ribs, the lower more medially on the sides of the bodies of the vertebrae. The first ganglion is often fused with the inferior cervical ganglion.

The trunk is joined to each intercostal nerve by a *white ramus communicans* and a *grey ramus communicans*. The white are preganglionic fibres and the grey are postganglionic. The preganglionic fibres have their cell bodies in the lateral horn of the thoracic spinal cord and leave the spinal cord in the ventral roots. They pass into the thoracic spinal nerves and then into their ventral rami which become the intercostal nerves. They leave the intercostal nerves as the white rami communicantes and join the ganglionated trunk. In the trunk they may (1) synapse in a ganglion at the same level; (2) pass upwards and synapse in a ganglion higher up, for example a cervical ganglion; (3) pass downwards and synapse in a ganglion at a lower level, for example a lumbar ganglion; (4) leave the trunk without synapsing (figure 52). The last are seen as the *splanchnic nerves* arising from the thoracic sympathetic trunk, the *greater* from the fifth to the ninth ganglia, the *lesser* from the tenth and eleventh and the *least* from the lowest ganglion (figure 49). These nerves pass downwards medial to the main trunk, enter the abdomen by piercing the crura of the diaphragm and join one of the abdominal sympathetic ganglia or suprarenal gland.

The second to the fifth ganglia give branches to the deep cardiac plexus and the second to the fourth to the pulmonary plexuses. The ascending aorta and arch of the aorta receive branches from the upper ganglia and the descending thoracic aorta from the lower ganglia.

The autonomic nerve plexuses in the thorax have already been referred to. There are two *cardiac plexuses*, a smaller superficial in the concavity of the arch of the aorta and a larger deep plexus behind the arch of the aorta on the bifurcation of the trachea. These plexuses are described on p. 40.

There are two *pulmonary plexuses* on each side, a larger *posterior* behind the hilum of the lung and a smaller *anterior* in front of the hilum. The posterior pulmonary plexus receives preganglionic branches from the vagus nerve and postganglionic branches from the second to the fourth or fifth thoracic sympathetic ganglia. The anterior pulmonary plexus receives branches from the vagus and the superficial and deep cardiac plexuses. Branches from the plexuses pass to the lungs along the bronchi and blood vessels and reach the visceral pleura. The motor vagal fibres cause the smooth muscle of the bronchi to contract and are secretomotor to the mucous glands. The motor sympathetic fibres cause the bronchial muscle to relax and are vasoconstrictor. There are also vagal and sympathetic sensory fibres to the lungs and visceral pleura.

The *oesophageal plexus* is mainly round the lower part of the oesophagus and is divided into an anterior and posterior part. The anterior part receives most of the left vagus and the posterior part most of the right vagus. The oesophageal plexuses continue into the abdomen, the anterior, mainly the left vagus, as the *anterior gastric nerves* (*anterior vagal trunk*), and the posterior mainly the right vagus, as the *posterior gastric nerves* (*posterior vagal trunk*). The oesophageal plexus also receives branches from the sympathetic trunk. The motor vagal fibres produce contraction of the smooth muscle of the oesophagus and are secretomotor to the oesophageal glands. The motor sympathetic fibres cause the circular muscle at the lower end of the oesophagus to contract.

The trachea, main bronchi and oesophagus

The *trachea* enters the thorax in the midline and lies much more deeply than it does in the neck where it is subcutaneous. The trachea is in front of the oesophagus but deviates a little to the right and divides at the level of the fourth or fifth thoracic vertebra into the right and left *principal* (*main*) *bronchi* (figure 49). This level is the same as that of the sternal angle anteriorly. The aortic arch is in front of the division of the trachea. Higher up, the brachiocephalic artery is on the right and the left common carotid artery on the left of the trachea.

The left brachiocephalic vein crosses from the left to the right in front of the trachea and the remains of the thymus separate the trachea from the sternum. The right vagus nerve lies on the right side of the trachea and the left recurrent laryngeal nerve runs upwards between the trachea and oesophagus. The tracheobronchial lymph nodes and the deep cardiac plexus are related to the division of the trachea.

The trachea consists of connective tissue in which there are about 20 C-shaped rings of hyaline cartilage with their open part posterior. The *carina*, a landmark in bronchoscopy, is a projection between the main bronchi which is formed by a backward hook-like process of the lower border of the last tracheal cartilage. Between the posterior ends of the cartilages there is smooth muscle supplied by the left recurrent laryngeal nerve which is also sensory to the trachea. The inferior thyroid artery supplies the trachea. Its lymphatic drainage is given in table 1, p. 54.

The *right main bronchus* is shorter, wider and more vertical than the left. Foreign bodies tend to go down into the right main bronchus because it is more vertical. The right bronchus, about 2.5 cm long, gives off the upper lobe bronchus before entering the lung. The main bronchus is behind the right pulmonary artery and superior vena cava and below the arch of the aorta. A pulmonary vein lies below the bronchus. The ascending aorta is in front of the pulmonary artery and main bronchus and the azygos vein is behind and then above the right bronchus. The *left main bronchus*, about 5 cm long, passes to the left lung behind the left pulmonary artery and in front of the descending thoracic aorta. Because the trachea deviates to the right of the oesophagus, the left bronchus is anterolateral to the oesophagus. Unlike the right, the left bronchus divides *after* it has entered the hilum of the lung. Each main bronchus has an autonomic plexus of nerves behind it. There are many lymph nodes related to the main bronchi.

The main bronchi have a similar structure to that of the trachea but the cartilage is often in the form of a short spiral. Vagal and sympathetic nerve fibres supply the bronchial muscle and glands, and extend along the bronchi to their subdivisions.

The *oesophagus* (figure 49) enters the thorax

slightly to the left of the midline and as it passes downwards moves towards the midline which it reaches at the level of the fifth thoracic vertebra. It then deviates to the left at the level of the seventh thoracic vertebra and passes through the right crus of the diaphragm about 2–3 cm to the left of the midline at the level of the tenth thoracic vertebra. The oesophagus lies in front of the vertebral column but at its lower end the descending thoracic aorta lies behind it. Anterior to the oesophagus is the trachea above and the left atrium below. Both the aortic arch and the left bronchus lie anteriorly and to the left of the oesophagus at the level of the fourth and fifth thoracic vertebrae. The descending thoracic aorta lies to the left of the oesophagus and then passes behind it to lie to its right above the diaphragm.

The thoracic duct as it passes upwards is behind the right border of the oesophagus. The duct crosses behind the oesophagus about the level of the fifth thoracic vertebra and continues upwards behind its left border. The right posterior intercostal arteries and the hemiazygos veins cross from left to right behind the oesophagus. The left recurrent laryngeal nerve lies on the left in the groove between the trachea and oesophagus. The vagus nerves form a plexus around the oesophagus in its lower part.

The oesophagus has the typical basic structure of the alimentary tract but is lined by non-keratinised stratified squamous epithelium. There are mucous glands in the submucosa. The muscle is skeletal in the upper third, mixed in the middle third and smooth in the lower third. Although there is no anatomical sphincter at the lower end of the oesophagus the circular muscle fibres can act like a sphincter. In a condition known as *achalasia* (*a = not*, *chalasis = relaxation*, Greek) this circular muscle goes into spasm, probably due to abnormal sympathetic stimulation, and interferes with swallowing.

The oesophagus is narrowed (1) where it begins at the sixth cervical vertebra as the continuation of the pharynx (15 cm from the incisor teeth); (2) where the arch of the aorta and the left bronchus are related to its left side about the level of the fourth and fifth thoracic vertebrae (20–25 cm from the incisor teeth); (3) at its lower end and where it passes through the diaphragm (40 cm from the incisor teeth). These constrictions are important and have to be kept in mind when passing tubes or instruments along the oesophagus. They are also the commonest sites of cancer and stricture.

The innervation of the upper end of the oesophagus is from the recurrent laryngeal nerves. Most of the thoracic part receives nerves from the vagus and sympathetic trunk (p. 50). The inferior thyroid artery supplies the upper part of the oesophagus, the descending thoracic aorta most of the thoracic part and the left gastric artery the lowest part. The veins correspond with the arterial supply and there is an important anastomosis between the systemic and portal system of veins at the lower end of the oesophagus (p. 104).

The lymphatic drainage of the oesophagus is given in table 1, p. 54.

In order to investigate the oesophagus radiologically it is necessary to introduce a radio-opaque material into its lumen. This is done by asking the patient to swallow a barium sulphate emulsion. An X-ray is taken while the patient is swallowing (figure 51). A more important part of the investigation is the use of a fluorescent screen by the radiologist so that the actual appearance and functioning of the organ can be observed. The oesophagus is constricted by the aorta, where it is crossed by the left bronchus and where it passes through the diaphragm. Diseased organs related to

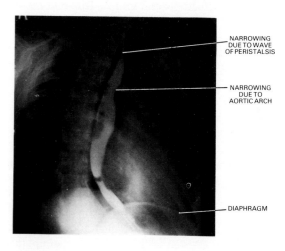

NARROWING DUE TO WAVE OF PERISTALSIS

NARROWING DUE TO AORTIC ARCH

DIAPHRAGM

Figure 51   An X-ray of the oesophagus (barium swallow).

the oesophagus may affect it. For example, an enlarged left atrium displaces the oesophagus backwards and to the right at the level of the sixth and seventh thoracic vertebrae.

By means of a flexible hollow tube containing lenses and a light (an *oesophagoscope*) the lining of the oesophagus can be examined and a small specimen can be removed by an instrument passed down the oesophagoscope.

The thoracic duct and lymph nodes of the thorax

The *thoracic duct* conveys all the lymph from the lower limbs, pelvis, abdomen, left side of the thorax and head and neck and left upper limb to the beginning of the left brachiocephalic vein (figure 53). The thoracic duct is the upward continuation of the cisterna chyli which is about 5 cm long and 1 cm wide and lies on the right side of the bodies of the first and second lumbar vertebrae below the diaphragm. The thoracic duct, about 3 mm in diameter, enters the thorax through the aortic opening of the diaphragm to the right of the aorta and as it passes upwards lies behind the right border of the oesophagus as far as the fifth thoracic

vertebra where it crosses behind the oesophagus to the left. The duct now passes upwards behind the left border of the oesophagus where it is crossed anteriorly by the aortic arch and enters the neck. The duct immediately arches forwards behind the carotid sheath and ends in the left brachiocephalic vein. The azygos vein is to the right of the thoracic duct for most of its course.

The thoracic duct has a number of valves which prevent lymph flowing downwards and give it a beaded appearance. There is a valve at its termination which prevents backflow of venous blood into the duct. The cisterna chyli receives the lymph from the lower limbs, abdominal and pelvic walls and the abdominal viscera. The thoracic duct receives the left bronchomediastinal lymph trunk in the thorax, and in the neck the left jugular and left subclavian lymph trunks from the left side of the head and neck and left upper limb respectively (figure 53). All of these lymph trunks can open independently into the left internal jugular or subclavian vein.

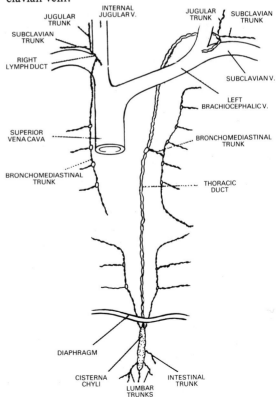

Figure 53   The main lymphatic ducts and trunks.

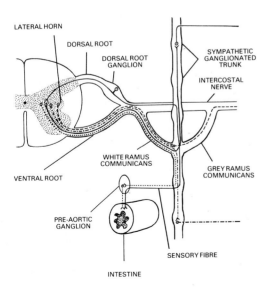

Figure 52   The possible pathways of the preganglionic sympathetic fibres.

The *lymph nodes of the thorax* are in groups related to the thoracic walls and the mediastinum. Those of the chest wall are anterior along the internal thoracic vessels at the anterior end of the intercostal spaces (*parasternal*), *intercostal* at the posterior ends of the intercostal spaces and *diaphragmatic* (*phrenic*). The most important afferent vessels to the parasternal nodes are from the medial half of the breast. These nodes also drain the deeper parts of the anterior chest wall. Their efferents form a trunk which joins the bronchomediastinal trunk. The intercostal nodes receive afferents from the deeper part of the chest wall posteriorly and their efferents go to the right lymph duct on the right and the thoracic duct on the left. The diaphragmatic nodes are round the periphery of the upper surface of the diaphragm and are *anterior*, *lateral* and *posterior*. The anterior group go to the parasternal nodes and the lateral and posterior to the posterior mediastinal nodes.

The most important mediastinal nodes are those round the division of the trachea and the main bronchi. These nodes also extend into the lung and are somewhat artificially divided into *pulmonary* (in the lung itself), *bronchopulmonary* (along the large bronchi) and *tracheobronchial* (round the division of the trachea). Their afferents come from the lung, bronchi and trachea and their efferents form the *bronchomediastinal lymph trunk* which joins the right lymph duct on the right and the thoracic duct on the left. On the left side these nodes lie near the recurrent laryngeal nerve which may be pressed on by enlarged nodes. This results in the voice being affected.

There are also *posterior mediastinal nodes* behind the heart. Their afferents come from the oesophagus and posterior part of the pericardium, and their efferents go to the thoracic duct. The *anterior mediastinal nodes* lie in front of the brachiocephalic veins. Their afferents come from the thymus, thyroid gland and anterior part of the pericardium. Their efferents go to the tracheo-bronchial nodes.

Cancer of the lung is common and it spreads along its lymphatic vessels to the nodes to which these vessels go. There is a superficial plexus of vessels deep to the visceral pleura and a deep plexus along the blood vessels. The bronchi have two plexuses, one is submucous and the other is more superficial. All these plexuses drain to the bronchial nodes. There are no lymph vessels round the alveoli. The lymph vessels of each lobe are separate but the bronchopulmonary segments have lymphatic communications with each other.

The lower part of the anterior thoracic wall has lymphatic connections with the upper part of the anterior abdominal wall. Cancer of the breast can spread along these connections to the abdominal cavity. The upper surface of the diaphragm has lymphatic communications with its lower surface. These vessels provide another channel for the spread of cancer from the thorax to the abdomen.

Table 1 is a summary of the lymphatic drainage of the thoracic walls and organs.

Table 1   Summary of the lymphatic drainage of the thoracic walls and organs

Structure	Nodes
Chest wall	
(a) Superficial	→ axillary → subclavian trunk
(b) Deep	
(1) Anterior	→ parasternal → bronchomediastinal trunk →
(2) Posterior	→ intercostal → right lymph duct or thoracic duct
Heart and pericardium	→ anterior and posterior mediastinal → bronchomediastinal trunk
Oesophagus	→ posterior mediastinal → thoracic duct
Pleura	
(a) Parietal	→ parasternal, intercostal, diaphragmatic
(b) Visceral	→ with lungs to tracheobronchial
Lungs	→ pulmonary, bronchopulmonary, tracheobronchial → bronchomediastinal trunk, right to right lymph duct left to thoracic duct
Diaphragm	
(a) Anterior	→ anterior diaphragmatic → parasternal → bronchomediastinal trunk
(b) Lateral and posterior	→ lateral and posterior diaphragmatic → posterior mediastinal → right lymph duct or thoracic duct

The thymus

This organ, which lies in the superior mediastinum, is present at birth but in the adult it is almost entirely replaced by fat and fibrous tissue. In the newborn it weighs about 15 g. It increases in size in the early years of life and almost doubles its weight before beginning to degenerate after puberty. It consists of two lobes each of which develops in the neck from the third pharyngeal pouch. The lobes have a distinct capsule. With the growth of the neck in the fetus the thymus comes to lie behind the manubrium of the sternum and in front of the arch of the aorta, its large ascending branches, the left brachiocephalic vein and the trachea. The thymus may extend upwards into the neck as far as the thyroid gland. Because of the deposition of fat after puberty the pink colour of the infant's thymus changes to yellow.

The role of the thymus in the defence mechanisms of the body has only been fully appreciated in recent years and although it degenerates at puberty its significance in the immune system of the body cannot be overestimated.

Part 2

The Abdomen

4

The Abdominal Wall

It is customary to consider the abdomen and pelvis separately but in many ways this is artificial since their walls, contents and cavities are continuous with each other. Their upper and lower limits are muscular. Above, where the abdominal cavity extends upwards within the rib cage, the diaphragm separates the abdominal from the thoracic cavity. Inferiorly the pelvic diaphragm separates the pelvic cavity from the perineum. A large part of the abdominal walls is muscular, especially anteriorly and laterally. Posteriorly the lumbar vertebrae are in the midline and there are muscles on each side of the vertebrae.

The pelvic walls are bony and are covered by muscles. The flared upper part of the pelvis forms the lateral walls of the lower part of the abdominal cavity (figure 101). The bony pelvis is formed anteriorly and laterally by the two hip bones which articulate in front at the *symphysis pubis*, a secondary cartilaginous joint, and behind by the sacrum, the part of the vertebral column wedged between the posterior parts of the hip bones. The articulations between the sacrum and iliac bone are called the *sacro-iliac joints* which are partly synovial (anteriorly) and partly fibrous (posteriorly). A plane through the upper anterior edge of the sacrum and upper edge of the symphysis pubis separates the upper *greater (false) pelvis* from the lower *lesser (true) pelvis*.

Within the abdominal and pelvic cavities there are the alimentary tract from the terminal part of the oesophagus to the rectum, almost the whole of the urinary tract, most of the female and part of the male genital tract, the lumbar and sacral nerve plexuses, autonomic nerves, the abdominal aorta and its branches, the inferior vena cava and its tributaries and lymph nodes and lymphatic vessels.

The Lumbar Vertebrae, Sacrum, Coccyx and Hip Bone

The lumbar vertebrae (figures 54, 55)

A *lumbar vertebra* (*lumbus = loin*, Latin) is recognised by the absence of a foramen in its transverse process (typical of a cervical vertebra) and the absence of a facet on the side of the body (typical of a thoracic vertebra). The *bodies* of the lumbar vertebrae are large relative to those of the vertebrae above them. The body has a large foramen on its posterior surface for the basivertebral vein emerging from its cancellous bone. The *vertebral arch* formed anteriorly by the diverging *pedicles* and posteriorly by the converging *laminae* show no special features. The backwardly projecting *spinous process* is approximately square and horizontal. A *transverse process* projects laterally on each side from the vertebral arch. That of the third lumbar vertebra is the longest. The *accessory process* is the tubercle on the medial part of the inferior border of the transverse process.

The paired *superior* and *inferior articular processes* project upwards and downwards from the vertebral arch. The plane of the synovial joint formed by the convex inferior articular process of one vertebra with the concave superior articular

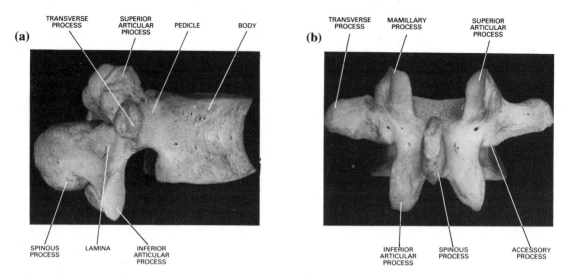

Figure 54   The first lumbar vertebra: (a) lateral view; (b) posterior view.

process of the one below is more or less sagittal although the adjacent surfaces are curved. The joint between the articular process of the twelfth thoracic and first lumbar vertebra is of this type (sagittal and curved) unlike the corresponding joints between the thoracic vertebrae which are more or less in the coronal plane and flat.

The joint between the bodies is a typical secondary cartilaginous joint with an intervertebral disc between the bony surfaces which are covered with hyaline cartilage. These discs are important because the highest incidence of prolapsed disc occurs in those between the fourth and fifth lumbar vertebrae and the fifth lumbar and first sacral vertebrae (65–70 per cent).

When the lumbar region of the vertebral column is examined as a whole (figure 55), it is seen to be curved with a posterior concavity often called the *lumbar lordosis*, although the term may be used only to describe an exaggerated curve (*lordos = curved with the convexity in front*, Greek). This curve varies with age (it is much more marked in infants learning to walk), sex (it is usually more marked in women) and race. It also becomes exaggerated in conditions which result in a more anterior position of the centre of gravity, for example in pregnancy — the increased lumbar curvature moves the centre of gravity backwards. The wedge shape of the discs, they are wider in front than behind, is

the main factor in producing the lumbar curvature.

The intervertebral foramina of the lumbar region are important. Anatomically they are similar to those of the rest of the vertebral column, that is they lie between the pedicles, behind the upper vertebral body and the intervertebral disc, and in front of the joint between the articular processes. The first lumbar spinal nerve emerges below the first lumbar vertebra and the fifth between the fifth lumbar and the first sacral vertebrae. The lumbar nerves, particularly the lowest two, are frequently pressed on as a result of narrowing of the intervertebral foramen associated with degeneration of the intervertebral disc, or by bony outgrowths due to disease of the joints in front of and behind them. Pressure on these nerves results in pain along their distribution in the hip region and lower limb, and also weakness of the muscles supplied by them.

The *fifth lumbar vertebra* has some distinctive features. Its transverse processes are much thicker than those of the rest of the lumbar vertebrae and are attached to the body of the vertebra as well as the vertebral arch. The weight of the body and upper limbs is transferred to the fifth lumbar vertebra and from there to the sacrum. The fifth lumbar vertebra tends to be pushed downwards and forwards. This is prevented by the strong *iliolumbar ligament* between the transverse process of the fifth lumbar vertebra and the iliac part of the

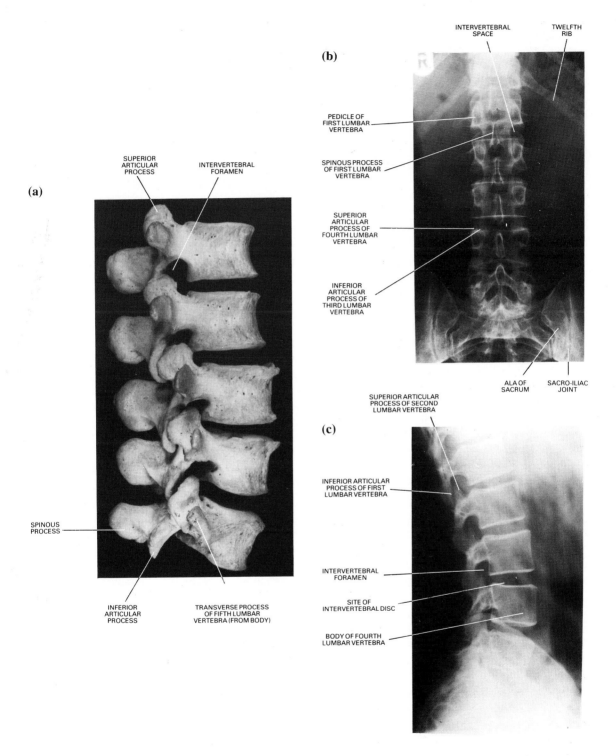

Figure 55   **(a) Lateral view of the lumbar vertebrae. (b) Anteroposterior X-ray of the lumbar vertebrae.
(c) Lateral X-ray of the lumbar vertebrae.**

hip bone and also by the change in the plane of the joints between the fifth lumbar vertebra and sacrum. This plane is much more coronal than sagittal as a rule.

The lumbar part of the vertebral canal is also of special importance because the spinal cord ends at about the level of the first lumbar vertebra and the roots of the lumbar and sacral spinal nerves accompanied by the meninges continue downwards as the *cauda equina* (= *horse's tail*, Latin) in the vertebral canal before forming the spinal nerves, each of which leaves through the appropriate intervertebral foramen. The meningeal space round the spinal cord roots containing the cerebrospinal fluid extends beyond the spinal cord to the level of the second sacral vertebra. It is possible to pass a hollow needle between the third and fourth lumbar vertebrae and enter this space without endangering the spinal cord. This procedure is called *lumbar puncture* and is used for obtaining cerebrospinal fluid or injecting drugs, for example in spinal anaesthesia.

Much more flexion and extension and lateral bending are possible in the lumbar part of the vertebral column than in the thoracic part, but rotation is more limited. This is due to the shape and plane of the joints between the articular processes and to the absence of ribs. The very extensive movements of the vertebral column seen in dancers and acrobats are largely due to increased mobility in the lumbar region.

The sacrum and coccyx

The sacrum (figure 56) consists of five fused vertebrae, is triangular in shape with the apex of the triangle inferior and is wedged between the posterior parts of the hip bones with which it articulates at the sacro-iliac joints. The *pelvic (anterior) surface* is concave and forms, with the coccyx below, the posterior wall of the pelvic cavity. There are four transverse ridges indicating the lines of fusion of the five vertebral bodies. Lateral to each ridge on each side is the *anterior sacral foramen*, which represents the anterior part of the intervertebral foramen.

The *dorsal (posterior) surface* is convex with a vertical midline row of tubercles which represent

the spinous processes. Lateral to these tubercles on each side there is a flat area representing the fused laminae. Usually the spinous processes and laminae of the fourth and fifth sacral vertebrae are absent so that the sacral canal is open. This opening is called the *sacral hiatus* and is used, for example during labour, for the insertion of a hollow needle or rubber tube through which an anaesthetic can be injected to anaesthetise the sacral nerves.

Lateral to the flat area there are two vertical rows of tubercles, a medial representing the articular processes, and a lateral representing the transverse processes. The former row is in line with the *sacral superior articular process* which articulates with the inferior articular process of the fifth lumbar vertebrae, and inferiorly with the *sacral cornua* (*cornu = horn*, Latin) which articulate with the coccyx. Between the two rows of tubercles are the *posterior sacral foramina*.

The *base (superior surface)* of the sacrum faces forwards as well as upwards and has a central area which is the upper surface of the first sacral vertebra. Its anterior border is called the *promontory* which is an important landmark in obstetrical anatomy. On each side of the superior surface there is a smooth area continuous with the iliac fossa of the hip bone.

The *lateral surface* of the sacrum is triangular with the apex below. The upper part of this surface is divided into an anterior pitted *auricular area* (shaped like an ear) which articulates with a similar area on the iliac part of the hip bone at the synovial sacro-iliac joint. The posterior part of this area is rough for ligaments. There is almost no movement at the sacro-iliac joints. The weight of the body transmitted from the fifth lumbar vertebra to the sacrum and thence through the sacro-iliac joint tends to push the sacrum directly downwards and forwards and also to rotate it in the same direction. This is prevented by powerful posterior ligaments.

The *ala* (*ala = wing*, Latin) of the sacrum refers to its upper lateral part and includes parts of the upper and pelvic surfaces. Reference is frequently made to structures passing over the ala of the sacrum into and out of the pelvis.

The female sacrum is shorter, wider and less curved in its upper part than the male sacrum. In the female the width of the body of the first sacral

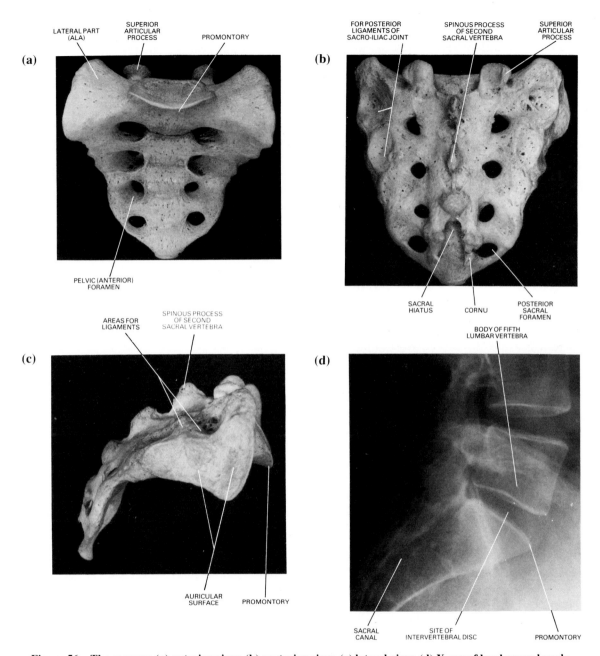

Figure 56 **The sacrum: (a) anterior view; (b) posterior view; (c) lateral view; (d) X-ray of lumbosacral angle.**

vertebra is equal to that of the ala; in the male the width of the body is greater than that of the ala.

A failure of fusion of the vertebral arches of the sacral and lumbar vertebrae results in a condition called *spina bifida*. If the abnormality is limited to the bones there may be no functional disturbance.

Not infrequently there are also abnormalities of the spinal cord and its coverings (the meninges). These babies usually have paralysed lower limbs and an incontinent bladder and bowel. Formerly they died within weeks or months but in recent years efforts have been made to keep these infants alive. Many of them, however, remain paralysed and incontinent. As a result the medical profession is faced with difficult ethical problems which are still being debated.

The basic ossification of the lumbar and sacral vertebrae is the same as that of the thoracic (p. 6). The individual sacral vertebrae fuse together to form one bone by about 25 years. Not uncommonly the fifth lumbar vertebra is partly or completely fused with the sacrum (*sacralised lumbar vertebra*). There may be six lumbar vertebrae and only four sacral vertebrae. In 10 per cent of skeletons the first lumbar vertebra has a rib or ribs.

Because *sacrum* means the *sacred bone* various explanations for the term have been put forward. It was suggested that as it was the last bone to disintegrate it was therefore the final place where the soul remained before leaving the body. Hence its name. It appears, however, that the Greek word for the bone, *os hieron*, although usually meaning *holy* or *sacred* also means the *best* bone in the sense that it was the *biggest*. The word was then translated into Latin as if the Greek word meant *sacred*.

The *coccyx* (*coccyx* = *cuckoo*, Greek; the bone resembles a cuckoo's beak) usually consists of four rudimentary vertebrae fused to form two pieces of bone which largely represent only the bodies. Superiorly the first coccygeal vertebra articulates by means of two *cornua* with the processes of the same name at the inferior end of the sacrum. The coccyx is bent forwards in continuity with the forward bend of the lower end of the sacrum.. The posterior wall of the vertebral canal of the coccyx is absent so that the sacral hiatus continues downwards over the back of the coccyx.

The coccyx can be fractured by a fall on the buttocks. The patient complains of chronic pain which is associated particularly with sitting and defaecation.

The hip bone (figure 57)

Because of its irregular shape the hip bone is also known as the *innominate bone*. It consists of three bones fused together. The upper part is the *ilium*, the posterior inferior part is the *ischium* and the anterior inferior part, the *pubis* (*ilium = groin* or *flank*, Latin; *ischion = hip joint*, Greek; *pubis = adult*, Latin, evidenced by the hair which appears in this region at puberty, hence the bone of this region). The three bones meet in the acetabulum, a deep hollow on the lateral surface of the hip bone for articulation with the head of the femur at the hip joint (*acetabulum = a little cup for holding vinegar*, Latin). The correct position of the hip bone in the erect body is obtained if the acetabulum is made to face laterally, and somewhat downwards and forwards. In this position the anterior superior iliac spine and the upper border of the symphysis pubis are in the same vertical plane.

The Ilium

The main part of the ilium (the *ala*) forms part of the lateral wall of the abdominal cavity. Its upper border is the *iliac crest* which ends anteriorly as the *anterior superior iliac spine* and posteriorly as the *posterior superior iliac spine*. The whole of the crest and the two spines can be palpated. On the outer border of the crest behind the anterior superior spine there is a prominence called the *iliac tubercle*. Below the anterior superior spine there is a notch bounded below by the *anterior inferior iliac spine*. Below the posterior superior spine is the *posterior inferior spine* and below that is the deep *greater sciatic notch*, the border of which becomes continuous with the ischium (*sciaticus* is a Latin modified form of the Greek *ischiadicos*).

The outer surface of the ala is called the *gluteal surface* and the inner surface the *iliac fossa*. Posterior to the fossa is the area for articulation with the sacrum. This area has an anterior *auricular part* for the synovial sacro-iliac joint and a posterior rough part for ligaments.

The iliac fossa is separated from the pelvic surface of the ilium by the *terminal (arcuate) line* which forms part of the *superior aperture (brim)* of the pelvis. The anterior part of this line has a distinct elevation, the *iliopubic eminence*, which marks the junction of the ilium with the pubis. The part of the ilium which takes part in the formation of the acetabulum is called the *body*.

The Ischium

The *body* of the ischium forms part of the acetabulum. The posterior border of the body is continuous above with the ilium where it forms the *greater sciatic notch*. Inferiorly this border ends as the prominent *ischial spine* below which there is a groove forming the *lesser sciatic notch*. The anterior border of the body forms superiorly the lower edge of the acetabulum and inferiorly the posterior edge of the obturator foramen. The pelvic surface of the body is continuous with the pelvic surface of the ilium and takes part in the formation of the lateral pelvic wall.

The *ischial tuberosity*, below and behind the body, is a mass of bone which can be felt if the thigh is flexed at the hip. The inferior part of the superficial surface of the tuberosity is that part of the pelvis on which one normally sits. The upper half has a number of muscles attached to it. The medial border of the tuberosity forms a sharp ridge and its posterior part, if followed upwards, is continuous with the ischial body. Anteriorly the tuberosity passes upwards as the *ischial ramus*, which is continuous with the inferior pubic ramus, thus forming the *ischiopubic ramus*.

The Pubis

The *body* is the anterior flat part forming the anterior wall of the pelvis which is more horizontal than vertical. Its medial border forms a secondary cartilaginous joint, the *symphysis pubis*, with the body of the pubis on the other side. Inferiorly the *inferior ramus* passes downwards and backwards from the body and joins the ischial ramus.

The superior part of the body has a *crest* extending laterally for about 1.5 cm and ending as the *pubic tubercle*, an important landmark which is palpable. Lateral to the tubercle the pubis forms the *superior ramus* and continues into the anterior part of the acetabulum. The *pectineal line* is on the upper surface of the superior ramus and is continuous laterally with the iliopubic eminence. (*Pecten = comb*, Latin, the line near the attachment of the pectineus muscle which resembles a comb.) The border of the superior aperture of the pelvis is formed by the symphysis pubis, the pubic crest, the pectineal line, the iliopubic eminence, the margin between the iliac fossa and pelvic surface of the ilium and the ala and promontory of the sacrum. The lower edge of the superior pubic ramus forms part of the boundary of the obturator foramen.

The inferior ramus of the pubis together with the ischial ramus forms part of the margin of the obturator foramen. The inferior edges of the two ischiopubic rami form the *pubic arch*.

The Obturator Foramen

This lies below and in front of the acetabulum and above the ischiopubic ramus. The *obturator membrane* closes the foramen except superiorly where there is an opening for the passage of the obturator vessels and nerve (*obturator = a structure which closes an opening*, Latin).

The Sciatic Foramina

The greater and lesser sciatic notches are converted into foramina by two ligaments (figure 104). The *sacrospinous ligament* is attached to the back of the sacrum and to the ischial spine and completes the *greater sciatic foramen*. The *sacrotuberous ligament* is attached to the back of the sacrum and to the ischial tuberosity and is posterior to the sacrospinous ligament. The *lesser sciatic foramen* is formed by the sacrospinous and sacrotuberous ligaments and the lesser sciatic notch. A large number of structures leave the pelvis through the greater sciatic foramen and enter the gluteal region. Some of them then pass through the lesser sciatic foramen into the perineum. The obturator internus muscle leaves the pelvis through the lesser sciatic foramen.

Ossification (figure 57 (c))

The hip bone ossifies in cartilage from three primary centres, one for the ilium at about 8 weeks, one for the ischium at about 12 weeks and one for the pubis at about 20 weeks of fetal life. At birth there is a Y-shaped (*triradiate*) *cartilage* in the

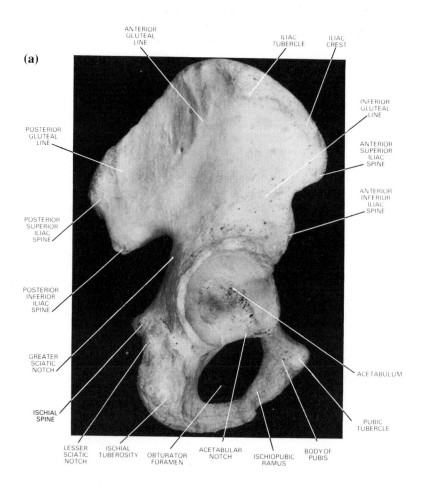

(a)

ANTERIOR GLUTEAL LINE

ILIAC TUBERCLE

ILIAC CREST

INFERIOR GLUTEAL LINE

ANTERIOR SUPERIOR ILIAC SPINE

ANTERIOR INFERIOR ILIAC SPINE

POSTERIOR GLUTEAL LINE

POSTERIOR SUPERIOR ILIAC SPINE

POSTERIOR INFERIOR ILIAC SPINE

GREATER SCIATIC NOTCH

ACETABULUM

ISCHIAL SPINE

PUBIC TUBERCLE

LESSER SCIATIC NOTCH

ISCHIAL TUBEROSITY

OBTURATOR FORAMEN

ACETABULAR NOTCH

ISCHIOPUBIC RAMUS

BODY OF PUBIS

Figure 57   The right hip bone: (a) lateral view.

acetabulum, where the three bones meet, and a cartilaginous union of the inferior ramus of the pubis and the ramus of the ischium. The ischiopubic ramus becomes wholly bone at about 5 years and the triradiate cartilage begins to ossify at puberty. Bony union is completed by 17 years.

There are several secondary ossification centres, for example on the iliac crest and the ischial tuberosity, appearing at puberty and fusing at about 20 years.

The Anterior Abdominal Wall

The skin

The *umbilicus* is an obvious landmark but although it is not recommended for use in surface anatomy because of its variable position, it is not infrequently used for this purpose, for example to indicate the position of the division of the abdominal aorta. The umbilicus usually lies about midway between the xiphoid process and the symphysis pubis.

Following a pregnancy the skin of the abdominal wall, especially inferiorly and laterally, usually shows a number of short, longitudinally running lines called *striae gravidarum* (= *the streaks of pregnant women*, Latin) which are due to the splitting of the deeper parts of the skin because of disten-

(b)

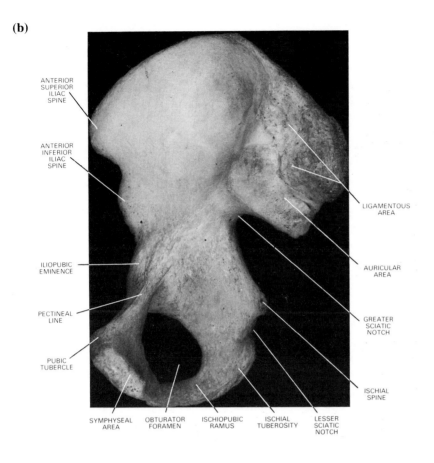

ANTERIOR
SUPERIOR
ILIAC
SPINE

ANTERIOR
INFERIOR
ILIAC
SPINE

ILIOPUBIC
EMINENCE

PECTINEAL
LINE

PUBIC
TUBERCLE

LIGAMENTOUS
AREA

AURICULAR
AREA

GREATER
SCIATIC
NOTCH

ISCHIAL
SPINE

SYMPHYSEAL
AREA

OBTURATOR
FORAMEN

ISCHIOPUBIC
RAMUS

ISCHIAL
TUBEROSITY

LESSER
SCIATIC
NOTCH

(c)

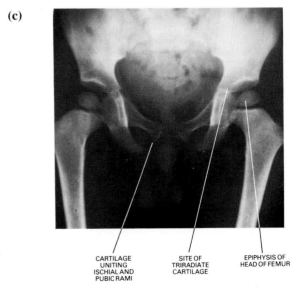

CARTILAGE
UNITING
ISCHIAL AND
PUBIC RAMI

SITE OF
TRIRADIATE
CARTILAGE

EPIPHYSIS OF
HEAD OF FEMUR

Figure 57   The right hip bone: (b) medial view. (c) Ossification as shown in an X-ray of the hip joints of a child about 1 year old.

sion. Similar striae appear in any condition involving gross stretching of the abdominal wall.

The skin is *innervated* by the lower intercostal (sixth or seventh to the eleventh thoracic spinal nerves), the subcostal (the twelfth thoracic spinal nerve) and the iliohypogastric and ilio-inguinal nerves (the first lumbar spinal nerve) (figure 9). The sixth or seventh thoracic dermatome is at the level of the xiphoid process, the tenth is at the level of the umbilicus, and the first lumbar is at the level of the symphysis pubis. Beyond the symphysis pubis in the region of the external genitalia the spinal nerve segment is the second sacral (compare this with the skin above and below the clavicle).

Certain bony features of the abdominal wall can be seen and/or felt (figure 58). The xiphoid process *and the* costal margin *form the upper limits of the anterior abdominal wall. Inferiorly and medially the* pubic tubercle *is palpable about 2–3 cm lateral to the midline. Laterally the* anterior superior iliac spine *can be felt and the* iliac crest *followed backwards to the* posterior superior iliac spine. *About 3–4 cm behind the anterior superior spine of the iliac crest there is an easily palpable lateral prominence, the* iliac tubercle.

The posterior superior spine is marked by a dimple and the line joining the right and left dimples crosses the spinous process of the second sacral vertebra. *A line joining the highest points of the iliac crests is usually at the level of the intervertebral disc between the third and fourth lumbar vertebrae. The line joining the iliac tubercles is at the level of the fourth lumbar vertebra. The lowest limit of the costal margin is at the level of the third lumbar vertebra and the xiphoid process is at the level of the ninth or tenth thoracic vertebra.*

For clinical purposes the abdominal wall can be divided into nine areas by two horizontal lines and two vertical lines (figure 58). The upper horizontal line is midway between the jugular notch of the sternum and the symphysis pubis. A horizontal plane through this line is called the transpyloric plane *because, as described by Addison, it passes through the pylorus of the stomach and is at the level of the first lumbar vertebra (C. Addison, later Lord, 1869–1951, London anatomist, later Minister of Health). This plane also lies approximately through a line midway between the xiphoid process and the umbilicus. The second horizontal line or plane is either the* intercristal *or the* intertubercular. *The former is at the level of the highest points of the iliac crests, the latter at the level of the iliac tubercles. The* vertical (lateral) lines *pass through the middle of the clavicle and are midway between the anterior superior iliac spine and the symphysis pubis on each side.*

The lateral six areas are from above downwards the right and left hypochondriac, lateral (lumbar) *and* inguinal (iliac). *The middle three areas are, from above downwards, the* epigastric, umbilical *and* pubic (hypogastric). *All these terms are used frequently in clinical medicine to indicate different parts of the abdomen.*

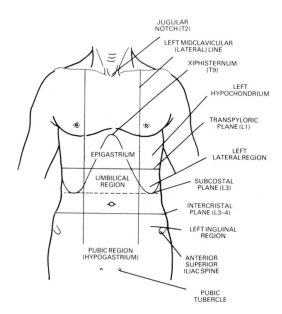

Figure 58   The surface bony markings, vertebral levels and areas of the abdominal wall.

The superficial fascia

This varies in thickness because of the variable amount of fat deposited in this part of the body. Inferior to the umbilicus the fascia is in two layers, a superficial fatty and a deep membranous layer. The membranous layer continues into the perineum beyond the symphysis pubis, surrounds the external genitalia and becomes attached to the ischiopubic rami. More laterally the membranous layer extends for about 1 cm beyond the inguinal ligament and fuses with the deep fascia of the thigh.

The muscles of the anterior abdominal wall

Laterally and anteriorly there are three muscles — the external oblique, the internal oblique and the transversus abdominis. The *external oblique* is attached by digitations to the outside of the lower eight ribs (figures 59, 60). The upper digitations interdigitate with those of the serratus anterior and the lower with those of the latissimus dorsi. Between the ribs and the iliac crest the external oblique has a posterior free edge. The lowest fibres of the external oblique pass downwards and forwards and are attached to the anterior half of the iliac crest. The muscle between the anterior superior spine and the pubic tubercle forms a fibrous structure called the *inguinal ligament*. The gap between the inguinal ligament and the hip bone is occupied by a number of structures which pass between the pelvis and thigh. The upper and

middle fibres of the muscle end in an aponeurosis which extends from the lowest costal cartilages to the body of the pubis. An *aponeurosis* is a flat wide tendon; *neuron* meant either a *sinew* or *nerve*. A large nerve was confused with a tendon so that the word meant *tendon* or *nerve* in Hebrew and Greek (see Jacob wrestling with the angel, Genesis XXXII, 23–33). The aponeurosis forms part of the anterior layer of the *rectus sheath* (p. 71) and meets the aponeurosis of the opposite external oblique in a dense fibrous tissue structure called the *linea alba* which extends in the midline from the xiphoid process to the pubic bone. The linea alba is wider above (1–2 cm) than below (3–4 mm).

There is a triangular opening in the aponeurosis of the external oblique in the region of the pubic tubercle (figure 60). The base of the triangle is medial to the tubercle and the sides of the opening (the *lateral* and *medial crura*) pass upwards and laterally so that the actual opening lies above the tubercle (*crus = leg*, Latin, or any structure like a leg, the part of the lower limb between the knee and the ankle). The opening is called the *superficial*

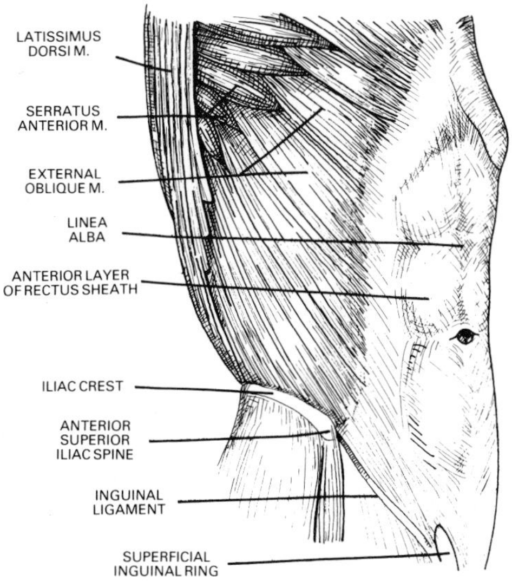

LATISSIMUS DORSI M.

SERRATUS ANTERIOR M.

EXTERNAL OBLIQUE M.

LINEA ALBA

ANTERIOR LAYER OF RECTUS SHEATH

ILIAC CREST

ANTERIOR SUPERIOR ILIAC SPINE

INGUINAL LIGAMENT

SUPERFICIAL INGUINAL RING

Figure 59   The external oblique muscle.

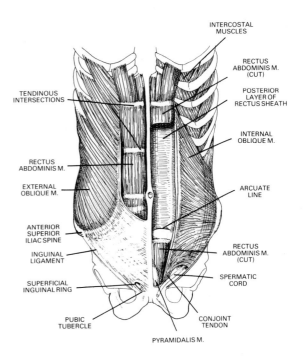

INTERCOSTAL MUSCLES

RECTUS ABDOMINIS M. (CUT)

POSTERIOR LAYER OF RECTUS SHEATH

INTERNAL OBLIQUE M.

ARCUATE LINE

RECTUS ABDOMINIS M. (CUT)

SPERMATIC CORD

CONJOINT TENDON

TENDINOUS INTERSECTIONS

RECTUS ABDOMINIS M.

EXTERNAL OBLIQUE M.

ANTERIOR SUPERIOR ILIAC SPINE

INGUINAL LIGAMENT

SUPERFICIAL INGUINAL RING

PUBIC TUBERCLE

PYRAMIDALIS M.

Figure 60   The muscles of the anterior abdominal wall.

inguinal ring and is the medial end of a canal in the anterior abdominal wall lying above the medial half of the inguinal ligament. The structures passing through the canal (the *spermatic cord* in the male and the *round ligament* in the female) evaginate the aponeurosis of the external oblique which continues as a covering (the *external spermatic fascia*) round the spermatic cord or round ligament into the scrotum, or female homologue, the labium majus.

There are three important structures at the medial end of the inguinal ligament (figure 61). The *lacunar or Gimbernat's ligament* (*lacuna = hollow* or *space*, Latin; A. de Gimbernat, 1734–1816, Spanish surgeon) is a triangular, horizontal, fibrous structure which lies in the angle between the medial end of the inguinal ligament and the pectineal line of the pubis. It has a lateral free edge which extends laterally along the pectineal line to form the *pectineal ligament* (of Cooper, p. 13). It becomes continuous with the fascia on the pectineus muscle. The *reflected part of the inguinal ligament* passes upwards and medially from the medial end of

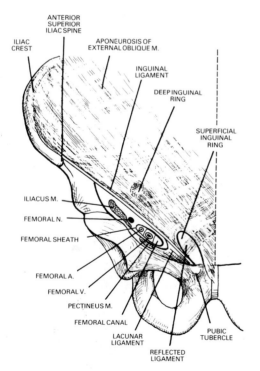

Figure 61   The structures associated with the medial end of the inguinal ligament.

the inguinal ligament behind the medial crus and spermatic cord or round ligament to the linea alba.

The *internal oblique muscle* (figure 60) passes obliquely upwards and inwards at right angles to the external oblique. The internal oblique is attached below to the anterior part of the iliac crest and the lateral two-thirds of the inguinal ligament and posteriorly to fascia which is attached to the lumbar and thoracic vertebrae (*thoracolumbar fascia*). The fibres of the internal oblique pass upwards and are attached to the outer surface of the lower ribs and to an aponeurosis which forms part of the rectus sheath. The right and left muscles meet in the linea alba.

The attachment of the internal oblique to the inguinal ligament is sufficiently medial for the spermatic cord to pass through the muscle and carry a covering with it into the scrotum. This consists of fibromuscular tissue and is called the *cremasteric fascia* and *cremaster muscle* (*cremastos = hangings or drapes*, Greek; the muscle fibres are in loops). The cremaster muscle is involved in the *cremasteric reflex* – when the inside of the upper part of the thigh is stroked the muscle contracts and pulls the testis upwards towards the inguinal canal. The skin area is supplied by the first and second lumbar nerves as is the cremaster muscle through the genital branch of the genitofemoral nerve.

The *transversus abdominis* (figure 62) has fibres which run horizontally. Below, the muscle is attached to the anterior part of the iliac crest and the lateral third of the inguinal ligament, posteriorly it is attached to the thoracolumbar fascia and superiorly it arises from the inner surface of the lower six costal cartilages interdigitating with the digitations of the diaphragm. As the muscle fibres pass forwards and medially they end in an aponeurosis which takes part in the formation of the rectus sheath and reaches the linea alba.

The *conjoint tendon* (figure 60) is formed by the lowest and most medial fibres of the internal oblique and transversus abdominis muscles, the fibres that are attached to the inguinal ligament. These fibres arch upwards and medially over the spermatic cord (or round ligament of the uterus) and pass downwards behind that structure to become attached to the crest of the pubis medial to the pubic tubercle. The conjoint tendon (most of it is muscular) comes to lie behind the medial end of the inguinal canal.

The *rectus abdominis muscle* (figure 60) is a flat rectangular muscle 6–7 cm wide, on either side of the midline, extending from the upper surface of the pubis to the anterior surface of the fifth, sixth and seventh costal cartilages. It has usually three transverse tendinous intersections which are (1) at the level of the umbilicus, (2) just below the xiphoid process, (3) midway between these two. Occasionally there may be another intersection between the umbilicus and the pubis. These intersections are attached to the anterior layer of the rectus sheath but not to the posterior layer. They indicate the segmental origin of the rectus abdominis.

Each rectus abdominis is enclosed in a dense sheet of fascia called the *rectus sheath* (figures 59–63). The anterior layer of the rectus sheath is formed by the aponeurosis of the external oblique and the anterior half of the aponeurosis of the internal oblique. The posterior layer is formed by the posterior half of the aponeurosis of the internal

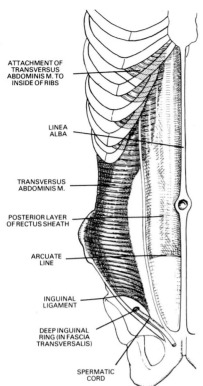

Figure 62 The transversus abdominis muscle.

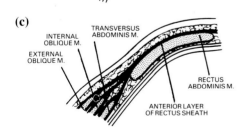

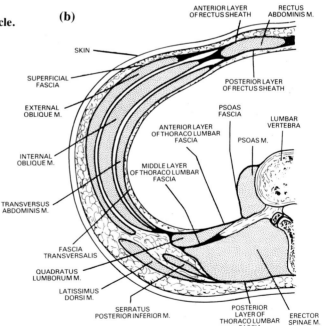

Figure 63 The thoracolumbar fascia and the formation of the rectus sheath: (a) a section through the lower end of the sternum; (b) a complete section through the second lumbar vertebra; (c) a section above the symphysis pubis.

oblique and the whole of the aponeurosis of the transversus abdominis. The anterior and posterior layers of the rectus sheath on both sides meet in the midline in the linea alba. Above the level of the costal margin only the aponeurosis of the external oblique is found and it forms the anterior layer of the rectus sheath in this region (figure 63). The posterior layer of the rectus sheath extends downwards only as far as a line midway between the umbilicus and symphysis pubis and ends as the *arcuate line* (fold of Douglas; J. Douglas, 1675–1742, Scottish anatomist and surgeon with at least seven structures associated with his name). Inferior to this line all the aponeuroses of the muscles pass in front of the rectus abdominis so that its posterior surface is in contact with the fascia transversalis.

The superior epigastric vessels from the thorax pass downwards between the posterior layer of the rectus sheath and the rectus abdominis and anastomose with the ascending inferior epigastric vessels which pass upwards posterior to the rectus abdominis and then anterior to the arcuate line (figure 65). The lower intercostal nerves end by passing medially between the posterior layer of the rectus sheath and the rectus abdominis and then anteriorly through the rectus abdominis which they supply before terminating in the skin near the midline.

The *pyramidalis muscle* lying between the anterior layer of the rectus sheath and the rectus abdominis (figure 60) is attached to the pubis near the midline and passes upwards for about 5–7 cm to become attached to the linea alba.

The muscles of the anterior abdominal wall are supplied by the lower six thoracic spinal nerves through the intercostal and subcostal nerves and by the first lumbar spinal nerve through the ilio-hypogastric and ilio-inguinal nerves.

The *functions* of the anterior abdominal muscles are (1) to retain the abdominal viscera within the abdominal cavity; (2) to keep the viscera in their normal position; (3) to increase the intra-abdominal pressure and assist the emptying of hollow viscera, for example in defaecation, micturition, parturition and vomiting; (4) to push the diaphragm upwards in deep expiration, and in coughing and sneezing; (5) to produce movements of the vertebral column such as flexion when lying on one's back or control-

ling extension of the trunk in the upright position or assisting in rotation of the trunk (the right external oblique and left internal oblique turn the trunk to the left) (figure 60); (6) to increase intra-abdominal pressure and relieve the strain on the vertebral column when lifting heavy weights.

It has been shown by means of electromyography that the oblique muscles and the transversus abdominis are used in expiration and not the recti unless expiration is very forced. The recti contract in normal flexion and extension movements of the vertebral column and the lateral muscles are not involved.

The arrangement of the muscles of the anterior abdominal wall is used by surgeons when planning incisions. A midline vertical incision of adequate length through the linea alba provides a comparatively bloodless approach to the abdominal cavity. A vertical incision 3–4 cm from the midline (parasagittal or paramedian) goes through the skin, superficial fascia and anterior layer of the rectus sheath. The rectus abdominis is pulled laterally and the posterior layer of the sheath is cut if the original incision is above the level of the arcuate line. If the original incision is high enough the anterior layer of the sheath has to be separated from the rectus muscle at its tendinous intersections. If the incision is in the region of the arcuate line, the inferior epigastric vessels usually have to be tied and cut. The rectus abdominis should not be cut longitudinally because the nerves supplying it run horizontally from the lateral to the medial side. A right-sided subcostal incision running parallel to and 2–5 cm below the costal margin from the midline is used for approaching the gall bladder. The rectus sheath and muscle are divided almost transversely. The cut edges of the rectus abdominis do not retract because of the fascial intersections. The vermiform appendix is approached on the right side by an oblique incision at right angles to the line joining the anterior iliac spine and the umbilicus. The incision is centred on the junction of the lateral and middle thirds of this line. The skin incision is parallel to the fibres of the external oblique which is split or cut in line with its fibres. The internal oblique and transversus are then split at right angles to the opening in the external oblique, that is in the line of their fibres. This is called the *gridiron* approach and permits access to the abdominal cavity without dividing the fibres of the muscles. This incision, however, is limited with regard to the size of the opening and the extent to which the abdominal cavity can be explored.

The fascia transversalis

There is a layer of fascia between the muscles of the abdominal and pelvic walls (posterior as well as anterior) and the peritoneum. In certain places this layer has specific names, usually that of the muscle next to which it lies. In the anterior abdominal wall it is called the *fascia transversalis* which is thicker just above the inguinal ligament than elsewhere. The *deep inguinal ring* is a round opening in the fascia transversalis 1 cm in diameter and 1 cm above the middle of the inguinal ligament. It is the lateral end of the inguinal canal and transmits the spermatic cord in the male and the round ligament in the female. The cord takes with it a covering of the fascia transversalis called the *internal spermatic fascia* which extends into the scrotum or labium majus.

The inguinal canal (figures 60, 61, 62, 64)

This is a canal lying just above the medial half of the inguinal ligament and passes from lateral to medial, slightly downwards and forwards. It is about 5 cm long. Its lateral opening in the fascia transversalis in the *deep inguinal ring* and its medial opening in the external oblique is the *superficial inguinal ring* (p. 69). The canal has an *anterior wall* which consists of the external oblique along its whole length and the internal oblique laterally. The fascia transversalis forms the *posterior wall* of the canal along its whole length. The conjoint tendon forms part of the posterior wall at its medial end. The whole of the *floor* of the canal is formed by the inguinal ligament with the lacunar ligament at the medial end. The attachment of the transversus abdominis to the inguinal ligament is too lateral for it to form part of the anterior wall but together with the internal oblique it forms the

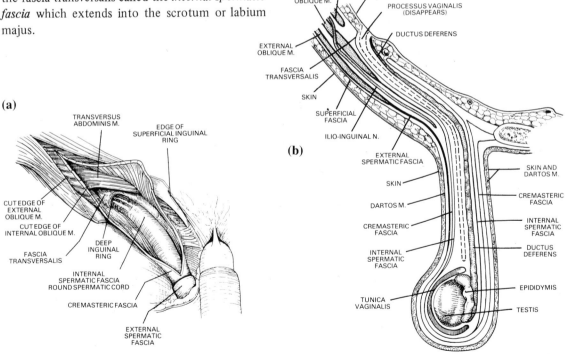

Figure 64 (a) A dissection of the walls of the inguinal canal. (b) The coverings of the spermatic cord and the development of the tunica vaginalis from the processus vaginalis.

conjoint tendon which arches over the canal from the lateral to the medial side. The contents of the canal take with them coverings from the fascia transversalis (internal spermatic fascia), internal oblique (cremasteric fascia) and external oblique (external spermatic fascia).

The *spermatic cord* is formed mainly by the structures passing to and from the testis which lies in the scrotum. The *ductus (vas) deferens* passes upwards from the testis and traverses the inguinal canal from the superficial to the deep ring. At the superficial ring it is medial to or just above the pubic tubercle. At the deep ring the ductus hooks round the lateral side of the inferior epigastric artery which passes upwards medial to the deep ring (figure 65). The ductus is about 3 mm in diameter and has a characteristic cordlike feel on palpation. The *testicular artery* from the abdominal aorta enters the deep ring and passes through the canal to the testis in the scrotum. The *testicular veins* begin as the pampiniform plexus (*pampinus = vine tendril*, Latin) in the scrotum which extends to the

superficial ring and emerges at the deep ring as the two testicular veins. These join and go to the inferior vena cava on the right and the left renal vein on the left.

There are two small arteries which enter the deep ring — an *artery to the vas* and an *artery to the cremaster muscle*. Postganglionic *sympathetic nerve fibres* accompany the testicular artery. The genital branch of the *genitofemoral nerve* enters the deep ring and supplies the cremaster muscle. The *ilio-inguinal nerve* which passes medially just above the inguinal ligament deep to the external oblique enters the canal and emerges through the superficial ring. The *lymphatic vessels* from the testis pass upwards through the canal to the lymph nodes in front of and at the sides of the abdominal aorta. This is in striking contrast with the lymphatic vessels of the skin of the scrotum which go to the superficial inguinal lymph nodes in the groin. These nodes are easily accessible to surgery but the aortic lymph nodes are not. In the female the *round ligament of the uterus* passes through the inguinal canal

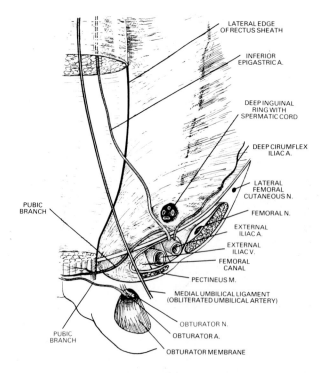

Figure 65   The deep aspect of right lower part of the anterior abdominal wall.

and ends in the labium majus. Some lymphatic vessels from the uterus accompany the round ligament and go to the inguinal nodes.

Inguinal and other hernias

The testis develops in the extraperitoneal tissue of the posterior abdominal wall and in the last month of pregnancy descends through the inguinal canal and into the scrotum, taking with it its blood vessels, lymphatics and nerve supply. As the testis passes through the inguinal canal it also takes with it prolongations of the walls of the canal which form the coverings of the cord (figure 64). There is also a tubular prolongation of the peritoneum lining the abdominal cavity, the *processus vaginalis*, which passes through the canal inside the coverings into the scrotum. Normally the testis invaginates this process so that the testis has a double layer of peritoneum covering it (the *tunica vaginalis*) and the rest of the processus vaginalis disappears from the upper pole of the testis to the deep inguinal ring.

Not infrequently the upper part of the processus vaginalis persists so that there is a peritoneal diverticulum extending through the deep inguinal ring into the inguinal canal and the scrotum. This diverticulum is not noticed until some part of the abdominal contents, most commonly a loop of the small intestine, passes into it in which case a swelling in the region of the groin appears. This constitutes a *hernia* which consists of a hernial sac, in this case the peritoneum, and its contents. (A *hernia* by definition consists of the protrusion of the lining membrane of any body cavity and some of its contents.) Depending on the extent of the diverticulum the swelling may be confined to the level of the superficial inguinal ring or may pass into the scrotum. What has been described is called a *congenital inguinal hernia* and because the canal is oblique it is called an *oblique hernia*. It is accepted that an oblique hernia can arise due to the peritoneum being pushed through the deep inguinal ring as a result of muscular effort causing increased intra-abdominal pressure, but it is likely that the peritoneal sac is congenital and a muscular strain pushes some part of the abdominal contents into the pre-existing sac. Usually this type of hernia is *reduced* when lying down, that is the contents go back into the abdominal cavity, and the swelling disappears. On standing the swelling reappears. If, however, the thumb is placed over the deep ring while the patient is lying down and the patient is asked to stand, the swelling will not reappear and an impulse can be felt against the thumb when the patient coughs, that is increases the intra-abdominal pressure.

In the female there is also a processus vaginalis which accompanies the round ligament into the perineum. Normally the whole processus up to the deep ring disappears. If it partly or wholly persists an inguinal hernia may develop.

The medial part of the posterior wall of the inguinal canal where it is formed by the conjoint tendon and fascia transversalis can become weakened with the result that the peritoneum projects forwards into the canal and, with some part of the abdominal organs, forms a *direct inguinal hernia*, that is a hernia passing directly through the wall of the canal. This type of hernia is always *acquired*. It appears at the superficial ring and does not pass downwards into the scrotum. It is also medial to the inferior epigastric artery whereas the oblique or indirect inguinal hernia because it passes through the deep ring is lateral to the artery (figure 65). The swelling due to a direct hernia disappears on lying down but if the thumb is placed over the deep ring it reappears on standing, unlike an oblique hernia. Because a direct hernia is associated with a weak abdominal wall it is much more difficult to treat surgically.

Another type of hernia, much less common than an inguinal hernia, appears in this region inferior to the medial part of the inguinal ligament and lateral to the lacunar ligament (p. 70). It is called a *femoral hernia* and produces a swelling below and lateral to the pubic tubercle as compared with the swelling of an inguinal hernia which is above and medial to the tubercle. This type of hernia is discussed in greater detail on p. 429.

Herniation of the peritoneum and some of the abdominal contents may occur in the region of the umbilicus. A true *umbilical hernia* occurs in infants either as a congenital condition through the umbilical opening or early in infancy due to weakness of the umbilical scar. An umbilical hernia in the adult is usually through the linea alba *near* the umbilicus (*para-umbilical*). An *incisional hernia* is due to a weak abdominal scar giving way and allowing the peritoneum and some of the abdominal contents to bulge through the separated edges of the scar.

The blood vessels and lymphatic drainage of the anterior abdominal wall

Laterally the main arteries are continuations of the lower posterior intercostal arteries which are derived from the descending thoracic aorta and accompany the lower intercostal nerves. On either side of the midline within the rectus sheath the superior epigastric artery, a branch of the internal thoracic, runs downwards and anastomoses with the inferior epigastric artery which runs upwards and is a branch of the external iliac artery.

Most of the intercostal veins end eventually in the azygos vein which is a tributary of the superior vena cava. The superior epigastric veins also end in veins which go to the superior vena cava. The inferior epigastric veins go to the external iliac veins which eventually reach the inferior vena cava. The veins of the anterior abdominal wall therefore constitute a connection between the superior and inferior venae cavae. The veins round the umbilicus have connections with the hepatic portal veins (p. 104).

For the purposes of describing its lymphatic drainage the whole trunk is divided into four parts by vertical and horizontal lines through the umbilicus. Each upper quadrant of the body wall is drained by lymphatic vessels which go to the axillary lymph nodes of its own side and each lower quadrant drains to the superficial inguinal nodes of its own side. Both the front and back of the trunk have lymphatic vessels which drain in this way. When asked in an examination which lymph nodes should be removed in a cancer of the umbilicus, the candidate was expected to answer the right and left axillary and right and left inguinal lymph nodes.

5

The Peritoneum

The peritoneum is the serous membrane (p. 23) lining the abdominal and pelvic cavities. Unlike the pleura and serous pericardium, its arrangement is complex due to the way in which the organs develop within the abdomen. It is possible, however, to follow its arrangement without a knowledge of the embryology which explains its post-natal complexities.

It must be emphasised that *all* organs lie *outside* the peritoneum, although if they invaginate it they can become almost wholly covered by peritoneum. The organ is then connected by a double fold of peritoneum to that lining the body wall. (Only the ovary is not covered by peritoneum. It, however, like all other organs, is extraperitoneal in the embryo but subsequently loses almost all its peritoneal covering.) These double folds of peritoneum are called *mesenteries* (they usually contain blood and lymphatic vessels and nerves) and *ligaments* (*mesos = middle, enteron = intestine*, Greek). Many mesenteries have special names which are related to the organ with which they are associated.

The *peritoneal cavity*, the main part of which used to be called the *greater sac*, has a diverticulum passing to the left from the upper part of its posterior wall. This diverticulum is much smaller than the main cavity and is called the *omental bursa* (or *lesser sac*). Before describing the peritoneum it is necessary to indicate the general arrangement of the abdominal and pelvic viscera (figure 66). The *oesophagus* and *stomach* are in the upper left part of the abdominal cavity below the diaphragm. The stomach usually ends just to the right of the mid-line at about the level of the first lumbar vertebra and continues into the *small intestine*, the first part of which curves round the second lumbar vertebra like a letter C and is called the *duodenum*. This leads into the second and third parts of the small intestine, the *jejunum* and *ileum*, which lie in coils in the middle of the abdomen. The end of the ileum passes upwards and to the right from the pelvis into the large intestine which more or less frames the small intestine with the *ascending colon* on the right, the *transverse colon* looping downwards from above and the *descending colon* on the left. The end of the large intestine passes towards the right to the midline and then downwards, ending as the *rectum* and *anal canal* in the posterior

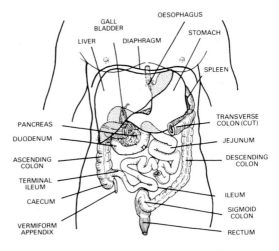

Figure 66   The general arrangement of the abdominal viscera.

part of the pelvis. The *liver* lies in the upper right part of the abdomen below the diaphragm, the *spleen* is to the left behind the stomach and the *pancreas* passes from the right to the left behind the stomach. The *kidneys* lie on the posterior wall to the right and left of the first three lumbar vertebrae. In the pelvis the *bladder* is behind the symphysis pubis. The *uterus* lies between the rectum and bladder.

The Arrangement of the Peritoneum in a Sagittal Section

The peritoneum is best described by following it in a longitudinal section of the abdomen and pelvis in a midline plane (figure 67). The peritoneum lines the anterior abdominal wall and passes upwards on to the inferior surface of the diaphragm from which it is reflected on to the upper surface of the liver. It passes over the anterior and inferior surfaces of the liver into a fissure on the inferior surface and

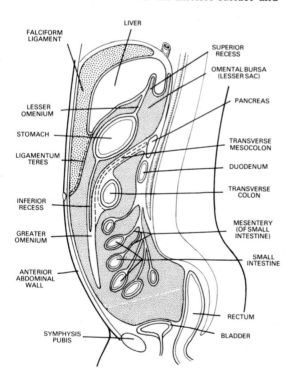

Figure 67   The arrangement of the peritoneum as seen in a sagittal section.

leaves the liver to continue downwards as the anterior layer of the *lesser omentum* (*omentum*, Latin = *epiploon*, Greek = *membrane*, especially one enclosing an internal organ). It passes on to the anterior surface of the stomach. At the inferior (left) border of the stomach, the peritoneum passes downwards for a considerable distance as the anterior layer of an apron-like fold called the *greater omentum*. At a variable level the peritoneum then turns upwards on itself to form the posterior layer of the greater omentum. This layer continues upwards behind the transverse colon as the posterior layer of its mesentery (the *transverse mesocolon*) and reaches the posterior abdominal wall at about the level of the middle of the pancreas. Originally the posterior layer of the greater omentum passed anterior to the transverse colon and after reaching the posterior abdominal wall turned downwards in front of and then upwards behind the transverse colon. It then passed to the posterior abdominal wall. The adjacent layers of the greater omentum and mesentery of the transverse colon fuse as indicated in figure 67 by the dotted lines.

The inferior layer of the transverse mesocolon continues downwards on the posterior abdominal wall and leaves it to form the mesentery of the small intestine (usually referred to as *the mesentery*). The inferior layer of this mesentery returns to the abdominal wall and after passing downwards lies in front of the rectum which it leaves to pass anteriorly on to the top of the bladder and continue on to the anterior abdominal wall. If there is a uterus the peritoneum leaves the rectum to pass on to the back of the upper part of the vagina and the whole of the back of the uterus, then down the front of the uterus and forwards on to the bladder. From the top of the bladder the peritoneum continues upwards on the anterior abdominal wall.

The peritoneum of the lesser sac lies behind the stomach. The opening into the lesser sac (the *epiploic foramen*) is above the duodenum between it and the liver. The lesser sac also extends upwards (*superior recess*) into the same fissure in the liver as the peritoneum of the greater sac to the left of its caudate lobe. The lesser sac also extends downwards (*inferior recess*) for a variable distance into the greater omentum. The anterior layer of the lesser sac forms the posterior layer of the lesser omentum. The posterior layer of the lesser sac fuses with the posterior layer of the greater omentum above the transverse colon and may be regarded as the upper (anterior) layer of the transverse mesocolon.

The Arrangement of the Peritoneum in Transverse Section

A transverse section of the abdomen at the level of the epiploic foramen, that is above the level of the duodenum, is shown in figure 68. The peritoneum of the lesser sac extends to the left behind the stomach as far as the spleen. The peritoneum of the greater sac lines the anterior abdominal wall. It passes to the left round the abdominal wall and posteriorly leaves the anterior aspect of the left kidney to enfold the spleen almost completely. It then passes to the right in front of the stomach. Continuing to the right it forms the anterior layer of the lesser omentum and then its right free edge. It becomes continuous with the posterior layer of the lesser omentum at the epiploic foramen. To the left of the opening the two layers of the lesser sac lie behind the stomach and become continuous with each other at the hilum of the spleen. The posterior peritoneum of the lesser sac continues to the right of the opening and beyond the opening becomes continuous with the posterior peritoneum of the greater sac. This passes to the right and then anteriorly to the anterior abdominal wall. At this level of the abdominal cavity the peritoneum in the midline is reflected on to the anterior surface of the liver as the *falciform ligament*.

The Ligaments and Mesenteries of the Peritoneum

Many of these have been referred to, but a brief description of the most important helps one to understand the arrangement of the peritoneum. The *falciform ligament* (*falx = sickle*, Latin) is a double fold of peritoneum in the sagittal plane extending from the anterior abdominal wall to the anterior and superior surfaces of the liver (figures 67, 68). It represents the fetal ventral mesogastrium in which the liver develops. It reaches as far inferiorly as the umbilicus and has a lower free edge which extends to the lower margin of the liver. A fibrous cord, the remains of the left umbilical vein, lies in this lower free edge, is called the *ligamentum*

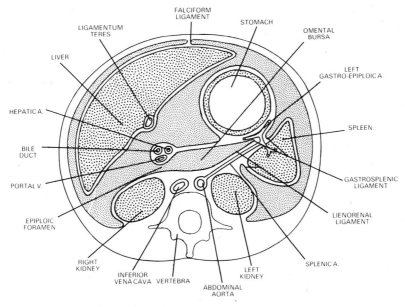

Figure 68   **The arrangement of the peritoneum in a transverse section of the abdomen above the level of the duodenum (viewed from below).**

teres (*teres = round*, Latin) and extends into a fissure on the inferior surface of the liver. The right and left leaves of the falciform ligament pass to the right and left over the liver.

The *right* and *left triangular ligaments* are double folds of peritoneum passing between the upper surface of the liver and the inferior surface of the diaphragm (figure 69). The two layers of the right triangular ligament pass to the left and as they do so they become separated and form the two layers of the coronary ligament. The result is that a considerable area of the upper and posterior surfaces of the right half of the liver is in direct contact with the diaphragm without the intervention of peritoneum. This is called the *bare area of the liver*. The superior layer of the coronary ligament is continuous with the right leaf of the falciform ligament. The inferior layer can be followed into the superior recess of the lesser sac as the posterior boundary of the epiploic foramen.

The two layers of the left triangular ligament remain close together as they pass to the right. The anterior layer becomes continuous with the left leaf of the falciform ligament. The posterior layer dips into a fissure on the inferior surface of the liver and becomes continuous with the anterior layer of the lesser omentum (figure 69).

The *lesser omentum* (figures 67, 68, 71, 82) is a double fold of peritoneum extending from the right border of the stomach (the lesser curvature) and the beginning of the duodenum to the inferior surface of the liver where some of the large blood vessels and hepatic duct enter or leave the liver (the *porta hepatis*). Between the layers lie the portal vein (posteriorly), the bile duct (to the right and anteriorly) and the hepatic artery (to the left and anteriorly). The layers of the lesser omentum are continuous with each other on the right where they form a free border which is the anterior boundary of the epiploic foramen. This opening, which lies between the liver and the beginning of the duodenum, has the following boundaries: anteriorly the right free edge of the lesser omentum, posteriorly the peritoneum covering the inferior vena cava, superiorly the liver (its caudate process) and inferiorly the beginning of the duodenum. As already described, the anterior layer of the lesser omentum passes to the left and is continuous with the posterior layer of the left triangular ligament. The posterior layer of the lesser omentum is continuous with the left edge of the superior recess of the lesser sac (figure 69).

The *greater omentum* is an apron-like fold of peritoneum suspended from the left border (greater curvature) of the stomach (figures 67, 71). Its anterior layer passes downwards for a varying distance to its lower free edge and turns upwards to pass behind the transverse colon beyond which it becomes the posterior layer of the transverse mesocolon. The greater omentum has a rich blood supply, is often loaded with fat and contains a large number of phagocytic cells. It is regarded as protective in function and is often found wrapped round an infective focus in the abdominal cavity thus limiting the spread of infection.

There are two double folds of peritoneum related to the spleen. The *lienorenal ligament* passes between the left kidney and the spleen (*lien = spleen*, Latin) and contains the splenic vessels (figure 68). Its posterior layer is peritoneum of the greater sac and its anterior layer is peritoneum of the lesser sac. The *gastrosplenic ligament* passes between the spleen and the stomach. Its anterior layer is peritoneum of the greater sac and its posterior layer is part of the wall of the lesser sac. It contains branches of the splenic artery to the stomach.

The *mesentery of the small intestine* (usually referred to as *the mesentery*) extends from the duodenojejunal flexure on the left of the second lumbar vertebra downwards to the right across the posterior abdominal wall to the right sacro-iliac joint (figures 67, 70). It is a remarkable structure

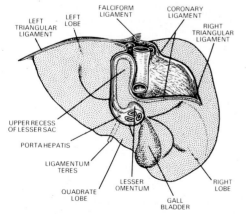

Figure 69   The peritoneal relations of the liver.

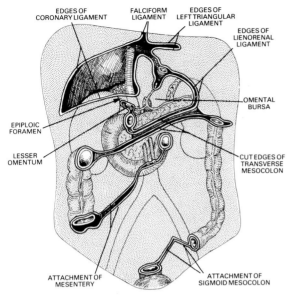

EDGES OF
CORONARY LIGAMENT

FALCIFORM
LIGAMENT

EDGES OF
LEFT TRIANGULAR
LIGAMENT

EDGES OF
LIENORENAL
LIGAMENT

OMENTAL
BURSA

EPIPLOIC
FORAMEN

LESSER
OMENTUM

CUT EDGES OF
TRANSVERSE
MESOCOLON

ATTACHMENT OF
MESENTERY

ATTACHMENT OF
SIGMOID MESOCOLON

Figure 70   The attachments of the peritoneum to the posterior abdominal wall.

in that at its abdominal attachment it is about 15 cm long and where it surrounds the small intestine it can be between 150 and 700 cm long, although it is never more than about 20 cm wide between these two attachments. It is much narrower at its left and right attachments to the abdominal wall. The mesentery contains blood and lymphatic vessels, autonomic nerves and a varying amount of fat.

The vermiform appendix has a short mesentery in which its blood and lymphatic vessels lie. It is called the *meso-appendix* and is attached to the right lower end of the mesentery of the small intestine behind the termination of the ileum.

The *transverse mesocolon* is the mesentery of the transverse colon and consists of two layers of peritoneum which are formed by the splitting of the posterior layer of the greater omentum (figures 67, 70). The posterior layer of the greater omentum consists of the fusion of its own posterior layer and the posterior layer of the inferior recess of the lesser sac. The transverse mesocolon is attached to the posterior abdominal wall along the middle of the pancreas and to the right crosses the second part of the duodenum. If the greater omentum is raised the transverse colon is raised with it. Entry to the lesser sac and the posterior wall of the stomach can be effected through the transverse mesocolon. The blood and lymphatic vessels and

the nerves of the transverse colon run in its mesentery.

The *sigmoid mesocolon* (figure 70) is a double fold of peritoneum suspending the sigmoid colon from the left pelvic wall. Its attachment is in the form of an inverted V, one limb of which runs along the brim of the pelvis to the left of the left sacro-iliac joint, where the two limbs of the V meet. The other limb passes downwards and medially to the middle of the third sacral vertebra.

The *broad ligament* is a double fold of peritoneum passing in the coronal plane from the lateral aspect of the uterus to the lateral pelvic wall. There is a large number of structures between the two layers of the broad ligament. The ovary is suspended from its posterior layer by a double fold of peritoneum called the *mesovarium* (p. 145).

The Peritoneal Spaces and Compartments

Because of the arrangement of the peritoneum, fluid in the abdominal cavity tends to collect and become localised in certain regions especially in relation to the liver. These are usually referred to as the *subphrenic spaces*. The *right* and *left subphrenic spaces* are between the diaphragm and the liver on either side of the falciform ligament. The right space is in front of the coronary ligament and the left space in front of the left triangular ligament.

The *right subhepatic space* lies below the liver between it and the right kidney. This is also called the *hepatorenal pouch* (of Morison; Rutherford Morison, 1853–1939, British surgeon) and is the lowest part of the abdominal cavity when lying flat on one's back. A groove lateral to the ascending colon (the right paracolic gutter) communicates with this space with the result that infection can spread from, for example, an inflamed appendix upwards to the hepatorenal pouch and also through the epiploic foramen. The *left subhepatic space* is the lesser sac which communicates with the right subhepatic space through the epiploic foramen.

There is also (1) a peritoneal compartment bounded above by the transverse mesocolon and below by the mesentery of the small intestine, (2) a compartment below and to the left of this mesentery (figure 70). These are called the *right* and *left infracolic spaces* respectively.

6

The Abdominal Alimentary Tract

The Abdominal Oesophagus

The *oesophagus* enters the abdominal cavity through the oesophageal opening in the right crus of the diaphragm as the crus crosses to the left (figure 71(a)). The opening is about 2 cm to the left of the midline at the level of the tenth thoracic vertebra. The oesophagus also passes forwards as it goes through the diaphragm and is accompanied by the right and left gastric nerves. In the abdomen the oesophagus is about 1.5 cm long and enters the stomach at the *cardiac orifice* (*cardia*). It lies in a groove on the upper part of the posterior aspect of the liver and is covered by peritoneum anteriorly and to the left.

The arteries to the abdominal oesophagus are derived from the left gastric artery as well as the abdominal aorta. The veins pass to the azygos vein (systemic) and left gastric vein (hepatic portal) and thus constitute a communication between the

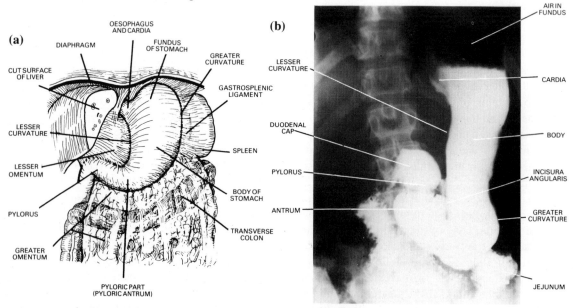

Figure 71 (a) **The abdominal oesophagus and the subdivisions of the stomach and its peritoneal relations. (b) The radiological appearance of the stomach after swallowing about 200 ml barium emulsion.**

systemic and portal venous systems. The nerves to the oesophagus are both parasympathetic (vagus) and sympathetic (thoracic sympathetic trunk and greater splanchnic nerves).

When the stomach contracts its contents do not normally pass back into the oesophagus. Many explanations are put forward to account for this:

(1) Although there is no thickening of the circular muscle of the oesophagus at its opening into the stomach and therefore no sphincter, contraction of this muscle would prevent regurgitation of the stomach contents.

(2) Circular muscle of the stomach may contract and produce the same effect.

(3) The acute angle at which the oesophagus enters the stomach could assist in closing the oesophagus.

(4) It has been suggested that the mucous membrane round the opening is thickened and can act like a valve.

(5) The intra-abdominal pressure closes the abdominal oesophagus.

(6) The fibres of the right crus of the diaphragm through which the oesophagus passes act like a sphincter.

(7) The oesophagus is twisted and under longitudinal tension. The result is that a pull by the contracting stomach causes the lumen of the oesophagus to close.

(8) A submucous pad of veins at the lower end of the oesophagus may contribute to its closure.

The Stomach

The Position, Form and Main Relations

The *stomach*, the most dilated part of the alimentary tract, is shaped like the letter J and lies in the upper left quadrant of the abdominal cavity. It varies considerably in its shape and position in different people, and also in the same individual with its state of distension, the position of the body and the state of the surrounding viscera. It has anterior and posterior surfaces and right and left borders (figure 71). The right border is called the *lesser curvature* and the left the *greater curvature*. The anterior surface is related above to the diaphragm and the left lobe of the liver, and below to the anterior abdominal wall. The posterior surface is related to a number of structures, often referred to as the *stomach bed* — inferiorly are the transverse colon and its mesocolon, above are the pancreas, left kidney and suprarenal gland and to the left are the splenic vessels and spleen which lies on the upper part of the left kidney (figure 72).

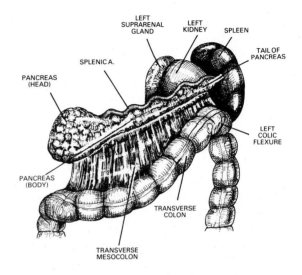

Figure 72   The posterior relations of the stomach (the stomach bed).

The stomach has two openings, the *cardiac orifice* where the oesophagus enters the stomach and the *pyloric orifice* in the pylorus where the stomach opens into the duodenum. *The cardiac orifice lies about 3 cm to the left of and below the xiphoid process and the pylorus is about 2 cm to the right of the midline on the transpyloric plane (p. 68) at the level of the first lumbar vertebra. The position of the pylorus, however, is much more variable than is suggested in most textbooks.*

The stomach is divided into the *fundus*, which is that part lying above the level of the cardiac orifice, the *body*, which is below the fundus, and the *pyloric part*, which is marked off from the body by the *angular notch* at the lower end of the lesser curvature (figure 71). The part next to the body is called the *pyloric antrum*. The circular muscle of the pylorus is thickened to form the *pyloric sphincter* which is marked on the surface by a groove in which a vein lies.

The lining of the stomach is ridged. The ridges are parallel along the lesser curvature but are more irregularly arranged elsewhere. A flexible instrument called a *gastroscope* can be passed from the mouth into the stomach and the mucous membrane examined. The folds can be seen and the lining appears to be reddish.

The Peritoneum (figures 67, 68, 71)

The peritoneum of the lesser omentum is attached to the lesser curvature and that of the greater omentum to the greater curvature (p. 80). The omental bursa extends to the left behind the stomach. The gastrosplenic ligament lies between the stomach and the spleen and contains the left gastro-epiploic and short gastric vessels.

The Blood Supply and Lymphatic Drainage (figure 73)

The stomach receives its blood supply from the *coeliac artery* or its branches. The coeliac artery is the *artery of the foregut* which extends to the middle of the descending (second) part of the duodenum. The term artery of the foregut is somewhat misleading because the foregut refers to the gut or enteron from the mouth to the middle of the duodenum. The coeliac artery supplies the gut only as far proximally as the abdominal oesophagus. It also supplies the derivatives of the foregut (the liver and pancreas) and the spleen, which develops in the dorsal mesogastrium and not from the foregut. The arteries to the stomach run along the curvatures, the left and right gastric arteries along the lesser and the left and right gastro-epiploic arteries along the greater. The left gastric artery is a direct branch of the coeliac artery and the right gastric is a branch of the common hepatic artery, which is a branch of the coeliac. The left gastro-epiploic artery is a branch of the splenic artery which arises from the coeliac and the right gastro-epiploic is a branch of the gastroduodenal, a branch of the common hepatic artery. There are also short gastric arteries which supply the fundus and come from the splenic artery.

The veins draining the stomach pass to the hepatic portal vein which goes to the liver. The hepatic portal vein is usually formed by the union of the splenic and superior mesenteric veins behind the neck of the pancreas. The right and left gastric veins go directly into the portal vein and the right gastro-epiploic veins to the superior mesenteric vein. The left gastro-epiploic and short gastric veins drain into the splenic vein (figure 87).

The lymphatic drainage of the stomach follows the pattern seen in the rest of the abdominal part of the alimentary tract. In the organ itself there are submucosal and muscular lymphatic plexuses which go to a subserous plexus of vessels. This plexus leaves the organ and passes to lymph nodes near the organ itself, which drain to nodes along the blood vessels. Most of these drain to nodes on the posterior abdominal wall. For its lymphatic drainage the stomach is conveniently divided into three parts as in figure 73(c). The right half of the stomach drains into nodes along the lesser curvature and thence to the coeliac nodes. The lymphatic vessels from the fundus and upper half of the left part of the stomach go to nodes along the greater curvature and thence to nodes along the splenic artery (pancreaticosplenic) and finally to the coeliac nodes. The lymphatic vessels from the lower half of the left part of the stomach go to nodes along the greater curvature and pylorus. From there the vessels may go to the coeliac nodes or to hepatic nodes near the liver. This connection with the hepatic nodes results in a lymphatic communication between the stomach and those hepatic lymphatic vessels which go to the mediastinum.

The Nerve Supply

The stomach has a parasymphathetic and sympathetic nerve supply. The parasympathetic nerves come from the gastric nerves. The anterior (mainly the left vagus nerve) supplies the cardia, lesser curvature and pyloric antrum. The posterior gastric nerve (mainly the right vagus) supplies the anterior and posterior walls of the body. The fibres of the gastric nerves are preganglionic and synapse with a ganglion cell in the wall of the stomach. The gastric (vagus) nerves are motor to the longitudinal muscle

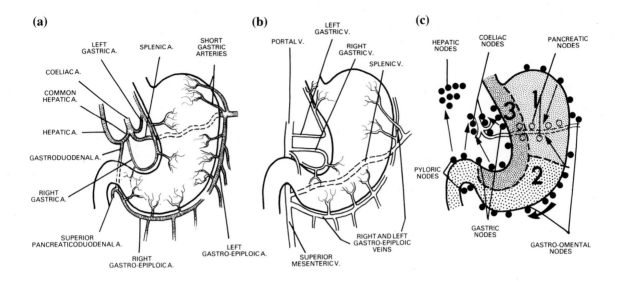

(a)

LEFT GASTRIC A.
SPLENIC A.
SHORT GASTRIC ARTERIES
COELIAC A.
COMMON HEPATIC A.
HEPATIC A.
GASTRODUODENAL A.
RIGHT GASTRIC A.
SUPERIOR PANCREATICODUODENAL A.
RIGHT GASTRO-EPIPLOIC A.
LEFT GASTRO-EPIPLOIC A.

(b)

PORTAL V.
LEFT GASTRIC V.
RIGHT GASTRIC V.
SPLENIC V.
RIGHT AND LEFT GASTRO-EPIPLOIC VEINS
SUPERIOR MESENTERIC V.

(c)

HEPATIC NODES
COELIAC NODES
PANCREATIC NODES
PYLORIC NODES
GASTRIC NODES
GASTRO-OMENTAL NODES

Figure 73 **(a) The arterial blood supply. (b) The venous drainage. (c) The lymphatic drainage of the stomach.**

and secretomotor to the glands. Cutting these nerves (*vagotomy*), an operation used in peptic ulcer, results in reduced motility and gastric secretion. The reduced motility may create a problem due to the stomach not being able to empty itself.

The sympathetic nerves to the stomach come from the coeliac plexus and are postganglionic. The preganglionic fibres to the coeliac plexus are mainly in the splanchnic nerves which come from the thoracic sympathetic trunk. The postganglionic fibres from the coeliac ganglia reach the stomach mainly as perivascular plexuses. The stomach also receives fibres from the upper lumbar sympathetic ganglia which contribute postganglionic fibres to the coeliac plexus. The sympathetic fibres inhibit peristalsis and gastric secretion and cause the circular muscle, especially the pyloric sphincter, to contract.

Both the parasympathetic and sympathetic nerves contain sensory fibres. The former are associated with gastric reflexes and the latter with pain.

The Coeliac Trunk (Artery)

This branch of the abdominal aorta arises just be-

low the crossing of the two crura of the diaphragm where the aorta enters the abdomen at the level of the upper part of the first lumbar vertebra. The artery is about 2 cm long and is surrounded by the autonomic coeliac ganglia and plexuses with the coeliac lymph nodes on either side. It usually divides into the left gastric, splenic and common hepatic arteries. There is considerable variation in the way in which the branches arise.

The *left gastric artery* passes upwards and to the left behind the omental bursa to the cardiac end of the stomach and turns downwards along the lesser curvature between the two layers of the lesser omentum towards the pylorus and anastomoses with the right gastric artery. It gives off oesophageal branches as well as branches to both surfaces of the stomach.

The *splenic artery* passes to the left behind the upper border of the pancreas with the splenic vein inferior to it. The artery crosses anterior to the left suprarenal gland and kidney behind the stomach and enters the lienorenal ligament in which it divides into five or six branches before entering the spleen.

The splenic artery is large and tortuous. It gives off pancreatic branches as it passes to the left. In the lienorenal ligament it gives off the *short gastric arteries* which pass in the gastrosplenic ligament to the fundus of the stomach, and the *left gastro-epiploic* which passes in the same ligament to the greater curvature of the stomach. The left gastro-epiploic artery runs to the right and anastomoses with the right gastro-epiploic artery. Both arteries supply the stomach and greater omentum.

The *common hepatic artery* runs to the right below the epiploic foramen to the upper border of the superior (first) part of the duodenum. It gives off the *right gastric artery* which passes to the left along the lesser curvature between the layers of the lesser omentum and anastomoses with the left gastric artery.

The common hepatic artery at the upper border of the superior part of the duodenum divides into the *hepatic* and *gastroduodenal arteries*. The hepatic artery runs upwards to the liver between the layers of the lesser omentum, anterior to the epiploic foramen, with the bile duct on its right and the portal vein posteriorly. The hepatic artery divides into the right and left hepatic arteries (p. 98). The *cystic artery* to the gall bladder arises most commonly from the right hepatic artery, although this occurs in less than 50 per cent of individuals.

The gastroduodenal artery passes downwards behind the superior part of the duodenum and head of the pancreas with the bile duct on its right. The artery divides into the *right gastro-epiploic* and *superior pancreaticoduodenal arteries*. The former runs along the greater curvature of the stomach to the left and anastomoses with the left gastro-epiploic artery. The superior pancreatico-duodenal artery runs downwards between the head of the pancreas and the descending (second) part of the duodenum and anastomoses with the inferior pancreaticoduodenal artery from the superior mesenteric artery.

The Small Intestine

This consists of the C-shaped *duodenum* which is retroperitoneal, that is directly related to the posterior abdominal wall, and the *jejunum* and the *ileum* which are suspended from the posterior abdominal wall by their *mesentery* (p. 80). The

duodenum is about 25 cm long. The jejunum and ileum are estimated to be from 1.5 m to 7 m long. This variation is due to the different methods used for measuring. In the living a radio-opaque tube can be swallowed and will pass to the end of the alimentary tract. In these circumstances the length of the jejunum and ileum is about 1.5 m. After death, before fixation by embalming, the length may be up to 7 m. The small intestine and its mesentery are folded like a concertina and can lengthen especially if the muscle of the wall is completely relaxed as in the cadaver.

The duodenum

Its name refers to its length, which is 12 fingers' breadth (*duodenum = duodenum digitorum = space of 12 fingers' breadth,* Latin). It is C-shaped and is related to the upper three lumbar vertebrae with the body of the second and the head of the pancreas in the concavity of the C. The duodenum begins at the pylorus about 2 cm to the right of the first lumbar vertebra and ends at the *duodeno-jejunal flexure* about 1.4 cm to the left of the second lumbar vertebra (figure 74). It is divided into four parts which used to be conveniently named *first*, *second*, *third* and *fourth*. The first part is now called the *superior*, the second the *descending*, the third the *horizontal* or *inferior*, and the fourth the *ascending*.

The *superior* (*first*) part is about 5 cm long and passes upwards to the right. It is anterior to the bile duct (right) and the gastroduodenal artery (left). These structures lie in front of the portal vein. The liver and gall bladder are anterior to this part of the duodenum.

The *descending* (*second*) part passes downwards and is about 7.5 cm long. It has a common opening on the middle of its posteromedial wall for the main pancreatic duct and bile duct. The opening is on a papilla. Within the wall the common opening is dilated and forms the *hepatopancreatic ampulla* (*of Vater*; A. Vater, 1684–1751, German anatomist), which is surrounded by the *ampullary sphincter* (*of Oddi*; R. Oddi, nineteenth century Italian surgeon). The descending part of the duodenum lies in front of the hilum of the right kidney and the renal vessels (figure 74). The transverse mesocolon crosses

(a)

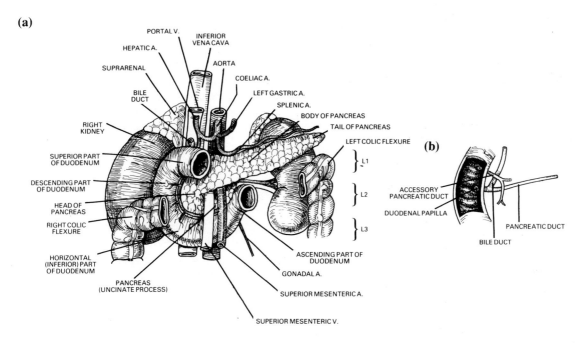

(b)

Figure 74   **(a) The main relations of the duodenum. (b) The common opening of the bile and main pancreatic ducts.**

anterior to this part of the duodenum (figure 70).

The *horizontal* (*third*) part, about 10 cm long, passes to the left anterior to the inferior vena cava and abdominal aorta as they lie in front of the lumbar vertebrae. The gonadal and inferior mesenteric arteries arise from the aorta behind this part of the duodenum which is crossed anteriorly by the superior mesenteric vessels.

The *ascending* (*fourth*) part, 2.5 cm long, passes upwards to the left of the second lumbar vertebra and bends forwards to become the jejunum at the duodenojejunal flexure. It lies to the left of the abdominal aorta and in front of the left renal and gonadal vessels.

The superior and ascending (first and fourth) parts have peritoneum on their anterior and posterior surfaces where they are adjacent to the stomach and jejunum respectively. The arrangement gives considerable mobility to these parts of the duodenum, especially the superior part. Elsewhere there is peritoneum only on the anterior surface of the duodenum. There are recesses of the peritoneum to the left of the ascending part of the duodenum (figure 80). The inferior mesenteric vein lies in the

fold forming the *paraduodenal fossa*. The *suspensory muscle of the duodenum* is a fibromuscular structure passing from the duodenojejunal flexure upwards behind the pancreas to the right crus of the diaphragm. This muscle is used by surgeons to identify the duodenojejunal junction. It may also kink the duodenum and cause obstruction.

The duodenum is derived from both the foregut and midgut, which meet just distal to the common opening for the bile and pancreatic ducts. Its blood supply comes from the coeliac artery through a branch of the gastroduodenal artery, the superior pancreaticoduodenal, and the inferior pancreaticoduodenal artery, a branch of the superior mesenteric, the artery of the midgut. These two arteries run vertically in the groove between the head of the pancreas and the duodenum (figure 74). This description of the arteries to the duodenum and head of the pancreas is an oversimplification, and supraduodenal, retroduodenal and anterior and posterior superior pancreaticoduodenal branches from the gastroduodenal artery are described.

The pancreaticoduodenal veins join the superior mesenteric vein which forms, with the splenic vein, the portal vein. The lymph nodes to which the lymphatic vessels from the duodenum drain lie between the head of the pancreas and the duodenum and these nodes drain into the pre-aortic nodes near the origin of the superior mesenteric artery.

The jejunum and ileum

These two parts of the small intestine are very similar in structure, although a part of the jejunum near the duodenum can be distinguished from a part of the ileum near its termination at the ileo-caecal opening. Reference has already been made to the mesentery of the jejunum and ileum (p. 80) and to the apparent variation in their length (p. 86). The jejunum and ileum lie in coils in the middle of the abdominal cavity framed by the large intestine (figure 66). The coils lie more or less in the middle of the abdominal cavity and hang down into the pelvis where they overlie the bladder and uterus. The terminal 10 cm of the ileum has a short mesentery and rises out of the pelvis to join the caecum.

A typical part of the jejunum has a thicker wall than the ileum and the folds on the lining (*plicae circulares*) are more marked and more numerous in the upper part of the jejunum. Near the termination of the ileum there are fewer folds. The mesentery of the upper part of the jejunum contains fewer arterial arcades than the mesentery of the lower part of the ileum and the jejunal arcades are nearer its margin (figure 75(b), (c)). The fat in the mesentery reaches the ileal margin but does not extend to the edge of the jejunum.

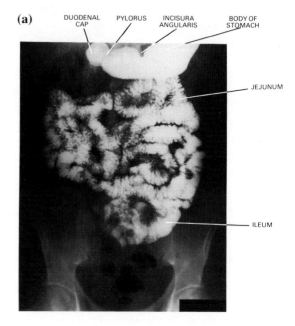

(a)   DUODENAL CAP   PYLORUS   INCISURA ANGULARIS   BODY OF STOMACH

JEJUNUM

ILEUM

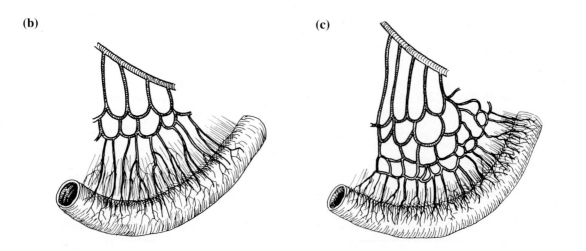

(b)   (c)

Figure 75   **(a) The radiological appearance of the jejunum and ileum 40 min after a barium meal. (b) The arterial arcades of the jejunum. (c) The arterial arcades of the ileum.**

The attachment of the mesentery to the posterior abdominal wall is called its *root*. The root crosses the abdominal aorta, the horizontal part of the duodenum and the right psoas muscle, ureter and gonadal vessels. The obliquity of the mesentery enables one to follow a loop of the small intestine either upwards to the left towards the duodenum or downwards to the right towards the caecum. The attachment of the mesentery produces two peritoneal spaces, a lower which communicates with the pelvis and an upper which is limited above by the transverse mesocolon (figure 70).

The circular folds of the lining of the jejunum and ileum are also present in the duodenum except for about 4 cm next to the pylorus (figure 75(a)). The surface of the folds looks like velvet due to the presence of *villi*. Lymph follicles are found throughout the whole alimentary tract but they become aggregated in a typical manner only in the ileum (*folliculi lymphatici aggregati*). The old eponymous name, *Peyer's patches*, seems to be a more convenient term (J.C. Peyer, 1653–1712, Swiss anatomist). These aggregations are not visible to the naked eye as a rule.

The Superior Mesenteric Artery and Vein

The arterial supply of the small intestine, except for the ascending part of the duodenum, is the *superior mesenteric artery*, which arises from the front of the aorta behind the body of the pancreas. At its origin the artery is crossed anteriorly by the splenic vein. The artery passes downwards in front of the left renal vein, the uncinate process of the pancreas and the horizontal part of the duodenum (figure 74) and enters the mesentery of the small intestine, in which it curves downwards and to the right.

From its left side it gives off a number of *jejunal* and *ileal* branches. From its right side above the third part of the duodenum it gives off the *inferior pancreaticoduodenal artery* which runs to the right and then upwards between the head of the pancreas and the descending part of the duodenum (figure 74). The superior mesenteric artery also gives off branches to the large intestine — the *middle colic* to the transverse colon, the *right colic* to the ascending

colon and the *ileocolic* to the caecum and terminal part of the ileum. All these arteries anastomose with each other (figure 76). The *caecal branches* are *anterior* and *posterior*, and the posterior caecal artery passes behind the end of the ileum and gives off the *appendicular artery* to the vermiform appendix. An *ileal branch* runs to the left and anastomoses with the termination of the superior mesenteric artery.

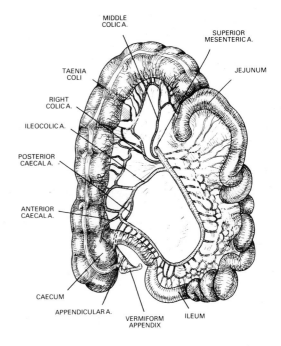

Figure 76   The superior mesenteric artery and its main branches

The superior mesenteric vein corresponds very closely with the artery in so far as it begins in the region of the ileocaecal junction, and receives tributaries corresponding to the branches of the artery as it passes upwards on the right of the artery in the mesentery of the small intestine. The vein lies in front of the horizontal part of the duodenum and deep to the neck of the pancreas. Here it unites with the splenic vein and forms the portal vein.

The superior mesenteric artery is the *artery of the midgut* which extends from just beyond the common opening of the bile and pancreatic ducts in the duodenum to the left colic flexure. That the transverse colon crosses the descending part of the

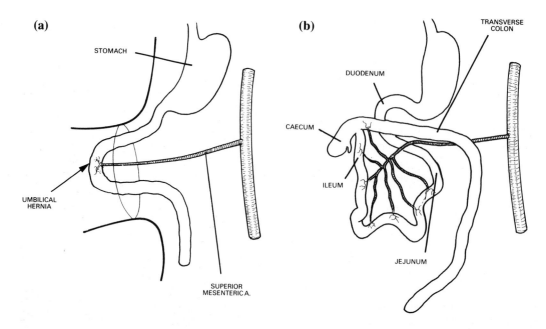

Figure 77   The rotation of the gut in the fetus: (a) the umbilical hernia; (b) the lower loop of the U rotates counterclockwise so that the colon crosses the descending part of the duodenum and the superior mesenteric vessels cross the inferior part of the duodenum.

duodenum and the superior mesenteric vessels cross the horizontal part is due to a complex process in the embryo referred to as the *rotation of the gut* (figure 77).

The alimentary tract or enteron develops from the yolk sac, part of which is enclosed in the embryo. For a time the enteron is continuous with the yolk sac through the vitello-intestinal duct. Normally this disappears but it may persist as a patent finger-like process communicating with the ileum. This is known as an *ileal* (*Meckel's*) *diverticulum* (J.F. Meckel, 1781–1833, German surgeon and anatomist). It is said to occur in 2 per cent of individuals, about 2 feet (60 cm) from the ileo-caecal junction and to be about 2 inches (5 cm) long. Its structure is similar to that of the ileum and it may be joined to the umbilicus by a fibrous cord.

The Large Intestine (figure 78)

This consists of the caecum and vermiform appendix, the ascending, transverse, descending and sigmoid (pelvic) colons and the rectum and anal canal (figure 66). Apart from that of the appendix and rectum the longitudinal muscle of the large intestine is arranged in three bands called *taeniae coli* (figure 76). Since they are shorter than the rest of the colon the taeniae produce characteristic sacculations of the wall called *haustra* (*taenia* = *band*, Latin; *haustrum* = *well bucket*, Latin). The wall of the large intestine has fatty projections, *appendices epiploicae*. They are covered by peritoneum and are not present on the caecum, appendix and rectum. One can distinguish the large intestine from the small by these three features — the taeniae, the sacculations and the appendices epiploicae. Although the large intestine has a greater diameter than the small this is an unreliable guide for distinguishing one from the other.

The Caecum

The caecum, a blind ending pouch about 10 cm long and 5 cm wide, is inferior to the entry of the ileum into the large intestine (*caecum = blind*,

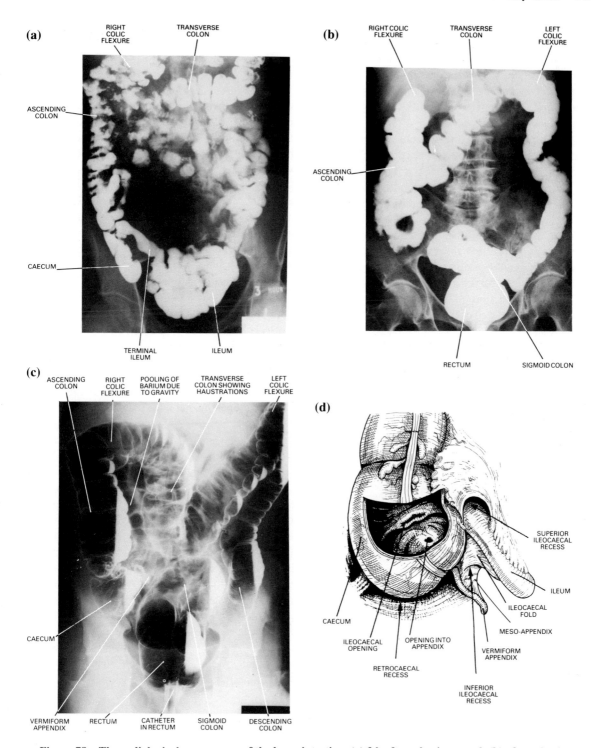

Figure 78 **The radiological appearance of the large intestine: (a) 3 h after a barium meal; (b) after a barium enema; (c) double contrast enema – a small quantity of barium followed by insufflation with air (left lateral position). (d) The vermiform appendix, caecum, related folds of the peritoneum, and ileocaecal opening**

Latin). It lies in the right iliac fossa on the iliacus and psoas muscles with the lateral femoral cutaneous and femoral nerves passing downwards and laterally behind it. *The caecum is above the lateral end of the inguinal ligament and lateral to the right lateral line*, and is related anteriorly to the anterior abdominal wall.

The peritoneum of the caecum is somewhat variable in its arrangement but usually it is almost surrounded by peritoneum so that it is fairly mobile with a recess passing upwards behind it, the *retrocaecal recess* in which the vermiform appendix often lies (figure 78(d)). There are superior and inferior folds of peritoneum between terminal parts of the ileum and the caecum. Appendicitis is common and when operating the surgeon must not mistake these folds for the meso-appendix.

The *ileocaecal opening* is transverse and is on the posteromedial wall of the caecum (figure 78(d)). It is bounded by two horizontal folds which project into the caecum, contain circular ileal muscle, and act like a valve. Intermittent relaxation of the valve allows the ileal contents to pass into the large intestine. The valve is not very effective in preventing a reflux of caecal contents into the ileum, especially when the caecum is distended by a barium enema.

The Vermiform Appendix (figure 78(d))

Of very variable length, 3–20 cm, and about 0.5–1 cm in width this structure is usually attached to the inferomedial aspect of the caecum. In the fetus it is at the apex of the caecum but although this may persist (3 per cent) the caecum usually grows more on its anterolateral side so that the site of origin of the appendix is moved medially and upwards. The three taeniae of the caecum always converge on to the appendix irrespective of its site of attachment.

The appendix is completely covered by peritoneum and has a mesentery (*meso-appendix*) which is attached to its proximal half and to the terminal part of the ileum and the posterior abdominal wall. The appendix is very mobile and its position very variable. Its two commonest sites are *retrocaecal* or *retrocolic* (65 per cent) and *pelvic* (20 per cent).

It can also be directed upwards and medially either behind or in front of the terminal ileum (1.5 per cent). Not all investigators would agree with these figures.

The signs and symptoms of appendicitis vary with these different positions. If retrocaecal, the iliacus and psoas muscles may go into spasm so that the right thigh is flexed. If pelvic, the rectum may be affected or in the female conditions associated with the female genital organs are simulated. Usually appendicitis begins with pain round the umbilicus because the pain is due to spasm of the inflamed organ and is referred to the abdominal wall which has the same segmental innervation. Later the pain is felt in the right iliac fossa, which is tender on palpation, because the inflammation has spread to the parietal peritoneum. The site of maximum tenderness is said to be at *McBurney's point* situated 1¾ inches (4.4 cm) from the anterior superior iliac spine on a line joining that spine to the umbilicus (C. McBurney, 1845–1913, American surgeon). This site of maximum tenderness must be more variable.

The opening into the appendix, 2 cm below the ileocaecal opening, has a fold of mucous membrane on one side but this has no valvular effect. In the infant the lumen of the appendix is patent along its whole length. Closure of the lumen begins at its tip and may be complete in old age.

The vermiform appendix has large masses of lymphoid tissue in its submucosa and its longitudinal muscle coat forms a more or less continuous layer unlike that of the rest of the large intestine. Because of its lymphoid tissue the appendix may be regarded as part of the homologue of the *bursa of Fabricius* in birds, in which case it may be an important organ in relation to the immune responses of the body (H. Fabricius, 1533–1619, Italian anatomist). On the other hand, because the appendix is a large lymphoid organ in herbivores, it is usually regarded as a vestigial structure in man with no particular significance.

The Ascending Colon

This extends from the ileocaecal orifice to the inferior surface of the right lobe of the liver at the level of the second lumbar vertebra where it turns to the left at the *right colic (hepatic) flexure*. Below the level of the liver the anterior abdominal wall and coils of small intestine are in front of the ascending colon *which lies to the right of the right lateral line*. Posteriorly are the iliacus and quadratus lumborum muscles with branches of the lumbar plexus of nerves intervening (the iliohypogastric and ilio-inguinal nerves). The right colic flexure (figure 74) is in front of the lower pole of the right kidney and to the right of the ascending part of the duodenum.

The ascending colon and right colic flexure usually lie directly on the posterior abdominal wall or directly on the organs to which they are related without any intervening peritoneum. They may have a mesentery (25 per cent of subjects). The right paracolic gutter has already been described (p. 81).

The Transverse Colon

This part of the colon extends from the right colic flexure across the abdomen to the *left colic (splenic) flexure* which is adjacent to the lower part of the visceral surface of the spleen. Beyond the right colic flexure the transverse colon is suspended from the posterior abdominal wall by the *transverse mesocolon* (p. 81) with the result that the colon hangs downwards to a very variable extent behind the greater omentum (figures 67, 71, 72). It can extend into the pelvis or lie behind the lower part of the stomach.

To the right, where the mesocolon is absent, the transverse colon is related posteriorly to the descending part of the duodenum and the head of the pancreas. Anteriorly it is related to the liver and gall bladder. The transverse colon when followed to the left lies behind the greater curvature of the stomach and in front of the small intestine and duodenojejunal flexure.

The left colic flexure is higher than the right and is the region where the transverse colon turns downwards and becomes the descending colon (figure 74). The left flexure is related posteriorly to the lower pole of the left kidney and antero-laterally to the lower part of the spleen. The flexure

is attached to the diaphragm near the eleventh and twelfth ribs by a fold of peritoneum, the *phrenico-colic ligament*.

The Descending Colon

This extends from the left colic flexure to the brim of the pelvis, where it becomes the sigmoid colon. It lies on the psoas and quadratus lumborum muscles and then on the psoas and iliacus muscles. *It is to the left of the left lateral line*.

Anteriorly the descending colon is related to coils of the small intestine and lower down to the anterior abdominal wall. Several structures pass downwards and laterally behind the descending colon – the left subcostal, iliohypogastric, ilio-inguinal, lateral femoral cutaneous and femoral nerves. At the brim of the pelvis the genitofemoral nerve and external iliac artery lie behind the descending colon.

Usually the peritoneum of this part of the colon covers only its front and sides, but there may be a short mesentery (35 per cent of subjects).

The Sigmoid (Pelvic) Colon

This is an S-shaped loop of variable length extending from the descending colon to the rectum which begins at the level of the third sacral vertebra. The sigmoid colon has a mesentery (the *sigmoid mesocolon*) which has two limbs (figure 70). One is attached to about 4 cm of the brim of the pelvis lateral to the left sacro-iliac joint and the other to the pelvic wall, from the joint downwards and medially to the middle of the sacrum. By picking up the pelvic colon and following the pelvic mesocolon to the apex of the two limbs one can find the left ureter as it crosses the division of the left common iliac artery in front of the sacro-iliac joint. There is often a recess of peritoneum extending upwards in front of the ureter.

The sigmoid colon hangs downwards into the pelvis in front of the rectum and behind the bladder or uterus. It will therefore be related to structures on the lateral wall of the pelvis such as the left ovary, or the ductus deferens, and the obturator nerve, and to structures on the posterior wall of the pelvis such as the internal iliac vessels, sacral plexus and piriformis.

The remainder of the large intestine, the rectum and anal canal, are described with the pelvis (p.134).

The Inferior Mesenteric Artery and Vein (figure 79)

This is the *artery of the hindgut*, which extends from the left colic flexure to the rectum. The artery arises from the abdominal aorta at the level of the third lumbar vertebra at the lower border of the horizontal part of the duodenum. As the artery passes downwards it moves to the left, crosses the left common iliac vessels and enters the pelvis behind the attachment of the pelvic mesocolon. It continues in the pelvis as the *superior rectal artery*. The inferior mesenteric vein runs to the left of the artery.

The blood supply of the caecum, appendix and ascending and most of the transverse colon comes from the superior mesenteric artery (p. 89). The inferior mesenteric artery gives off the *left colic artery* which passes to the left in front of the psoas

muscle, ureter and gonadal vessels, and supplies by ascending and descending branches part of the transverse colon, the left colic flexure and the descending colon. These branches anastomose above with the middle colic artery and below with the next branches of the inferior mesenteric artery, the *sigmoid arteries*. These supply the lowest part of the descending colon and the sigmoid colon and anastomose below with the superior rectal artery.

The inferior mesenteric vein corresponds closely with the artery. It begins as the superior rectal vein which passes upwards to become the inferior mesenteric vein. It receives the sigmoid and left colic veins and behind the body of the pancreas ends in the splenic vein which takes part in the formation of the portal vein.

To the left of the duodenojejunal flexure the inferior mesenteric vein often lies in a peritoneal fold behind which there may be a peritoneal recess to the left, the *paraduodenal fossa* (figure 80). A loop of small intestine may form an impacted internal hernia in this recess and the presence of the vein in the anterior wall of its opening has to be kept in mind if an attempt is made to release the hernia by cutting the opening.

The communications between the superior rectal veins and the rest of the veins of the rectum constitute one of the *portal-systemic anastomoses*. These are referred to more fully on p. 87.

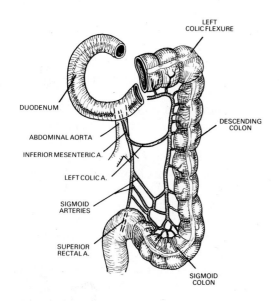

Figure 79   The distribution of the inferior mesenteric artery.

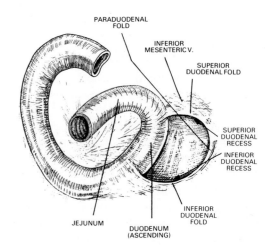

Figure 80   The peritoneal fossae related to the ascending (fourth) part of the duodenum.

The Lymphatic Drainage and Nerve Supply of the Small and Large Intestine

The arrangement of the lymphatic vessels and lymph nodes is the same for both the large and small intestine. There are submucous and subserous plexuses of vessels which drain to lymph nodes along the intestinal wall (figure 99). These nodes drain to nodes along the blood vessels and these in turn to nodes on the front and at the sides of the aorta and inferior vena cava. Most of the nodes are named after vessels to which they are related — *superior* and *inferior mesenteric, ileocolic, right colic*, etc. *Intestinal lymph trunks* are formed and go to the cisterna chyli which is the beginning of the thoracic duct and lies to the right of the abdominal aorta just below the diaphragm.

The villi of the small intestine contain a lymph vessel called a *lacteal*. These lacteals pass to the submucous plexus. They are called lacteals because they are filled with a milky fluid (absorbed fat) after a meal.

Cancer of the colon is fairly common and spreads along the lymphatic vessels to the nodes. It can also spread to the liver via the tributaries of the hepatic portal vein.

Both the small and large intestine have a sympathetic and parasympathetic innervation. The *sympathetic innervation* is from the plexuses on the front and sides of the aorta, mainly the *superior mesenteric, intermesenteric* and *inferior mesenteric plexuses*. These fibres are postganglionic and go to the gut wall as plexuses round the arteries. The preganglionic fibres are in the greater and lesser splanchnic nerves which go to the coeliac plexuses and extend downwards in front of the aorta. Some of the postganglionic fibres come from the lumbar sympathetic ganglia. The sympathetic fibres inhibit peristalsis and cause contraction of the ileocaecal sphincter and vasoconstriction.

The *parasympathetic fibres* to the small intestine and the large intestine as far as the left colic flexure come from the vagus (gastric) nerves which go to the coeliac plexuses and pass downwards to the bifurcation of the aorta and beyond. These parasympathetic fibres are preganglionic, reach the gut wall by passing along the arteries, and synapse with ganglion cells in the intestinal wall itself.

From the left colic flexure to the rectum the preganglionic parasympathetic fibres come from the *pelvic splanchnic nerves* (contained in the second, third and fourth sacral spinal nerves) which go to plexuses in the pelvis and pass upwards into the abdomen either along the superior rectal and then the inferior mesenteric arteries or independently in the retroperitoneal tissues. Stimulation of the parasympathetic nerves produces peristalsis and glandular secretion.

The sensory fibres from the small and large intestine are both sympathetic and parasympathetic, and when stimulated by stretching (distension) of the gut or spasm produce the painful sensations described as *abdominal colic*. Cutting or burning the gut wall does not produce pain since these sensory fibres apparently do not respond to this type of stimulus.

The Radiology of the Alimentary Tract

By means of a barium meal the stomach and small and large intestines can be made radio-opaque and visualised radiologically. About 200 ml of an emulsion containing 50 per cent w/v of barium are swallowed and the stomach is examined by the radiologist using a fluoroscopic screen. An X-ray can be taken and a typical appearance of the stomach is shown in figure 71(b). There is considerable variation, however, in the size, form and position of the organ and the variations are related to the body build, the position of the body, respiration, the gastric contents and the state of closely related organs.

Only the superior (first) part of the duodenum is clearly outlined by the barium. The rest of the duodenum is broken up by the mucosal folds and is not clearly seen. The superior part of the duodenum is referred to as the *duodenal cap* because it often is seen as a triangle with the base next to the pylorus. A peptic ulcer, a very common condition, can affect any of the walls of the superior part of the duodenum. It is therefore examined from different angles so that various parts of the cap can be visualised.

The jejunum and ileum are visible (figure 75(a)) after about 40 min. This procedure is called a *barium follow-through* and is sometimes used to examine the large intestine. The barium in the small intestine is moved very rapidly and broken up by the mucosal folds with the result that the jejunum and ileum present the serrated appearance seen in the figure. The terminal part of the ileum, less active and with fewer folds, often appears as an opaque cylinder with a smooth outline running upwards and to the right from the pelvis.

After about 3 h the outline of the large intestine can be seen (figure 78(a)), but this part of the alimentary tract is usually investigated by means of a barium enema (figure 78(b)). Typically the colon shows sacculations (haustrations) due to transverse bands of contraction. Their absence in some parts of the colon is due to one part of the colon overlapping another.

Immediately after evacuation of the barium the large intestine is again examined because more details of the lining may sometimes be seen. A *double contrast enema*, in which a small amount of barium emulsion is followed by insufflation of the large intestine with some air, is used to obtain a detailed view of the mucosa (figure 78(c)). The barium levels seen are due to the X-ray being taken with the subject in the left lateral position.

7

The Liver, Bile Passages, Pancreas and Spleen

The liver and pancreas develop from the caudal end of the foregut to which they remain attached through the bile duct from the liver and the pancreatic ducts. The spleen develops in the dorsal mesogastrium and all three organs are supplied by the artery of the foregut, the coeliac, and are drained by veins which join the portal vein.

The Liver

The Form and Position

The liver is a large, reddish-brown, glandular organ weighing about 1.5 kg, firm to touch but easily torn. It lies in the upper right quadrant of the abdominal cavity (figure 66) and is pyramidal in shape with the base to the right and the apex to the left. Its thick fibrous capsule sends incomplete septa into its substance and there is also a fibrous tissue framework derived from the connective tissue coverings of the blood vessels and bile ducts. Superiorly, anteriorly, posteriorly and to the right it is related to the diaphragm (*diaphragmatic surface*). Its *inferior (visceral) surface* faces backwards, downwards and to the left. The *falciform ligament* (p. 79) divides the liver into two lobes, a large right and a much smaller left. *The left lobe extends to the left of the midline for about 8 cm. The upper surface of the liver is at the level of the anterior end of the fifth or sixth intercostal space. Its lower edge runs upwards to the left and corresponds with the right costal margin. In the midline*

it is about 3 cm below the level of the xiphoid process. Normally the lower edge of the liver is not palpable below the costal margin. By percussion below the xiphoid process one can demonstrate that the liver moves downwards on inspiration and upwards on expiration.

The Peritoneum (figure 81(a))

The relations of the peritoneum to the liver have already been described (p. 80). These include the *falciform ligament* between the anterior abdominal wall and the diaphragm and liver, the *right* and *left triangular* and the *coronary ligaments* between the diaphragm and the liver, the upper part of the *lesser omentum* round the edges of the porta hepatis (p. 80) and the *upper recess of the lesser sac* in the fissure for the ligamentum venosum (p. 78). The liver is covered by peritoneum except for the bare area which is between the two layers of the coronary ligament. Here the liver is in direct contact with the diaphragm.

The Lobes and Main Relations (figure 81)

The visceral surface is divided into a number of lobes. The right and left lobes are separated by two deep fissures. The lower is the *fissure for the ligamentum teres*. It contains the *ligamentum teres* which runs in the lower free border of the falciform ligament and is the remains of the fetal *left*

(a)

(b)

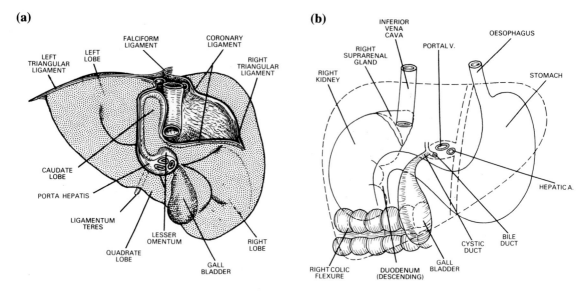

Figure 81   **(a) The peritoneal relations of the liver. (b) The posterior relations of the liver.**

umbilical vein. The upper fissure is the *fissure for the ligamentum venosum* in which lies the ligament of that name. This ligament is the remains of the fetal *ductus venosus* which joined the left umbilical vein to the inferior vena cava via the left portal vein and left hepatic vein.

The inferior vena cava lies behind the liver on the posterior part of the diaphragmatic surface about 3 cm to the right of the midline and marks off the *caudate lobe* which lies between the inferior vena cava and the fissure for the ligamentum venosum (figure 81(a)). This fissure extends to the right between the caudate lobe and the main part of the liver and contains the superior recess of the lesser sac.

The *quadrate lobe* is that part of the right lobe lying between the fissure for the ligamentum teres and the gall bladder which lies on the inferior surface of the right lobe about 3 cm to the right of the fissure for the ligamentum teres. The *porta hepatis*, where the portal vein and hepatic artery enter the liver and the common hepatic duct leaves it, lies between the caudate lobe and the quadrate lobe.

The organs related to the visceral surface are shown in figure 81(b). Above and to the right are the right kidney and suprarenal gland. Below and to the right is the right colic flexure. The descend-

ing part of the duodenum is to the left of the renal area and lateral to the porta hepatis. The stomach is in contact with the left lobe, and the oesophagus lies in a notch to the left of the fissure for the ligamentum venosum.

The Blood Vessels and Hepatic Ducts

The liver receives blood from the *hepatic artery* and *hepatic portal vein* (figure 82). The *hepatic artery* is a continuation of the common hepatic, a branch of the coeliac artery, and passes upwards in the lesser omentum to the porta hepatis where it divides into right and left branches. The *portal vein* receives the venous blood from the alimentary tract (from the oesophagus to the rectum), the spleen and the pancreas and is formed behind the neck of the pancreas by the union of the splenic and superior mesenteric veins. The portal vein passes upwards in the lesser omentum behind the hepatic artery and bile duct and at the porta hepatis divides into right and left branches. Within the liver the right and left branches of the artery and vein are not distributed to the right and left lobes (figure 83). The left portal vein and hepatic artery go to the quadrate lobe and half of the caudate lobe as well as the left lobe. The right branches go

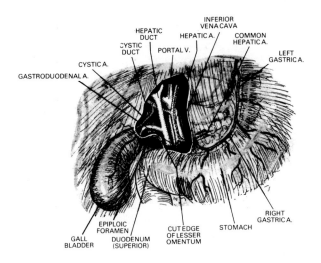

Figure 82   The structures entering and leaving the porta hepatis.

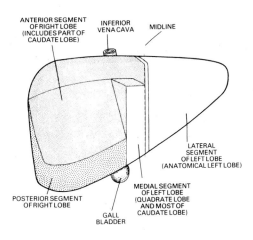

Figure 83   The segments of the liver.

to the rest of the right lobe and half of the caudate lobe.

The liver is now regarded as being divided into four segments — a *left lateral* which is equivalent to the left lobe, a *left medial* which is formed by the quadrate lobe and half of the caudate lobe and *anterior* and *posterior right segments* divided by a transverse plane passing obliquely upwards and backwards in the right lobe (figure 83). These segments correspond with the subdivisions of the portal vein and hepatic artery.

The *common hepatic duct* is formed by the union of the *right* and *left hepatic ducts* which are formed by *segmental ducts* in a manner parallel to the way in which the portal vein and hepatic artery subdivide. The common hepatic duct passes downwards in the lesser omentum in front of the portal vein and to the right of the hepatic artery. It is joined by the cystic duct about 3 cm below the porta hepatis and beyond this junction is called the *bile duct*.

Within the liver a small branch of the portal vein, hepatic artery and hepatic duct (a *portal triad*) together with a lymphatic vessel lie at the angles of the subdivisions of the lobes called the lobules. From these the blood passes between the liver cells in *sinusoids* (a special type of capillary) and goes to the central vein in the middle of the

lobule. Bile secreted by the liver cells passes in the opposite direction to the blood flow in the sinusoids, and goes to the *bile ductule* of the portal triad.

The blood leaves the liver by the *hepatic veins*. These are formed by the union of smaller veins which lie in the middle of the lobules of the liver (*central veins*). The hepatic veins are not segmental in their arrangement. All of these veins open into the inferior vena cava as it lies adjacent to or sometimes almost embedded in the right lobe of the liver. It is thought that these veins hold the liver in position in the abdomen and that the peritoneal ligaments are functionally unimportant in this respect.

The Lymphatic Vessels and Nerves

Superficial lymphatic vessels from the diaphragmatic surface of the liver pass through the diaphragm and go to thoracic lymph nodes along the internal thoracic vessels. Lymphatic vessels from the inferior surface go to nodes at the porta hepatis. Deep lymphatic vessels may go to nodes near the upper part of the inferior vena cava and thence to thoracic nodes on the upper surface of the diaphragm or to the nodes at the porta hepatis and thence to the

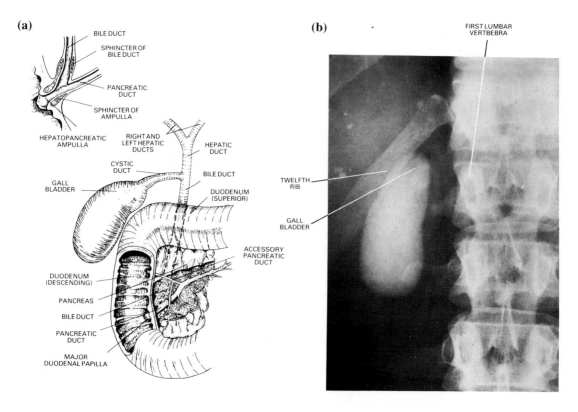

Figure 84   **(a) The extrahepatic bile passages. (b) A cholecystogram.**

coeliac nodes on the aorta.

The *nerves* supplying the liver are both sympathetic and parasympathetic and are derived from a plexus round the hepatic artery. The plexus is an extension of the coeliac plexus but it also receives a large branch from the anterior gastric (vagus) nerve. The sympathetic fibres are vasoconstrictor but the functions of the other fibres in relation to the liver are not known.

The Bile Passages

The bile passages (figure 84) include the *gall bladder*, the *cystic duct*, the *common hepatic duct* and the *bile duct*. The *gall bladder* is about 10 cm long and is pear-shaped. It lies in a hollow on the inferior surface of the liver *with its lower wider end (the* fundus*) projecting beyond the edge of the liver at the tip of the right ninth costal cartilage. This corresponds with the transpyloric plane (p. 68)*

and with the crossing of the costal margin by the linea semilunaris, which is formed by the right border of the rectus muscle and sheath.

The gall bladder is subdivided into the *fundus*, *body* and *neck* as it passes upwards and somewhat backwards and to the left. It is usually loosely attached to the liver by connective tissue but it may be almost embedded in the liver or hang from it by a short mesentery. The posterior surface is covered by peritoneum and is related inferiorly to the right end of the transverse colon and superiorly to the descending and superior parts of the duodenum (figure 81 (b)).

The neck of the gall bladder continues into the *cystic duct* which arches towards the left and joins the common hepatic duct to form the bile duct. The mucous membrane of the cystic duct and part of the neck forms a spiral ridge called the *spiral valve*.

The bile duct, about 7 cm long and 1 cm wide, runs downwards in the lesser omentum in front of the epiploic foramen with the hepatic artery on its left and the portal vein posteriorly (figure 82). At the upper border of the superior part of the duodenum the hepatic artery is replaced by its descending branch, the gastroduodenal artery which with the bile duct passes downwards behind the superior part of the duodenum and head of the pancreas. The bile duct passes to the right in front of the right renal vein and enters the posteromedial wall of the descending part of the duodenum in which it runs for about 2 cm before entering a dilatation (the *hepaticopancreatic ampulla*). The pancreatic duct also enters this ampulla which opens into the duodenum on the *duodenal papilla* (figure 84). The ampulla is surrounded by the *hepaticopancreatic sphincter* (of Oddi). The sphincter may also surround the terminal parts of the bile and pancreatic ducts.

The gall bladder and upper part of the bile duct are supplied by the *cystic artery* which most commonly arises from the right hepatic artery and passes to the gall bladder behind the cystic duct. The *veins* from the gall bladder and bile duct pass into the liver itself and into the portal vein. Its *lymphatics* go to the hepatic nodes. The *nerve supply* of the muscle of the gall bladder is sympathetic and parasympathetic from the coeliac plexus and reaches the gall bladder via the hepatic and cystic arteries. Stimulation of the parasympathetic causes the gall bladder to contract and the ampullary sphincter to relax but hormonal control of the muscle of gall bladder and any smooth muscle in the bile duct is more important. The sympathetic fibres are vasoconstrictor and may also be sensory. The right phrenic nerve supplies fibres to the peritoneum over the gall bladder and these may be important in producing pain referred to the shoulder if the gall bladder is inflamed.

The gall bladder stores bile and concentrates it. About 1500 ml of bile are produced each day. By concentrating the bile about 10 times the capacity of the gall bladder need be only about 50 ml, which are passed into the duodenum three times each day.

The gall bladder can be made opaque to X-rays by giving an iodine-containing compound by mouth on the previous evening (oral cholecystography) or by administering a similar compound intravenously about 30 min prior to the radiological examination. The liver secretes the contrast medium in the bile and the gall bladder can be seen in an X-ray. Typically it appears on the right as a pear-shaped structure between the twelfth rib and the first lumbar vertebra (figure 84(b)). There is considerable variation in its shape and position. If a fatty meal is given and the subject X-rayed about 20 min later, the gall bladder is seen to be emptying and the contrast medium outlines the cystic duct and bile duct (*cholangiography*).

The foregoing description of the gall bladder, ducts and blood supply is the most frequent arrangement of these structures but there is considerable variation. Examples of these variations are as follows: (1) the cystic artery may arise from the left hepatic artery or the hepatic artery before it divides; (2) the cystic artery may be anterior to the cystic duct; (3) the cystic duct may have a long course downwards before joining the bile duct; (4) the cystic duct may be short and join the right hepatic duct. It should be added that there is considerable variation in the origin of the common hepatic artery and there is also the possibility of there being accessory right and left hepatic arteries.

The Pancreas

The pancreas is a pinkish glandular structure about 12 cm long lying transversely behind the peritoneum on the posterior abdominal wall and extending from the concavity of the duodenum on the right to the spleen on the left. It has a head, neck, body and tail from right to left (figure 85). The *uncinate process* is an extension of the lower part of the head towards the left and below the neck. As the pancreas passes to the left it lies behind the stomach separated from it by the omental bursa. The two layers of the transverse mesocolon are attached to the anterior surface of the pancreas and the right end of the transverse colon, where its mesocolon is short, lies in front of the head.

As the pancreas passes to the left it is also oblique so that the tail is higher than the head. It also projects forwards as it crosses the vertebral column. Many of the structures lying behind the pancreas have already been mentioned. The bile

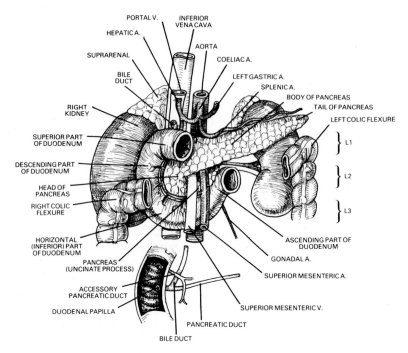

Figure 85   The relations of the pancreas.

duct runs downwards posterior to the head and may be embedded in it. Behind the neck the portal vein is formed by the union of the superior mesenteric and splenic veins. The splenic vein runs to the right from the spleen and is joined behind the body by the inferior mesenteric vein. The splenic artery runs to the left along the upper border of the pancreas. The inferior vena cava with the termination of the renal veins runs upwards behind the head and the aorta with the origin of the superior mesenteric artery lies behind the neck. The superior mesenteric vessels lie in front of the uncinate process. The left kidney and suprarenal gland are crossed anteriorly by the body of the pancreas.

The pancreas is surrounded by a fibrous tissue capsule from which septa pass into the substance of the gland so that it is markedly lobulated. The lobes are subdivided into lobules from which small ducts arise and enter the *main pancreatic duct*. This begins in the tail and passes to the right through the body, neck and head in which it turns somewhat downwards. It meets the bile duct which lies on its right and both ducts pass through the posteromedial wall of the descending part of the duodenum

(figure 84) and open into the hepaticopancreatic ampulla, which has already been described (p. 101). There may be an *accessory pancreatic duct* which begins in the lower part of the head, runs upwards in front of the main duct with which it communicates and turning to the right opens into the duodenum about 2 cm proximal to the common opening of the bile and main pancreatic ducts.

The *arteries* to the pancreas come from the superior and inferior pancreaticoduodenal (to the head) and splenic arteries (to the neck, body and tail). The *veins* eventually go to the portal vein. The *lymphatic vessels* from the pancreas go to nodes along its upper border (pancreaticosplenic) which drain to the coeliac nodes. In the region of the head of the pancreas the lymph vessels go to nodes along the arteries supplying it. Some of these nodes drain into the superior mesenteric nodes.

The Spleen

The spleen (figure 86) is a soft, dark purplish organ about 12 cm long, 6 cm wide and 3 cm thick and

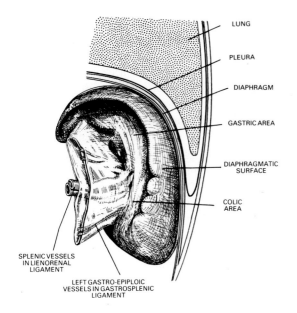

LUNG

PLEURA

DIAPHRAGM

GASTRIC AREA

DIAPHRAGMATIC
SURFACE

COLIC
AREA

SPLENIC VESSELS
IN LIENORENAL
LIGAMENT

LEFT GASTRO-EPIPLOIC
VESSELS IN GASTROSPLENIC
LIGAMENT

Figure 86   The relations of the spleen.

is approximately oval in shape. It lies in the upper left posterior part of the abdominal cavity with its inner (visceral) surface wedged between the left kidney which is posterior and the stomach which is anterior. Its smooth outer (diaphragmatic) surface is next to the diaphragm. *The spleen lies with its long axis along the line of the posterior part of the tenth rib and extends upwards as far as the ninth and downwards as far as the eleventh rib. Its upper posterior end (pole) is about 4 cm from the midline and its lower anterior end (pole) reaches as far as the midaxillary line.*

The lower lateral part of the visceral surface is related to the left colic flexure. The hilum where the splenic vessels enter and leave is between the areas related to the stomach and kidney and the tail of the pancreas reaches the spleen next to the hilum. The diaphragmatic surface of the upper third of the spleen is related indirectly to the lung, and the upper two-thirds to the pleura (costodiaphragmatic recess). If specimens of splenic tissue (splenic pulp) are required (*splenic puncture*), it is important to insert the needle into its lower third where only the diaphragm is external to the spleen (figure 86).

The spleen has upper and lower borders. The upper is usually notched, a relic of the fetal lobulation. If the spleen enlarges, the superior border moves downwards and inwards and the notch is a palpable diagnostic landmark.

The spleen is almost completely covered by peritoneum. The *lienorenal ligament* passes from the kidney to the spleen (p. 80) and contains the splenic vessels and tail of the pancreas. The *gastrosplenic ligament* goes from the spleen to the greater curvature of the stomach (p. 80) and contains branches of the splenic vessels to and from the stomach (the left gastro-epiploic and short gastric vessels). Inside the peritoneal coat the spleen is enclosed in a fibrous capsule from which trabeculae pass into the spleen and provide a pathway for the large vessels and a framework for the splenic pulp.

On the cut surface of the spleen white dots are visible. These are aggregations of lymphocytes and constitute the *white pulp*. The rest of the spleen contains a variable number of red blood corpuscles in sinusoids and is called the *red pulp*.

The size of the spleen and its external appearance vary considerably. The former is influenced by the quantity of blood in the spleen and the latter by the surrounding organs, particularly the stomach and colic flexure. In many animals there are smooth muscle fibres in the capsule and trabeculae but in man there are very few. The muscle fibres can squeeze blood from the spleen where it is stored. It is thought that in man contraction of the walls of the blood vessels produces the same effect.

The splenic artery is a branch of the coeliac artery. It is a large tortuous vessel passing along the upper border of the pancreas to the hilum of the spleen where it breaks up into a number of branches. The splenic vein is formed by the union of a number of veins at the hilum and passes to the right behind the body of the pancreas inferior to the artery. It receives the inferior mesenteric vein and with the superior mesenteric vein forms the portal vein behind the neck of the pancreas.

Although the spleen is a lymphoid organ, its lymphatic vessels drain the capsule and trabeculae and are not found in the splenic pulp. In other words the lymphocytes produced by the spleen pass straight into its blood vessels.

An *accessory spleen* or *spleens* in the lienorenal

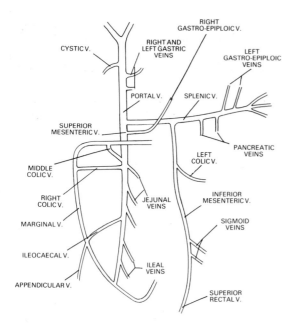

Figure 87 The tributaries of the portal vein.

and gastrosplenic ligaments, the tail of the pancreas, the greater omentum and mesentery of the small bowel are not infrequent and have to be considered when the spleen is removed for certain blood diseases.

Rupture of the spleen as a result of violence to the upper left part of the abdomen and/or the lower left ribs is not uncommon and produces a massive intraperitoneal haemorrhage. This possibility has to be kept in mind in any injury to this part of the body.

The Hepatic Portal Vein and its Tributaries

The term *portal* is used to describe a venous system which passes through two sets of capillaries before returning to the circulation. Originally the term referred to the veins returning blood from the alimentary tract in the abdomen, spleen and pancreas as the word *portal* itself indicates – the vein which entered the porta hepatis (*porta = entrance*, Latin). When other systems of veins passing through two sets of capillaries were described, for example the hypophyseal veins, the term portal was used. The word *hepatic* is added to distinguish the alimentary

veins from other portal systems.

Most of the vessels forming and entering the portal vein have been described and only a brief summary is given here (figure 87). The portal vein is usually formed deep to the neck of the pancreas by the union of the superior mesenteric and splenic veins. It passes upwards behind the superior part of the duodenum and goes to the liver in the lesser omentum anterior to the inferior vena cava and posterior to the bile duct (on the right) and hepatic artery (on the left). (The gastroduodenal artery replaces the hepatic behind the superior part of the duodenum.) The portal vein usually receives directly the right and left gastric veins and the pre-pyloric and cystic veins. The superior mesenteric vein is described on p. 89 and the inferior mesenteric on p. 94. The splenic vein (p. 103) receives veins from the spleen and pancreas as well as the short gastric and left gastro-epiploic veins.

The portal vein divides into the right and left portal branches at the porta hepatis. These branches divide into segmental branches as described on p. 98. The ligamentum teres from the umbilicus joins the left branch of the portal vein. The ligamentum venosum joins the left branch to the inferior vena cava (p. 98).

The portal vein and its tributaries have no valves. Obstruction to the flow of blood through the portal vein or through the liver results in the blood in the portal system entering the systemic veins where there are anastomoses between them. The most important sites are in the abdominal oesophagus (the left gastric vein which goes to the portal vein and the oesophageal veins to the hemiazygos vein) and the rectum (the superior rectal to the inferior mesenteric and the inferior rectal which goes to the internal pudendal) (p. 136). The oesophageal veins enlarge and form oesophageal varices which may rupture and cause a serious haemorrhage. Other sites are where the bare area of the liver is in contact with the diaphragm, and round the umbilicus where veins in the abdominal wall are connected with the portal vein by veins passing along the ligamentum teres. The enlarged radiating veins round the umbilicus reputedly produce an appearance called a *caput medusae*, a somewhat uncommon condition, since few people seem to have seen it. Other possible sites of anastomoses are places where the alimentary tract is in direct contact with the abdominal wall, for example the ascending and descending colons.

Among the conditions which can cause obstruction are cirrhosis of the liver (increased fibrous tissue pressing on the branches of the portal vein in the liver; *cirrhos = orange-coloured*, Greek; the appearance of the cut surface of the liver in this condition), cancer of the head of the pancreas, primary and secondary cancer of the liver, and enlarged cancerous nodes at the porta hepatis. Obstruction to the return of blood in the portal vein also causes *ascites* (fluid in the abdominal cavity; *ascos = bladder, belly*; *-ites = condition of*, Greek; the original term was *ascites hydrops* and in time the *hydrops* was omitted) due to fluid passing through the capillaries of the serous (peritoneal) coat of the abdominal organs.

8

The Posterior Abdominal Wall and Related Structures

The posterior abdominal wall consists of the five lumbar vertebrae in the midline and the psoas and quadratus lumborum muscles on either side. The forward curvature of the lumbar vertebrae brings the posterior wall very near to the anterior abdominal wall and in a thin individual the abdominal aorta can be seen pulsating near the umbilicus. The posterior part of the diaphragm with its crura also forms part of the posterior abdominal wall, and, lateral to the quadratus lumborum, the transversus abdominis is attached to the fascia related to that muscle (figures 63, 88). The kidneys with the suprarenal glands on their upper poles lie on either side on the muscles and extend above and below the level of the twelfth rib. The ureters run downwards at approximately the level of the tips of the transverse processes of the lumbar vertebrae, and the inferior vena cava and abdominal aorta lie to the right and left respectively of the bodies of the lumbar vertebrae. The branches of the lumbar plexus emerge from the psoas muscle and the autonomic nerves and lymph nodes are related mainly to the aorta.

The Muscles and Fascia (figure 88)

The Psoas Muscles. In 60 per cent of individuals there are two psoas muscles, major and minor. The *psoas major* is attached to the transverse processes and to the upper and lower borders of the bodies of the lumbar vertebrae and the adjacent intervertebral discs. The latter attachments come from a series of fibrous arches which are related to the middle of the bodies. The muscle passes downwards to the pelvic brim, sweeps round its outer edge and enters the thigh behind the inguinal ligament. Its tendon lies in front of the capsule of the hip joint, from which it is separated by a bursa, and is attached to the lesser trochanter of the femur.

The most important relations of the psoas major are the kidney with its blood vessels and ureter which are anterior, the branches of the lumbar plexus some of which are lateral and some medial, and the inferior vena cava (on the right) and abdominal aorta (on the left) which are medial.

The nerve supply of the muscle comes from the ventral rami of the first three lumbar nerves. Its main action is, with the iliacus, to flex the thigh at the hip or the trunk on the thigh from the supine position.

The *psoas minor* is attached above to the twelfth thoracic and first lumbar vertebrae, passes downwards anterior to the psoas major and ends in a tendon which blends with the fascia on the anterior part of the brim of the pelvis. It is innervated by the first lumbar nerve and assists the psoas major in flexion of the trunk.

The Quadratus Lumborum. This muscle is attached to the twelfth rib and below to the iliac crest and also has an attachment to the tips of the transverse processes of the lumbar vertebrae. Its nerve supply is from the ventral rami of the first three lumbar nerves. Its actions are not very well understood. It may fix the twelfth rib when the diaphragm con-

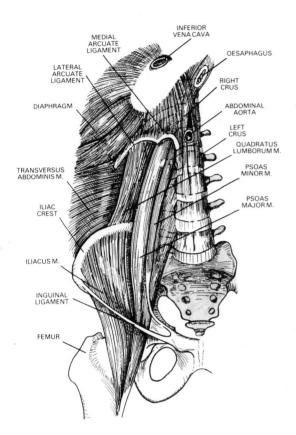

Figure 88   The muscles of the posterior abdominal wall.

LABELS (on figure):
MEDIAL ARCUATE LIGAMENT
INFERIOR VENA CAVA
OESAPHAGUS
LATERAL ARCUATE LIGAMENT
RIGHT CRUS
DIAPHRAGM
ABDOMINAL AORTA
LEFT CRUS
QUADRATUS LUMBORUM M.
TRANSVERSUS ABDOMINIS M.
PSOAS MINOR M.
ILIAC CREST
PSOAS MAJOR M.
ILIACUS M.
INGUINAL LIGAMENT
FEMUR

tracts. From its attachments one assumes that the right quadratus lumborum pulls the vertebral column to the right, a movement called lateral flexion or bending.

The Iliacus. The iliacus is attached to the iliac fossa and passes downwards and medially on the lateral side of the psoas major into the thigh deep to the inguinal ligament. It joins the psoas tendon to form the iliopsoas tendon and is attached to the lesser trochanter. It is supplied by the femoral nerve (the ventral rami of the second, third and fourth lumbar nerves) and it flexes the thigh at the hip or the trunk on the thigh.

The Fascia of the Posterior Abdominal Wall. The muscles are covered by fascia which is the same

fascia lining the abdominal wall elsewhere (fascia transversalis). Over the psoas it is called the *psoas fascia* and over the iliacus, the *fascia iliaca*. The upper border of the psoas fascia forms the *medial arcuate ligament* and that of the fascia over the quadratus lumborum the *lateral arcuate ligament*. Both ligaments have fibres of the diaphragm attached to them (p. 17). Although nowadays almost unknown in this country, tuberculosis of the vertebral bodies, particularly the lower thoracic and upper lumbar, was not uncommon. This often resulted in an abscess which tracked downwards deep to the psoas fascia and appeared in the upper medial part of the thigh. The fascia in front of the quadratus lumborum forms the anterior layer of the thoracolumbar fascia which laterally fuses with the middle and posterior layers (figure 63).

The Kidneys, Suprarenal Glands and Ureters

The kidneys and ureters are part of the urinary system. The suprarenal glands, which are endocrine in function, are also called the *adrenal* glands, a name which is used to describe one of its secretions (*adrenalin*). In many animals the suprarenal gland is not as close to the kidney as it is in man.

The kidneys

These are paired, reddish-brown organs of a characteristic shape. Each kidney lies at the side of the twelfth thoracic and upper lumbar vertebrae and has upper and lower poles, anterior and posterior surfaces and lateral and medial borders. The upper pole is nearer the midline than the lower and the anterior surface faces laterally as well as forwards. On the medial border is the hilum where the blood vessels and ureter enter and leave the kidney. An average kidney is about 12 cm long, 6 cm wide and 3 cm thick, and weighs about 150 g.

The surface markings of the kidneys are important (figure 89). From the front, the hilum is approximately at the level of the transpyloric plane, about 5 cm lateral to the midline. This corresponds with the first lumbar vertebra. The right

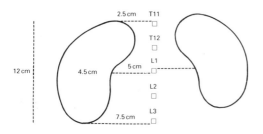

Figure 89   The surface markings of the kidneys from in front.

kidney is somewhat lower than the left because of the liver. The upper pole is about 6 cm above this plane and 2.5 cm from the midline, and the lower pole is 6 cm below this plane, and 7 cm from the midline. From behind, the guide to the kidney is the twelfth rib, which crosses obliquely downwards and laterally, posterior to the kidney. The hilum is opposite the spinous process of the first lumbar vertebra 5 cm from the midline. Since the left kidney is somewhat higher it is crossed by the eleventh rib. The positions of the upper and lower poles are determined in the same way as on the anterior abdominal wall.

There are three connective tissue coverings of the kidney (figure 90). It is enclosed in the *renal fascia* the two layers of which are fused superiorly and laterally but not inferiorly. Medially both layers merge with the tunica adventitia of the renal vessels. A perinephric abscess will therefore only spread downwards where the two layers of the renal fascia are not fused.

Surrounding the kidney within the renal fascia is the *adipose capsule* (*perinephric fat*). This fat is said to be the only fat in the body which is solid at body temperature and is thus responsible for maintaining the position of the kidney. In wasting diseases this fat disappears and the kidney can then move downwards. If this happens the suprarenal gland remains in position because it is enclosed in its own compartment of renal fascia (figure 90). The kidney has its own *fibrous tissue capsule* which normally strips off easily but becomes adherent in many diseases of the kidney. There is also a variable amount of fat behind the kidney outside the renal fascia (the *pararenal fatty body*).

The anterior relations of the right and left kidneys are shown in figure 91(a). This is probably the most useful diagram for understanding the relations of almost all the organs in the upper half of the abdominal cavity. The duodenum (on the right), the colic flexures, suprarenals and pancreas (on the left) are directly related to the kidneys without intervening peritoneum.

The posterior relations are shown in figure 91(b). Placing the twelfth (and eleventh) ribs in position is the first essential. The diaphragm is superior to the twelfth rib and the three abdominal muscles are inferior. The three nerves passing laterally between the kidney and quadratus lumborum can then be placed in position.

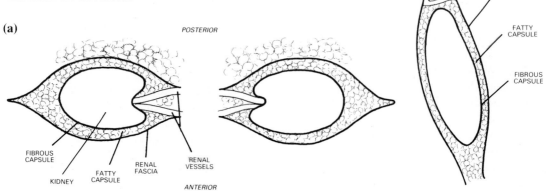

Figure 90   The connective tissue structures round the kidneys: (a) transverse section; (b) longitudinal section.

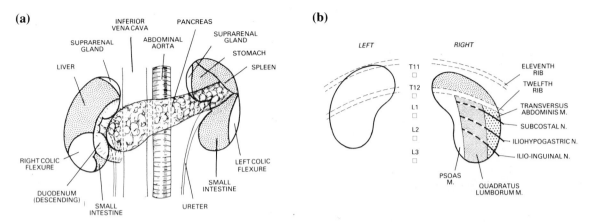

(a)

INFERIOR VENA CAVA
PANCREAS
ABDOMINAL AORTA
SUPRARENAL GLAND
STOMACH
SUPRARENAL GLAND
SPLEEN
LIVER
RIGHT COLIC FLEXURE
LEFT COLIC FLEXURE
DUODENUM (DESCENDING)
SMALL INTESTINE
SMALL INTESTINE
URETER

(b)

LEFT
RIGHT
T11
T12
L1
L2
L3
ELEVENTH RIB
TWELFTH RIB
TRANSVERSUS ABDOMINIS M.
SUBCOSTAL N.
ILIOHYPOGASTRIC N.
ILIO-INGUINAL N.
PSOAS M.
QUADRATUS LUMBORUM M.

Figure 91 **(a) The anterior relations of the kidneys. (b) The posterior relations of the kidneys.**

The hilum of the kidney leads into a space called the *renal sinus* in which there are the renal artery and vein, lymphatic vessels, nerves and the expanded upper end of the ureter, the *renal pelvis*. This is frequently referred to as the *pelvis of the ureter*. At the hilum the vein is anterior to the artery which is anterior to the ureter. Very frequently the artery breaks up in the sinus into its large branches and one of these passes posterior to the ureter.

The renal pelvis is formed by the union of two or three *major calices* each of which is formed by the union of three to six *minor calices*. These can be seen in a section of a kidney cut parallel to the surfaces from the lateral to the medial border (figure 92). On the surface of this section there are also the darker *renal pyramids*, the apices of which project into the minor calices. The *collecting ducts* of the kidney open on to the apices. That part of the kidney external to the bases of the pyramids is called the *cortex* and the part internal to the bases, the *medulla*. Each pyramid and the cortex overlying it constitutes a *lobe* of the kidney. The *renal columns* are the extensions of cortical tissue which pass between the pyramids towards the hilum.

The Renal Artery and Vein. The renal arteries come from the aorta just below the origin of the superior mesenteric artery. The right artery passes horizontally behind the inferior vena cava, the right renal vein, the head of the pancreas and the

descending part of the duodenum and enters the hilum. The left artery runs to the left kidney behind the left renal vein, the body of the pancreas and the splenic vein. Each artery gives off a branch to the suprarenal gland and the upper part of the

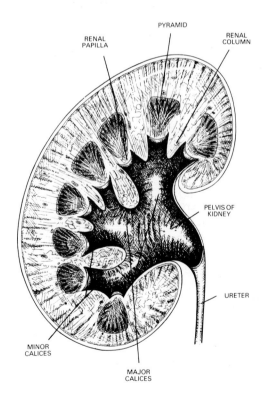

PYRAMID
RENAL PAPILLA
RENAL COLUMN
PELVIS OF KIDNEY
URETER
MINOR CALICES
MAJOR CALICES

Figure 92 **Longitudinal section of the kidney.**

(a)   **(b)**

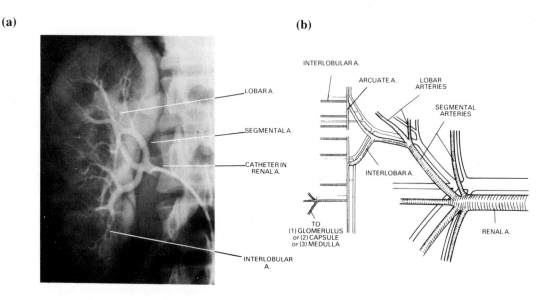

Figure 93   (a) A renal arteriogram. (b) The larger branches of the renal artery.

ureter. In 30 per cent of individuals there are additional right or left arteries from the aorta (*accessory* or *aberrant renal arteries*) usually to the upper or lower pole. These are thought to be persistent lateral splanchnic arteries of the embryo which supply the kidney as it is pushed upwards from its original pelvic position during fetal growth. An accessory renal artery to the lower pole of a kidney is usually anterior to the ureter and it is thought that it may press on the ureter and obstruct it. Usually an accessory artery is an end-artery and necrosis of a segment of a kidney may result from tying it.

A renal artery divides into *segmental arteries*, each of which is an end-artery. Figure 93(a) shows a renal arteriogram which is obtained by introducing a catheter into the femoral artery in the upper part of the thigh and passing it upwards through the iliac arteries into the abdominal aorta. The catheter is then passed into the renal artery and radio-opaque material is injected into the artery. The segmental arteries can be seen but there is some argument as to how the segments are arranged in the kidney and whether there are more than five. Each segmental artery divides into a number of *lobar arteries* (figure 93(b)). A lobar artery divides into two *interlobar arteries* which pass

between the pyramids. At the junction of the medulla and cortex each interlobar artery divides into *arcuate arteries* which run at right angles to the parent trunk. From the arcuate arteries *interlobular arteries* supply the lobules which are subsections of a lobe consisting of several nephrons, the functioning units of the kidney. The further distribution of the interlobular arteries is not considered here but there is a separate arterial supply to the glomeruli and convoluted tubules, to the loop of Henle and to the subcapsular region. From these three sources the blood is returned to the *interlobular*, *arcuate*, *interlobar* and *segmental veins*. These unite in the renal sinus and emerge from the hilum as the renal vein. The right vein passes posterior to the descending part of the duodenum, and enters the inferior vena cava. The left renal vein receives the suprarenal and gonadal veins and passes to the right behind the body of the pancreas and in front of the aorta to the inferior vena cava.

The Renal Nerve Supply and Lymphatic Drainage. The plexus of nerves accompanying the renal artery into the kidney is derived from the coeliac and aortic plexuses, the lowest splanchnic nerve from the thorax and the first lumbar ganglion. The fibres are mainly postganglionic sympathetic but the preganglionic splanchnic fibres synapse in ganglion cells in the plexus at the hilum. There are also some parasympathetic fibres. The autonomic fibres are almost entirely vasomotor. Some are sensory and convey painful sensations from the renal pelvis and upper part of the ureter.

The lymphatic vessels drain to the nodes at the side of the aorta near the origin of the renal artery. The vessels come from a plexus within the kidney and a subcapsular plexus.

Malformations and Anomalies. These are not uncommon and are more liable to become diseased. One kidney may have a *double ureter* or there may be *three ureters* with an extra kidney. One kidney may be much smaller than the other or remain in the pelvis. The two kidneys may be united across the midline inferiorly, in front of the inferior vena cava and aorta (*horseshoe kidney*). The failure of union between the tubules derived from the ureteric bud and those derived from the metanephrogenic blastema results in one or more *congenital cysts. Surface fetal lobulation* may persist in the adult.

The suprarenal glands

Each suprarenal gland lies on the upper pole of a kidney, the right being triangular and the left crescentic in shape, and weighs about 5 g. It is about 5 cm vertically, 3 cm transversely and 1 cm antero-posteriorly. At birth it is about one-quarter the size of the kidney and is relatively much larger than it is in the adult in whom it is about one-thirtieth of the size of the kidney. Shortly after birth the glands decrease in size and then increase again. Each gland is enclosed in a compartment of renal fascia.

The right gland lies on the diaphragm lateral to the right crus and behind the inferior vena cava (figure 74). More laterally the gland is in contact anteriorly with the bare area of the liver. The left gland lies on the left crus of the diaphragm, and anteriorly is related to the stomach, near the cardia, and the pancreas.

The suprarenals consist of an outer *cortex* and inner *medulla*, the latter being about one-tenth the weight of the whole gland. Developmentally, structurally and functionally the cortex and medulla are different. The medullary cells have an affinity for salts of chromic acid and form part of the *chromaffin system* which includes small masses of cells found among the ganglia and autonomic plexuses of the sympathetic nervous system, and the *para-aortic bodies* which lie alongside the abdominal aorta near the inferior mesenteric artery. Chromaffin tissue secretes noradrenalin and adrenalin.

Each suprarenal gland has a rich blood supply derived from the inferior phrenic artery, the abdominal aorta and the renal artery. A single large vein leaves the medial border of the gland and on the right goes to the inferior vena cava and on the left to the left renal vein.

The nerves of the glands are derived mainly from the coeliac plexus and can be traced back to the greater splanchnic nerve from the thorax. These fibres are preganglionic and end by synapsing with the medullary cells which may be regarded as sympathetic ganglion cells.

The ureter

This is a muscular tube about 25 cm long and 0.3 cm wide passing downwards on the psoas muscle from the kidney. It enters the pelvis and passes to the bladder which lies in the front of the pelvis. The dilated upper end of the ureter is called the *renal pelvis* (p. 109). At the junction of the renal pelvis with the abdominal part of the ureter it is usually slightly constricted.

As it lies on the psoas the ureter is crossed anteriorly by the gonadal vessels and is itself anterior to the genitofemoral nerve (figure 94). The right ureter is lateral to the inferior vena cava and passes behind the root of the mesentery and its vessels to the brim of the pelvis which it crosses at the level of the sacro-iliac joint anterior to the division of the common iliac artery. The abdominal part of the left ureter is posterior to the apex of the sigmoid mesocolon at the superior aperture of the pelvis in front of the division of the common iliac

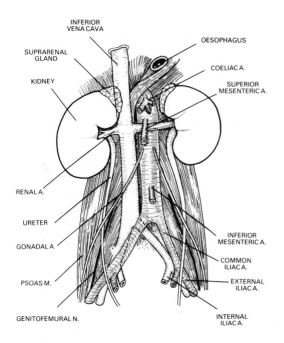

INFERIOR
VENA CAVA

OESOPHAGUS

SUPRARENAL
GLAND

COELIAC A.

KIDNEY

SUPERIOR
MESENTERIC A.

RENAL A.

URETER

INFERIOR
MESENTERIC A.

GONADAL A

COMMON
ILIAC A.

EXTERNAL
ILIAC A.

PSOAS M.

GENITOFEMURAL N.

INTERNAL
ILIAC A.

Figure 94   The abdominal part of the ureter.

artery. The pelvic part of the ureter is described on p. 140.

In addition to its constriction just beyond the renal pelvis, the ureter is narrowed where it crosses the pelvic brim and where it enters the bladder. These three sites of narrowing are the places where a renal stone is liable to become impacted. This is associated with severe pain due to spasm of the ureteric muscle. The pain usually begins in the loin and is referred along the distribution of the eleventh thoracic to second lumbar spinal nerves, that is to the anterior abdominal wall, the groin and scrotum (or labium majus) and the upper medial part of the front of the thigh. The *nerve supply* of the abdominal part of the ureter is from the plexuses along the abdominal aorta. These sympathetic preganglionic fibres are from the lowest three thoracic and first lumbar spinal segments. Many of the sympathetic fibres are sensory.

The *arterial blood supply* of the upper part of the ureter is derived from the renal artery, of the middle part from the gonadal artery and of the lowest part from the vesical artery. These vessels form a longitudinal anastomosis along the length of the ureter. The vessels are attached to the peri-

toneum behind which the ureter lies and if the peritoneum is picked up the ureter comes with it. Stripping the peritoneum off the ureter may deprive it of its blood supply and result in its necrosis.

The *lymphatic vessels* from the abdominal part of the ureter pass to the nodes along the aorta and common iliac artery. From the pelvic part the vessels go to the nodes along the large arteries — the external and internal iliac.

The ureter is related to the following bony points. The renal pelvis is at the level of the first or second lumbar vertebra (the transpyloric plane indicates the approximate level) 5 cm from the midline. The abdominal part of the ureter is said to lie in front of the tips of the transverse process of the lumbar vertebrae. Frequently it lies nearer the bodies. The ureter is in front of the sacro-iliac joint at the superior aperture of the pelvis and crosses the ischial spine within the pelvis. These relations are seen in an X-ray investigation called *pyelography* .in which the calices, renal pelvis and ureter can be seen (figure 95). This can be done by injecting an iodine-containing compound into a vein (*intravenous pyelogram*). The contrast medium used has an iodine content of 420 mg ml^{-1} and the amount of iodine given is related to the weight of the subject (0.25 g iodine kg^{-1}). The compound is excreted by the kidney very soon after the injection. X-rays are taken at intervals of 5 min and the calices, renal pelvis and upper part of the ureter can be seen in about 5 min on both sides (figure 95(b)). The investigation is always preceded by an X-ray of the abdomen which is used as a control (figure 95(a)). After 20 min the bladder can be seen (figure 95(b)).

Another technique involves passing a cystoscope into the bladder through the urethra and then by direct vision passing into each ureter a catheter through which a radio-opaque substance is injected (*retrograde pyelogram*) (figure 95(c)). The latter method has the advantage of enabling the investigator to obtain a separate sample of urine from each kidney. It is, however, a much more troublesome procedure for the patient.

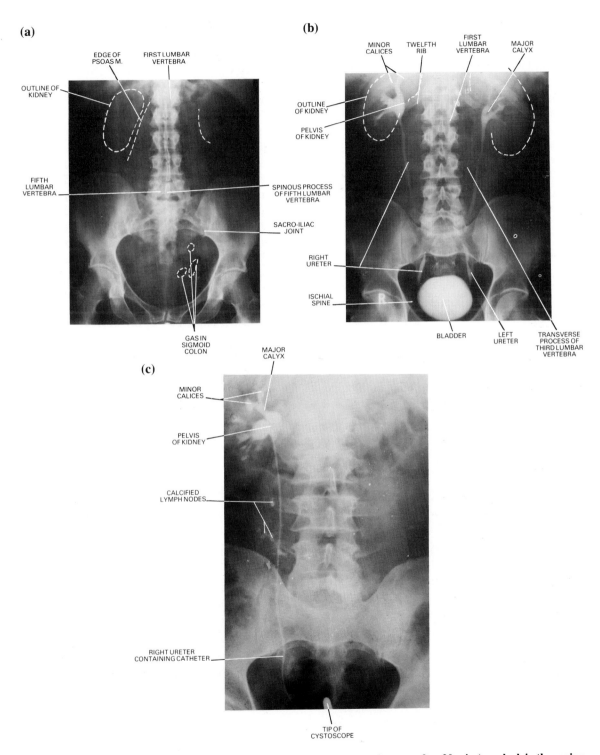

Figure 95 (a) A control X-ray of the abdomen. (b) An intravenous pyelogram after 20 min (see clock in the region of the twelfth thoracic vertebra). (c) A retrograde pyelogram (note the shadow of the cystoscope).

The Abdominal Aorta, Inferior Vena Cava, Autonomic Nerves and Lymph Nodes

It should be appreciated that much of the description of these structures is a repetition of what has already been described or referred to in previous sections. The abdominal aorta to the left and the inferior vena cava to the right run more or less vertically in front of the lumbar vertebral column. The autonomic plexuses and ganglia lie on the front and at the sides of the aorta and the lymph nodes although irregularly arranged lie alongside the aorta.

The abdominal aorta

This is a continuation of the thoracic aorta beyond the diaphragm and begins in the midline between the twelfth thoracic and first lumbar vertebrae. The abdominal aorta descends in front of the lumbar vertebrae and moving slightly to the left divides into its terminal branches, the right and left common iliac arteries, at the level of the fourth lumbar vertebra. *The surface marking of this division is 2.5 cm below and to the left of the umbilicus.* In front of the aorta from above downwards are the omental bursa and lesser omentum, the left renal vein, the body of the pancreas and splenic vein, the horizontal part of the duodenum and the mesentery of the small intestine (figure 74).

Just below the diaphragm a crus and a coeliac ganglion lie on either side of the aorta. On the left below the crus there are the duodenojejunal flexure and, running longitudinally, the sympathetic trunk and inferior mesenteric vessels. Near the diaphragm on the right there are the cisterna chyli and azygos vein and inferior to these the inferior vena cava.

The abdominal aorta and some of its branches can be seen following the injection of a radio-opaque substance into the aorta. This may be carried out by means of a needle inserted through the back or a catheter inserted into the femoral artery in the upper part of the thigh as described on p. 110 for obtaining a renal artery arteriogram. Figure 83(b) is taken from the same subject as figure 96(b) and makes it easier to distinguish the different branches of the aorta.

The branches (figure 96) are in three groups:

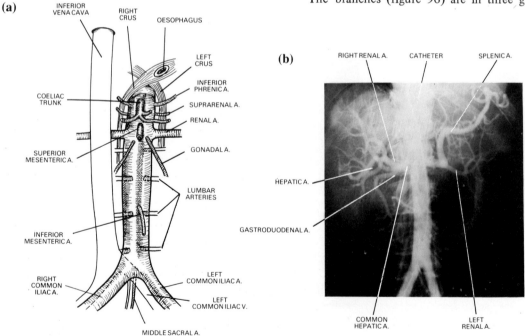

Figure 96   (a) The abdominal aorta and its branches. (b) An aortic arteriogram.

(1) anterior unpaired splanchnic to the alimentary tract, liver, pancreas and spleen; (2) lateral paired splanchnic to other viscera (the suprarenal glands, kidneys and gonads); (3) paired segmental (including the vertically running unpaired median sacral artery which arises from the back of the aorta just above its bifurcation).

The Anterior Splanchnic Branches. The *coeliac trunk* about 1 cm long arises just below the diaphragm, passes horizontally above the body of the pancreas and divides into the left gastric, splenic and common hepatic arteries. The *left gastric* runs to the left behind the omental bursa towards the abdominal oesophagus and turns downwards along the lesser curvature of the stomach (p. 85). It supplies the lower end of the oesophagus and part of the stomach.

The *common hepatic artery* runs to the right along the upper border of the superior part of the duodenum and divides into the *hepatic artery* which passes upwards in the right border of the lesser omentum and the *gastroduodenal artery* which runs downwards behind the superior part of the duodenum (pp. 86 and 98).

The *splenic artery* runs to the left along the upper border of the pancreas behind the stomach, and crosses the kidney to enter the lienorenal ligament and reach the spleen (p. 85).

The next anterior unpaired branch is the *superior mesenteric artery* which is described on p. 89 and the third the *inferior mesenteric artery* (p. 94). *The Lateral Splanchnic Branches.* The *suprarenal (middle)* and *renal branches* of the aorta have been described (p. 109). The *testicular or ovarian arteries* (figure 94) arise just below the origin of the renal arteries and run downwards and slightly laterally on the psoas muscle. They are anterior to the ureter and genitofemoral nerve and posterior to the alimentary tract and its vessels and mesenteries. The right artery is anterior to the inferior vena cava. The testicular artery leaves the psoas and goes to the deep inguinal ring where it becomes part of the spermatic cord (p. 74). The ovarian artery crosses the external iliac vessels and the brim of the pelvis to enter the lateral end of the upper edge of the broad ligament of the uterus (p. 142) (the suspensory ligament of the ovary).

Its further course in the broad ligament and its distribution are described on p. 145. The branches of the gonadal artery to the ureter have already been referred to (p. 112).

The Segmental Parietal Branches. The *inferior phrenic arteries* leave the aorta just below where it emerges from behind the diaphragm. They may arise from the coeliac artery. Each artery runs laterally across the crus, supplies the diaphragm and anastomoses with the terminal branches of the internal thoracic artery. The inferior phrenic artery gives off a branch to the suprarenal gland.

There are four or five paired *segmental lumbar arteries* which pass laterally across the crura of the diaphragm, go deep to the psoas and quadratus lumborum muscles and are distributed to the body wall. The lumbar arteries give off a posterior branch, which passes backwards to the muscles and skin of the back, and also a spinal branch which enters the vertebral canal through an intervertebral foramen and supplies the meninges, spinal nerves and roots, and spinal cord.

The *median sacral artery* passes downwards into the pelvis on the front of the sacrum and supplies the coccygeal body, a cellular vascular mass in front of the coccyx.

The common iliac arteries and their branches

These arteries extend from the division of the abdominal aorta on the left side of the body of the fourth lumbar vertebra to the sacro-iliac joint at the brim of the pelvis where they divide into the external and internal iliac arteries. The *right common iliac artery*, about 5 cm long, lies in front of the fourth and fifth lumbar vertebrae and the common iliac veins where they join to form the inferior vena cava. Most of the structures entering the pelvis are posterior to the artery – the sympathetic trunk, the obturator nerve and the lumbosacral trunk. The ureter, however, is anterior to its bifurcation.

The *left common iliac artery*, about 4 cm long, lies in front of and lateral to the left common iliac vein. Its relations are similar to those of the right artery. In addition the pre-aortic autonomic plexus and the superior rectal artery are anterior to it as they pass into the pelvis.

The *external iliac artery* runs round the brim of the pelvis medial to the psoas muscle from the sacro-iliac joint to its entry into the thigh deep to the inguinal ligament at a point midway between the anterior superior iliac spine and the symphysis pubis. Beyond the inguinal ligament the external iliac artery becomes the *femoral artery*, the artery of the lower limb. The external iliac vein if followed backwards from the inguinal ligament is medial and then posterior to the artery. The ovarian vessels as they enter the pelvis cross the artery which is also crossed by the round ligament of the uterus as it leaves the pelvis and passes towards the deep inguinal ring. The ductus deferens enters the pelvis by crossing the external iliac vessels.

The external iliac artery has two large branches both of which arise just proximal to the inguinal ligament (figure 65). The *inferior epigastric artery* passes upwards medial to the deep inguinal ring and ductus deferens and passes anterior to the arcuate line and posterior layer of the rectus sheath. It anastomoses with the superior epigastric artery, a branch of the internal thoracic, and the lower intercostal arteries. The inferior epigastric gives off the *cremasteric artery* which enters the spermatic cord, and *pubic branches* which go to the back of the body of the pubis where they anastomose with branches of the obturator artery. One of the branches of the inferior epigastric artery may be large enough to replace the obturator artery. This *abnormal obturator artery*, as it passes to the obturator canal, may be lateral or medial to the femoral ring. It is in danger, especially if medial, in operations for a femoral hernia. The relation of an indirect and direct inguinal hernia to the inferior epigastric artery has already been discussed (p. 78).

The other branch of the external iliac artery is the *deep circumflex iliac artery* which passes laterally along the deep surface of the inguinal ligament to the anterior superior iliac spine and then along the iliac crest. It ends by entering the abdominal wall. This artery anastomoses with arteries of the lower limb as well as arteries of the anterior and posterior abdominal walls.

The inferior vena cava and its tributaries (figure 97)

The *inferior vena cava* is formed by the union of the common iliac veins to the right of the midline at the level of the body of the fifth lumbar vertebra. As it passes almost vertically upwards the inferior vena cava lies behind the mesentery of the small intestine, the inferior part of the duodenum, the head of the pancreas, the superior part of the duodenum, the lesser omentum from which it is separated by the epiploic foramen and the liver in which it may be deeply embedded (figure 74). The lesser omentum contains the portal vein, bile duct and hepatic artery. Where the inferior vena cava lies on the right crus of the diaphragm, the right suprarenal gland and coeliac ganglion lie behind it and the right renal, inferior phrenic and suprarenal arteries pass to the right behind it. The sympathetic trunk runs downwards posterior to the inferior vena cava, and the abdominal aorta is on its left.

At the diaphragm the inferior vena cava passes upwards through its tendinous part to the right of the midline at the level of the eighth thoracic vertebra in a plane anterior to that of the opening for

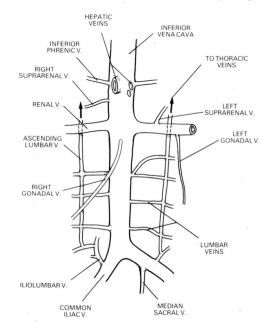

Figure 97   The inferior vena cava and its tributaries.

the oesophagus, and enters the posterior part of the right atrium from below. *This can be indicated on the surface by the anterior end of the sixth right costal cartilage. The surface marking of the beginning of the inferior vena cava is on the transtubercular plane 2.5 cm to the right of the midline.*

The tributaries of the inferior vena cava are the common iliac, lumbar, right gonadal, renal, right suprarenal, inferior phrenic and hepatic veins. The *lumbar veins*, four on each side, are important in that they effect a communication with the superior vena cava (1) through the veins of the abdominal wall and (2) through the azygos veins. This alternative venous circulation opens up if the inferior vena cava is blocked. The lumbar veins also communicate with the vertebral plexus of veins which extends from the pelvis to the skull (p. 336).

The course of the gonadal veins is similar to that of the gonadal arteries. The *testicular vein* on each side emerges from the deep inguinal ring usually as two veins which join to form one vein before ending on the right in the inferior vena cava and on the left in the left renal vein. On both sides they lie behind the alimentary tract and its mesenteries and blood vessels. Each *ovarian vein* emerges from the broad ligament, crosses the external iliac vessels and runs upwards on the posterior abdominal wall.

The *left renal vein* is about 7.5 cm long, the *right* about 2.5 cm long. Each vein lies in front of its artery. The left renal vein receives the left gonadal and left suprarenal veins.

There is one large *suprarenal vein* which on the right joins the inferior vena cava and on the left the left renal vein. The *inferior phrenic veins* correspond with the arteries of the same name.

The *hepatic veins* (p. 99) are in two groups. The upper group consists of three large veins, a right, middle (from the caudate lobe) and left. The lower group consists of smaller veins and come from the right and caudate lobes.

The *common iliac veins* are formed at the sacroiliac joints at the brim of the pelvis by the union of the external and internal iliac veins. The *right common iliac* vein is behind and then lateral to its artery. The *left common iliac* vein is medial to its artery and passes behind the right common iliac artery to join the right common iliac vein.

The *external iliac vein* is the upward continuation of the femoral vein above the inguinal ligament. The right vein runs at first medial to and then behind the external iliac artery. The left remains medial to its artery along its whole course. Both veins are medial to the psoas muscle as it runs round lateral to the brim of the pelvis and are crossed by the ovarian vein and either the round ligament of the uterus or the ductus deferens. The external iliac vein receives the *inferior epigastric* and *deep circumflex iliac veins*. These veins communicate with veins in the abdominal wall which communicate with veins in the thoracic wall and in this way with the superior vena cava.

The lumbar plexus of nerves

This plexus is often described with the sacral plexus but it is much simpler to deal with the two plexuses separately. It is also more convenient to relate its branches to the psoas muscle as in figure 98. The nerves contributing to the plexus are the ventral rami of the five lumbar spinal nerves. The middle three rami (second, third and fourth) form both

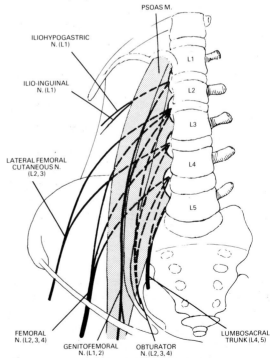

Figure 98   A diagram of the formation of the lumbar plexus.

the *femoral nerve*, which emerges laterally from the psoas, and the *obturator nerve* which emerges medially. Each has a nerve associated with it; the *lateral femoral cutaneous nerve* (second and third) emerges laterally above the femoral nerve and the *accessory obturator* (third and fourth) emerges from the medial border of the psoas muscle.

The *femoral* and *lateral femoral cutaneous nerves* pass laterally and downwards, the former between the iliacus and psoas muscles and the latter on the iliacus. They pass into the thigh deep to the inguinal ligament, the femoral nerve lateral to the femoral vessels but outside their sheath and the lateral femoral cutaneous nerve about 2 cm medial to the anterior superior iliac spine. The femoral nerve gives a branch to the iliacus and is distributed in the thigh to the skin anteriorly and medially, and to the flexor muscles of the thigh at the hip and extensor muscles of the leg at the knee.

The *obturator nerve* after emerging from the psoas muscle passes behind the common iliac vessels and runs round the lateral wall of the pelvis 1 cm below the brim with the obturator vessels below it. The nerve leaves the pelvis through the obturator canal in the upper part of the obturator foramen and is distributed mainly to the adductor muscles of the thigh at the hip. It also has some sensory branches. The *accessory obturator* (present in only 30 per cent of individuals) passes deep to the inguinal ligament and supplies the pectineus muscle.

The remaining branches of the lumbar plexus are as follows: (1) the *iliohypogastric* and *ilio-inguinal nerves* which arise from the first lumbar nerve and pass laterally from the psoas behind the kidney on the quadratus lumborum muscle into the abdominal wall; (2) the *genitofemoral nerve* which arises from the first and second lumbar nerves and runs downwards on the psoas; (3) the *lumbosacral trunk* which is formed by the fourth and fifth lumbar nerves, emerges medial to the psoas and runs downwards into the pelvis behind the common iliac vessels to join the sacral plexus. The *iliohypogastric* and *ilio-inguinal nerves* are largely sensory and are distributed to the skin of the lateral side of the buttock and anterior abdominal wall above the inguinal ligament (p. 69). The

ilio-inguinal nerve also supplies the skin on the upper medial side of the thigh and the skin of the external genitalia near the symphysis pubis. It is important to appreciate that the cutaneous spinal nerve segments over the symphysis pubis and just below it are the twelfth thoracic and first lumbar and the the next cutaneous segment in the perineum is supplied by the second sacral spinal nerve.

The *genitofemoral nerve*, as its name implies, divides into a *genital branch* which enters the deep inguinal ring and supplies the cremaster muscle and the skin of the scrotum or labium majus, and a *femoral branch* which enters the femoral sheath and passes behind the inguinal ligament to supply the skin over the upper medial part of the thigh.

The *lumbosacral trunk* passes downwards behind the common iliac vessels, enters the pelvis and joins the sacral plexus. Two further points about the plexus may be made. The ventral rami divide into ventral and dorsal divisions and the femoral and lateral femoral cutaneous nerves are formed by the dorsal divisions. All the other nerves are from the ventral divisions. Secondly, the ventral rami of the lumbar spinal nerves, mainly the second and third, supply the quadratus lumborum and the psoas major muscles.

The autonomic plexuses and ganglia of the abdomen

These consist mainly of two parts. One is formed by the *right* and *left lumbar ganglionated sympathetic trunks* which lie on the front of the lumbar vertebrae behind the inferior vena cava on the right and the abdominal aorta on the left and are continuations of the right and left thoracic ganglionated trunks which pass downwards posterior to the medial arcuate ligaments. There are four or five ganglia on each trunk from which grey rami communicantes containing postganglionic fibres go (1) to the ventral rami of the lumbar spinal nerves to be distributed through branches of the lumbar plexus, (2) to the plexuses on the front of the aorta. The preganglionic fibres are from the lower three thoracic and upper two lumbar segments of the cord and reach the lumbar sympathetic trunk either by passing down in the thoracic sympathetic trunk or come from the upper two lumbar ventral rami. The postganglionic fibres are distributed (1) to the lower limb through the nerves supplying it or as plexuses round the arteries, (2) to the viscera through the plexuses around the branches of the abdominal aorta. The lumbar ganglionated trunk passes behind the common iliac vessels and enters the pelvis.

The second arrangement of the autonomic nerves of the abdomen takes the form of ganglia and plexuses of nerves in front and at the sides of the abdominal aorta. The ganglia are related mainly to the single branches of the aorta — the coeliac trunk and the superior and inferior mesenteric arteries. There are therefore *coeliac ganglia*, a *superior mesenteric ganglion* and an *inferior mesenteric ganglion*. There are also *renal ganglia*. Plexuses surround the branches of the aorta and their branches — coeliac, hepatic, gastric, splenic, testicular, ovarian, etc.

The abdominal aortic plexuses and ganglia are both sympathetic and parasympathetic. The sympathetic preganglionic fibres are in the splanchnic nerves from the thoracic sympathetic trunk (greater, lesser and lowest, which is often called least but *ima = lowest*). These go mainly to the coeliac ganglia but the lowest go to the renal ganglia. There are also postganglionic fibres from the lumbar ganglionated trunk. The parasympathetic fibres are in the vagus nerves which enter the abdomen through the oesophageal opening in the diaphragm as the gastric nerves. These are preganglionic fibres most of which pass through the abdominal aortic plexuses and synapse in the wall of the organ which they supply.

The *sacral parasympathetic nerves* from the second, third and fourth sacral nerves pass upwards either as a plexus round the inferior mesenteric artery or as independent nerves and supply the left colic flexure and descending and pelvic colons.

The abdominal aortic plexus continues downwards beyond the bifurcation of the aorta anterior to the fifth lumbar vertebra and the sacrum as the *superior hypogastric plexus* or *presacral nerve*.

The postganglionic sympathetic fibres innervate the smooth muscle of the blood vessels of the organs in the abdominal cavity so that their main effects are produced by altering the blood supply

and circulation in these organs. In addition to their vascular effects, the sympathetic fibres cause contraction of the pyloric and ileocaecal sphincters and may be inhibitory to the longitudinal muscle of the gut. Many postganglionic fibres from the lumbar ganglia go to the lower limb in the femoral and obturator nerves and round the femoral artery. The preganglionic fibres to the suprarenal medulla have already been mentioned.

The parasympathetic fibres are motor to the muscle of the alimentary tract, gall bladder and biliary ducts, and secretomotor to its glands. They are inhibitory to the pyloric, ileocaecal and ampullary sphincters.

There are sensory fibres in both the sympathetic and parasympathetic nerves to the viscera. The sympathetic fibres are associated with the sensation of pain and go to the same spinal segments as those from which the preganglionic motor fibres originate. Pain is often referred to the somatic structures supplied by the same spinal nerve segments. Reference has already been made to the umbilical pain associated with early appendicitis (the tenth thoracic segment supplies both the umbilical region of the body wall and the appendix) and the pain in the groin and thigh associated with ureteric colic (the first and second lumbar segments supply both the groin and ureter). There are also parasympathetic sensory fibres from the stomach and intestine which when stimulated produce a sensation of pain, for example colic. The sensations of hunger and nausea are thought to be mediated through vagal sensory fibres from the stomach.

The lymph nodes of the abdomen (figures 99, 100, table 2)

The lymph nodes are arranged in two groups: (1) the nodes along the large blood vessels — the external, internal and common iliac, the inferior vena cava and the abdominal aorta; (2) the nodes which drain the viscera and are arranged along their blood vessels.

(1) There are nodes along the external iliac vessels which receive the lymphatic vessels from the lower limb as well as the buttock and the external genitalia via the inguinal lymph nodes (p. 427). The

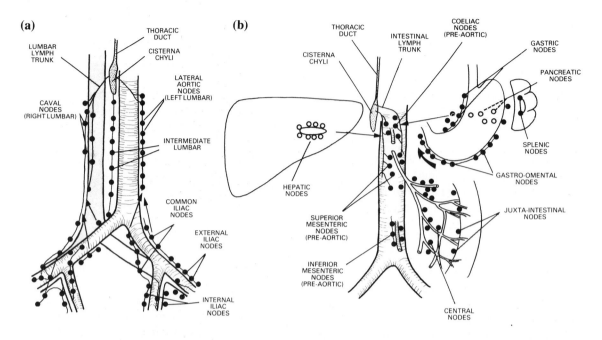

(a)

LUMBAR
LYMPH
TRUNK

THORACIC
DUCT

CISTERNA
CHYLI

LATERAL
AORTIC
NODES
(LEFT LUMBAR)

CAVAL
NODES
(RIGHT LUMBAR)

INTERMEDIATE
LUMBAR

COMMON
ILIAC
NODES

EXTERNAL
ILIAC
NODES

INTERNAL
ILIAC
NODES

(b)

THORACIC
DUCT

CISTERNA
CHYLI

INTESTINAL
LYMPH
TRUNK

COELIAC
NODES
(PRE-AORTIC)

GASTRIC
NODES

PANCREATIC
NODES

HEPATIC
NODES

SUPERIOR
MESENTERIC
NODES
(PRE-AORTIC)

INFERIOR
MESENTERIC
NODES
(PRE-AORTIC)

SPLENIC
NODES

GASTRO-OMENTAL
NODES

JUXTA-INTESTINAL
NODES

CENTRAL
NODES

Figure 99   The abdominal lymph nodes: (a) the lumbar (aortic) nodes; (b) the nodes associated with the alimentary tract.

external iliac nodes drain into the common iliac nodes which also receive the vessels from the internal iliac nodes of the pelvis. The common iliac nodes drain into nodes along the aorta and the inferior vena cava. These aortic and caval nodes are drained by *left* and *right lumbar lymph trunks* which enter the cisterna chyli (p. 122). These nodes also receive the lymphatic vessels from the posterior abdominal wall and the kidneys, suprarenal glands, uterus and gonads.

(2) The lymphatic vessels draining the alimentary tract usually pass through two or three groups of nodes: (a) near the organ itself; (b) along the vessels supplying the organ; and (c) near the aorta at the origin of the vessel supplying the organ. The stomach has nodes along the lesser curvature (*gastric*), along the greater curvature (*gastro-omental*) and around the pylorus (*pyloric*). The lymphatic vessels from these nodes eventually drain into the coeliac nodes round the coeliac trunk (for the lymphatic drainage of the stomach, *see* p. 84). The duodenum, jejunum, ileum, caecum, appendix and colon have nodes adjacent to their wall, from which lymphatic vessels pass to nodes along the

arteries supplying them. These nodes drain into *superior mesenteric* and *inferior mesenteric nodes* around the origin of the arteries of these names. There are nodes near the hilum of the spleen and nodes along the upper and lower borders of the pancreas. These drain into the coeliac nodes. There are *hepatic nodes* at the porta hepatis and these drain to the coeliac. All the nodes in front of the aorta drain eventually by one or two *intestinal lymph trunks* into the cisterna chyli.

Radio-opaque compounds can be injected into a lymphatic vessel made visible by subcutaneous injection of a blue dye which is taken up by the lymphatic vessels. If this is done in the region of the ankle joint the radio-opaque material can be followed by means of X-rays as it moves upwards to the nodes of the inguinal region and the nodes along the external and common iliac vessels which are reached after about 45 min (figure 100(a)). From there the radio-opaque lymph goes to the nodes along the abdominal aorta, at first to the nodes on the same side but eventually to the nodes on both sides, and in front of and behind the aorta. Figure 100(b) shows the appearance of the aortic

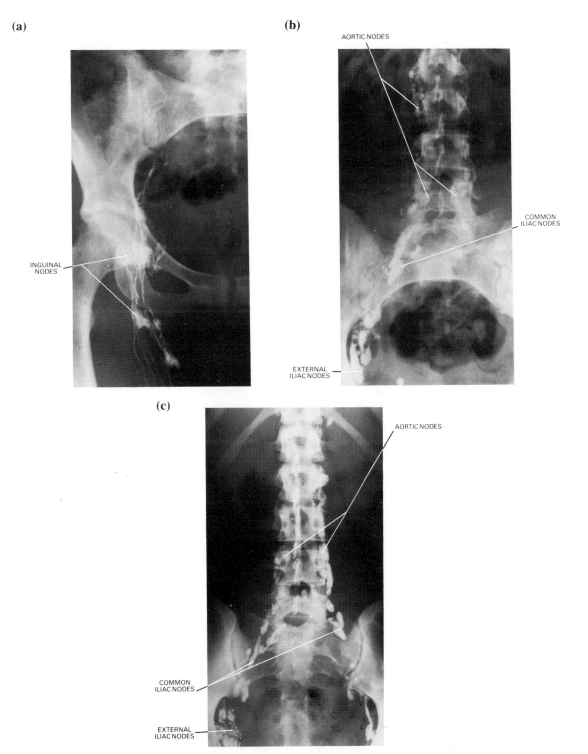

Figure 100 Lymphangiography: (a) the nodes and lymphatic vessels in the inguinal region; (b) the right iliac and some of the aortic nodes; (c) the iliac and aortic nodes of both sides.

**Table 2   Summary of the lymphatic drainage of the
abdominal organs**

Organ	Nodes
Abdominal oesophagus	→ left gastric → coeliac (pre-aortic)

Stomach
   (a) Right part
   (b) Upper left part
      including fundus
      and most of body
   (c) Lower left part
   (d) Pylorus
	→ lesser curvature → left gastric
	→ pancreaticosplenic
	
	→ right gastro-epiploic → pyloric
	→ left gastric and hepatic ⎫ coeliac
	                 → (pre-aortic)

Duodenum	→ pyloric → hepatic and superior mesenteric

Jejunum, ileum, caecum,
  vermiform appendix,
  ascending and transverse
  colon
	→ adjacent to wall → intermediate along blood
	vessels → superior mesenteric (pre-aortic)

Descending and sigmoid colon	→ adjacent to wall → intermediate along blood vessels → inferior mesenteric (pre-aortic)
Upper half of rectum	→ pararectal → intermediate along blood vessels → inferior mesenteric (pre-aortic)

Lower half of rectum
  and anal canal above
  mucocutaneous junction
	→ along middle rectal vessels → internal iliac

Anal canal below mucocutaneous junction	→ superficial inguinal

Liver
   (a) Superficial
   (b) Deep
	→ caval, hepatic (porta hepatis) and coeliac
	→ inferior diaphragmatic → parasternal or
	hepatic (porta hepatis)

Gall bladder and bile ducts	→ hepatic (porta hepatis)
Pancreas	→ pancreaticosplenic → coeliac (pre-aortic) → superior mesenteric (pre-aortic)

nodes 5 h after the injection. The iliac and aortic nodes of both sides are seen in figure 100(c) after the injection of radio-opaque material into lymphatic vessels in the ankle region of both limbs.

The Cisterna Chyli

This structure has already been referred to (p. 53). It is a thin-walled sac about 3 cm long and 0.5 cm wide lying on the right crus of the diaphragm near the right coeliac ganglion to the right of the commencement of the abdominal aorta. Its upward continuation is the thoracic duct which enters the thorax with the azygos vein through the opening for the aorta. The size of the cisterna chyli and the arrangement of the lymph trunks opening into it are subject to considerable variation and even its conventional description as a dilated sac has recently been questioned. As has been indicated, the cisterna chyli receives lumbar and intestinal lymph trunks through which passes all the lymph from the lower limbs, posterior abdominal walls and abdominal and pelvic organs. The cisterna may also receive lymph from structures in the lowest part of the thoracic cavity.

Part 3

The Pelvis and Perineum

9

The Pelvis

The pelvis is divided into the *greater* (*false*) and the *lesser* (*true*) pelvis by an approximately circular opening described variously as the *superior aperture*, *brim*, or *inlet* which is outlined by the promontory of the sacrum (upper anterior border of the body of the first sacral vertebra), the ala of the sacrum, the terminal (arcuate) line of the ilium, the iliopubic eminence, the pectineal line, the pubic crest and the upper border of the symphysis pubis (figure 101). The greater pelvis consists largely of the ala of the ilium on each side where it extends upwards and laterally above the superior aperture. Actually the greater pelvis forms the lower lateral walls of the abdominal cavity. It is proposed therefore to use the word *pelvis* to describe the *lesser pelvis* unless further definition is required.

It is convenient to consider the walls of the greater and lesser pelvis as consisting of bones, joints and ligaments lined by muscles which are covered by fascia. The fascia is lined by peritoneum and the organs project into the cavity of the pelvis so that they acquire a fascial (often thin) and peritoneal covering or lie outside the peritoneum (figure 102). The nerves of the pelvis are outside the fascia and the blood vessels are either embedded in the fascia or internal to it. The floor of the pelvis is in the form of a muscular diaphragm. The contents of the pelvis are as follows: (1) the termination of the alimentary tract posteriorly; (2) the bladder and termination of the urinary tract anteriorly; (3) the internal female genitalia between (1) and (2) or parts of the male genitalia; (4) the internal iliac vessels and their branches; (5) the obturator nerve

and the sacral plexus which is joined by the lumbosacral trunk from the fourth and fifth lumbar nerves; (6) sympathetic and parasympathetic autonomic ganglia and nerves; (7) lymph nodes.

It is important to appreciate that the cavity of the lesser pelvis is divided into a superior part which is above the pelvic diaphragm (mainly the levator ani muscles) and an inferior part which is below the diaphragm (figures 102, 118, 122). The latter is called the *perineum*. If looked at from below the perineum is divided by a line joining the ischial tuberosities into an anterior *urogenital triangle* and a posterior *anal triangle (figure 103(a))*.

The Pelvic Bones, Ligaments and Joints

As already described on p. 59 the bony pelvis consists of the hip bones and sacrum. The outline of the superior aperture has already been described above. The back wall of the cavity of the lesser pelvis consists of the concave sacrum and coccyx. The front wall is formed by the symphysis pubis and internal surface of the body of the pubis on each side of the symphysis. The side walls are formed by the ilium, ischium and pubis (figure 57(b)) and contain the obturator foramen.

The *inferior aperture* or *outlet* of the pelvis is bounded anteriorly by the lower border of the symphysis pubis, posteriorly by the tip of the coccyx or the lower edge of the sacrum (because of the mobility of the coccyx the sacrum is used for this purpose) and laterally by the ischial tuber-

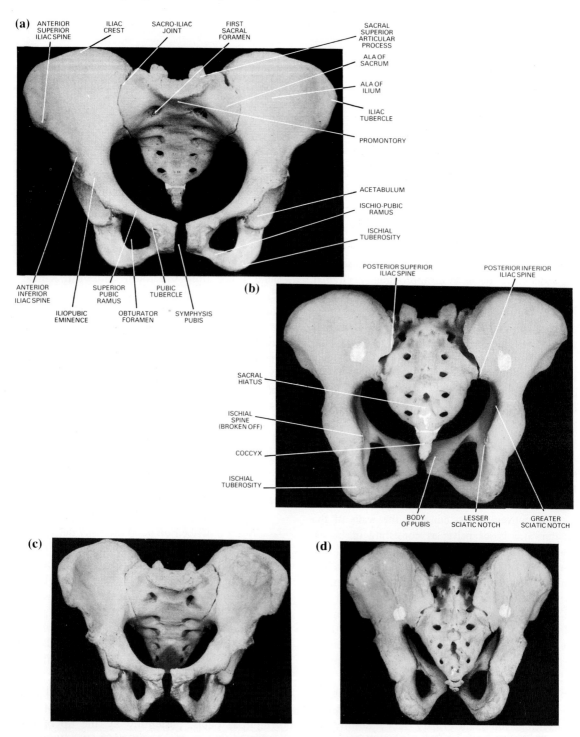

Figure 101   The female pelvis: (a) anterior view; (b) posterior view. The male pelvis: (c) anterior view; (d) posterior view. (The sacrum in both pelvises has five foramina on each side due to the fusion of the first piece of the coccyx with the sacrum.)

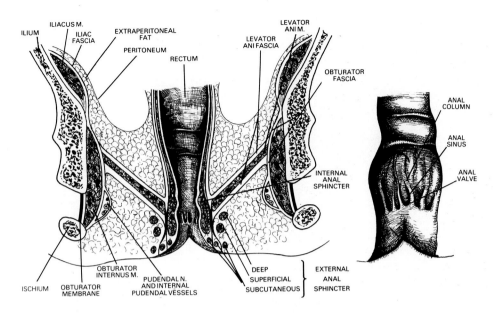

Figure 102   A coronal section through the posterior half of the pelvis to indicate the structures forming its walls and also the structures in the anal triangle.

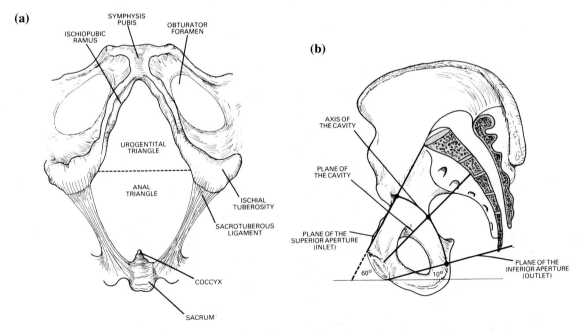

Figure 103   (a) An inferior view of the pelvis to indicate the perineum and its subdivisions. (b) The planes of the pelvic inlet, cavity and outlet and the axis of the pelvic cavity.

osities (figure 103(a)). The outlet is not in one plane since the lateral boundaries anteriorly are formed by the ischiopubic rami and posteriorly by the sacrotuberous ligaments.

The plane of the superior aperture is about 60° above the horizontal and the plane through the lower edge of the symphysis pubis and coccyx is about 10° above the horizontal (figure 103(b)).

(a)

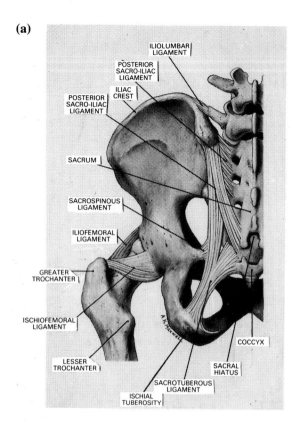

(b)

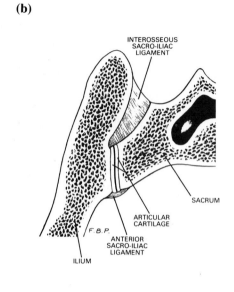

Figuree 104   The sacro-iliac joint: (a) a posterior view; (b) a coronal section through the second sacral vertebra (reproduced from *Hamilton's Textbook of Human Anatomy* **by courtesy of the editors and the Macmillan Press).**

The ligaments of the pelvis apart from those of the joints are the sacrospinous, sacrotuberous and inguinal and the obturator membrane. These together with bony margins form entrances and exits into and out of the pelvis. The sacrospinous ligament from the back of the sacrum to the ischial spine and the greater sciatic notch form the *greater sciatic foramen*. The sacrotuberous ligament from the back of the sacrum to the inner edge of the ischial tuberosity, the sacrospinous ligament and the lesser sciatic notch form the *lesser sciatic foramen* (figure 104(a)). There is a space between the inguinal ligament (p. 69), attached to the anterior superior iliac spine and the pubic tubercle, and the iliac and pubic bones. The obturator membrane almost fills the obturator foramen but there is a gap (the *obturator canal*) in the upper part of the membrane.

The *sacro-iliac joint* is a synovial joint formed by the articulation between the auricular area of the anterior lateral surface of the sacrum and a similar area on the sacral surface of the ilium. Since the surfaces behind the synovial joint are united by powerful interosseous ligaments, one may regard the sacro-iliac joint as being both synovial and fibrous. This synovial joint shows partial bony fusion in older people. The irregular surfaces of the joint lock together and reduce movement to a minimum. There are also strong posterior and weak anterior sacro-iliac ligaments.

The weight of the body tends to displace the sacrum downwards and this is prevented by the structure of the joint and the arrangement of its ligaments. In addition a coronal section through the second and third segment of the sacrum shows that the sacrum in this region is wedge-shaped with the narrower part of the wedge anterior (figure 104(b)). The result is that the weight of the body wedges the sacrum between the two iliac bones. The upper part of the sacrum also tends to tilt downwards and forwards but this is prevented by the sacrotuberous and sacrospinous ligaments. Investigations have shown two types of movement at these joints. One is a tilting of the upper part downwards and forwards of about 5° when standing as compared with lying, and another is a downward movement of the whole sacrum of about 2 mm when standing as compared with lying.

These joints are important clinically. Sudden bending can result in tearing the posterior ligaments or even minor dislocation of the adjacent joint surfaces. Both conditions are extremely painful in flexion movements of the trunk and can be very disabling. Treatment is often difficult and not infrequently manipulation **produces** a successful result.

The symphysis pubis is a secondary cartilaginous joint between the medial surfaces of the bodies of the two pubic bones. The adjacent surfaces of the bones are covered by hyaline cartilage and a disc of fibrocartilage, firmly attached to the hyaline cartilage, fills the gap between the two bones. Above, below and in front of the joint there are thickenings of fibrous tissue forming ligaments. These, together with the structure of the joint itself, produces an immobile joint which resists separation of the hip bones.

During pregnancy the ligaments of the joints of the pelvis are softened and some movement at the sacro-iliac joints may occur. More important there occurs some separation at the symphysis pubis so that the circumference of the superior aperture is increased. The order of separation is about 2 mm and, although small, may make it easier for the fetal head to pass through the pelvic cavity. The bone adjacent to the joint is sometimes absorbed and this also assists separation at the symphysis. The marked loosening of and separation at the joint leading to instability of the pelvis during walking described in some textbooks are very rare.

Sex Differences in the Bony Pelvis (figure 101)

These differences are mainly related to the requirements of childbirth. Other differences due to the greater weight and muscularity of the male are also described and these result in a bony pelvis with more distinct muscular and ligamentous markings and in the bones on the whole being heavier. In the male the iliac crest is thicker and curves inwards more markedly at its anterior end than in the female. These differences are, however, relative and not particularly reliable for determining the sex of a pelvis.

The main differences to look for are as follows: (1) the subpubic angle in the female is about 85° as compared with 55° in the male; (2) the diameter of the acetabulum in the female is less than the distance between the anterior border of the acetabulum and the symphysis pubis (in the male they are equal); (3) the greater sciatic notch in the female forms an angle of about 75° and in the male an angle of about 50°.

Other differences are (1) the obturator foramen is triangular in the female, and oval in the male; (2) the ischial spines (usually broken off in a skeleton) turn inwards more in the male than in the female; (3) the medial edges of the ischiopubic rami in the male are much more roughened and everted for the attachment of the crus of the penis and its overlying muscle as compared with the edges of the rami in the female (these also are often broken in a skeleton); (4) in the female there is a sulcus on the ilium in front of its auricular area (*pre-auricular sulcus*).

Most of these differences can be identified on a single hip bone. The sacrum also shows sex differences. In the female the transverse diameter of the upper surface of the body of the first sacral vertebra is less than one-third of the total transverse diameter. In the male it is more than one-third. The female sacrum is shorter and less curved than the male. The sacro-iliac joint in the female is said to extend over only the first and second sacral segments but in the male the third segment is usually involved. This has been questioned.

Further differences between the sexes in the superior aperture, cavity and inferior aperture of the bony pelvis are discussed in the next section.

The Obstetric Pelvis

Since the fetus has to pass through the bony pelvis

the pelvic dimensions are very important. The superior aperture (inlet) of the female pelvis is rounded with the sacral promontory projecting into it from behind. It is therefore often described as heart-shaped. In the male it is more triangular.

The important *diameters* of the inlet are the *transverse*, the maximum diameter which can be measured (average female 13 cm) and the *antero-posterior*, the distance between the middle of the promontory and the middle of the upper edge of the symphysis pubis (average female 11 cm). Both diameters in the male are 0.5–1.0 cm less.

The anteroposterior diameter is called the *true conjugate* and indirect methods of measuring this are used in obstetrics. The *diagonal conjugate* can be measured per vaginam and is the distance between the promontory and the lower edge of the symphysis pubis. It is about 1.5 cm greater than the true conjugate. Much of the information about the dimensions of the brim and other parts of the pelvis was obtained by means of X-rays but it is now realised that any unessential X-raying, especially in the early weeks of pregnancy, must be avoided. Many radiological investigations, however, were carried out before the dangers were realised.

Of the dimensions of the fetus those of the head are the most important because it is relatively large and the least compressible part. In a normal birth the long diameter of the baby's head enters the transverse diameter of the pelvic brim, that is the occiput is to the right or left. It was taught at one time that the head entered with its greatest diameter in the *oblique diameter* of the brim (the distance between the sacro-iliac joint at the brim and the opposite iliopubic eminence). Since this is not the case the oblique diameter of the brim is of little obstetrical importance.

There are similar diameters, anteroposterior, transverse and oblique, for the pelvic cavity but they are not of the same significance as those of the brim. The *plane of greatest pelvic dimensions* passes through the middle of the symphysis pubis and the middle of the third segment of the sacrum (figure 104). The *axes of the pelvic brim* and *outlet* are lines at right angles to the middle of their planes. The *axis of the cavity* is a similar line through the plane of greatest pelvic dimensions. A curved line joining these three axes is the *axis of*

the pelvic cavity. The transverse diameter between the ischial spines is important because in the male type of pelvis this diameter is reduced. As the fetal head descends it normally rotates so that the occiput becomes anterior. A narrowing of the pelvic cavity at this level may interfere with the further progress of labour.

The anteroposterior diameter of the outlet in the female is about 13.5 cm and is greater than the transverse diameter which is the distance between the ischial tuberosities and measures about 11.5 cm. Because the male pelvic cavity is longer and narrows much more than the female, these diameters in the male are much smaller — the anteroposterior is about 8 cm and the transverse about 8.5 cm. Normally the baby is born with the long diameter of the head in the larger anteroposterior diameter of the pelvic outlet.

Pelvises can be classified according to the shape of the brim which may be approximately round, triangular, transversely oval or anteroposteriorly oval. Caldwell and Moloy in 1933 and 1940 introduced a classification which included many other features of the pelvis besides the shape of the brim. This classification is widely accepted. The terms used are (1) *gynaecoid* which shows the typical female features of the pelvis as described above; (2) *android* which shows the typical features of the male pelvis; (3) *anthropoid* in which the brim is oval anteroposteriorly; (4) *platypelloid* in which the brim is transversely oval (*platus = wide, flat*; *pella = wooden bowl*, Greek).

Anthropologists are also very interested in the shape and size of the different parts of the pelvis because of the changes produced by the upright posture and bipedal gait of man as compared with the pelvic characteristics of the primates.

The Pelvic Muscles and Fascia

The Psoas and Iliacus Muscles and Fasciae

The iliacus (p. 107) and psoas (p. 106) muscles have already been described. These muscles merge as they pass deep to the inguinal ligament and form a common iliopsoas tendon which is attached to the lesser trochanter of the femur. The iliacus and psoas are covered by the *fascia iliaca* and *psoas*

(a)   **(b)**

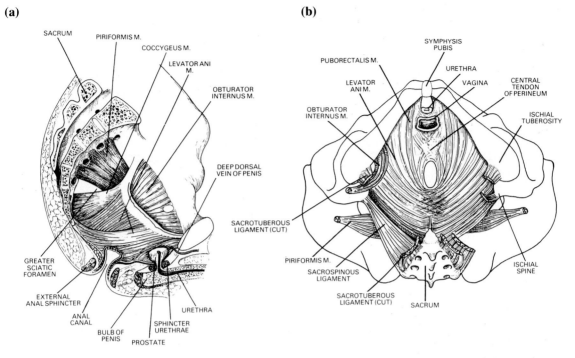

Figure 105   The pelvic muscles: (a) superior view; (b) inferior view.

fascia respectively. The latter has been described on p. 107. The fascia iliaca continues into the thigh as the posterior layer of the femoral sheath which surrounds the femoral vessels and is considered in detail with the lower limb (p. 429).

The Piriformis Muscle (figure 105)

The piriformis is attached to the pelvic surface of the middle three segments of the sacrum, passes laterally out of the pelvis through the greater sciatic foramen and is attached to the upper border of the greater trochanter of the femur. It is a lateral rotator of the thigh at the hip joint and is supplied by the second and third sacral nerves.

The Obturator Internus Muscle and Fascia (figures 102, 105, 118, 123)

The *obturator internus* lines the lateral wall of the pelvis and is attached to the obturator membrane and the bone surrounding the obturator foramen.

Inferiorly the tendon of the muscle turns laterally at a right angle, leaves the pelvis through the lesser sciatic foramen and is attached to the upper edge of the greater trochanter of the femur. The muscle is a lateral rotator of the thigh at the hip joint and is innervated by its own nerve from the sacral plexus (L5, S1, 2). This nerve leaves the pelvis through the greater sciatic foramen, crosses the ischial spine and passes through the lesser sciatic foramen before supplying the muscle. The obturator internus is covered by the *obturator fascia* to which a large part of the levator ani is attached.

The Levator Ani Muscles and Fascia (figures 102, 105, 118, 119, 121)

The *levator ani* muscles form the main part of the floor or diaphragm of the pelvis. Each muscle is attached to bone anteriorly and posteriorly — to the back of the body of the pubis and to the ischial spine. Between these bony attachments it arises from the obturator fascia. Since the muscle is attached medially to the coccyx it is more or less in the plane of the pelvic outlet, that is it is almost horizontal. Its fibres pass backwards and medially and meet the fibres of the opposite levator ani except where the two muscles surround the structures passing through them in the midline — the rectum, vagina and urethra. The anterior medial edges of the two levatores ani do not meet and this narrow gap is occupied by fascia. This fascia is formed by the fusion of the fasciae on the upper and lower surfaces of the levator ani (figures 118, 121). In the female the urethra lies just behind this fascia and in the male the prostate containing the urethra lies on it.

When viewed from below the two levator ani muscles if followed forwards in the midline are attached to the coccyx and the *anococcygeal body* (the fibrous tissue between the coccyx and anal canal), surround the anal canal, and are attached to the *perineal body* (p.   ). In the male the anterior borders then slightly diverge. In the female the muscles surround the vagina and then separate slightly.

Several parts of the levator ani are described. The *pubococcygeus* is that part which runs backwards from the body of the pubis to the coccyx. In the male, it is attached to the prostate (*levator prostatae*) and in the female to the urethra and vagina (*pubovaginalis*). Behind the prostate (or the vagina) some of its fibres insert into the perineal body. Some of the inferior fibres on each side from the body of the pubis pass backwards and form a sling at the level of the junction of the rectum and anal canal (the *puborectalis*). The most inferior of these fibres join the deepest part of the external anal sphincter (p. 135).

The part of the muscle from the obturator fascia is called the *iliococcygeus* and goes mainly to the coccyx and anococcygeal body. The *coccygeus muscle* which can be regarded as the most posterior part of the levator ani is attached to the spine of the ischium and to the coccyx and lower part of the sacrum. These muscles are the tailwaggers of other animals and have acquired different attachments and functions in man.

The nerve supply of the levator ani is derived from the third, fourth and possibly fifth sacral nerves on its superior surface and also on its inferior surface from the branches of the pudendal nerve to the anal canal and perineum (S2, 3, 4).

The functions of the levator ani muscles are important but there are differences of opinion about them. It is agreed that they form a muscular pelvic diaphragm supporting the pelvic viscera. They function in conjunction with the thoracic diaphragm and the anterior abdominal muscles in response to changes in intra-abdominal pressure. In strong muscular effort all these muscles contract. In defaecation, micturition and labour, the abdominal muscles and thoracic diaphragm contract and the pelvic diaphragm relaxes. In coughing, the abdominal muscles and pelvic diaphragm contract and the thoracic diaphragm relaxes.

Some of the fibres of the levator ani muscles act as sphincters to the urethra, vagina and anal canal. Other fibres are said to pull the urethra, vagina and anal canal open and contribute to the fall in pressure in the anal canal and urethra associated with the initiation of defaecation and micturition respectively.

During childbirth the levator ani muscles are frequently torn and support of the pelvic viscera is decreased. This contributes to the descent of the pelvic viscera mainly involving the uterus in the condition known as *prolapse*. The bladder, urethra and rectum may also be involved. In a condition called *stress incontinence* usually associated with prolapse the increase in intra-abdominal pressure in coughing results in the expulsion of a small quantity of urine because the sphincteric mechanism of the torn levator ani muscles is defective.

The Pelvic Peritoneum

The fascia related to the pelvic viscera is described with the organs, the general arrangement of which is shown in figures 106, 107. It can be seen that the rectum and anal canal are posterior, the bladder is anterior and in the female the uterus and vagina lie between the bladder and rectum. In the male the peritoneum posteriorly passes downwards in front of the upper two-thirds of the rectum and then forwards on to the upper edge of the back of the bladder. From there it covers the upper surface of the bladder and then runs upwards on the anterior abdominal wall. The space between the rectum and bladder is called the *rectovesical pouch* and

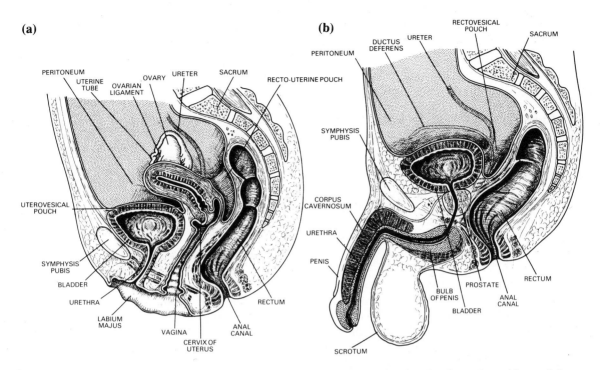

Figure 106   **A hemisection of (a) the female and (b) the male pelvis showing the viscera in position and the arrangement of the peritoneum.**

usually contains loops of small intestine.

In the female the peritoneum leaves the rectum and passes forward on to the posterior aspect of the upper third of the vagina. From there it runs upwards over the posterior surface and fundus of the uterus. It passes downwards on the front of the upper two-thirds of the uterus and then forwards and is related to the bladder and anterior abdominal wall in the same way as in the male. There are two pouches in the female, the deep *recto-uterine pouch* between the rectum and uterus and the more shallow *uterovesical pouch* between the uterus and bladder.

There is an anteroposterior fold of peritoneum on each side of the recto-uterine pouch forming its lateral margins (*recto-uterine folds*). On either side of the uterus a double fold of peritoneum passes from its lateral border to the lateral wall of the pelvis. This is called the *broad ligament*. The uterine tube lies in the medial four-fifths of its upper border and the ovary is attached to its posterior surface. The broad ligament is described in more detail on p. 144.

Pelvic peritonitis which is more common in women than in men may cause an abscess in the recto-uterine pouch. This can be drained through the upper part of the posterior wall of the vagina.

When the bladder enlarges it passes upwards between the peritoneum and the anterior abdominal wall. This has to be kept in mind when making an incision into the lower part of the abdominal wall but it also makes it possible to operate on the bladder and prostate without entering the peritoneal cavity.

10

The Pelvic Organs

The Rectum and Anal Canal

The Form, Position and General Relations

The rectum is about 12 cm long and is continuous with the sigmoid colon at the level of the third sacral vertebra. It is curved with an anterior concavity as it lies in the hollow of the sacrum (figure 106). At its lower end the rectum bends backwards at almost a right angle to become continuous with the *anal canal* at about the level and 2.5 cm in front of the coccyx. The rectum has less marked lateral curves, an upper and lower to the right and a middle to the left. Perhaps *rectum*, which means *straight* (Latin), is a misnomer. The lower end is somewhat dilated (the *ampulla*) as compared with the upper end which is about 4 cm in diameter.

The peritoneum covers the front and sides of the upper third of the rectum and only the front of its middle third. The lowest third is below the level of the peritoneum which passes forwards on to either the bladder or the vagina and uterus.

The main structures lying behind the rectum in addition to the sacrum are the superior rectal and median sacral vessels. Posteriorly and laterally on each side there are the piriformis, coccygeus and levator ani muscles, the ventral rami of the middle sacral nerves and the pelvic autonomic nerves. In the male the base of the bladder with the terminal part of the ureter, and a ductus deferens and seminal vesicle on each side, and more inferiorly, in the middle, the prostate are anterior (figure 107). In the female the uterus and vagina are anterior. The

rectovesical or recto-uterine pouch in front of the rectum usually contains loops of the small intestine and the sigmoid colon.

The rectum is unlike the main part of the large intestine in that it has no appendices epiploicae, sacculations nor taeniae coli. The longitudinal muscle forms an almost complete layer and is deficient only at the lateral edges. Internally the rectal lining has a number of horizontal folds which do not extend round the whole circumference. They are permanent and of variable structure in that some contain only the circular muscle and others the longitudinal muscle as well. The most important is the middle fold (there are usually three) which is on the anterior and right walls. It is immediately above the ampulla and is thought to divide the rectum into an upper part which contains faeces and a lower part (the ampulla) which is normally empty. Other authorities maintain that the whole rectum is normally empty and the faeces collect in the sigmoid colon. Distention of the rectum due to downward movement of the faeces produces the desire to defaecate. Probably the commonest cause of constipation is a habitual ignoring of this reflex which in time ceases to function.

The anal canal is about 4 cm long and extends from the ampulla of the rectum to the *anus*. It is much narrower than the ampulla and normally the lateral walls are in contact so that the lumen forms an anteroposterior slit. Behind the anal canal there is a mass of fibrous and muscular tissue called the *anococcygeal ligament* (*body*) and in front is the *perineal body*, another fibromuscular structure which separates the anal canal from the vagina in the female and the membranous urethra and beginning of the prostatic urethra in the male (figure 106). Laterally on each side is the ischiorectal fossa (p. 156).

The Anal and Rectal Sphincters (figure 102)

The wall of the anal canal contains the internal and external anal sphincters which receive a contribution from the levator ani muscles. The *internal sphincter* is a thickening of the circular smooth muscle surrounding the upper two-thirds of the anal canal and has an autonomic nerve supply — the sympathetic nerves cause it to contract and the parasympathetic nerves inhibit its action.

The *external sphincter* consists of skeletal muscle and extends along the whole of the anal canal. It has three parts. The *subcutaneous part* is immediately under the skin round the anus. Deep to the subcutaneous part are the *superficial* and *deep parts* which surround the internal sphincter. All three parts have fibres which enter the anococcygeal ligament posteriorly and the perineal body anteriorly. Only the superficial part is attached to bone posteriorly. Two further details are (1) the deepest fibres of the deep part are joined by fibres from the puborectalis muscle (p. 132); (2) some of the fibres of the puborectalis muscle join the longitudinal smooth muscle of the rectum and continue downwards with it to form septa which split the subcutaneous part of the external sphincter and become attached to the skin (figure 102). The most peripheral of these separate off a space round the terminal part of the anal canal (the *peri-anal space*). Infection in this space does not spread laterally but circumferentially. The external sphincter is supplied by the pudendal nerve (second and third sacral nerves) and the fourth sacral nerve (perineal branch).

Normally the anal canal is kept closed by the sphincters, which relax during defaecation. Incontinence occurs if all three parts of the sphincter mechanism, the puborectalis and external and internal sphincters, are cut in the region of the anorectal junction. Incontinence is unlikely if the sphincters are cut below this level.

The Lining of the Anal Canal

The lining of the anal canal has a number of important features (figure 102). The upper part, developed from the *cloaca* (*cluere* = *to cleanse*; *cloaca* = *sewer*, Latin) and therefore endodermal in origin, is lined by a variable but mainly mucous columnar epithelium. The lower part, developed from a depression from the exterior (the *proctodeum*; *proctos*, Greek = *anus* and also denotes *rectum*) and therefore ectodermal in origin, is lined by stratified squamous epithelium and contains sebaceous and sweat glands. The upper half has a number of longitudinal folds which are called the *anal columns* and are formed by terminal branches of the superior rectal artery and vein. The *anal valves* are crescentic folds of mucous membrane joining the lower ends of the columns. Opposite each valve is a recess forming an *anal sinus*. Mucous glands extending a variable distance into the wall and muscle, open on to the sinuses. The line formed by the attached edges of the anal valves (the *pectinate line*) is regarded as the junction between the endodermal and ectodermal parts of the anal canal. This has been disputed. An intermediate zone below the anal valves is described and is called the *pecten*. It is covered by stratified epithelium which is thinner than that covering the lowest part of the anal canal and does not contain sweat glands. The lower limit of this is marked by what is called the *white line* and this is said to be the dividing line between the ectodermal and endodermal parts of the anal canal. This line marks the lower limit of the internal sphincter and the upper edge of the subcutaneous part of the external sphincter and the *anal intersphincteric groove* can be palpated at this level on digital examination of the anal canal.

The difference between the sensory innervation of the lining of the upper half of the anal canal and that of the lower half is important. The upper half with its autonomic innervation does not respond to the usual stimuli producing pain. The lower half is extremely sensitive. This is evidenced by the marked pain in the condition called *fissure in ano* in which there is a longitudinal splitting of the lining of the lower half of the anal canal.

The Arteries, Veins, Lymphatics and Nerve Supply

Although strictly speaking the rectum and anal canal are described as separate parts of the large intestine and the anal canal is below the level of the floor of the pelvic cavity and therefore in the perineum, the term *rectal* is used frequently to include the anal canal. Thus the arterial blood supply, venous and lymphatic drainage, nerve supply and development of the rectum usually refer to both structures.

The *superior, middle* and *inferior rectal arteries* supply the rectum and anal canal. The superior rectal artery is a continuation of the inferior mesenteric. Its terminal branches run eventually in the submucosa of the anal canal and extend as far as the anal valves. Each middle rectal artery is a branch of the internal iliac but is distributed mainly to the muscle and forms few anastomoses with the superior and inferior arteries. The connective tissue in which it runs on either side of the rectum forms the *lateral ligament of the rectum*. The inferior rectal artery comes from the internal pudendal in the ischiorectal fossa and anastomoses with the superior rectal.

The *superior rectal vein* is formed by the union of about six large submucous veins which begin in the anal columns. The *middle rectal vein* on each side goes to the internal iliac vein and the *inferior rectal vein* to the internal pudendal vein. These veins constitute an important communication between the systemic and hepatic portal veins (p. 104). Internal haemorrhoids are the enlarged, distended (*varicose*), submucosal veins in the anal columns and especially affect the left lateral and right anterior and posterior veins. Although it is easy to understand how haemorrhoids can occur in conditions associated with increased portal venous pressure or in pregnancy, in which there is increased pressure on the pelvic veins due to the fetal head, this condition most commonly occurs for no obvious reason. It has been said to be due to constipation associated with straining during defaecation. The lack of submucosal connective tissue supporting the veins may be an important factor. This explains why haemorrhage from and descent of the haemorrhoids is common. Obviously everyone lacks this connective tissue but haemorrhoids are

not universal. Perhaps some people have more connective tissue in this site than others.

The *lymphatic vessels* of the upper half of the rectum drain upwards along the superior rectal vessels. They pass through nodes at the side of the rectum and along the vessels to nodes at the origin of the inferior mesenteric artery. The vessels from the lower half of the rectum and upper part of the anal canal (down to the mucocutaneous junction) pass with the middle rectal vessels to the nodes along the internal iliac vessels. The lymphatic vessels from the lowest part of the anal canal, the part lined by skin, go to the superficial inguinal lymph nodes.

The *motor* and *sensory nerve supply* to the rectum and anal canal has already been referred to (p. 119). Sensory impulses setting up reflexes due to distension of the rectum are mediated through parasympathetic fibres which come from the pelvic splanchnic nerves (the second, third and fourth sacral nerves) via the inferior hypogastric plexus which lies on each side of the rectum close to its lateral wall. This close relationship has to be kept in mind by the surgeon when removing the rectum. Otherwise the parasympathetic motor nerves to the bladder may be cut. Both sympathetic and parasympathetic fibres are associated with pain arising from the rectum and upper part of the anal canal.

Rectal Examination

The anal canal and lower part of the rectum are frequently examined by means of the gloved index finger (*rectal examination* – another example of the inclusion of the anal canal with the rectum). It is important to remember that the anal canal passes upwards and forwards from below. The anal canal is normally empty. The lining is palpated and one or more of the transverse rectal folds can be reached. The state of the sphincters can be estimated. Through the posterior wall the sacrum and coccyx are palpated. *In the male* anteriorly the main structure to be felt is the prostate, inferior to which are the membranous part of the urethra and bulb of the penis. The base of the bladder and seminal vesicles lie above the prostate and are normally not palpable. *In the female* anteriorly the upper part of the vagina and the cervix of the uterus can be palpated. A pathological ovary, uterine tube or broad ligament may be felt laterally. An inflamed pelvic appendix in the recto-uterine or rectovesical pouch may cause tenderness on rectal examination. Most of these anterior and lateral structures cannot be palpated unless they are enlarged. If inflamed, rectal examination will reveal that they are tender.

Although in the female a vaginal examination is more informative regarding many of the organs in the pelvis, in certain circumstances, for example in a virgin, a rectal examination may be necessary or preferable.

The *proctoscope* and *sigmoidoscope* are instruments which permit the direct visual examination for a distance of up to 25 cm of the anal canal, rectum and part of the sigmoid colon. A flexible *colonoscope*, 180 cm long, makes it possible to examine the whole lining of the large intestine.

Abnormalities

Some of the congenital abnormalities associated with the rectum and anal canal are readily appreciated if one knows that they develop from the posterior part of the cloaca, which is the caudal end of the hindgut (the bladder and the urethra or part of it develop from the anterior part), and from the downgrowth of ectoderm which forms the proctodeum. One type of *imperforate anus* results from a failure of the membrane between the proctodeum and hindgut to break down. This is a relatively simple problem since the membrane can be incised. The hindgut may fail to meet the proctodeum. If the hindgut is near the proctodeum they can be joined but if they are widely separated joining them may be impossible. Both types present problems of sphincter control. The third type of problem is due to an incomplete separation of the anterior from the posterior parts of the cloaca so that there are communications between the rectum and bladder. If everything else is normal the difficult operation of closing off the bladder from the rectum may be successful.

The Urinary Bladder (figure 106)

The Form, Position and Relations

The urinary bladder is a hollow organ lying in the front of the pelvis, of varying size and shape depending on the amount of urine it contains. In the

(a)

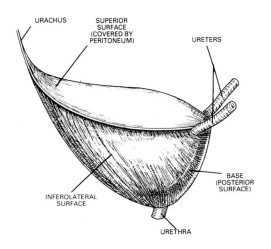

(b)

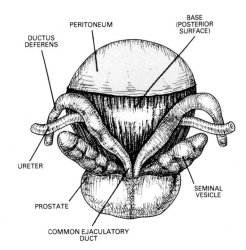

Figure 107 **The bladder: (a) its shape and surfaces; (b) its posterior surface (base).**

adult when empty it is described as having four triangular sides (figure 107). The *base* is posterior and the other three sides meet anteriorly at the *apex*. It has a superior and two inferolateral surfaces. When the bladder enlarges it becomes more globular in shape and rises about 6 cm above the symphysis pubis when full. If the outflow of urine is obstructed the bladder may reach as high as the umbilicus. As the bladder enlarges it passes upwards between the peritoneum and the anterior abdominal wall (p. 133). In the infant the bladder is higher comparatively than in the adult and is an abdominal organ. It becomes pelvic at about 5 years of age but its final position is related to changes at puberty.

The peritoneal relations have been described (p. 133). Coils of the small intestine lie on the upper surface of the bladder and become posterior as the bladder enlarges. The entrances of the ureters mark off the posterior angles of the superior surface. The remains of the *urachus* (*ourachos = urinary canal of a fetus*; *ouron = urine*, *echein = to hold*, Greek) extend from the anterior apex to the umbilicus and form the *median umbilical ligament* on the deep aspect of the midline of the anterior abdominal wall.

The inferolateral surfaces are related to the pubis anteriorly from which they are separated by fat (retropubic pad of fat) containing thickenings of connective tissue passing backwards from the pubis to the prostate (*puboprostatic ligaments*) or in the female to the bladder (*pubovesical ligaments*).

The triangular base, which faces downwards as well as backwards, is demarcated superolaterally by the entrance of the ureters into the bladder and inferiorly by the urethra at the *neck* of the bladder. In the male the neck lies on the prostate and in the female on the pelvic fascia. The neck is the most fixed part of the bladder. In the male, the base of the bladder is related to the rectum, separated above by the rectovesical pouch of peritoneum and inferolaterally on each side by a ductus deferens and seminal vesicle (figure 107). In the female, the base of the bladder is immediately in front of the upper part of the vagina and supravaginal cervix (figure 106).

The Ligaments

The peritoneum forms a lateral fold on each side of the bladder and posterior folds passing backwards to the sacrum. These folds are called the *false ligaments* (*lateral* and *posterior*) of the bladder. The *true ligaments* of the bladder are condensations of fascia: (1) anteriorly between the pubis and bladder in the female (*pubovesical ligaments*); (2) laterally from the obturator fascia to the side of the bladder; (3) posteriorly round the vesical plexus of veins from the base of the bladder to the internal iliac veins. They are true ligaments because they support its position.

The Interior

The lining of the bladder is loosely attached to the underlying tissue and is folded when empty, except for a triangular area (the *trigone*) which is smooth. As the bladder fills the whole lining becomes smooth. The trigone is outlined by the two ureteric orifices at its superolateral angles and the urethral opening in the midline inferiorly. The sides of the trigone in an empty bladder measure about 2.5 cm and in a full bladder increase to about 5 cm. There is a ridge between the ureteric orifices (the *interureteric fold*) which can be seen on cystoscopy, and is a guide to the slit-like openings of the ureters. The interureteric ridge is formed by a continuation of the longitudinal muscle of the ureters into the wall of the bladder. The internal urethral opening is crescentic in outline, is the lowest part of the bladder and is about 3 cm behind the middle of the symphysis pubis. Behind this opening, especially in older men, there is usually a projection formed by the prostate gland. It is called the *uvula vesicae*.

The interior of the bladder in the living can be examined by means of a hollow instrument with lenses and a light, a *cystoscope*, which is introduced into the bladder via the urethra. This instrument also makes it possible to pass into each ureter a catheter by means of which separate samples of urine from the two kidneys can be obtained and radio-opaque material injected into the pelvis and calices of the kidney (figure 95). Radio-opaque material (20 per cent sodium iodide) can be introduced into the bladder for investigation by X-rays. In addition, by screening, the emptying of the bladder can be observed (*voiding micturating cystogram*).

The smooth muscle of the bladder (the *detrusor muscle*) is arranged as an outer longitudinal layer which runs on its superior surface, over the apex, downwards and backwards on the inferolateral surfaces and finally along the base. Some of the fibres pass backwards in the posterior ligament of the bladder towards the rectum (*rectovesical muscle*) and some pass forwards towards the pubis in the puboprostatic or pubovesical ligaments (*pubovesical muscle*). A middle circular layer is irregular in its distribution and is most prominent round the internal urethral orifice (*sphincter vesicae*). It also extends into the proximal part of the urethra. There is a thin inner longitudinal layer which is arranged like the outer. It extends into the proximal part of the urethra. Recent work describes a complex arrangement of muscle and tissue in the region of the trigone.

When the bladder contains about 300–400 ml of urine an individual becomes aware of a desire to empty it. It can hold about 600 ml in some people but there is a point at which it will empty involuntarily. The voluntary act of micturition involves the contraction of the detrusor muscle and the relaxation of the sphincter mechanisms which function at the proximal part of the male urethra and along most of the urethra in the female. The essential parts of this mechanism are (1) the change in the region of the trigone from being flat to its becoming like a funnel; (2) the relaxation of the sphincter of the urethra. The first stage of voluntary micturition involves contraction of the anterior abdominal muscles and thoracic diaphragm so that the intra-abdominal pressure is increased. This is followed by relaxation of the voluntary sphincter of the urethra and a concomitant relaxation of the sphincter vesicae and contraction of the detrusor muscle. Towards the end of micturition the abdominal muscles contract again and increase the intra-abdominal pressure. They then relax. Finally the detrusor muscle relaxes and the sphincter vesicae contracts so that the region of the trigone becomes flat again. This is followed by contraction of the sphincter of the urethra.

It has been suggested that the change in shape at the neck of the bladder is due to relaxation of the pelvic floor, particularly the pubovesical part of the levator ani, and that this is the essential precursor to micturition. After childbirth, if the muscles are torn, this ability to lift up the neck of the bladder is lost and the smooth muscle of the sphincter vesicae cannot prevent urine being expelled if intra-abdominal pressure is increased (stress incontinence).

The Nerves, Blood Vessels and Lymphatics

There is a vesical autonomic plexus at the side of the bladder which is both sympathetic and parasympathetic. The preganglionic motor sympathetic fibres are from the eleventh and twelfth thoracic and first and second lumbar segments and synapse in the hypogastric plexuses. The postganglionic sympathetic fibres are motor to the sphincter vesicae and may be inhibitory to the detrusor muscle. The preganglionic parasympathetic motor fibres come from the second, third and fourth sacral segments and synapse in or near the walls of the bladder with the postganglionic neurons which are motor to the detrusor muscle and inhibitory to the sphincters.

There are both sympathetic and parasympathetic sensory fibres. The former reach the spinal cord via the first and second lumbar spinal nerves and the latter via the second, third and fourth sacral nerves. The sensory fibres function as stretch receptors which are mainly parasympathetic and are responsible for the sensations associated with distension and reflex emptying of the bladder. There are also sympathetic and parasympathetic fibres associated with pain which may be elicited by overdistension or spasm of the muscle or pathological conditions such as a stone or inflammation.

The arteries are the *superior* and *inferior vesical* from the internal iliac. In the fetus the internal iliac artery continues on each side as the umbilical artery which after birth becomes obliterated and forms the *medial umbilical ligament*. The superior vesical artery arises just proximal to the obliteration and supplies the upper part of the bladder.

The inferior vesical artery supplies the base of the bladder and also neighbouring structures such as the prostate and seminal vesicles. The veins of the bladder form a plexus on its inferolateral surface and drain backwards to the internal iliac veins. The lymphatic vessels pass mainly to the nodes along the external iliac vessels.

Abnormalities

The urachus may remain patent up to the umbilicus with the result that the baby is born with a *urinary fistula* (*fistula* = a communication between two epithelial surfaces). This can be treated by tying and excision. In *ectopia vesicae* the anterior wall of the abdomen and the bladder do not develop and the baby is born with the inside of the bladder and ureteric and urethral orifices exposed on the surface. This is difficult to treat and is fortunately a rare condition.

The Ureter in the Pelvis

The total length of the ureter is about 25 cm and half of it lies in the pelvis. It crosses the brim of the pelvis at the level of the sacro-iliac joint anterior to the division of the common iliac artery. The ureter passes downwards and backwards anterolateral to the internal iliac artery on the obturator internus and lies medial to the obliterated umbilical artery and obturator vessels and nerve. At the level of the spine of the ischium it turns medially on to the levator ani. In the male (figure 108(b)) it is crossed above and anteriorly by the ductus deferens, enters the upper lateral angle of the base of the bladder obliquely and opens into it at the upper lateral angle of the trigone. It runs in the bladder wall for about 2 cm, with the result that when the muscle of the bladder contracts the ureter is closed and urine does not pass into the ureter.

In the female (figure 108(a)) the ureter lies behind the ovary on the lateral pelvic wall and below the broad ligament about 1.5 cm lateral to the cervix of the uterus. Here it lies in the thickened connective tissue at the side of the cervix and is crossed anteriorly and superiorly by the uterine artery. The ureter passes medially in front of the lateral border of the vagina and enters the bladder.

The arteries, lymphatic drainage and nerve supply of the whole ureter are described on p. 112, where reference is made to its constrictions and the radiological methods of investigating the ureter. It

(a)

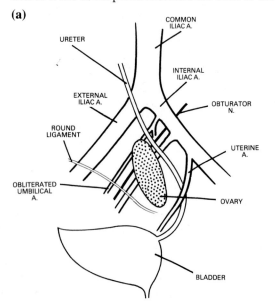

(b)

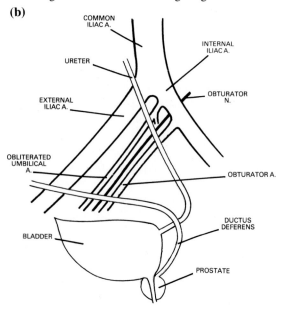

Figure 108   The ureter in the pelvis: (a) female; (b) male.

should be added that the urine is transmitted along the ureter by peristaltic waves which occur at intervals varying from 10 to 40 s. The ureter can undergo considerable distension and hypertrophy if there is chronic obstruction to the passage of urine in the ureter or urethra.

The Female Pelvic Genital Organs (figures 109, 110)

These include the ovaries, uterine tubes, uterus and vagina. The lower part of the vagina passes through the pelvic floor and lies in the perineum.

The ovary

This is one of a pair of organs producing the oöcytes and important hormones which act on the uterus.

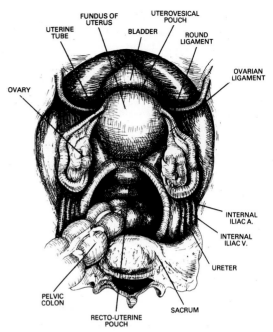

Figure 109   The female pelvic organs seen from above.

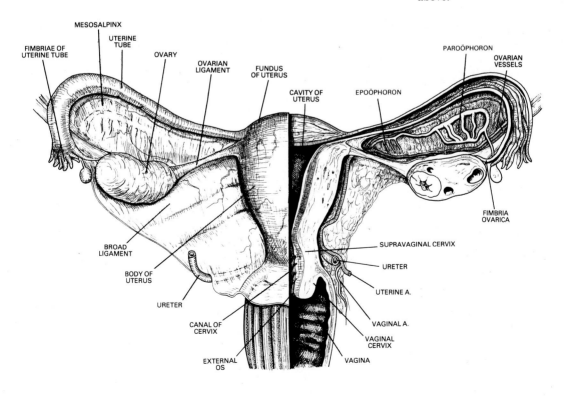

Figure 110   The uterus and broad ligament.

In the fertile, adult woman it is almond-shaped and about 3 cm long, 2 cm wide and 1 cm thick. Its position is variable but it may lie in the *ovarian fossa* on the lateral wall of the pelvis bounded posteriorly by the ureter and the internal iliac artery and anteriorly by the obliterated umbilical artery (figure 108(a)). When the ovary lies in the fossa, it is separated from the obturator vessels and nerve by peritoneum. The ovary is suspended from the posterior (superior) layer of the broad ligament by the short *mesovarium*, a double fold of peritoneum which originally continued round the ovary but subsequently almost completely disappears leaving only one layer of cells on the surface. The blood and lymphatic vessels and autonomic nerves of the ovary run in the mesovarium to and from the ovary.

The ovary has a medial (uterine) and lateral (tubal) end. A fibrous cord, the *ovarian ligament*, is attached to the uterine end and also to the upper lateral part of the uterus. The tubal end of the ovary is closely related to the lateral end of the uterine tube, one of whose fimbriae (the *fimbria ovarica*; *fimbria = fringe*, Latin) is attached to the lateral pole of the ovary. The *suspensory ligament of the ovary* is the name given to the fold of peritoneum passing from the lateral wall of the pelvis to the lateral part of the ovary in the region of the opening of the uterine tube. It contains the ovarian blood and lymphatic vessels as they pass towards the mesovarium. This ligament is the lateral fifth or quarter of the upper border of the broad ligament.

The ovary develops on the posterior abdominal wall and for some years after birth it lies in the iliac fossa. It becomes a pelvic organ at about 6 years of age and in the nulliparous woman lies almost vertically with its tubal end higher than its uterine end, and its lateral surface on the peritoneum covering the ovarian fossa. During pregnancy it is pulled upwards with the enlarging uterus and returns to the pelvis after the baby is born, but its position is now very variable and it is no longer vertical. In a child the surface is smooth. After puberty the surface becomes more and more irregular due to successive ovulations which result in the formation of areas of fibrous tissue. The ovary tends to become smaller after the meno-pause.

The *ovarian artery* (figure 110) is a branch of the abdominal aorta (p. 115) and passes downwards anterior to most of the structures on the posterior abdominal wall. The artery runs in the suspensory ligament of the ovary, that is in the lateral part of the upper border of the broad ligament and then inferior to the uterine tube towards the uterus. It gives off branches which go in the mesovarium to the ovary, and then anastomoses with branches of the uterine artery running laterally below the uterine tube in the broad ligament. There is a plexus of veins round the ovary from which arise two *ovarian veins*. The two veins unite and form one vein which joins the inferior vena cava on the right and the left renal vein on the left. The *lymphatic vessels* of the ovary follow the same course as the blood vessels and end in the nodes on the posterior abdominal wall (lumbar or aortic).

The *nerves* to the ovary are postganglionic sympathetic and usually end in the walls of the blood vessels.

The uterine tube

There is a *uterine tube* on each side of the uterus. It is about 10 cm long and lies in the medial three-quarters of the upper border of the broad ligament. The medial end passes through the lateral wall of the uterus and opens into the upper lateral angle of the uterine cavity. At the lateral end of the tube its lumen opens on to the peritoneal cavity near the ovary. The tube is related to the mesovarium and extends on to the medial surface of the ovary.

The tube is divided into four parts. The narrowest is the *intramural part* which lies in the wall of the uterus and is about 1–2 mm in diameter. Next to the uterine wall is the *isthmus* which is also narrow. The widest part, about 4 mm in diameter, is further laterally and is called the *ampulla*, which is also thin walled and tortuous. Near the ovary the tube is funnel-shaped and forms the *infundibulum*. The lateral opening (*ostium*) is surrounded by finger-like processes called the *fimbriae*, one of which is attached to the ovary, the *fimbria ovarica*.

The lining of the tube is continuous with the lining of the peritoneal cavity, so that the peritoneal cavity in a female is continuous with the exterior via the tubes, uterus and vagina. There thus exists in the female a communication between the exterior and the pelvic peritoneum which may become infected by this route.

When an ovum is released by the ovary at ovulation, it is thought that the lateral end of the tube more or less wraps itself round the ovary so that the ovum passes straight into the tube and does not have to enter the tube via the peritoneal cavity. The smooth muscles in the fimbriae enable them to move to some extent. However, it is also known that there is a capillary-like movement of fluid from the peritoneal cavity towards and into the tube due to the action of its ciliated epithelial lining. This can carry an ovum into its lumen. There are many more ciliated cells in the lateral part of the tube than in its medial part.

The ovum is usually fertilised at the lateral end of the tube and it takes about 4 days for it to reach the uterine cavity. The fertilised ovum is moved by the contraction of the smooth muscle in the wall of the tube as well as by the action of the cilia. Delay in the passage of the dividing fertilised ovum may result in its embedding in the wall of the tube (*tubal pregnancy*). The commonest sequel to this is a rupture of the tube about 4–6 weeks after fertilisation accompanied by a dangerous haemorrhage.

The hormonal changes during the menstrual cycle produce changes in the lining of the tubes, their motility and their vascularity.

The tubal arterial blood supply comes from the ovarian and uterine arteries, its veins drain to the veins of the same name and its lymphatic drainage runs mainly with the ovarian lymphatic vessels. Some lymph from the uterine end of the tube drains to the superficial inguinal nodes along the round ligament.

The uterus

The Form, Position and Relations

The uterus is the organ in which the embryo and fetus normally develop and grow. It is usually described as being shaped like an inverted pear and in the nulliparous woman is about 7.5 cm long, 5.0 cm wide and 2.5 cm thick. It is slightly flattened anteroposteriorly so that it has anterior (vesical) and posterior (intestinal) surfaces and right and left borders. It is divided into an upper part, the *body*, and a lower part, the *cervix*, separated by a slightly constricted part called the *isthmus* which is about 1 cm long. The part of the body above the entrance of the uterine tubes is called the *fundus*. The *cornu* of the uterus is where the tube joins the body. The cervix is divided into a lower *vaginal part* which projects into the vagina and an upper *supravaginal part* above the level of the attachment of the vagina.

The proportions of the different parts of the uterus vary with age. Before puberty the cervix is longer than the body. At puberty the uterus enlarges and the body eventually becomes twice as long as the cervix.

The normal position of the uterus in the adult is such that the whole uterus is bent forwards at a right angle to the vagina (figure 106(a)). This is called *anteversion*. (It is important to appreciate that the vagina passes upwards and backwards, at an angle of 60° to the horizontal.) The body is also bent forwards on the cervix. This is called *anteflexion*. The result is that the anterior surface of the uterus lies on the upper surface of the bladder. When the bladder fills the uterus is partially straightened. A uterus in which the body is bent to some extent backwards on the cervix (*retroflexion*) and is itself bent backwards relative to the vagina (*retroversion*) is quite common (20 per cent of women) and although many ailments, such as pain on menstruation (dysmenorrhoea), pain on intercourse (dyspareunia), sterility, spontaneous abortion and backache, may be due to this condition, it can exist without any signs or symptoms. Before puberty anteversion and anteflexion are much less marked and the body of the uterus, cervix and vagina are much more in line with each other.

The main relations of the uterus are the bladder anteriorly, separated by the uterovesical pouch, and the rectum posteriorly, separated by the much deeper uterorectal pouch in which there are usually the sigmoid colon and some coils of the small intestine. Laterally the broad ligament, a double fold of peritoneum, extends from the lateral margin of the uterus to the lateral wall of the pelvis. This ligament is described below. The peritoneum covers the front of the uterus as far as the junction of the body and the cervix and posteriorly extends as far as the upper third of the vagina. At the cornu of the uterus the uterine tube passes through its wall and opens into its cavity. The ovarian ligament is attached to the uterus just behind the tube and is continuous below the tube with the round ligament which is attached anterior to the tube.

The Cervix and Isthmus

The supravaginal part of the cervix is more cylindrical than the body and is related laterally to the connective tissue inferior to the broad ligament. This connective tissue extends round the whole cervix and is called the *parametrium*. The ureter passes forwards in the parametrium to the bladder about 1.5 cm lateral to the cervix. Here the uterine artery which is running medially to the side of the cervix lies above and in front of the ureter.

The vaginal part of the cervix is circular and has an opening called the *os of the uterus* (*external cervical os*). The cervix projects into the vagina so that there is a gap between it and the upper part of the vaginal wall. This is called the *fornix* (*fornix = arch*, Latin; it also = *brothel*, hence the word *fornicate*) which is divided into anterior, posterior and two lateral fornices for purposes of description. In a woman who has had a child the os is usually transverse and presents an anterior and posterior lip. In the nulliparous woman the os is more circular and feels harder on palpation. The change in shape is due to the tearing of the cervix during childbirth. Due to the forward bending of the uterus the os is in contact with the posterior vaginal wall.

The *isthmus* is about 1 cm long and includes that part of the cervix adjacent to the body. Although structurally somewhat different from the rest of the body it is much more like the body than the cervix. During pregnancy it is included in the body, *taken up* is the term used, and constitutes the *lower uterine segment* of obstetrics. It lies below the level of the line of reflection of the peritoneum from the uterus to the bladder . In a caesarean section, following separation of the peritoneum a transverse incision through this segment is used much more often than the classical vertical incision through the body of the uterus.

The main differences between the cervix and the body of the uterus are as follows.

(1) There is much more fibrous tissue in the wall of the cervix than in that of the body, which consists almost entirely of smooth muscle.

(2) Although both undergo cyclical changes the lining of the cervix shows different and less marked changes and is not shed.

(3) The glands of the cervix are different in that they produce a secretion which forms a suitable medium for the spermatozoa to swim through. This secretion is normally less viscid at ovulation. An abnormal secretion is a possible cause of sterility. The glands of the body of the uterus produce a secretion for the nourishment of the fertilised ovum if pregnancy occurs.

(4) The cervix takes no part in the expulsion of the fetus during labour and apparently disappears during the first stage of labour, which extends from the onset of true labour pains to the full dilatation and taking up of the cervix.

The Uterine Cavity

The cavity of the uterus is small because of the thickness of its wall. Anteroposteriorly it is merely a slit. Transversely it is triangular in shape with the base superiorly. The cavity narrows below and becomes continuous with the canal of the cervix. Where they are continuous is often referred to as the *internal cervical os*. The cervical canal is spindle-shaped and has oblique ridges (the *palmate folds*) radiating from the midline on its anterior and posterior walls often referred to as an *arbor vitae*.

The Uterine Ligaments

The various ligaments of the uterus have very different functions and origins and although they are called *ligaments* they probably have only one feature in common — they all consist of some form of connective tissue. The *broad ligament* is the double fold of peritoneum extending on each side from the lateral margin of the uterus to the lateral wall of the pelvis (figure 110). Because of the ante-version of the uterus the ligament has superior (posterior) and inferior (anterior) surfaces. The uterine tube lies in the medial three-quarters of its upper edge. The lateral end of the tube opens on to the peritoneal cavity and the peritoneum of the broad ligament is continuous with the lining of the tube. The ovary is suspended from the lateral part of the superior surface of the broad ligament by the mesovarium. That part of the ligament between the tube and the mesovarium is called the *mesosalpinx*. In it there are the ovarian vessels and the terminal parts of the uterine vessels. The rest of the broad ligament is called the mesometrium (*metra = womb*, Greek; *uterus = womb*, Latin; *hysteron = womb*, Greek). (Webster's Dictionary lists no less than 38 medical terms beginning with *metro-*. Hysteria, by no means confined to women, was thought to originate in the womb. The use of different words meaning *womb* is largely due to the anathema with which classical scholars regarded hybrid words, words with both a Latin and Greek origin. Hence *hysterectomy* and not *uterectomy*, etc., and *autokineton* in Greece instead of *automobile*.)

The uterine artery runs upwards between the layers of the broad ligament adjacent to the uterus, turns laterally below the uterine tube and anastomoses with the ovarian artery. The ovarian vessels having crossed the brim of the pelvis run medially in the suspensory ligament of the ovary (that part of the broad ligament between the lateral end of the uterine tube and the lateral pelvic wall) then below the uterine tube towards the uterus. It gives off branches which go in the mesovarium to the ovary and in the mesosalpinx to the tube.

The *ovarian ligament* runs from the uterine pole of the ovary to the cornu of the uterus and is visible as a ridge on the superior layer of the broad ligament. The *round ligament*, continuous with the ovarian ligament below the uterine tube, is visible as a ridge on the inferior surface of the broad ligament as it passes downwards and anteriorly towards the deep inguinal ring.

Inferior to the broad ligament at the side of the cervix the ureter passes forwards below the uterine artery as it passes medially to the side of the uterus.

Between the two layers of the broad ligament there are tubules which are the remnants of the mesonephros and the mesonephric duct. They are called the *epoöphoron* laterally, and the *paroöphoron* medially. The tubules may be joined by a longitudinal duct, usually called the *duct of Gartner* (*longitudinal duct of the epoöphoron*) (H.T. Gartner, 1785–1827, Danish anatomist) which may continue medially and downwards in the lateral wall of the cervix and vagina. These tubules or the duct may become cystic in adult life.

The broad ligament is essentially a mesentery for the ovary, uterine tube and uterus and moves readily with the uterus when it changes its position. It plays no part in maintaining the normal position of the uterus.

The ovarian and round ligaments have been described. They are regarded as the remains of the *gubernaculum ovarii* which in the embryo is attached to one pole of the ovary, passes along the posterior abdominal wall and across the pelvis to the anterior abdominal wall. It then traverses the inguinal canal to end in the labium majus. (Compare this with a description of the gubernaculum testis, substituting *testis* for *ovary* and *scrotum* for *labium majus*.) Unlike the testis the ovary descends only as far as the pelvis. The round ligament on its way to the deep inguinal ring crosses medial to the obturator vessels and nerves, the obliterated umbilical artery and the external iliac vessels. At the deep inguinal ring it is lateral to the inferior epigastric artery.

The round ligament has a considerable amount of smooth muscle in it, especially near the uterus. It is not regarded, nor is the ovarian ligament, as playing any important part in maintaining the anteverted position of the uterus, although shortening the round ligaments is used as a means of converting a retroverted into an anteverted uterus, if all the other structures supporting the uterus are normal. In the fetus an extension of the peritoneum passes with the round ligament into the inguinal canal and labium majus. This is comparable with the processus vaginalis in the male and if it persists can give rise to an indirect congenital inguinal hernia (p. 75).

The *parametrium*, the connective tissue round the cervix, has already been referred to (p. 144). Thickenings of this tissue pass laterally from the

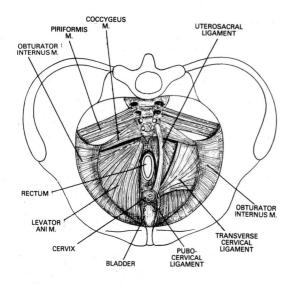

Figure 111 The fascial ligaments of the uterus.

cervix and upper part of the vagina to the lateral pelvic wall and are called the *transverse cervical ligaments* (*ligaments of Mackenrodt, cardinal ligaments*; A.K. Mackenrodt, 1859–1925, German gynaecologist; *cardo = hinge*; *cardinal = important*, *principal*, Latin; it is interesting that *hinge* may be used in English in the same sense). These spread out as they pass laterally, have a wide attachment to the pelvic wall, and are regarded as among the main structures maintaining the position of the uterus in the pelvis (figure 111). The ureter and uterine vessels lie in the upper part of the ligament. The *pubocervical ligaments* extend from the body of the pubis on each side to the anterior part of the cervix and the *uterosacral ligaments* pass backwards from the back of the cervix on either side of the rectum to the sacrum. All these ligaments contain a variable amount of smooth muscle. The position of the vault of the vagina (the region of the fornices) and cervix is maintained by these ligaments and stretching and tearing them in childbirth results in a descent of the vault of the vagina and of the uterus, a condition called *prolapse*. As the uterus descends through the pelvic floor it becomes less anteverted. This, however, is secondary to the basic cause of the condition.

The muscles forming the floor of the pelvis, particularly that part which passes backwards from the pubis to the vagina (the pubovaginalis) and that part which is inserted into the perineal body (p. 170) lying between the vagina and anal canal, play a very important role in maintaining the position of the uterus. During childbirth both may be torn so that their muscular support is lost. In addition the pubovaginalis supports the neck of the bladder and the perineal body supports the rectum. As a result of the tearing the bladder and rectum can bulge into the vagina (*cystocele* and *rectocele* respectively). The sphincter mechanism of the urethra adjacent to the bladder may also be defective. Surgery involving bringing the lateral cervical ligaments in front of the cervix and repairing the torn muscular floor of the pelvis usually restores the uterus to its normal position and the bladder to its normal functioning.

The Changes in the Uterus During and After Pregnancy

During pregnancy the uterus increases in size and weight. From being a pelvic organ it enlarges upwards and reaches the symphysis pubis by 12 weeks, the umbilicus by 24 weeks and the xiphisternum by 36 weeks. During the last 4 weeks the fetal head may descend into the pelvis (the *engagement of the head*) and the fundus may descend to some extent. This is more common in the first pregnancy than in subsequent pregnancies.

The uterus increases in weight from about 40 g to 1000 g and this is largely due to an increase in the size and length of its muscle fibres and their multiplication. In addition the connective tissue elements increase in quantity and the blood vessels become thickened. The thickness of the uterine wall is reduced from about 12 mm to 4 mm during the second half of the pregnancy.

The cervix apart from an increase in its secretion does not undergo any hypertrophy. If anything it is reduced in length because its upper part together with the isthmus forms the lower uterine segment (p. 144).

After the end of labour the uterus returns to approximately its former size in about 6 weeks, but it remains about 1 cm greater in all its dimensions. The uterus loses about half its weight during the first week after labour.

The Blood and Lymphatic Vessels and Nerve Supply of the Uterus

Each *uterine artery* is a branch of the corresponding internal iliac artery and is the main blood supply to the uterus. There is a considerable anastomosis with the ovarian artery in the broad ligament and with the vaginal artery near the cervix through its vaginal branch. The uterine artery passes medially across the levator ani into the connective tissue below the broad ligament where it runs anterior to and above the ureter about 1.5 cm lateral to the cervix. The uterine artery pursues a tortuous course upwards along the lateral margin of the uterus between the two layers of the broad ligament. At the junction of the uterine tube with the uterus the artery turns laterally below the tube and reaches the region of the mesovarium. The uterine artery gives branches to the uterine tube and round ligament. The *uterine vein* corresponds with the artery and ends in the internal iliac vein. The uterine veins (systemic) are connected with the superior rectal veins (hepatic portal) by vessels which pass below the peritoneum of the recto-uterine pouch.

The *lymphatic vessels* from the fundus, upper part of the body and cornu run with the vessels from the tube and ovary along the ovarian vessels to the nodes on the posterior abdominal wall (lumbar or aortic). The lymphatic vessels from the rest of the body and the cervix go to the external and internal iliac and sacral nodes. There is a node in the connective tissue alongside the cervix which is the first to be affected by the spread of cancer from the cervix, a cancer which is fairly common. Lymphatic vessels from the region of the cornu pass along the round ligament and end in the superficial inguinal nodes, although gynaecologists claim that they have never seen secondary cancer from the body of the uterus in these nodes.

The *nerves* of the uterus are sympathetic and parasympathetic, motor and sensory. The sympathetic motor preganglionic fibres have their cell bodies in the eleventh and twelfth thoracic and first and second lumbar spinal cord segments. They reach the pelvis mainly through the hypogastric plexuses where they synapse, but some synapse in the sacral sympathetic ganglia. The latter reach the uterus via the plexus round the blood vessels or via the plexus at the side of the cervix. The parasympathetic motor preganglionic fibres arise from the second, third and fourth sacral nerves and go via the inferior hypogastric plexuses to the paracervical plexus where they synapse. There appears to be little evidence of parasympathetic innervation of the muscle of the body of the uterus. The sympathetic fibres are thought to cause contraction of the muscle fibres, especially the circular fibres near the cervix. It should be emphasised that the uterine muscle responds readily to hormonal changes.

The sympathetic sensory fibres end in the lowest thoracic and upper lumbar spinal cord segments. Pulling on or dilatation of the cervix produces pain which is referred along the distribution of the twelfth thoracic and first lumbar spinal nerves. There are also sensory fibres from the cervix in the parasympathetic nerves from the second, third and fourth sacral spinal segments. Pain can be referred to the lower part of the back through these nerves.

Methods of Investigating the Uterus

An enlarged uterus can be palpated through the abdominal wall. The cervix can be felt by rectal examination (p. 137). *Vaginal examination* is usually bimanual with two fingers of one hand in the vagina and the other hand on the lower abdominal wall above the pubic bone. The upper part of the vagina, and the cervix and body of the uterus, can be palpated and their size and position determined. Anteriorly the urethra and bladder and posteriorly the contents of the rectum and any abnormal masses in the recto-uterine pouch can be felt. Laterally the ureters, ovaries and uterine tubes may be palpated, especially if enlarged. A speculum introduced into the vagina permits direct visual examination of the cervix as well as the vagina.

The cavities of the uterus and uterine tubes can be outlined by radio-opaque material injected into the cervix (*hysterosalpingography*) (figure 112). The main objective as a rule is to determine the patency of the tubes and the cause of their obstruction if possible. It is simpler to test the patency of

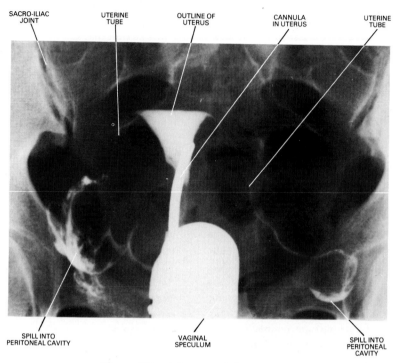

SACRO-ILIAC JOINT   UTERINE TUBE   OUTLINE OF UTERUS   CANNULA IN UTERUS   UTERINE TUBE

SPILL INTO PERITONEAL CAVITY   VAGINAL SPECULUM   SPILL INTO PERITONEAL CAVITY

Figure 112   A hysterosalpingogram.

the tubes by *insufflation* in which air (or carbon dioxide) is injected into the canal of the cervix by means of an apparatus which registers the pressure of the injected air. *Laparoscopy (lapara = flank, abdominal wall*, Greek) which involves the insertion of a tube with lenses and a light through the anterior abdominal wall makes it possible to examine the interior of the pelvic cavity and also the interior of the abdominal cavity. Sterilisation by tying the uterine tubes can be carried out through the same instrument.

The Main Congenital Abnormalities of the Uterus

These arise because of the failure of complete fusion of the two paramesonephric ducts from which the uterus develops. There may be two separate bodies, cervices and even vaginas; there may be two uterine cavities and one cervical canal; there may be a sagittal septum within the cavity of the body so that the uterus appears to have two horns.

The vagina (figure 106(a))

The *vagina* is a tubular structure about 7.5 cm long and 4 cm wide, but capable of elongation and widening. It extends from the cervix of the uterus, which projects into it, to the vulva and opens between the labia minora at the vestibule (p. 165). The vagina is parallel to the brim of the pelvis, that is its long axis is about 60° above the horizontal. The space between the cervix and vagina is called the *fornix*, which is usually divided into an anterior, posterior and two lateral parts. The posterior wall of the vagina is longer than the anterior so that the posterior fornix is deeper than the anterior. In the region of the cervix the vagina is circular, about its middle it forms a transverse slit, and inferiorly it is H-shaped in cross-section.

Anteriorly there are the base of the bladder and the urethra which opens into the vestibule anterior to the vaginal opening. The urethra is adherent to the anterior vaginal wall. Posteriorly the upper third of the vagina forms the anterior wall of the recto-uterine pouch and is covered by peritoneum.

11

The Pelvic Blood Vessels, Nerves and Lymph Nodes

The Internal Iliac Artery and Vein

The *internal iliac artery* is one of the two terminal branches of the common iliac artery and extends from the brim of the pelvis at the sacro-iliac joint downwards and backwards for about 3 cm. Although commonly described as dividing into ventral and dorsal divisions, it is probably true to say that the branches of the internal iliac artery show more variation in their origin from the parent trunk than those of any other artery. As it lies in front of the sacro-iliac joint on the wall of the pelvis, the artery is anterolateral to the internal iliac vein and lumbosacral trunk and medial to the external iliac vein, psoas muscle and obturator nerve. The ureter is anterior to the artery at its commencement.

Its branches (figures 113, 114) are best considered grouped into *parietal* and *visceral*. The *iliolumbar artery* is the first parietal branch, runs upwards and laterally in the iliac fossa and supplies the iliacus (iliac branch) and psoas (lumbar branch). The *lateral sacral arteries*, usually two, are segmental arteries, which divide to form four and enter the pelvic sacral foramina.

The parietal arteries which leave the pelvis posteriorly are the *superior gluteal* (above the piriformis and between the lumbosacral trunk and the first sacral nerve), the *inferior gluteal* (below the piriformis and between the first and second sacral nerves) and the *internal pudendal* (below the piriformis more medially). The gluteal arteries are distributed to the buttock (p. 437). The internal pudendal artery with the pudendal nerve medial to it crosses the spine of the ischium and enters the perineum through the lesser sciatic foramen to run forwards on the medial side of the ischial tuberosity in the pudendal canal with the pudendal nerve. The *obturator artery*, unlike the previous three branches, passes downwards and forwards with the obturator nerve which lies above it and leaves the pelvis through a gap in the obturator membrane in the upper part of the obturator foramen. It forms a circle of arteries on the outer surface of the membrane deep to the obturator externus muscle.

The visceral branches of the internal iliac artery include the *umbilical artery* which is a continuation of the internal iliac artery for a short distance on the lateral wall of the pelvis below and lateral to the bladder. In the fetus this artery is the main vessel on each side which returns the fetal blood

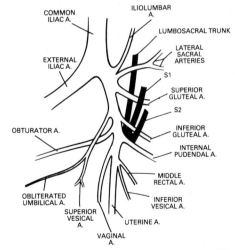

Figure 113   The right internal iliac artery and its branches.

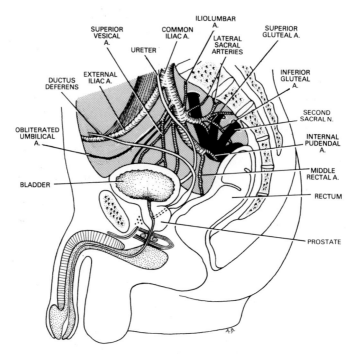

Figure 114   The structures on the lateral wall of the male pelvis.

to the placenta. After birth, most of it forms a fibrous cord passing forwards in the pelvis and then upwards on the deep surface of the anterior abdominal wall to the umbilicus. It forms the *medial umbilical fold* of peritoneum. From the small part which remains patent the *superior vesical artery* and *artery to the ductus deferens* arise, although the latter is often a branch of the former.

The *uterine artery* runs downwards, forwards and medially, and then below the broad ligament where it crosses anterior to and above the ureter, about 1.5 cm from the lateral vaginal fornix. Its further course and distribution in the broad ligament is described on p. 147. The *vaginal artery* may arise from the uterine artery. It runs downwards lateral to the vagina and gives off horizontal branches to the vagina as it does so.

The *middle rectal artery*, the smallest of the three rectal arteries, runs medially to the rectum in a thickening of fascia which forms the *lateral rectal ligament*.

The *internal iliac vein* is formed by tributaries which are similar to the branches of the artery. The vein lies posteromedial to the artery and joins the external iliac vein behind the beginning of the

common iliac artery to form the common iliac vein.

Before forming one or two main veins the veins related to the viscera form *plexuses* in the fascia around each viscus — *rectal*, *uterine*, *vesical* and *prostatic*. These plexuses of veins which have thin walls and few valves communicate with each other. They also communicate with a sacral plexus of veins behind the rectum which has anastomatic connections with the veins of the posterior abdominal and thoracic walls. Furthermore the pelvic veins communicate with the plexus of veins within the vertebral canal and thus with veins along the length of the vertebral column and the inside of the skull. Infection and thrombi can therefore spread very widely from the pelvis.

The venous plexus of the rectum constitutes one of the connections between the systemic and hepatic portal venous systems.

The Sacral Plexus of Nerves (figures 113, 114, 249)

The *sacral plexus* is formed by the ventral rami of

the first four sacral nerves and is joined by the lumbosacral trunk from the fourth and fifth lumbar nerves. The plexus lies on the piriformis where most of its branches are formed. They leave the pelvis through the greater sciatic foramen, inferior to the piriformis to be distributed to the buttock and lower limb. The exception is the *superior gluteal nerve* (L4, 5, S1) which with the superior gluteal vessels passes into the buttock above the piriformis muscle.

The largest nerve of the plexus, and of the body, is the *sciatic nerve* which is formed by L4, 5, S1, 2, 3. The *posterior femoral cutaneous nerve* (S1, 2, 3) leaves the pelvis with the sciatic nerve. More medially the *pudendal nerve* (S2, 3, 4), and the *nerve to the obturator internus* (L5, S1, 2), with the internal pudendal artery between them, leave the pelvis together. The pudendal nerve is medial to the artery. They all cross the ischial spine or sacrospinous ligament and enter the perineum. The *inferior gluteal nerve* (L5, S1, 2), posterior to the sciatic nerve, leaves with the inferior gluteal vessels. The last of the nerves leaving through the greater sciatic foramen is the *nerve to the quadratus femoris* (L4, 5, S1).

The segmental value of these nerves may be summarised as follows:

L4, 5, S1, 2, 3	sciatic nerve
L4, 5, S1	superior gluteal nerve
L4, 5, S1	nerve to quadratus femoris
L5, S1, 2	inferior gluteal nerve
L5, S1, 2	nerve to obturator internus
S1, 2, 3	posterior femoral cutaneous nerve
S2, 3, 4	pudendal nerve

There are in addition the nerves to the piriformis (S1, 2) and the levator ani (S3, 4). A branch of the second and third sacral nerves which pierces the sacrotuberous ligament and supplies the skin over the medial part of the fold of the buttock is variable and there is usually a branch of the fourth sacral nerve which pierces the coccygeus muscle and runs forwards in the ischiorectal fossa. It gives a branch to the external anal sphincter and is sensory to the skin over the ischiorectal fossa.

The ventral ramus of the *coccygeal nerve* pierces the coccygeus muscle and is joined by branches from the ventral rami of the fourth and fifth sacral nerves to form a plexus on the coccygeus muscle. A few fine nerves, sensory in function, arise from this plexus and after piercing the sacrotuberous ligament are distributed to the sacrococcygeal joint and the skin over the coccyx.

The Pelvic Autonomic Nerves and Plexuses

These come from three main sources.

(1) The abdominal aortic plexus continues downwards over the fifth lumbar vertebra and promontary of the sacrum into the concavity of that bone as the *superior hypogastric plexus* (often referred to as the *presacral nerve*). It consists largely of postganglionic motor sympathetic fibres whose preganglionic fibres arise from the eleventh and twelfth thoracic and first and second lumbar spinal cord segments. The synapses are in the preaortic ganglia. Some of the postganglionic fibres come from the lower ganglia of the lumbar part of the ganglionated sympathetic trunk. There are no vagus nerve fibres in the superior hypogastric plexus.

(2) *The sacral part of the ganglionated sympathetic trunk*, a continuation of the lumbar part of the trunk which enters the pelvis over the ala of the sacrum, consists of four or five ganglia lying near the pelvic sacral foramina.

(3) Parasympathetic branches arise from the *second, third and fourth sacral nerves*.

All three sources contain sensory fibres as well as motor.

The superior hypogastric plexus divides into *right* and *left hypogastric nerves*. Each hypogastric nerve joins an *inferior hypogastric plexus* which lies at the side of the rectum. In the male the plexus extends forwards to the side of the bladder and prostate. In the female it extends forwards to the side of the cervix and vagina and then to the side of the bladder. The inferior hypogastric plexuses receive postganglionic sympathetic fibres from (1) and (2) above and preganglionic parasympathetic fibres from (3). They also contain sensory fibres which pass through the lower thoracic and upper lumbar spinal cord segments (sympathetic) and sacral segments (parasympathetic).

The branches of the inferior hypogastric plexuses go to the rectum and bladder, and either the uterus, vagina and uterine tubes, or the prostate, seminal vesicles and deferent ducts. The branches go either directly to the organs or as plexuses round the arteries.

The innervation of each of these organs has already been discussed. Briefly, the rectum receives preganglionic parasympathetic fibres which synapse in its wall and produce expulsive movements and relaxation of the internal sphincter. The postganglionic sympathetic fibres to the rectum inhibit the longitudinal muscle and cause contraction of the internal sphincter. The sensory fibres are associated with painful sensations and, probably more important, the sensations of fullness which precede defaecation.

The bladder receives parasympathetic fibres which are motor to its detrusor muscle and inhibitory to its sphincter and are responsible for the emptying of the bladder. Parasympathetic sensory fibres respond to the tension produced by the filling of the bladder. The sympathetic fibres may be inhibitory to the detrusor muscle, motor to the sphincter and sensory to the trigone.

Although the body and cervix of the uterus and

Table 3   Summary of the lymphatic drainage of the pelvic organs

Organ	Nodes
Rectum	
Upper part	⟶ superior rectal ⟶ inferior mesenteric ⟶ aortic
Lower part	⟶ internal iliac directly or via sacral and pararectal
Anal canal	
Upper part	⟶ internal iliac
Lower part	⟶ superficial inguinal
Uterus	
Fundus	⟶ caval and aortic with ovarian lymphatic vessels
Body	⟶ internal iliac
Cervix	⟶ internal iliac directly or via node at side of cervix
Cornu	⟶ superficial inguinal
Vagina	
Upper two-thirds	⟶ internal iliac
Lower third	⟶ superficial inguinal
Ovary and uterine tube	⟶ caval and aortic
Seminal vesicle and ductus deferens	⟶ external iliac
Prostate	⟶ internal iliac directly or via sacral
Bladder	
Main part	⟶ external iliac directly or via nodes adjacent to bladder
Base	⟶ internal iliac
Pelvic part of ureter	⟶ external and internal iliac

vagina receive an autonomic innervation its effects are not fully understood. Parasympathetic branches go to the erectile tissue of the clitoris and vestibular bulb and are responsible for vasodilatation of these structures. Sympathetic fibres to these structures produce a vasoconstriction.

The plexus of nerves round the prostate is distributed to the neighbouring structures. It is thought that the seminal vesicles and ejaculatory ducts contract due to sympathetic stimulation which at the same time causes contraction of the sphincter of the bladder. The result is that the seminal fluid is prevented from passing into the bladder.

Parasympathetic fibres also go to the genital erectile tissue and are responsible for vasodilatation of its blood vessels. For this reason, although this is only one of the functions of the sacral parasympathetic nerves, they have been called the *nervi erigentes* (*erigentes* = *erecting*, Latin).

The sacral parasympathetic nerves also pass upwards from the pelvis into the abdomen through the superior hypogastric plexus to the abdominal aortic plexus and then to the plexus round the origin of the inferior mesenteric artery. They supply the pelvic and descending colons and left colic flexure either as plexuses round the branches of the inferior mesenteric artery or as separate retroperitoneal nerves.

The Pelvic Lymph Nodes

These are nodes along the external, internal and common iliac vessels. The *external iliac nodes* receive lymphatic vessels from (1) the inguinal nodes which lie distal to the medial part of the inguinal ligament; (2) the deeper layers of the lower part of the abdominal wall; (3) the urinary bladder; (4) the cervix of the uterus and the upper part of the vagina. The efferent vessels from the external lymph nodes go to the common iliac nodes.

The *internal iliac nodes* receive afferent lymphatic vessels from the pelvic viscera — the pelvic part of the ureter, the lower part of the bladder, the prostate, the ductus deferens, the seminal vesicle, the uterus, the rectum and the upper part of the anal canal. The efferent vessels from the internal iliac nodes go to the common iliac nodes. The *common iliac nodes* drain to the *caval* or *aortic nodes*.

There are also some nodes at the side of and behind the rectum in the hollow of the sacrum. These receive lymphatic vessels from the rectum and prostate and their efferents go to the internal and common iliac nodes.

The lymphatic drainage of individual organs (already given) are summarised in table 3.

12

The Perineum, Including The External Genitalia

The *perineum* is defined anatomically as the region inferior to the pelvic diaphragm bounded anteriorly by the lower border of the symphysis pubis, posteriorly by the tip of the coccyx and laterally by the ischial tuberosities (figure 103). The region is diamond-shaped, the diverging ischiopubic rami forming its anterior boundaries and the sacrotuberous ligaments its posterior boundaries. In obstetrics the perineum refers to the small region between the anterior edge of the anus and the posterior edge of the vagina. In anatomy the fibromuscular tissue of this region is called the *tendinous centre of the perineum* and is also known as the *perineal body*. A transverse line between the anterior parts of the ischial tuberosities divides the perineum into a posterior *anal triangle* and anterior *urogenital triangle*. For purposes of description the scrotum, penis, testis and urethra are described with the male urogenital triangle.

The Anal Triangle

The anal canal opens on to the exterior at the *anus* in the middle of the triangle. The edges of the anus have radiating folds probably due to the tonic contraction of the external anal sphincter (the folds disappear during defaecation) and not to the presence of a special subcutaneous muscle called the *corrugator cutis ani*. Some longitudinal muscle fibres from the rectum and the levator ani pass downwards to the skin and may constitute this muscle and produce the folds.

The *natal cleft* extends in the midline to the posterior edge of the anus. Anteriorly in the midline there is a raphe in the skin which in the male is continuous with the midline raphe of the scrotal skin. In the female the raphe extends to the posterior edge of the vagina. The skin is innervated by the fourth and fifth sacral and coccygeal nerves.

The ischiorectal fossa

On either side of the anal canal (p. 135) there is a fat-filled space called the *ischiorectal fossa* which is wedge-shaped with the base of the wedge on the superficial surface, that is the skin (figure 102). The lateral wall of the fossa is formed by the lower part of the obturator internus muscle and fascia and the ischial tuberosity. The medial wall, formed by the inferior surface of the levator ani covered with fascia, slopes upwards and outwards to meet the lateral wall at the edge of the wedge where the levator and obturator fasciae are continuous. Below the level of the levator ani the external anal sphincter lies medially.

The pudendal nerve and internal pudendal vessels enter the perineum through the lesser sciatic foramen and run forwards in a fascial canal on the lateral wall of the ischiorectal fossa medial to the ischial tuberosity and obturator internus towards the anterior part of the perineum. Both the nerve and artery give off inferior rectal branches to the anal canal. The nerve supplies the external anal sphincter and the artery the wall of the anal canal from which veins pass to the internal pudendal vein. The ischiorectal fossa also contains the perineal branch of the fourth sacral nerve which is sensory to the skin and motor to the external sphincter.

Infection in the fossa is common and may affect only the lateral part which is separated from the more medial peri-anal part by one of the vertically running septa which are extensions of the longitudinal muscle coat of the rectum (p. 135). A peri-anal infection may spread from one side posteriorly round the anal canal. Infection in the lateral part of the ischiorectal fossa may spread forwards into an extension of the fossa above the urogenital diaphragm almost to the symphysis pubis (figure 123) or backwards between the sacrotuberous and sacrospinous ligaments.

Infection of the lining of the anal canal may track through its wall into the ischiorectal fossa and may open through the skin on to the surface at the side of the anus. This condition results in a *fistula-in-ano* which usually becomes chronic and requires surgical treatment.

The Male External Genitalia

The *penis* and *scrotum* are the male external genitalia. The scrotum contains the *testes* and the beginning of the *ductus deferentes* and their blood and lymphatic vessels and nerves. The *urethra* running longitudinally in the penis is the common channel to the exterior for the urine and seminal fluid.

The penis

This organ consists of three cylinders of erectile tissue, the *corpus spongiosum* which is median and anterior and the *corpora cavernosa* which are on either side of the midline and posterior (figure 115). The corpus spongiosum is enlarged at both its ends. At the distal free end it forms the *glans of the penis* which fits like a cap on the free ends of the corpora cavernosa. The edge of the glans is raised (*corona of the glans*) and is separated from the shaft of the penis by the *neck of the glans*. The proximal attached end of the corpus spongiosum is enlarged and forms the *bulb of the penis* (or *of the corpus spongiosum*). The corpora cavernosa diverge when followed backwards and form the *crura* (singular *crus*) *of the penis* (or *of the corpora cavernosa*) each of which is attached to the edge of an ischiopubic ramus. The bulb and crura form the *root of the penis*.

The penis is covered by skin which is thin, dark and movable over the underlying fascia. This fascia

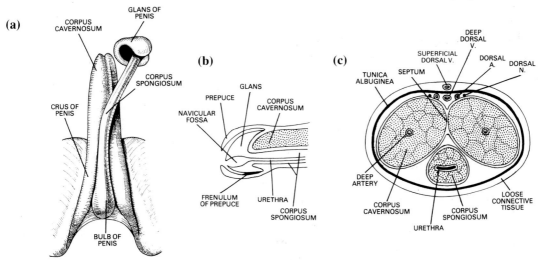

Figure 115   The penis: (a) the corpus spongiosum and corpora cavernosa; (b) a sagittal section to show the structure of the prepuce; (c) a transverse section.

is a continuation of the deeper membranous layer of the superficial fascia of the abdominal wall and is continuous with a similar layer deep to the skin of the scrotum and extending into the urogenital triangle. On the penis the fascia ends at the neck of the glans. The corpora cavernosa are surrounded by another more dense layer of fascia (the *tunica albuginea*) extending into the substance of the corpora cavernosa as trabeculae which divide the corpora into large blood spaces (figure 115(c)). A similar arrangement of sheath and trabeculae is found in the corpus spongiosum. The trabeculae consist of collagen, smooth muscle and elastin and contain blood vessels and nerves.

The skin of the body of the penis is attached to the neck of the glans beyond which it forms a double fold called the *prepuce* (figure 115(b)). The inner layer of the prepuce passes back to the neck and is continuous with the skin over the glans. At the neck there are some glands which produce a white secretion called *smegma*. Unlike the skin surrounding the body of the penis this skin is firmly adherent to the underlying tissue. There is a midline fold of skin on the inferior surface of the glans between the glans and the prepuce called the *frenulum of the prepuce.*

The urethra passes along the length of the corpus spongiosum and opens on to the exterior at the *external urethral orifice* where its lining is continuous with the skin over the glans.

The dorsal artery and nerve and deep dorsal vein of the penis pass along its length on its dorsal surface in the tunica albuginea of the corpora cavernosa (figure 115(c)). (The term *dorsal* to describe this surface is applicable if the penis is pointing upwards.) Outside the tunica albuginea there is a more superficial dorsal vein which eventually joins the femoral vein. The deep dorsal vein passes inferior to the symphysis pubis and ends in the prostatic plexus of veins. There are also deep arteries of the penis which pass through the middle of the corpora cavernosa and an artery to the bulb which extends into the corpus spongiosum. These arteries and the dorsal artery are branches of the internal pudendal artery.

The dorsal nerve of the penis supplies its skin. Deep perineal nerves which enter the bulb supply the urethra. Both are branches of the pudendal nerve. The skin of the penis near the root is supplied by the ilio-inguinal nerve. Since the pudendal nerve comes from the second, third and fourth sacral nerves and the ilio-inguinal from the first lumbar, there is a considerable gap in the segmental innervation of the skin of the penis. (The same applies to the scrotum.) The intervening nerve segments innervate the lower limb.

Autonomic nerves, both sympathetic and parasympathetic, supply the smooth muscle of the walls of the cavernous tissue and the blood vessels of the corpora cavernosa and corpus spongiosum. These nerves go to the penis either directly from the prostatic plexus of nerves by passing from the pelvis inferior to the pubic arch or in the pudendal nerve and its branches. In erection of the penis the parasympathetic fibres by causing vasodilation of the arteries of the corpora produce engorgement of the cavernous spaces. This engorgement presses on the veins and prevents emptying of the spaces. After ejaculation the parasympathetic stimulation ceases and with sympathetic stimulation producing vasoconstriction of their arteries the cavernous spaces empty.

The scrotum

This is a bag of skin containing the testes and associated structures (figure 64(b)). It is usually divided into two by a septum. The skin is continuous with that of the penis and abdominal wall and is usually wrinkled and somewhat pigmented. It has scattered hairs and large sebaceous and sweat glands. Inferiorly the skin has a midline raphe which is continuous posteriorly with the raphe of the perineum and anteriorly with that of the penis. The wrinkling of the skin is due to its elasticity and the underlying *dartos muscle*. Its fibres are smooth and are readily activated by stimuli such as cold or stroking. In old men the skin of the scrotum is usually smooth due to the loss of elastic fibres.

The scrotum has no subcutaneous fat. Deep to the dartos there is a layer of loose fascia continuous with the superficial fascia of the penis and the perineum. The three fascial layers of the spermatic cord (p. 74) spread out and line the scrotum (figure 64(b)). The outer layer of the tunica vaginalis of the testis is loosely attached to the innermost layer of the coverings of the spermatic cord, the internal spermatic fascia. The septum consists of all the layers of the scrotum except the skin.

The nerve supply of the scrotum anteriorly is from the ilio-inguinal nerve and the femoral branch of the genitofemoral nerve (the first lumbar spinal cord segment) and posteriorly from the scrotal branches of the perineal nerve, a branch of the pudendal (the second, third and fourth sacral spinal cord segments). The arteries anteriorly come from a branch of the femoral artery and posteriorly from the scrotal branches of the internal pudendal artery and also from the cremasteric artery in the spermatic cord. The veins correspond with the arteries and the lymphatic vessels go to the superficial inguinal lymph nodes.

Because of its dependent position fluid readily collects in the loose connective tissue of the scrotum in conditions in which excess fluid is retained in the body.

The testis and epididymis

The external position of the testes somewhat belies their classification with the internal genital organs.

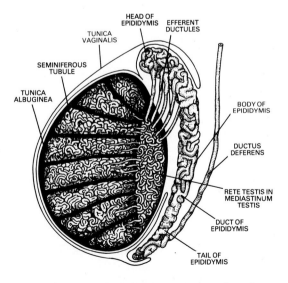

Figure 116   The structure of the testis and epididymis.

In fact they would not function properly if they remained inside the abdominal cavity. Each testis lies in one half of the scrotum, is supported by the scrotal wall and is more or less suspended from the structures entering and leaving it (the spermatic cord). The testis is oval and about 4–5 cm long, 3 cm wide and 3 cm anteroposteriorly. Along the posterior border of the testis lies a comma-shaped structure called the *epididymis* (figure 116). Because the ductus deferens and the blood vessels enter and leave the lower posterior part of the testis and epididymis the testis hangs obliquely so that its lower part is more posterior than its upper. The left testis is usually about 1 cm lower than the right in right-handed men.

The testis is covered by a double layer of peritoneum called the *tunica vaginalis* (figure 116). The outer layer is loosely attached to the internal spermatic fascia, the innermost layer of the scrotal wall. The inner layer is attached to the fibrous tissue covering of the testis, the *tunica albuginea*. The inner and outer layers of the tunica vaginalis are continuous with each other posteriorly so that the posterior borders of the testis and epididymis are not covered by the tunica vaginalis. The blood vessels and ductus deferens enter and leave in this gap where the inner layer is reflected on to the outer layer. On the lateral side the inner layer dips into the space between the testis and epididymis and forms the *sinus of the epididymis*. The tunica vaginalis is the persisting distal end of the peritoneal processus vaginalis which in the fetus accompanies the testis when it descends through the inguinal canal into the scrotum. Usually the processus vaginalis from the deep inguinal ring to the upper pole of the testis disappears. If this part persists an indirect inguinal hernia may develop (p. 75).

The tunica albuginea is the dense fibrous covering of the testis. It is thickened posteriorly to form the *mediastinum testis* from which septa radiate into the testis and divide it into about 250 lobules (figure 116). The mediastinum testis contains the blood and lymphatic vessels and the ducts going to and leaving the rest of the testis. Each lobule contains one to three *seminiferous tubules* which are coiled. If teased out each tubule is about 75 cm long. The coiled part of a tubule ends in a straight tubule which goes to the mediastinum testis in which there is a network of tubules called the *rete testis*. This network ends in about 15 *efferent ductules* which pass upwards into the upper end (head) of the epididymis.

The *epididymis* (*epi* = *on*, *didymos* = *twin* or *testis*, Greek; perhaps *twin* was a euphemism for the organ which is also called *orchis* in Greek, as in *orchitis* = *inflammation of the testis*) lies along the posterior margin of the testis and extends over its lateral surface which is separated from the epididymis by the sinus of the epididymis. The upper end is called the *head* which contains about 15 lobules in the form of conical masses each of which is a convoluted extension of an efferent ductule and about 15 cm long. All the ductules open into the upper end of the coiled duct of the epididymis which is about 6 m long and forms its *body* and *tail*. In the tail the duct becomes thicker and straighter and emerges posteriorly as the *ductus deferens* which passes upwards behind the epididymis through the scrotal sac to the superficial inguinal ring. As it does so it forms together with blood and lymphatic vessels and nerves the spermatic cord (p. 74).

The blood supply of the testis is the testicular artery from the abdominal aorta (pp. 74 and 115). It runs down the posterior border of the testis medial to the epididymis and gives off branches which also supply the epididymis. They penetrate the tunica albuginea deep to which they form a vascular coat (*tunica vasculosa*). Branches from this coat pass between the lobules in the septa and supply the seminiferous tubules. The artery to the ductus anastomoses with the testicular artery. The veins from the testis form the *pampiniform plexus* which passes upwards as part of the spermatic cord. Below the superficial inguinal ring the plexus forms three or four veins which enter the inguinal canal. The lymphatic vessels from the testis go directly to the aortic nodes on the posterior abdominal wall.

The nerve supply of the testis and epididymis is mainly sympathetic and is both motor and sensory. The preganglionic fibres come from the tenth and eleventh thoracic segments of the spinal cord and reach the testis mainly as a plexus round the testicular artery. The motor fibres supply the blood vessels and smooth muscle found in the coverings of the testis. The smooth muscle of the ductules of the head, the duct in the tail and the ductus have a greater innervation than that of the rest of the duct of the epididymis. This may be related to the much more marked contractions of these structures in ejaculation as compared with the contractions of the duct in the body of the epididymis. Painful sensations of a characteristic nature, usually described as very severe and sickening, result from blows or squeezing of the testes. Pain due to other conditions affecting the testis may be referred to the lower part of the abdominal wall.

Various remnants of the mesonephros may persist in relation to the testis and epididymis, for example the *appendix of the epididymis* at its upper end. A remnant of the paramesonephric duct may be found at the upper end of the testis (the *appendix of the testis*).

Persistence of the processus vaginalis and its relation to oblique inguinal hernia has already been referred to (p. 75). *Hydrocele* is a condition in which fluid collects between the two layers of the tunica vaginalis. Although the processus may be closed off at the deep inguinal ring it may remain as an upward extension of the tunica vaginalis. In these circumstances the fluid in the hydrocele extends upwards towards the superficial ring. Sometimes an unobliterated part of the processus vaginalis remains along the spermatic cord, shut off from the peritoneal cavity and the tunica vaginalis. If fluid collects in this the condition is called an *encysted hydrocele of the cord*. Occasionally the whole processus vaginalis remains so that fluid in a hydrocele can pass into the peritoneal cavity.

The testis in its descent follows a fibromuscular cord, the *gubernaculum testis*, which is attached to the lower pole of the testis and to the lowest part of the scrotum. Normally the testis follows the gubernaculum although its descent is thought to be due to hormones (gonadotrophins and androgens). A testis which is arrested somewhere along its normal path, for example in the abdomen, in the inguinal canal, or at either the deep or superficial inguinal ring, is called an *undescended testis*. A testis which ends somewhere other than along its normal path, for example in the abdominal wall just above the medial part of the inguinal ligament, in the perineum or in the upper part of the thigh, is called an *ectopic testis*. Not infrequently an undescended testis passes into the scrotum at puberty due to normal hormonal stimulation. If, however, a testis does not reach the scrotum, spermatogenesis does not take place or is very much reduced. The undescended testis, however, does produce androgens at puberty, although in reduced quantities. Bilateral undescended testes will result in sterility. The temperature in the scrotum, lower by about 3°C than that in the abdominal cavity, is necessary for normal spermatogenesis. One of the ways in which the temperature of the testis is kept below that of the rest of the body is by *countercurrent flows*. In this situation heat from the testicular artery is lost to the vessels of the pampiniform plexus so that the blood reaching the testis is at a lower temperature than that of the blood of the rest of the body.

The Urethra in the Male

The *urethra* extends from the *internal urethral orifice* at the neck of the bladder to the *external urethral orifice* (*meatus*) at the end of the penis. The urethra is divided into a *prostatic* part about 3 cm long, a *membranous* part about 1 cm long which passes through a fascial space called the deep perineal pouch (figure 118), and a *penile* or *spongiose* part about 15–20 cm long which passes

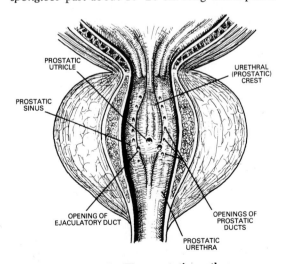

PROSTATIC UTRICLE

URETHRAL (PROSTATIC) CREST

PROSTATIC SINUS

OPENING OF EJACULATORY DUCT

OPENINGS OF PROSTATIC DUCTS

PROSTATIC URETHRA

Figure 117   The prostatic urethra.

through the corpus spongiosum of the penis (figure 115). The prostatic part is almost vertical and semilunar in section with the concavity posteriorly and the membranous part is ridged longitudinally and curves forwards. The part of the urethra in the bulb of the corpus spongiosum continues to curve forwards and in a penis hanging downwards the urethra then curves downwards through the corpus spongiosum in which it is a transverse slit but becomes a sagittal slit at the external meatus.

The *prostatic urethra* is the widest and most dilatable part of the urethra (figure 117). On the posterior wall there is a longitudinal elevation of variable length, the *urethral crest*, on each side of which there is a depression, the *prostatic sinus*, into which the ducts of the prostatic glands open. Opening on to the middle of the urethral crest is the *prostatic utricle*, which extends upwards deep to the crest and produces an elevation of the upper half of the crest called the *colliculus seminalis*. On each side of the opening of the prostatic utricle there is the opening of an ejaculatory duct. The utricle is a persistent part of the paramesonephric ducts, is about 5 mm long and has small glands in its fibromuscular wall. When the middle lobe of the prostate enlarges it pushes forwards the posterior wall of the prostatic urethra and obstructs its lumen.

The *membranous urethra*, the narrowest and least dilatable part, is surrounded by the (*external*) *sphincter of the urethra*, which consists of skeletal muscle (figure 118). The sphincter is attached to the ischiopubic rami and to a layer of fascia deep in the muscle, the perineal membrane, which in turn is attached to the rami. This part of the urethra is the least mobile and may be torn in injuries to the bony pelvis. On each side of the urethra a *bulbo-urethral gland* (*of Cowper*; W. Cowper, 1666–1709, London surgeon) is embedded in the sphincter. Its duct perforates the perineal membrane and opens into the part of the urethra which is in the bulb of the corpus spongiosum (figure 118).

The *spongiose* (*spongy, penile*) *urethra* has two enlargements, one within the bulb and one within the glans proximal to the external orifice. The urethra is in the middle of the corpus spongiosum along most of its length but next to the perineal membrane there is no erectile tissue anteriorly for

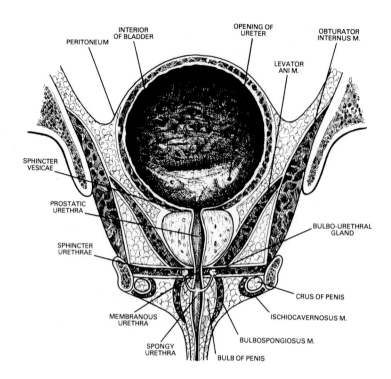

Figure 118   A coronal section through the male urogenital triangle (diagrammatic).

about 0.5 cm and in the glans there is little or no erectile tissue next to the floor of the urethra. The enlargement in the glans is called *the navicular fossa* (*fossa terminalis*) (figure 115(b)) in the roof of which there is a recess extending backwards. Between the recess and the lumen of the urethra there is often a fold of mucous membrane in which the tip of an instrument passed along the urethra may be caught. In addition, along the length of the urethra there are also smaller recesses into which urethral glands open. The external orifice and the membranous urethra are the narrowest parts of the urethra so that an instrument, for example a catheter, which can pass through the orifice, normally passes along the rest of the urethra. A catheter in the urethra can be felt through the inferior wall of the corpus spongiosum and in the membranous urethra behind the scrotum.

Acute and chronic infection of the urethral glands, the bulbo-urethral glands, the seminal vesicles and the prostate often occur as complications of gonorrhoea which begins as a urethritis.

The blood supply of the urethra is from prostatic and penile arteries. The veins pass to the prostatic plexus or to the internal pudendal veins. The urethral lymphatic vessels pass mainly to the external and internal iliac lymph nodes although some vessels from the penile urethra go to the deep inguinal nodes. There are motor and sensory autonomic nerves to the smooth muscle and lining of the urethra. The nerves are both parasympathetic from the sacral outflow through the nerves from the prostatic plexus, and sympathetic through the pudendal nerve. The sphincter of the membranous part is innervated by the somatic part of the pudendal nerve.

The Urogenital Triangle in the Male

This is the anterior part of the perineum and is demarcated posteriorly by a transverse line between the anterior parts of the ischial tuberosities. If the scrotum and penis are pulled forwards and upwards

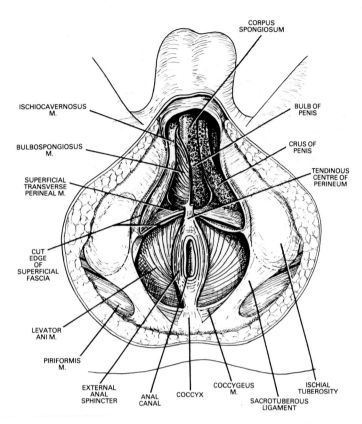

Figure 119   The male superficial perineal pouch.

the skin of this region, supplied by the third and fourth sacral nerves, is seen to have a midline raphe. Deep to the skin there is the *superficial perineal fascia*. Its deep part forms a membrane attached to the ischiopubic rami laterally. (This was known as *Colles' fascia*; A. Colles, 1773–1843, Dublin surgeon.) Anteriorly it is continuous with a similar layer deep to the skin of the scrotum and the shaft of the penis, and with the membranous layer of the superficial fascia of the abdominal wall (figure 120).

The bulb of the corpus spongiosum and the crura of the corpora cavernosa are deep to this layer of fascia. Deep to these structures there is another layer of fascia called the *inferior fascia of the urogenital diaphragm* or *perineal membrane*. This is attached to the ischiopubic rami laterally and fuses posteriorly with the posterior edge of the superficial perineal fascia.

The space between these two layers of fascia is called the *superficial perineal pouch* (figure 119). The perineal membrane does not reach anteriorly as far as the symphysis pubis and the dorsal vein of the penis passes through this gap to the prostatic plexus of veins. In the superficial perineal pouch are the bulb of the corpus spongiosum, covered by a muscle, the *bulbospongiosus*, and laterally on each side a crus covered by the *ischiocavernosus* muscle. All these structures are attached to the perineal membrane. The bulbospongiosus is also attached to the perineal body posteriorly and the ischiocavernosus is attached to the ischiopubic ramus. It is thought that these muscles contract in ejaculation, especially the bulbospongiosus, and are not responsible for erection of the penis. The bulbospongiosus expels the last drops of urine from the urethra. The *superficial transverse perineal muscles* are attached to the inner surface of the ischial tuberosity and pass behind the bulb to become attached to the perineal body. The urethra

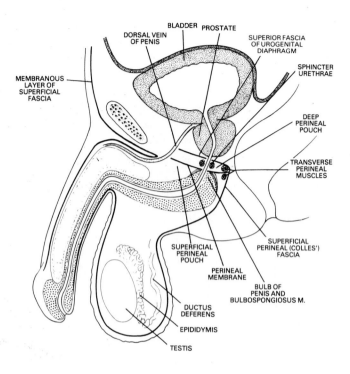

DORSAL VEIN OF PENIS

BLADDER PROSTATE

SUPERIOR FASCIA OF UROGENITAL DIAPHRAGM

SPHINCTER URETHRAE

MEMBRANOUS LAYER OF SUPERFICIAL FASCIA

DEEP PERINEAL POUCH

TRANSVERSE PERINEAL MUSCLES

SUPERFICIAL PERINEAL POUCH

SUPERFICIAL PERINEAL (COLLES') FASCIA

PERINEAL MEMBRANE

BULB OF PENIS AND BULBOSPONGIOSUS M.

DUCTUS DEFERENS

EPIDIDYMIS

TESTIS

Figure 120   A sagittal section of the male pelvis to show the fasciae.

passes through the perineal membrane to enter the bulb. On each side the duct of a bulbo-urethral gland perforates the perineal membrane lateral to the urethra, enters the bulb and opens into the spongy urethra.

The muscles are innervated by the pudendal nerve through its deep perineal branch. The arteries which supply the structures in the superficial perineal pouch come from the internal pudendal artery and continue into the scrotum. The bulb and the crura also receive arteries which enter these structures in the superficial pouch. The artery in the bulb continues into the corpus spongiosum and the arteries in the crura continue into the corpora cavernosa. They are the arteries involved in distending their cavernous spaces in erection.

Deep to the perineal membrane there is a space, the *deep perineal pouch*, containing the (external) sphincter of the urethra and the two bulbo-urethral glands (figure 118). The deep limit of this space is formed by the *superior fascia of the urogenital diaphragm* which is attached laterally

to the ischiopubic rami and posteriorly to the perineal membrane and membranous superficial fascia. Anteriorly it does not reach the symphysis pubis so that there is a gap for the passage of the deep dorsal vein of the penis.

The *sphincter urethrae* is attached laterally to the ischiopubic rami and passes medially to surround the membranous urethra. Posteriorly some of its fibres enter the perineal body. It is a voluntary muscle supplied by the pudendal nerve through a branch which continues as the dorsal nerve of the penis. The muscle can be contracted voluntarily to interrupt micturition and may be involved in expelling the last drops of urine. If damaged, control of micturition is not markedly interfered with, provided the mechanism at the internal urethral orifice and trigone of the bladder remains intact. Some of the fibres of the muscle which extend upwards towards the lower part of the prostatic urethra are thought to open the urethra in ejaculation while the sphincter mechanism at the internal orifice remains closed so that there is no reflux of seminal fluid into the bladder. The *deep transverse perineal muscles* behind the sphincter pass from the rami of the ischium to the midline where they are attached to the perineal body. The *urogenital diaphragm* is defined as the two layers of fascia forming the deep perineal pouch, and its enclosed muscles.

The two round *bulbo-urethral glands*, about 1 cm in diameter, are embedded in the sphincter urethrae on each side of the membranous urethra. Its duct, about 3 cm long, perforates the perineal membrane, enters the bulb of the penis and opens into the floor of the penile urethra. The glands secrete a form of mucus the function of which is not known.

Near the midline the superior fascia of the urogenital diaphragm fuses with the fascia of the prostate and with the fascia between the levatores ani. More laterally it is separated from the inferior surface of the levator ani, which slopes upwards, by the forward extension of the ischiorectal fossa (figure 118).

The *tendinous centre of the perineum (perineal body)* is a fibromuscular mass of tissue lying in front of the anal canal and behind the urogenital diaphragm to which it is attached. The muscles which are partly attached to it are the levator ani, the sphincter urethrae and deep transverse perineal muscles, the bulbospongiosus and superficial transverse perineal muscles and the sphincter ani externus. Some smooth muscle fibres from the longitudinal muscle of the rectum pass forwards and downwards into the perineal body.

The Female External Genitalia

Collectively these form the *vulva* or *female pudendum* and extend from the front of the symphysis pubis to the tendinous centre of the perineum (perineal body). The vagina (p. 148) opens externally in this region into the *vestibule of the vagina*.

The mons pubis, labia majora and labia minora (figure 121)

The *mons pubis* (formerly the *mons Veneris*) is the prominence in front of the symphysis pubis and is due to the underlying subcutaneous fat. (In a laudable desire to eliminate eponymous nomenclature even the name of *Venus* had to be sacrificed for the more mundane term *pubis*.) At puberty the mons becomes covered with coarse hair which has a crescentic upper border just superior to the pubic symphysis, unlike the hair in the male which extends to the umbilicus and has a triangular outline.

The *labia majora* (the homologues of the male scrotum) are two prominent folds of skin on either side of the pudendal cleft into which the vagina opens. After puberty, when the labia enlarge, hairs grow on their outer surface. There are no hairs on their inner surface but both surfaces have sebaceous glands. Each labium contains the termination of a round ligament of the uterus and fatty tissue, which anteriorly is continuous with that of the mons pubis. In the fetus a peritoneal processus vaginalis, the *canal of Nuck* (Anton Nuck, 1650–92, Leyden physician and anatomist) extends into the labium majus and normally disappears. If it persists a congenital inguinal hernia may develop. Normally the medial edges of the labia are in contact with each other but after the menopause the labia atrophy and may become separated.

The *labia minora* are folds of skin which lie within the labia majora. They are non-hairy, have sebaceous glands and do not contain any fat. Anteriorly the edge of each labium divides and the two divisions extend forwards in front of and behind the clitoris. The anterior form the *prepuce of the clitoris* and the posterior its *frenulum*. The labia minora are regarded as the homologue of the inferior (ventral) part of the penis. Posteriorly the labia minora fuse and form the *frenulum of the labia (fourchette)* which is present only in a virgin.

The vestibule (figure 121)

This is the cleft between the labia minora where the vagina opens on to the exterior. The urethra opens on to the anterior part of the vestibule just in front of the vaginal opening. Many small glands open on to the surface of the wall of the vestibule (*lesser vestibular glands*). The *greater vestibular glands of Bartholin* (Caspar Bartholin, 1655–1738,

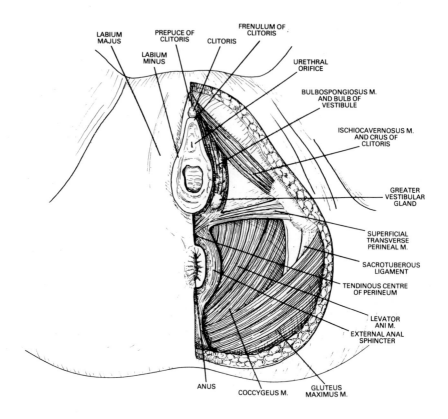

Figure 121   The female superifical perineal pouch.

Copenhagen anatomist) lie on either side of the vestibule posteriorly. Each gland is round and about 1 cm in diameter. Its duct opens laterally between the labia minora and the vaginal hymen or its remains.

The *bulbs of the vestibule* are two masses of erectile tissue about 3 cm long lying on each side of the vaginal opening. They are homologues of the bulb of the penis but the presence of the vagina results in there being two structures. The bulbs are continuous with each other anteriorly in front of the vagina (the *commissure of the bulbs*) and extend towards the glans of the clitoris (comparable with the corpus spongiosum of the penis). Posteriorly the bulbs are enlarged and related to the greater vestibular glands. Superficially each bulb is covered by a *bulbospongiosus muscle*.

The clitoris

This is the homologue of the penis. It is about 2 cm long and consists of two cylinders of erectile tissue called the *corpora cavernosa of the clitoris*. The free end of the clitoris is enlarged and forms the *glans of the clitoris*. This also consists of erectile tissue. The glans has a *prepuce* and a *frenulum* formed by the division and subsequent fusion of the anterior ends of the labia minora (p. 165). The corpora cavernosa diverge as they pass backwards and form the *crura* which are attached one on each side to the ischiopubic ramus. The *ischiocavernosus* surrounds the crus and is attached to the ramus. The clitoris is surrounded by a dense layer of fascia continuous with the membranous layer of the superficial fascia of the abdominal wall and

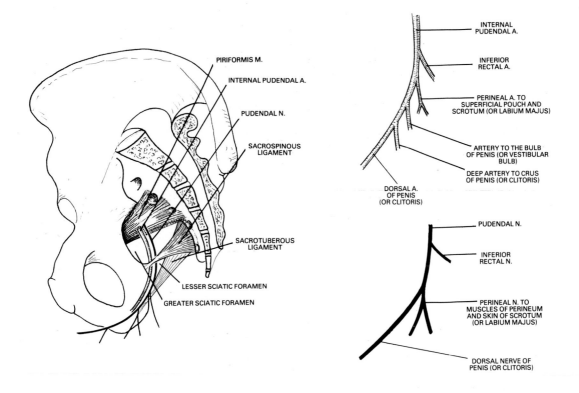

Figure 122   The pudendal nerve and the internal pudendal artery

posteriorly with a superficial fascial layer in the urogenital triangle.

The blood and nerve supply and lymphatic drainage of the female external genitalia

The *arteries* to the external genitalia are derived mainly from the internal pudendal (figure 122) but there are also branches from the femoral arteries (the *deep* and *superficial external pudendal arteries*). The branches from the internal pudendal are (1) the *posterior labial*; (2) the *artery to the bulb*; (3) the *deep* and *dorsal arteries to the clitoris*. A *perineal branch* supplies the muscles and skin which also receive branches from the labial arteries. The clitoris and bulbs of the vestibule consist of

special erectile tissue. Their cavernous spaces become filled with blood which is retained by the contraction of the ischiocavernosus and bulbospongiosus muscles.

The *veins* of the external genitalia correspond with the arteries. Most of them drain into the internal pudendal vein but the veins of the clitoris drain mainly to the pelvic venous plexuses (vaginal and uterine) by passing inferior to the symphysis pubis. Some veins go to the tributaries of the femoral vein. The *lymphatic vessels* from the vulva drain to the superficial inguinal lymph nodes.

The *nerves* to the skin of the external genitalia come mainly from the pudendal nerve (the second, third and fourth sacral nerves). The posterior femoral cutaneous nerve (S1, 2, 3) gives off some perineal branches. The segmental innervation of the skin, however, is mainly the third and fourth sacral nerves. The most anterior part of the skin of the labia majora and the skin near the symphysis pubis is supplied by the ilio-inguinal nerve (L1). The perineal branch of the pudendal nerve supplies the muscles.

The sacral parasympathetic nerves supply dilator fibres to the arterioles of the erectile tissue. These fibres are mainly derived from the peri-arterial plexuses round the vaginal arteries but some travel in the pudendal nerve. The clitoris and labia minora have a rich sensory nerve supply which is specially related to sexual stimulation and erection of the vascular tissue of the region.

The Urethra in the Female (figure 106(a))

The *urethra* is about 4 cm long and passes downwards and forwards from the *internal urethral orifice* of the bladder to the *external urethral orifice (meatus)* which is in front of the vaginal opening and between the anterior ends of the labia minora. Most of the urethra is adherent to or almost embedded in the anterior vaginal wall. The internal orifice is about 3 cm behind the middle of the symphysis pubis and the external orifice is about 1 cm behind the lower border of the symphysis. Although the external orifice is an anteroposterior slit, the anterior and posterior walls of the rest of the urethra are in apposition and the lining has longitudinal folds. A prominent posterior fold is called the *urethral crest*. The diameter of the urethra is about 5 mm but it can be dilated to about 1 cm by an instrument.

There are many small *urethral glands* along the length of the urethra and near the external orifice a group of these glands open by a common duct (the *para-urethral duct*) on either side of the orifice. These glands (often called *Skene's tubules*; A.J.C. Skene, 1838–1900, New York gynaecologist) are regarded as homologous with the prostate. The female urethra is equivalent to that part of the prostatic urethra extending from the bladder to the opening of the prostatic utricle. The female urethra passes through the urogenital diaphragm, where it is surrounded by the striated *sphincter urethrae* supplied by the pudendal nerve. The

internal orifice is surrounded by smooth circular muscle, the *internal sphincter* or *sphincter vesicae*, which is supplied by sympathetic nerve fibres. It operates in the way described on p. 139. The sphincter mechanism involving the pubovesicalis part of the levator ani may be damaged as a result of trauma in childbirth so that stress incontinence occurs (p. 139).

The arterial blood supply comes mainly from the vaginal arteries. There is an erectile plexus of veins along the length of the urethra continuous with the erectile tissue of the vestibular bulb. The veins drain into the internal iliac and internal pudendal veins. The urethra receives autonomic nerve fibres, both sympathetic and parasympathetic, from the plexus round the vaginal arteries and its distal part is innervated by the pudendal nerve.

The Urogenital Triangle in the Female

The main external features of this region have already been described in the previous section (the female external genitalia). The fascial arrangements are similar to those in the male and will be briefly referred to. Deep to the skin there is a layer of superficial fascia, the superficial part of which is fatty and is seen in the labia majora and mons pubis. The deep layer is membranous and surrounds the clitoris. It can be followed forwards on to the anterior abdominal wall and ends posteriorly at the level of the anterior part of the ischial tuberosities.

The *superficial perineal pouch* (figures 121, 123, 124) is between the *superficial membranous fascia* and the *inferior fascia of the urogenital diaphragm (the perineal membrane)*. Passing through the pouch are the vagina and the urethra. On each side of the vagina in the pouch are a bulb of the vestibule with a bulbospongiosus muscle and a greater vestibular gland. More laterally on each side the crus of the clitoris and the ischiocavernosus muscle are attached to the ischiopubic ramus. The posterior edge of the perineal membrane fuses with the posterior edge of the superficial membranous fascia behind the superficial transverse perineal muscles. The anterior edge of the perineal membrane does

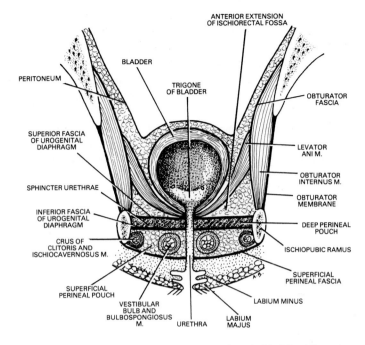

Figure 123   A coronal section through the female bladder (diagrammatic).

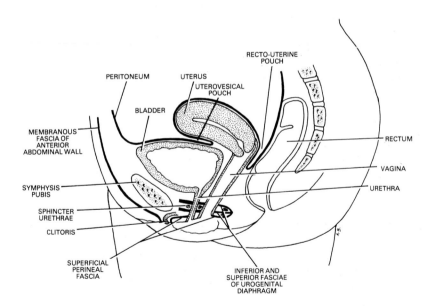

Figure 124   A sagittal section of the female pelvis to show the fasciae.

not reach the symphysis pubis so that there is a gap through which veins pass into the pelvis.

The *deep perineal pouch* (figure 123) is between the *inferior* and *superior fascial layers of the urogenital diaphragm*. The vagina and urethra pass through the pouch in which the sphincter urethrae lies. The posterior edges of the two fascial layers of the urogenital diaphragm fuse behind the deep transverse perineal muscles. Their anterior edges do not reach the symphysis pubis.

The arteries and veins of this region come from and go to the internal pudendal vessels. It is innervated by the pudendal nerve and receives sympathetic and parasympathetic nerve fibres.

The tendinous centre of the perineum in the female (the perineal body or obstetrical perineum)

This structure and the muscles which are partly attached to it have already been described in the male (p. 165). In the female it lies between the anterior wall of the anal canal and the posterior wall of the vagina. It is frequently torn during childbirth and to prevent the tear extending into the rectum an *episiotomy*, an incision directed posterolaterally from the middle of the posterior edge of the vagina, is made deliberately (*episeion = region of the pubis or vulva*, Greek). The deeper parts of such an incision (or of a tear) must be carefully sewn together in order to restore the continuity of the levator ani muscles, as well as all the other muscles which enter the perineal body. An intact perineal body is an important factor in maintaining the position of the uterus and the vault of the vagina in the pelvis.

Part 4

The Head and Neck

13

The Skull and the Cervical Vertebrae

The skeleton of the head is the skull, which may be regarded as a number of bony cavities associated with the nervous system and the beginnings of the respiratory and alimentary systems. The largest of these is the cranial cavity, which contains the brain and the beginnings or ends of the cranial nerves. The nasal cavity is associated with respiration and smell and the oral cavity with taste, sucking, chewing, swallowing and respiration. Both cavities are involved in speech. The orbit contains the eyeball and all its associated structures. Cavities in the temporal bone contain the organs associated with balance and hearing. Many of the bones of the skull have cavities the functions of which in man are somewhat obscure.

The muscles attached to the skull are related either to movements of the head in space or chewing and swallowing, or to facial expression. The muscles in the last named group have retained in some cases their original functions of opening and closing the entrances to the cavities to which they are related, for example the orbit and the mouth, but in others, for example the muscles related to the nasal apertures, this function has been largely lost. Many of the muscles whose functions are alimentary and respiratory are used in speech, for example the muscles of the lips, cheeks, tongue and palate.

The skeleton of the neck is formed by the cervical vertebrae and their functions are similar to those of the rest of the vertebral column — movement, weight transmission and protection of the spinal cord. The structures of the rest of the neck are (1) continuations downwards of the alimentary and respiratory tracts; (2) vessels and nerves which pass upwards or downwards from or to the thorax; (3) cervical segmental spinal nerves. The upper spinal nerves remain mainly in the neck, and the lower form the brachial plexus which supplies the upper limb. The larynx, primarily associated with respiration, is also responsible for controlling the egressive air stream required for normal speech. Many of the muscles of the neck produce movement of the vertebral column but some are involved indirectly in respiration, chewing, swallowing and speech.

The Skull

General

The skull consists of the *cranium* and the *mandible* and the cranium is subdivided into an upper box-like part, the *calvaria* containing the brain, and a lower anterior part consisting of the *facial skeleton* (*calvus* = bald, *calvaria* = bare skull, Latin; the word calvaria has the same derivation as Calvary where Jesus was crucified; it was called Calvary because the site, not the Church of the Holy Sepulchre, looked like a skull-shaped rock or hillock; in Hebrew it was called *Goulgoleth*, the word for a *skull*, which was translated into the Greek *Golgatha* and Latin *Calvaria* or *Calvary*). Almost all the bones of the skull articulate with each other by fibrous joints called *sutures* at which in the adult there is

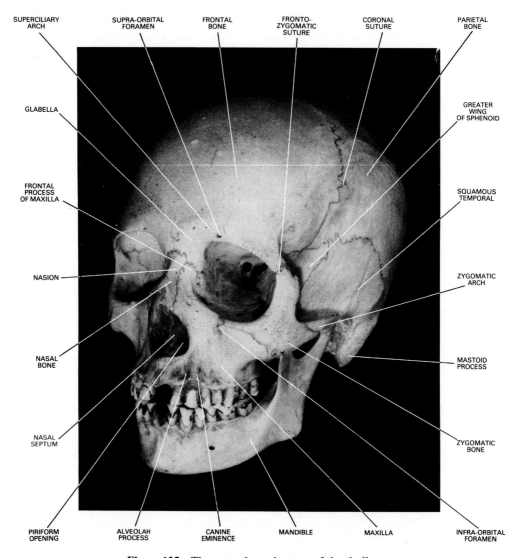

Figure 125   The anterolateral aspect of the skull.

no movement. The edges of the joint may be *serrated* or straight or overlapping (*squamous suture*). In the fetus and at birth there is a considerable quantity of fibrous tissue between the edges of the bones of the vault of the skull and this permits a certain amount of movement. The mandible articulates with the base of the skull by means of a condyloid synovial joint at which there is considerable movement. Two of the bones forming part of the middle of the base of the skull (the occipital and sphenoid) articulate with each other by a cartilaginous joint which becomes bony at about 25 years.

Many of the bones forming the sutures eventually become united by bone (*synostosis*).

The anterior aspect of the skull (figure 125)

The *frontal bone* forms the anterior part of the dome of the calvaria and the upper margin of the orbital opening. Laterally the frontal bone articulates with the *zygomatic* (*cheek, malar*) *bone* and medially with the *frontal process* of the *maxilla*. The *fronto-zygomatic* suture can be felt as a depression on the lateral edge of the orbital opening. Above the medial part of the orbital opening there is a prominence of varying size called the *superciliary arch*. About 2.5 cm from the midline there is the *supra-orbital notch* or *foramen* on the upper border of the orbital margin.

Below the orbits the two *maxillae* form most of the skeleton of the face. They meet in the midline below the *piriform* (pear-shaped) *opening* of the nasal cavity and form an upward projecting *anterior nasal spine* just above the suture. Superiorly the maxillae are separated by the two *nasal bones*. Each nasal bone articulates laterally with the maxilla and superiorly with the frontal bone. The nasal bones meet in the midline and form the bridge of the nose above which there is a depression called the *nasion*. The projection above the nasion is called the *glabella* (*glaber = smooth*, Latin) and is used for making measurements on the skull.

The lateral and adjacent part of the inferior margin of the orbital opening is formed by the zygomatic bone which forms the prominence of the cheek. The rest of the inferior margin and the medial margin is formed by the maxilla. About 1 cm below the inferior margin and 2.5 cm from the midline there is the *infra-orbital foramen*.

Below the zygomatic bones the narrow part of the face is formed by the *alveolar processes* of the maxillae (*alveus = a hollow*, Latin) the lower borders of which form the *alveolar arch* containing the sockets for the teeth. There are elevations on the surface of the maxilla; the most prominent of these is the *canine eminence* about 2 cm from the midline overlying the tooth of that name.

Within the nasal cavity the *nasal septum* can be seen, usually deviated to one side. There are also very thin plates of bone projecting medially and downwards from the lateral wall. These are the *conchae* (*concha = shell*, Latin) or *turbinate bones* (*turbo = scroll-like*, Latin).

The *mandible* (described separately) forms the lower part of the front of the skull.

The lateral aspect of the skull (figure 126)

The *vault* of the skull is formed by the *occipital*, *parietal* and *frontal bones* from behind forwards.

The occipital bone articulates with the parietal at the serrated *lambdoidal suture* (*lambda = the Greek letter L*; when looked at from behind the suture on both sides forms this Greek letter, shaped thus Λ). The serrated *coronal (frontal) suture* is between the parietal and frontal bones. Inferior to the parietal bone, the temporal bone forms the side of the skull (*temporal = related to time*, Latin; possibly the greying of the hair at the temple indicates the passage of time). This is the *squamous part* of the temporal bone and it articulates with the parietal at the *squamosal suture* at which the bones overlap (*squama = scale*, Latin). In front of the squamous temporal bone a part of the greater wing of the sphenoid bone articulates with three bones — the parietal, temporal and frontal — at an H-shaped suture called the *pterion* (*sphen = wedge*, Greek; *pterux = wing*, Greek).

The *zygomatic process* of the squamous temporal bone projects forwards and articulates with the zygomatic bone to form the *zygomatic arch* (*zygon = yoke*, Greek). The space between the arch and the side of the skull is called the *temporal fossa*. Behind the root of the zygomatic process the *tympanic part* of the temporal bone forms a cylinder which is the bony part of the external acoustic meatus. The cylinder is defective postero-superiorly. Behind the meatus the *mastoid process* projects downwards in front of the occipital bone (*mastus = breast*, Latin; psychologists would be interested in the number of structures thought by anatomists to be shaped like a breast or nipple). This process is continuous medially with the petrous part of the temporal bone (*petros = stone*, Greek). In front of the meatus the *mandibular fossa* for the condyle of the mandible extends into the base of the skull. It is part of the squamous temporal. The fourth part of the temporal bone, the *styloid process*, projects downwards and forwards. It is embedded in the petrous temporal behind the tympanic part (*stylus = stake* or *pole*, later a *pencil* or *pen*, Latin).

If the mandible is removed and the skull held so that the lower border of the orbital opening and the middle of the external acoustic meatuses are in the same horizontal plane, the facial skeleton is seen to extend below the level of the posterior part of the skull. The *body* of the maxilla is below

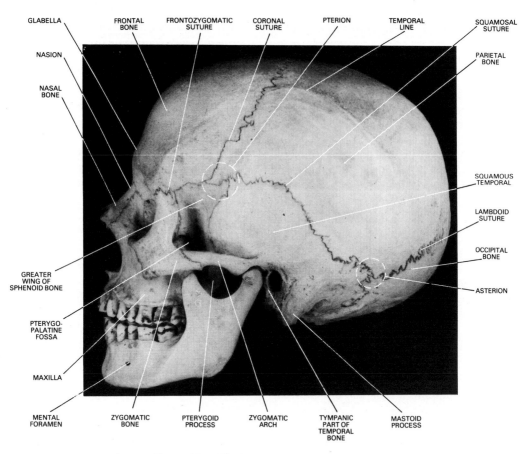

Figure 126   The lateral aspect of the skull.

and in a deeper plane than the zygomatic bone. Behind the maxilla the *pterygoid process* of the sphenoid bone projects downwards and is separated from the back of the maxilla by a space called the *pterygopalatine fossa* (the pterygoid process has two flat plates projecting backwards like wings). The pterygoid process is in a deeper plane than that of the lateral surface of the maxilla. The *greater wing* of the sphenoid bone has a horizontal part as well as the vertical part on the lateral wall of the skull. The *infratemporal fossa* is the space bounded anteriorly by the back of the maxilla, posteriorly by the temporomandibular joint, superiorly by the greater wing of the sphenoid bone and medially by the pterygoid process.

At the back of the skull there is a prominence on the occipital bone called the *external occipital protuberance* which can be felt on one's own skull.

The petrous temporal bone articulates with the occipital and parietal bones at the *occipitomastoid* and *parietomastoid sutures* respectively. The *asterion* is where the lambdoid suture meets these two sutures.

The posterior aspect of the skull (figure 127)

The most posterior part of the skull is formed by the *occipital bone* which extends upwards into the vault of the skull (the *squamous part* of the occipital bone) and forwards into its base. The external occipital protuberance is a palpable prominence in the midline of the squamous part and is called the *inion*. The *superior* and *highest nuchal lines* extend laterally from the prominence. The *external occipital crest* extends downwards from the prominence

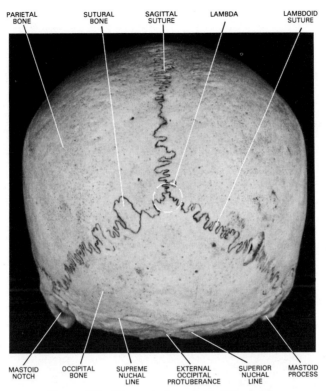

PARIETAL BONE   SUTURAL BONE   SAGITTAL SUTURE   LAMBDA   LAMBDOID SUTURE

MASTOID NOTCH   OCCIPITAL BONE   SUPREME NUCHAL LINE   EXTERNAL OCCIPITAL PROTUBERANCE   SUPERIOR NUCHAL LINE   MASTOID PROCESS

Figure 127   The posterior aspect of the skull.

in the midline to the *foramen magnum*, which lies in the basal part of the occipital bone. The *condyles* are nearer the anterior part of the foramen magnum and are directed anteromedially. The *basilar part* of the occipital bone is in front of the foramen magnum.

The posterior end of the sagittal suture between the parietal bones meets the lambdoid suture at the *lambda*. This is the commonest site for small additional bones to be found (*sutural* or *Wormian bones*; O. Wormius, 1588–1654, Danish anatomist). The occipitomastoid and parietomastoid sutures are lateral and a mastoid process projects downwards on each side. A deep groove, the *mastoid notch*, is medial to the mastoid process. There is usually a large *mastoid foramen* medial to and above the mastoid process.

The superior aspect of the skull (figure 128)

The smooth outline of the calvaria is usually oval with the anteroposterior diameter greater than the transverse, but there is considerable variation in the shape, and the skull may be nearly round. The ratio of one diameter to the other is used for classifying skulls. The precision with which a certain type of skull can be assigned to a large group of people (a race) or a smaller group (a tribe) waxes and wanes with the enthusiasm of the observer and the refinement of measuring and statistical techniques.

The *sagittal suture* lies between the two parietal bones. The coronal and lambdoid sutures are between the frontal and parietal and parietal and occipital bones respectively. The bregma (*bregma = front of the head*, Greek) is where the sagittal and coronal sutures meet. The highest point of the skull is called the *vertex*. On either side of the sagittal suture about 3 cm anterior to the lambda there is a *parietal foramen*. There may be a persistent suture between the two halves of the frontal bones (*metopic suture*). This is always present at birth and usually disappears by 7 years of age (*metopon = forehead*, Greek).

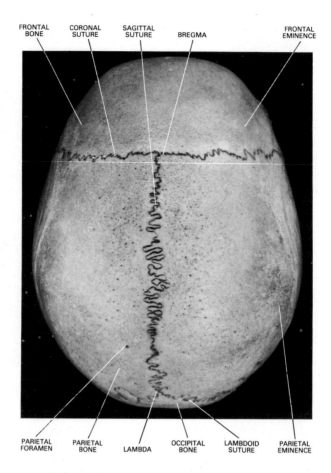

FRONTAL BONE   CORONAL SUTURE   SAGITTAL SUTURE   BREGMA   FRONTAL EMINENCE

PARIETAL FORAMEN   PARIETAL BONE   LAMBDA   OCCIPITAL BONE   LAMBDOID SUTURE   PARIETAL EMINENCE

Figure 128   The superior aspect of the skull.

From this aspect of the skull the *parietal* and *frontal eminences* are seen as bulges on each side of the bones. They are related to the mode of ossification of the bones, although together with less regular prominences of other bones they formed the basis of the discredited pseudoscience of phrenology, the study of the conformation of the skull as indicative of mental faculties and character. The diameter between the parietal eminences is usually the largest transverse diameter and these eminences obscure the zygomatic arches when the skull is viewed from above.

The inferior aspect of the skull (figure 129)

Many of the features of the *occipital bone* have already been described — the external occipital protuberance, the external occipital crest, the foramen magnum, the occipital condyles, and the basilar part of the occipital bone. Posterior to the occipital condyle there is the *condyloid foramen* and superolateral to it is the opening of the *hypoglossal canal*. The *jugular foramen* between the occipital and petrous temporal bones is lateral to the occipital condyle. On each side of the foramen the occipital and petrous temporal bones articulate with each other. The *pharyngeal tubercle* is in the midline on the basilar part of the occipital bone 1 cm anterior to the edge of the foramen magnum.

Anterolateral to the occipital bone the petromastoid part of the temporal bone projects forwards and medially towards the body of the

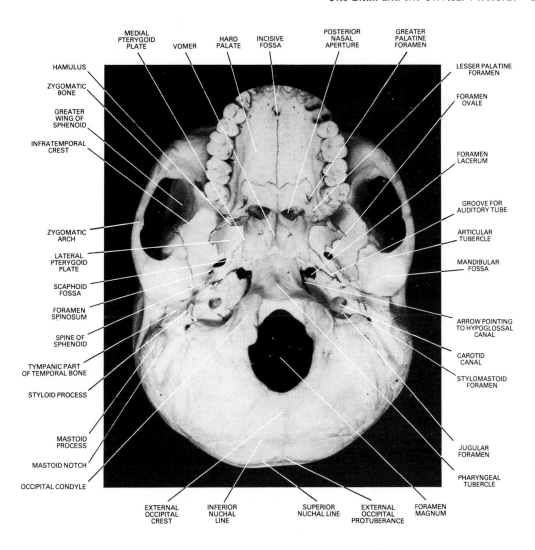

Figure 129   The inferior aspect of the skull.

sphenoid bone from which it is separated by the *foramen lacerum*. This foramen in the living is closed in its lower part by fibrocartilage. The mastoid process and mastoid notch are on the lateral part of the petrous temporal bone. About 1 cm medial to the mastoid process, the styloid process projects downwards and forwards. The *stylomastoid foramen* is behind the styloid process. The *carotid canal* is anteromedial to the stylomastoid foramen and is in front of the jugular foramen.

The inferior surface of the tympanic part of the temporal bone is in front of and lateral to the styloid process. The mandibular fossa is in front of the tympanic part and is limited anteriorly by the *articular tubercle* which forms part of the temporomandibular joint. Between the tympanic part and the mandibular fossa there is a fissure. The zygomatic arch extends forwards from the articular tubercle.

The *body of the sphenoid bone* is continuous with the basilar part of the occipital bone in the midline. It forms the anterior 5 mm of this part of the base of the skull and continues forwards as the roof of the *choanae* (the *posterior nasal apertures*). The posterior edge of the *nasal septum*, formed by the *vomer*, separates the choanae (*choane = funnel*, Greek). The *hard palate* forms the lower edge of the openings. On each side of the choanae the pterygoid process of the sphenoid bone projects downwards. It consists of the more or less vertical *medial* and *lateral pterygoid plates* with a hollow, the *pterygoid fossa*, between them. The posterior border of the medial plate is prolonged downwards and laterally as the *pterygoid hamulus* (*hamulus = a little hook*, Latin). The medial pterygoid plate is in the same plane as the posterior part of the lateral wall of the nasal cavity.

The greater wing of the sphenoid bone is lateral to the upper end of the pterygoid process. If followed laterally its anterior part bends upwards and forms part of the lateral wall of the skull. In the horizontal part in the base the *foramen ovale* is lateral to the pterygoid process and the *foramen spinosum* is posterolateral to the foramen ovale. The latter foramen is named after the *spine of the sphenoid bone* which is posterolateral to the foramen. In front of the greater wing of the sphenoid the *inferior orbital fissure* leads into the orbit. Laterally the greater wing articulates with the squamous part of the temporal bone and posteriorly with the petrous part. Posterior to this articulation the *groove for the auditory (Eustachian) tube* passes laterally and backwards into a canal in the petrous part of the temporal bone.

At a lower level than the rest of the base of the skull, the hard palate is in line with the lower border of the choanae. The anterior three-quarters of the hard palate are formed by the palatine processes of the maxillae and the posterior quarter by the horizontal plates of the palatine bones. The hard palate is bounded anteriorly and laterally by the alveolar processes of the maxillae. The inferior surface of the processes form the alveolar arch which contains the sockets for the teeth. In the midline just behind the anterior part of the arch there is a depression called the *incisive fossa* into which several foramina open. Posterolaterally the *greater* and *lesser palatine foramina* open on to the palate.

The mandible (figure 130)

The *mandible* (*mandire = to chew*, Latin) consists

of a *body* and two *rami*. The body is the horizontal, horseshoe-shaped part in front and each ramus is the vertical part at the posterior end of the body. The middle of the body anteriorly is called the *mental symphysis* (*mentum = chin*, Latin). At birth the mandible is in two pieces, united by fibrous tissue in the midline at the symphysis (*syn = together*, *phyo = to grow*, Greek). By the end of the first year the two halves are united by bone. The triangular elevation on the front of the lower half of the external surface is called the *mental protuberance*.

The *mental foramen* is about 2.5 cm lateral to the symphysis about midway between the upper and lower borders of the body. The opening faces upwards and backwards. The *oblique line* passes upwards and backwards from the mental foramen and is continuous with the anterior border of the ramus. The lower border is thickened as compared with the rest of the body. The upper alveolar part of the body forms an arch in which are the alveoli (sockets) for the teeth. The posterior end of the arch is medial to the posterior end of the body.

The *digastric fossa* is a small depression near the midline on the lower border. The *mylohyoid line* passes upwards and backwards on the internal surface of the body and extends as far as the socket for the third molar tooth (*mylo = millstone*, Greek, referring to the crushing functions of the molar teeth). The *submandibular fossa* is below and the *sublingual fossa* above the line. The groove above the posterior end of the mylohyoid line at the level of the third molar tooth is for the lingual nerve. The *mylohyoid groove* is a narrower and longer groove which passes downwards and forwards below the mylohyoid line. On either side of the midline on the inner surface of the symphysis there are four tubercles, two on each side one above the other. They are collectively called the *mental spine* but were known as the *right* and *left*, *superior* and *inferior genial tubercles* (*geneion = chin*, Greek; the word is still retained for the muscles attached to them — genioglossus and geniohyoid).

The quadrilateral ramus has two *processes* on its upper border, a posterior *condylar* and an anterior *coronoid*. The *mandibular notch* is between the two processes. The condylar process has an upper *head* whose axis passes medially and backwards

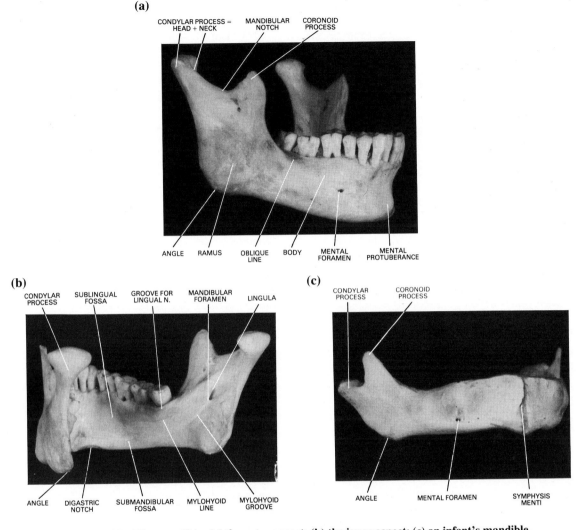

(a)

CONDYLAR PROCESS = HEAD + NECK   MANDIBULAR NOTCH   CORONOID PROCESS

ANGLE   RAMUS   OBLIQUE LINE   BODY   MENTAL FORAMEN   MENTAL PROTUBERANCE

(b)

CONDYLAR PROCESS   SUBLINGUAL FOSSA   GROOVE FOR LINGUAL N.   MANDIBULAR FORAMEN   LINGULA

ANGLE   DIGASTRIC NOTCH   SUBMANDIBULAR FOSSA   MYLOHYOID LINE   MYLOHYOID GROOVE

(c)

CONDYLAR PROCESS   CORONOID PROCESS

ANGLE   MENTAL FORAMEN   SYMPHYSIS MENTI

Figure 130   The mandible: (a) the outer aspect; (b) the inner aspect; (c) an infant's mandible.

and a lower narrower *neck* with an anteromedial pit. The lateral end of the head can be felt below the posterior end of the zygomatic arch especially on opening and closing the jaw. The coronoid process is triangular and is deep to the zygomatic arch when the mouth is closed. The posterior and inferior borders of the ramus meet at the *angle of the mandible*.

On the middle of the inner surface of the ramus the *mandibular foramen* leads into the *mandibular canal* which runs downwards and forwards in the body. The *lingula (small tongue)* is an upward projection of bone above and medial to the foramen.

There is a thickened ridge of bone on the inner surface of the ramus extending from the medial end of the condylar process to the mandibular foramen. This is a bony strut which resists compressive forces produced by bringing the jaws together.

Note

In the preceding description of the skull, the structure of the bony walls of the orbit and the nasal cavity and of the inside of the skull has been omitted. These regions will be dealt with in due course.

As a result of these omissions many small bones have not been mentioned, for example the *lacrimal*, or have been only referred to, for example the *palatine*. A detailed description of all the bones of the skull will not be given and is not considered necessary for understanding the anatomy of the head and neck. However, the following three sections give some basic information about the structure, ossification and growth of the skull.

The structure of the bones of the skull

Most of the bones of the skull consist of two plates of compact bone containing a layer of cancellous bone. The bones of the vault are on the whole of a uniform thickness although the ratio of cancellous bone to compact bone is somewhat variable. The cancellous bone is called *diploe* (*diplöos = double*, Greek; this refers to the two layers of compact bone) and contains the *diploic veins*. These veins have very thin walls, show small dilatations along their course and are about 3 mm wide when seen in an X-ray of the skull. They are found in the frontal, parietal, squamous temporal and occipital bones and communicate with the intracranial and extracranial veins. They begin to develop at about the age of 2 years.

Some bones or parts of the bones of the skull are very thin and are so reduced in thickness that they consist of only one thin plate of bone, for example the nasal and lacrimal bones and the orbital plate of the frontal bone. In other situations the amount of compact bone is increased and replaces the cancellous bone. This is seen in the zygomatic process of the frontal bone and the medial part of the petrous temporal bone. Different parts of a bone are subjected to different pressures and therefore have varied thicknesses; for example the structure of the mandible and maxilla reflects the forces which act on them while biting and chewing.

Because the bones of the vault of the adult skull within certain limits possess elasticity, a blow on the side of the head may result in a fracture of the inner plate while the outer plate of bone remains intact. This is due to the outer plate being subjected to compression forces which are resisted more easily than the tensile forces to which the inner plate is subjected.

The type of fracture seen in the skull or mandible due to direct blows is related to the structure of the different parts of the skull. The mandible usually fractures at the neck of the condylar process or in the body near the canine tooth where the bone is thinnest. Thin bone such as the squamous temporal may be protected by overlying muscle. Violence to the vault of the skull often produces linear fractures which radiate from the site of the blow along the lines of least resistance. In the base of the skull the thick petrous temporal bone usually resists fracture but the thin bone of the greater wing of the sphenoid in front of the petrous temporal breaks.

The vault of an infant's skull, which is more elastic than that of an adult, may become indented and remain in this state without being fractured (*pond fracture*).

The ossification of the bones of the skull

The details of the ossification of the individual bones are complex but some generalisations can be made. Two groups of bones ossify in cartilage (endochondral ossification) and form the chondocranium. These are the bones forming the base of the skull and the bones developing in the olfactory (nasal) capsule. The two groups which ossify in membrane (membranous ossification) are those forming the vault of the skull and those forming the facial skeleton. Table 4 summarises this. The term *neurocranium* includes the bones forming the braincase (the endochondral base and the membranous vault) and those developing in relation to the organs of hearing and smell (endochondral).

The *frontal bone* ossifies in membrane from two primary centres, one for each lateral half of the bone appearing at about the eighth week of intra-uterine life. The frontal eminence indicates the site of the centre. At birth the bone is in two halves (figure 131(a)). The midline (metopic) suture begins to disappear during the first year and has gone as a rule by about the seventh year.

The *parietal bone* ossifies in membrane from two primary centres which appear about the eighth

Table 4

Type of ossification	Region of skull	
Membranous	*Vault:* occipital above highest nuchal line, squamous temporal, parietal, frontal, greater wing of sphenoid	*Face:* maxilla, zygomatic bone, lacrimal, palatine, vomer
Cartilaginous	*Base:* occipital below highest nuchal line, petromastoid and styloid process of temporal, body and lesser wing of sphenoid	*In olfactory capsule:* ethmoid, inferior concha, sphenoidal concha

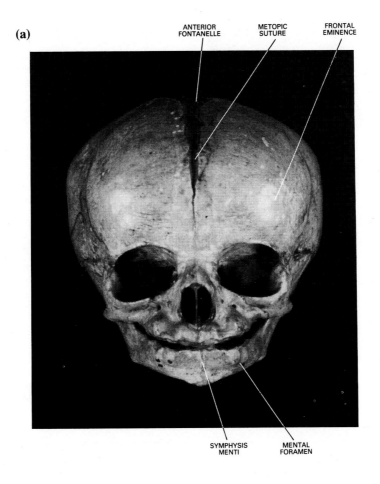

Figure 131   The infant skull: (a) from in front.

(b)

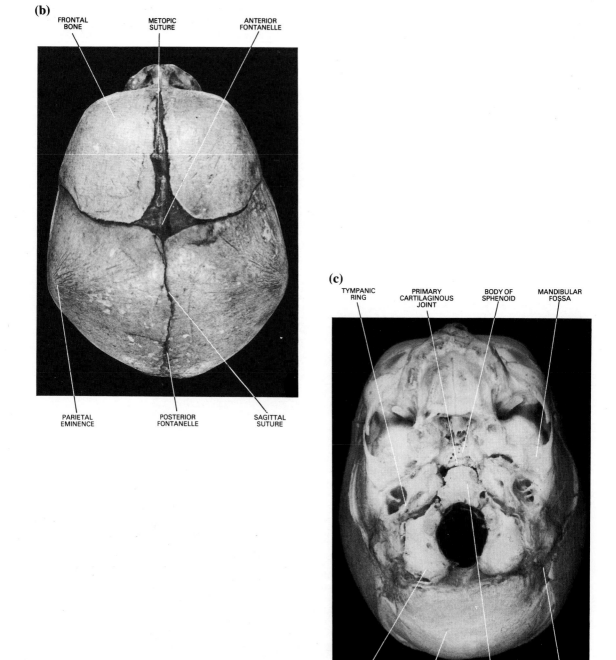

Figure 131   **The infant skull: (b) from above; (c) from below.**

week of intra-uterine life. The parietal eminence also indicates the centre of ossification.

Of the four parts of the *temporal bone*, the squamous part ossifies in membrane and has a primary centre of ossification which appears about the eighth week of intra-uterine life. The tympanic part ossifies in membrane from a centre which appears about the 12th week of intra-uterine life. The petromastoid part ossifies in cartilage from a large number of centres which appear at about the 20th week and fuse together at about the 24th week of intra-uterine life. The styloid process ossifies in cartilage from two centres, an upper appearing just before birth and a lower just after birth.

At birth the tympanic part, in the form of a ring, is fused with the squamous part (figure 131 (c)). During the first year all the four parts fuse together except for the distal part of the styloid process which fuses with the proximal part at about puberty. The mastoid process does not develop until the second year and the tympanic ring deepens into a canal during the early years of childhood so that the tympanic membrane comes to lie at the inner end of the external acoustic meatus.

At birth the mandibular fossa is shallow and faces laterally. During infancy and the early years of childhood it becomes deeper and faces downwards and the squamous temporal grows downwards behind the tympanic ring and fuses with the petrous part. The growth of the mastoid process results in the facial nerve lying much more deeply and the *mastoid antrum*, a cavity in the bone, becoming separated from the surface by nearly 15 mm of bone instead of only 5 mm. By puberty the extension of spaces from the antrum into the mastoid process form the *mastoid air cells*.

The squamous part of the *occipital bone* ossifies in membrane (upper part) and cartilage (lower part). The four centres of the upper part appear at about the eighth week of intra-uterine life. By the 12th week all four centres have fused. Each condylar part and the basilar part ossify separately in cartilage. These appear about the eighth week of intra-uterine life. The condylar part meets the basilar part in the middle of the condyle. At birth there are four parts to the occipital bone (figure 131(c)). They all fuse at about 5 years of age. The occipital bone fuses with the sphenoid at about the 25th year.

The *sphenoid bone* ossifies partly in membrane and partly in cartilage from a large number of centres of ossification appearing about the eighth week of intra-uterine life. At birth the sphenoid consists of three parts, the body and the lesser wings forming one part, and on each side there are a greater wing and pterygoid process. These three parts fuse during the first year after birth.

The *mandible* ossifies in membrane from the mesenchyme of the mandibular (first) branchial arch on the outer side of *Meckel's cartilage* which forms part of the skeleton of that arch (J.H. Meckel, 1781–1833, German anatomist). Ossification begins in the sixth week in a centre for each half. Meckel's cartilage does not undergo ossification except possibly for the part below the incisor teeth. Accessory pieces of cartilage appear near the coronoid and condylar processes and the mental symphysis. At these sites endochondral ossification may occur and contribute to the growth of the bone. The state of the mandible at birth and its subsequent changes are described on p. 186.

The growth of the skull

In the newborn the head is about one-quarter of the height of the child. This is due to the large size of the brain and of the neurocranium. If a horizontal line is drawn at the level of the lower border of the orbital openings the facial skeleton is about one-third of the height of the skull as compared with one-half in the adult. The bones of the vault are separated by fibrous tissue and the edges of the sutures are not serrated. At the four angles of the parietal bones there is a considerable amount of fibrous tissue forming *fontanelles* (figure 131(b)). The largest is the diamond-shaped *anterior fontanelle* between the two halves of the frontal bone and the two parietal bones. The *posterior fontanelle* is triangular and lies between the occipital bone and the two parietal bones where the sagittal suture meets the lambdoid suture. The *sphenoidal fontanelle* is anterolateral at the pterion, and the *mastoid fontanelle* is posterolateral where the parietal and occipital bones meet the petrous temporal bone (figure 131(c)). The orbits of the newborn are proportionately larger than in the adult.

The brain and skull grow most rapidly in the first 6 years at which time the brain is about 90 per cent of its adult size. Growth is most marked in the first year. During this time the parietal eminence becomes much less prominent. Growth of the skull is due to bone being added at the sutures and also to the outside of the skull while it is removed from the inside. Growth of the skull ceases at about 16 years. All the fontanelles are closed by the end of the first year except the anterior which closes between 18 and 24 months after birth. By this time the edges of the sutures are serrated.

The base of the skull grows in length, mainly at the cartilaginous junction between the occipital and sphenoid bones. This growth ceases at about 25 years when the bony union between the bones occurs. This is related to the eruption of the teeth. The third molar (wisdom) tooth does not erupt after 25 years.

The sutures of the vault begin to disappear and become bony after 30 years of age, a process which commences on the inside of the skull at first and affects the sagittal, coronal and the lambdoid suture in that order.

The facial skeleton grows most markedly during the eruption of the second dentition, that is from 8 to 14 years when the maxilla and mandible increase in size. There is also a downward and forward growth of the bones surrounding the nasal cavity so that the palate lies at a much lower level. The air sinuses in the maxilla, body of the sphenoid and frontal bone all become enlarged during the eruption of the second dentition. The growth of the maxillary sinus is a major factor in the increase in the size of the facial skeleton.

The mandible is small at birth and is in two halves which become united by the end of the first year (figure 130(c)). At birth the angle between the body and the ramus is large, about 160°, with the result that the coronoid process is higher than the condylar. The mental foramen is near the lower border of the mandible. Growth takes place during the eruption of the deciduous teeth, especially in the lower part of the body, so that the mental foramen is further from the lower border. The angle between the body and ramus decreases so that the coronoid and condylar processes are almost at the same level. During the eruption of the permanent teeth there is considerable growth especially of the body in an anteroposterior direction. This growth takes place by the deposition of bone on the back and removal of bone from the front of the ramus. The mental foramen comes to lie midway between the upper and lower borders, and the coronoid and condylar processes are at the same level.

With the loss of the teeth, the bone on the alveolar margin is absorbed so that the mental foramen lies nearer the upper border. The angle between the ramus and the body increases and the coronoid process is higher than the condylar.

The growth changes in the temporal bone are described on p. 185.

The Cervical Vertebrae (figure 132)

All cervical vertebrae have a foramen transversarium in the transverse process. The first and second cervical vertebrae (the atlas and axis respectively) are obviously different from the others and the seventh has some individual features.

Typically the *body* of a cervical vertebrae is small relative to the bodies of the thoracic and lumbar vertebrae and is oval with its long axis transverse. The anterior edge of the lower surface of the body projects downwards and the lateral edges of the upper surface project upwards. The projections fit into corresponding depressions on the neighbouring vertebrae. There is usually a joint on each side between the adjacent lateral parts of the bodies. These joints are immediately anterior to the intervertebral foramen in which lies a spinal nerve.

The *pedicles* of the *vertebral arch* are small and their attachment to the body is lower than that of the pedicles in the thoracic and lumbar region. The *laminae* are in the form of flat plates which overlap each other between neighbouring vertebrae. The vertebral foramen is large and triangular. The *spinous process* projects backwards and somewhat downwards and is bifid except for that of the atlas which is only a tubercle and that of the seventh

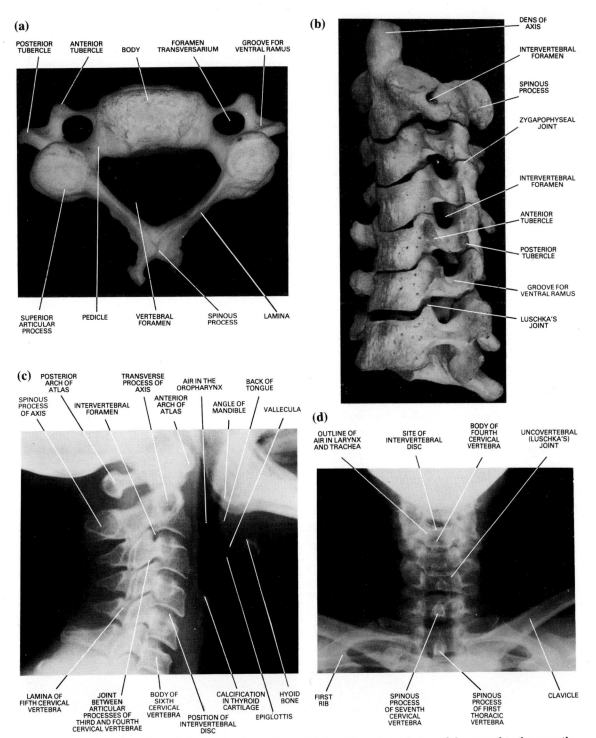

Figure 132 (a) A typical cervical vertebra from above. (b) An oblique lateral view of the second to the seventh cervical vertebrae. (c) A lateral X-ray of the cervical vertebrae. (d) An anteroposterior X-ray of the cervical vertebrae.

cervical vertebra. The *superior articular process* faces upwards as well as backwards and the *inferior* downwards as well as forwards. These processes are on a comparatively stout piece of bone so that when the cervical vertebrae are articulated together the articular processes form a bony pillar which is weight-bearing in a way not seen in the thoracic and lumbar regions of the vertebral column.

A *transverse process* consists of two roots, one from the body and one from the region of the articular processes, and a *costotransverse bar* which joins the two roots. The lateral ends of the roots project beyond the bar as *anterior* and *posterior tubercles*. There is a deep groove on the upper surface of the bar. The anterior tubercle of the transverse process of the sixth cervical vertebra is enlarged and is called the *carotid tubercle* because the common carotid artery lies in front of and can be compressed against it.

The Atlas. The first cervical vertebra, the *atlas*, has no body and no spinous process (figure 133). It consists of a bony ring divided into a smaller *anterior arch* and larger *posterior arch* by a *lateral mass* on each side. The posterior arch has a *posterior tubercle* instead of a spinous process. Near the lateral mass the arch is flattened from above downwards and forms a groove which may be converted into a

foramen by bone passing from the lateral mass medially and arching over the groove. The anterior arch is flattened anteroposteriorly and has a facet on its concave posterior surface for the anterior surface of the dens of the axis, and a tubercle on its convex anterior surface.

The lateral mass is a thick piece of bone which is weight-bearing. It is directed forwards and medially and has on its superior surface an elongated concave facet for the occipital condyle. The shape of the articular area is very variable, but frequently it is narrowed on one or both sides in its middle. It may even be completely divided into two articular areas. The facet on the inferior surface is flat and rounded or oval and faces downwards and medially. On the medial side of the lateral mass there is a tubercle to which a transverse ligament is attached. Together with the anterior arch this ligament completes a ring in which the dens of the axis rotates. The atlas is the widest of the cervical vertebrae due to the lateral mass on each side and the elongated transverse processes. *The process can be palpated midway between the angle of the mandible and mastoid process.*

The Axis. The second cervical vertebra, the *axis*, has projecting upwards from its body, the *dens* (*odontoid process*) (figure 132(b)). The dens is the

(a)   **(b)**

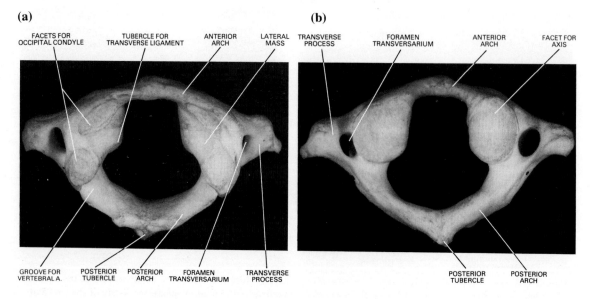

Figure 133   The atlas: (a) from above; (b) from below.

body of the atlas fused to the body of the axis. Between the dens and body there is a groove in which lies the transverse ligament already referred to. On the anterior surface of the dens there is a facet for the anterior arch of the atlas. The facet for the lateral mass of the atlas is round and flat and faces upwards and laterally. The *spinous process* is the largest of the cervical spinous processes. The *foramen transversarium* is directed laterally as well as upwards because of the width of the atlas.

The Seventh Cervical Vertebra. This vertebra has a small *foramen transversarium* because the vertebral artery passes upwards by entering the foramen of the sixth vertebra and not that of the seventh. The *spinous process* is not bifid but is sufficiently elongated to be seen projecting in the midline deep to the skin. Although the seventh cervical vertebra is called the *vertebra prominens* it is not as a rule the vertebra with the most prominent spinous process. That of the first thoracic is more frequently the most prominent. The anterior part of the *transverse process* of the seventh cervical vertebra may be separate and form a *cervical rib*. This can be of a varied length and may form a complete rib articulating through a costal cartilage with the manubrium of the sternum. More frequently it is attached by fibrous tissue to the sternum or ends blindly in the anterior muscles of the neck. The branch of the first thoracic spinal nerve which goes to the upper limb in the brachial plexus has to pass over a cervical rib and pressure on this nerve may result. This produces vascular effects because of pressure on the postganglionic sympathetic fibres which are vasoconstrictor. The muscles of the hand, supplied by the first thoracic spinal nerve, are also affected.

The Joints of the Cervical Vertebrae. The cervical vertebrae when articulated together form a curve with its convexity forwards. The joints between the vertebrae, except for those between the occiput and atlas and atlas and axis, are those found elsewhere in the vertebral column — secondary cartilaginous joints between the bodies, and synovial joints between the articular processes. In addition there are joints laterally between the adjacent bevelled edges of the bodies. The projecting edge of the body is called the *uncus* (*uncus* = *hook*,

Latin) and the joint the *uncovertebral joint* or more commonly the *joints of Luschka* (H. Von Luschka, 1820–75, German anatomist). It is agreed that these joints are not synovial and between the bodies, but splits in the adjacent lateral part of the intervertebral disc.

The intervertebral foramina transmit the cervical spinal nerves of which there are eight, the first lying above the atlas and the eighth below the seventh cervical vertebra. While lying in the foramen the nerve is closely related anteromedially to the cartilaginous joint between the bodies, posteriorly to the joint between the articular process and anteriorly to the uncovertebral joint. Narrowing of the spaces between the bodies due to degeneration of the intervertebral discs and hence narrowing of the intervertebral foramina, most commonly between the fifth and sixth, and sixth and seventh cervical vertebrae results in pressure on the nerve with pain radiating into the upper limb along the distribution of the sixth and seventh cervical nerves. A prolapsed disc or disease of the other joints resulting in projections of bone (*osteophytes*) may press on the cervical spinal nerves.

The movements which take place between the cervical vertebrae are flexion and extension, rotation to the right and left and lateral flexion or bending to the right and left. As compared with the rest of the cervical part of the vertebral column there is much more flexion and extension between the occipital bone and atlas and much more rotation between the atlas and axis than elsewhere. The special joints involved are described with the vertebral column as a whole (p. 329). The movements are also considered in more detail, but it can be said that the cervical region has as great a range of movement in all directions as any part of the vertebral column.

Ossification. A typical cervical vertebra ossifies in the same way as other typical vertebrae — three primary centres, one for the body (centrum) and one for each half of the neural arch. These appear at about the eighth week of intra-uterine life. There are five secondary centres, one for each transverse process, one on each surface of the body and one for the spinous process. These appear during the 15th year and unite with the rest of the vertebra at about 25 years.

The atlas has three primary centres, one for the anterior arch and one for each lateral mass and half of the posterior arch. The centre for each lateral mass appears about the seventh week and they unite posteriorly at about 3 years. That for the anterior arch appears at about 1 year and unites with the lateral mass at about 7 years.

The axis ossifies in a typical manner but has in addition a primary centre for the dens which appears at about the 26th week of intra-uterine life. The apex of the dens ossifies from a separate centre at about 2 years. It fuses with the rest of the dens at puberty or later but the dens itself is separated by cartilage from the body of the axis until late in life.

14

The Face, Scalp and Parotid Gland

Surface Features

The skin of the face is attached to the underlying tissue, in which there are many subcutaneous muscles. In the scalp the skin is attached to a broad sheet of connective tissue. The red margin of the lips meet laterally at the *angle of the mouth* and the *philtrum* is the shallow vertical groove between the nose and red margin (*philtron = love potion, the groove on the upper lip*, Greek; the site where such a potion could be placed and act as an aphrodisiac).

Characteristically with advancing age lines appear in various parts of the face, transverse in the forehead, downwards and lateral from the attachment of the external nose to the angle of the mouth (*nasiolabial furrow*) and vertical from the angle of the mouth towards but not reaching the lower border of the mandible. These creases are due to the loss of elastic tissue in the deeper layer of the skin and can be reduced or eliminated by cosmetic surgery known as *face lifting*. This is almost literal in that incisions which are hidden by the hair are used to enable the surgeon to pull up the skin and so eliminate or reduce the lines.

The surface features of the eyelids and auricle are described with the eye (p. 266) and ear (p. 277). The depression of the bridge of the nose (nasion) and projection of the glabella *above it can be felt as can the* superciliary ridges *above the eyebrows. The bony edge of the orbit is palpable with its supra-orbital notch 2.5 cm from the midline. On the lateral side of the* boundary of the orbit, *there is a depression above the prominence of the cheek bone. This is the site of the* frontozygomatic suture. *Passing backwards from the cheekbone the* horizontal zygomatic arch *can be felt. This leads to the opening of the* external acoustic meatus *and the* auricle. *The posterior and inferior borders of the* ramus of the jaw *meet at the* angle *and behind and above the angle the* mastoid process *is palpable. In the midline at the back, just above the level of the mastoid process, the* external occipital protuberance *can be felt. The lower border of the mandible can be followed forwards and then towards the midline to the* prominence of the chin.

The Arteries, Nerves and Veins of the Face and Scalp (figures 134, 135)

The skin of both the scalp and face has a rich blood and nerve supply. *The* facial artery *can be felt pulsating as it crosses the lower border of the mandible 4 cm in front of its angle.* The artery runs towards the angle of the mouth then towards the junction of the nostril with the face and finally towards the inner angle of the eye. It gives off branches to the lips and the side of the nose and its terminal part is called the *angular artery*. The branches of the two facial arteries anastomose across the midline. Because of the rich blood supply, wounds of the face bleed freely and also heal readily without infection.

The scalp is supplied anteriorly by the *frontal artery* which comes from the orbit, laterally by the

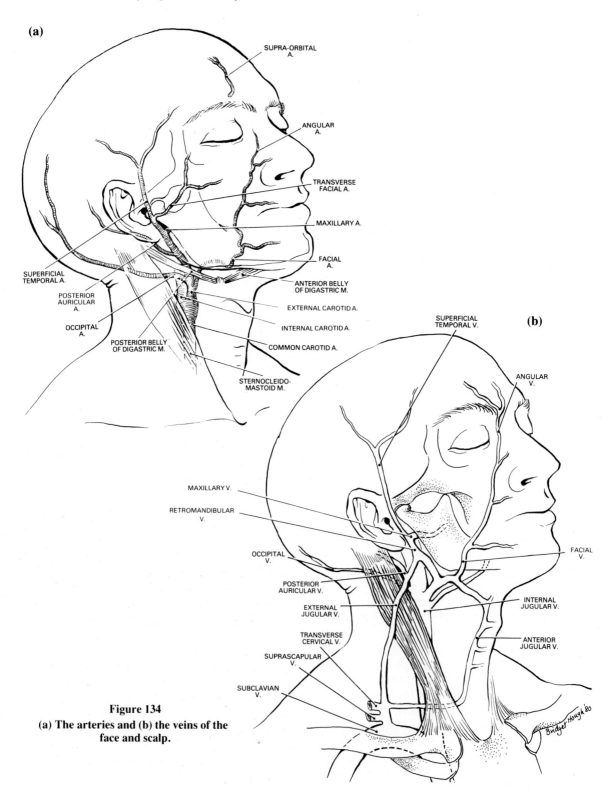

(a)

SUPRA-ORBITAL A.

ANGULAR A.

TRANSVERSE FACIAL A.

MAXILLARY A.

FACIAL A.

ANTERIOR BELLY OF DIGASTRIC M.

EXTERNAL CAROTID A.

INTERNAL CAROTID A.

COMMON CAROTID A.

STERNOCLEIDO-MASTOID M.

SUPERFICIAL TEMPORAL A.

POSTERIOR AURICULAR A.

OCCIPITAL A.

POSTERIOR BELLY OF DIGASTRIC M.

(b)

SUPERFICIAL TEMPORAL V.

ANGULAR V.

MAXILLARY V.

RETROMANDIBULAR V.

OCCIPITAL V.

POSTERIOR AURICULAR V.

EXTERNAL JUGULAR V.

TRANSVERSE CERVICAL V.

SUPRASCAPULAR V.

SUBCLAVIAN V.

FACIAL V.

INTERNAL JUGULAR V.

ANTERIOR JUGULAR V.

Figure 134
**(a) The arteries and (b) the veins of the
face and scalp.**

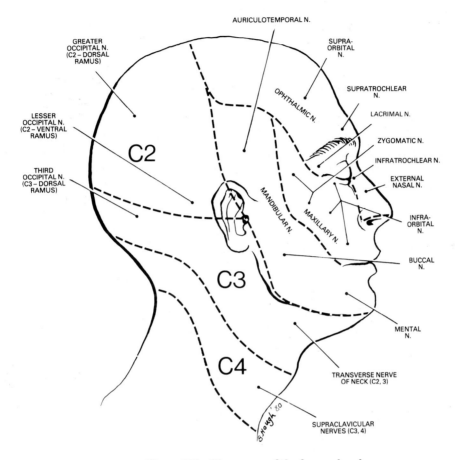

Figure 135   The nerves of the face and scalp.

superficial temporal and *posterior auricular arteries* and posteriorly by the *occipital artery*. The last three arteries are branches of the external carotid artery. *The superficial temporal artery can be felt pulsating as it crosses the posterior end of the zygomatic arch and may be seen wending its tortuous way upwards in the scalp*. It also gives off a *transverse facial branch* which runs forwards below the zygomatic arch.

The *trigeminal (fifth cranial) nerve* supplies the skin of the front and side of the scalp as far back as a line corresponding approximately to the auricle and all the skin of the forehead, eyelids, external nose, cheeks, lips and chin. The *ophthalmic nerve*, a major division of the trigeminal, supplies the skin of the front of the scalp as far back as the vertex through the *supra-orbital nerve* and more medially the *supratrochlear nerve*, the skin of the upper

eyelid and the conjunctiva through the *lacrimal nerve* laterally and the *infratrochlear nerve* medially, and the skin of the side of the nose except the edge of the naris (the external nasal aperture) by the *infratrochlear* and *external nasal nerves*. The *maxillary nerve*, the second division of the trigeminal, supplies the side of the scalp and the skin over the cheek bone (zygoma) through the *zygomatic nerve*, and the skin of the lower eyelid, anterior part of the cheek, edge of the naris and upper lip through the *infra-orbital nerve*. The *mandibular nerve*, the third division of the trigeminal, supplies the skin of the scalp above the auricle and the lateral surface of the auricle through the *auriculotemporal nerve*, the skin of the posterior part of the cheek through the *buccal nerve* and the skin of the lower lip and chin through the *mental nerve*.

The scalp behind the back of the auricle is supplied by ventral rami of the second and third cervical spinal nerves (the *great auricular* and the *lesser occipital nerves*) and the posterior part of the scalp is supplied by the dorsal rami of the second and third cervical spinal nerves (the *greater* and *third occipital nerves*). The great auricular nerve also supplies part of the lateral surface of the auricle.

The veins of the face and scalp correspond to some extent with the arteries but can take two routes to the main venous channels of the head and neck. The straight *facial vein* posterior to the tortuous facial artery is joined by a large anterior tributary from the *retromandibular vein* which as the name suggests lies behind the ramus of the mandible. The facial vein then runs into the neck and joins the *internal jugular vein*. The retromandibular vein itself is formed in the space deep to the ramus of the mandible by the union of the *superficial temporal* with the deep *maxillary vein*. In the parotid gland which lies behind the mandible the retromandibular vein divides into anterior and posterior branches. The posterior branch joins the *posterior auricular vein* and forms the *external jugular* vein which runs downwards as a superficial vein in the neck.

The veins of the front of the scalp and the facial vein communicate with the veins of the orbit and through these veins make connection with the veins (venous sinuses) inside the cranium. There are also many connections, *emissary veins*, between the veins of the scalp and the diploic veins and intracranial veins through foramina in the skull bones. Infection can therefore spread from the scalp and face to the intracranial region.

The Muscles of the Face and Scalp (figure 136)

They are usually referred to as the *muscles of facial expression* because this is one of their main functions. It is also a useful term because one of the muscles of mastication on the outer surface of the ramus of the mandible, the *masseter*, is in a literal sense a muscle of the face. The facial muscles are related to the openings of the orbit, mouth,

nasal cavity and external ear. Many of the muscles open or close these orifices. However, the function of the small muscles of the auricle, usually lost in man, is to move the auricle in order to direct sound waves into the external acoustic meatus. The muscles of the external nose retain their opening and closing functions to some extent. They were called the *dilatator naris* and *compressor naris* respectively but now have new names. The dilator muscle is seen to function in deep inspiration in many people, and inspiratory dilatation of the nostrils is seen in children with bronchopneumonia. Dilatation of the nostrils also occurs in some emotional states and is frequently used to express deep emotion in acting. Compression of the nostrils resulting in their closure may be very useful to a camel in a sandstorm.

The *orbicularis oculi* is an important muscle. Most of its fibres are arranged in a circular manner outside the edge of the opening of the orbit and in the eyelids. The outer *orbital part* is attached to the frontal bone and maxilla medially and sweeps round the orbital opening without bony attachment elsewhere. Some of the upper fibres are attached to the skin of the eyebrows. The fibres of the orbital part are coarser than those of the *palpebral part* (*palpebra* = *eyelid*, Latin) which is attached to the bone medially and in the eyelid lies in front of its connective tissue layer. Some fibres of the orbicularis oculi on the medial side (the *lacrimal part*) are attached to the bone behind the lacrimal sac. The sac lies in the nasolacrimal groove in the anterior part of the medial wall of the orbit. The palpebral part closes the eyes gently and voluntarily or in the involuntary act of blinking, and the orbital part closes the eyes firmly. The orbital part also pulls medially the skin of the forehead, temple and cheek adjacent to the orbit and produces radiating lines from the lateral angle of the eyelids. These frequently become visible as a result of sunbathing and become permanent with age. The lacrimal part can pull the eyelids medially and may open the lacrimal sac so that tears are sucked into the sac.

The *orbicularis oris* is a complex muscle surrounding and radiating from the opening into the mouth and forms the main substance of the lips and cheeks. If grouped, the different parts of the

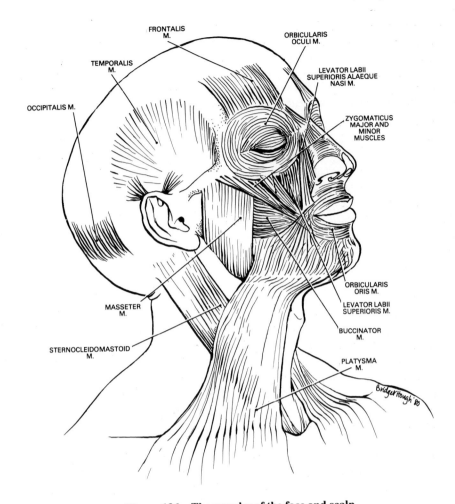

FRONTALIS M.

ORBICULARIS OCULI M.

TEMPORALIS M.

LEVATOR LABII SUPERIORIS ALAEQUE NASI M.

OCCIPITALIS M.

ZYGOMATICUS MAJOR AND MINOR MUSCLES

ORBICULARIS ORIS M.

LEVATOR LABII SUPERIORIS M.

MASSETER M.

BUCCINATOR M.

STERNOCLEIDOMASTOID M.

PLATYSMA M.

Bridger Hough '80

Figure 136   The muscles of the face and scalp.

muscle are more easily remembered.

(1) There are circular fibres which pass completely round the opening of the mouth in the lips and are regarded as the orbicularis oris muscle itself.

(2) There is an elevator of the upper lip (*levator labii superioris*) and of the angle of the mouth (*levator anguli oris*). These are attached to the maxilla. Three additional muscles assist in elevating the upper lip, one of which is attached to the side of the external nose as well (*levator labii superioris alaeque nasi*). The other two are attached to the zygomatic bone (*zygomaticus major* and *minor*).

(3) There is a depressor of the lower lip (*depressor labii inferioris*) and of the angle of the mouth

(*depressor anguli oris*). These are attached to the body of the mandible.

(4) There are three muscles which enter the angle of the mouth. The smallest is the *risorius*, which is placed more or less horizontally and extends backwards into the cheek for a variable distance. The *platysma* is a subcutaneous muscle of the neck which forms a wide, flat sheet and extends upwards over the mandible to the angle of the mouth (*platysma = flat sheet*, Greek). The *buccinator* is the deepest and most important of these muscles. Its main posterior attachment is to the *pterygomandibular raphe*, which extends from the hamulus of the medial pterygoid plate to the posterior end of the mylohyoid line. The buccinator is also attached to the outer surfaces of the

maxilla and mandible opposite the molar teeth. Posteriorly the muscle is deep to the ramus of the mandible but as it passes forwards it becomes more superficial and forms the main muscle of the cheek. It continues into the lips, with the central fibres crossing so that the lower fibres enter the upper lip and the upper fibres the lower lip.

There are also slips of muscle radiating from the incisive fossae of the maxillae and mandible towards the angles of the mouth, and a vertical muscle near the midline passing downwards into the lower lip towards the chin (*mentalis*).

There are two pairs of muscles in the scalp at the front and back of its aponeurotic layer. The *occipitalis muscles* are attached posteriorly to the highest nuchal lines of the occipital bone but the *frontalis muscles* over the frontal bone have no bony attachment.

The nerve supply and functions of the muscles

The *facial* (*seventh cranial*) *nerve* supplies all the muscles of the face and scalp (figure 137(a)). The nerve leaves the skull through the stylomastoid foramen in the temporal bone and runs forwards lateral to the styloid process into the parotid gland. Before entering the parotid gland it gives off a branch which runs upwards behind the ear and supplies some of the auricular muscles and the occipitalis. Five branches emerge from the edge of the parotid gland. An upper *temporal branch* runs upwards and supplies the frontalis and orbicularis oculi and a *zygomatic branch* runs anteriorly and superiorly and supplies the orbicularis oculi and some of the muscles entering the upper lip. The *buccal branch* runs forwards in the cheek and supplies the buccinator and muscles entering the upper lip. The *mandibular branch* runs below the angle and lower border of the mandible and then ascends and supplies the muscles entering the lower lip. The *cervical branch* runs downwards deep to the platysma and supplies it. All these branches communicate with the sensory branches of the trigeminal nerve of the face.

The functions of the orbicularis oculi and the nasal muscles have already been referred to. The muscles of the lips are involved in all their motor functions such as sucking, chewing, swallowing and speech. A baby born with a bilateral *cleft (hare) lip* cannot form a seal round a nipple or teat and requires at least a temporary operation to enable it to do so. Socially speaking it is unfortunate that it is possible to chew with the lips separated but luckily this is interrupted because it is difficult to swallow with the lips apart. Sounds in speech such as *b, p, ph, m*, require the use of the lips in various ways and the muscles of the lips produce the different shapes required for different vowel sounds.

The muscles of facial expression are aptly named when one considers the use of the forehead muscles for surprise, disapproval and anxiety, the eyes and mouth for smiling, the mouth for sadness and derision. The buccinator (*buccinator = trumpeter*, Latin) is used to expel air from the mouth but one of its most important functions is to push the food back between the teeth during chewing. The buccinators are obviously used in blowing the trumpet but the lips also function in a variety of skilful ways for playing different types of wind instrument.

Paralysis of the facial muscles follows damage to the facial nerve. This condition, known as *facial* or *Bell's palsy* (C. Bell, 1774–1842, Scottish surgeon and physiologist), occurs spontaneously, although it has been suggested that it may be due to the nerve swelling in the bony canal in which it fits tightly with the result that its blood supply is cut off. Why the nerve swells is not known. In Bell's palsy the face is pulled to the unaffected side because of the unopposed action of the normal muscles of the opposite side of the face. On the paralysed side the eyebrow cannot be raised, the forehead wrinkled, the eye closed, nor the nose twitched, and the patient cannot smile, whistle or snarl on the affected side (the platysma is involved in pulling the angle of the mouth downwards and raising vertical folds in the neck). Sleep is possible because the eyeball is pulled upwards and outwards so that the cornea (clear part of the eye) is covered. Food collects between the gum and the cheek because the buccinator is paralysed. Full recovery occurs in about 50 per cent of cases and anything from a minor to a complete paralysis may persist.

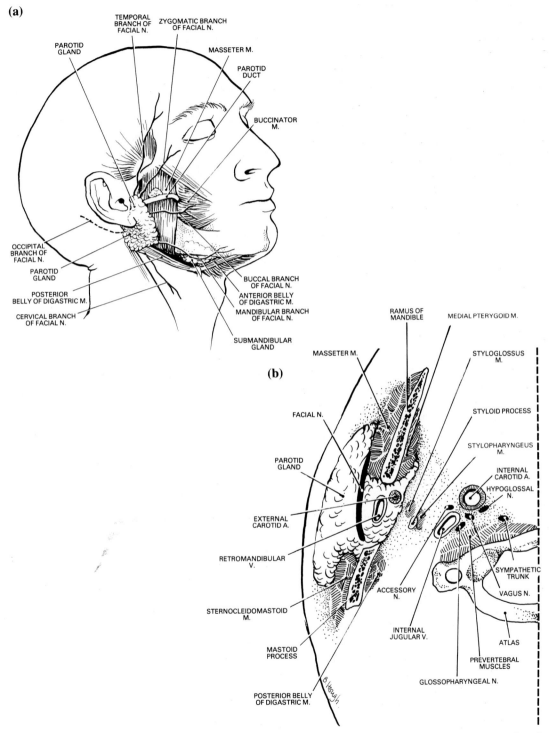

(a)

PAROTID
GLAND

TEMPORAL
BRANCH OF
FACIAL N.

ZYGOMATIC BRANCH
OF FACIAL N.

MASSETER M.

PAROTID
DUCT

BUCCINATOR
M.

OCCIPITAL
BRANCH OF
FACIAL N.

PAROTID
GLAND

POSTERIOR
BELLY OF DIGASTRIC M.

CERVICAL BRANCH
OF FACIAL N.

BUCCAL BRANCH
OF FACIAL N.

ANTERIOR BELLY
OF DIGASTRIC M.

MANDIBULAR BRANCH
OF FACIAL N.

SUBMANDIBULAR
GLAND

(b)

MASSETER M.

FACIAL N.

PAROTID
GLAND

EXTERNAL
CAROTID A.

RETROMANDIBULAR
V.

STERNOCLEIDOMASTOID
M.

MASTOID
PROCESS

POSTERIOR BELLY
OF DIGASTRIC M.

RAMUS OF
MANDIBLE

MEDIAL PTERYGOID M.

STYLOGLOSSUS
M.

STYLOID PROCESS

STYLOPHARYNGEUS
M.

INTERNAL
CAROTID A.

HYPOGLOSSAL
N.

SYMPATHETIC
TRUNK

VAGUS N.

ATLAS

PREVERTEBRAL
MUSCLES

GLOSSOPHARYNGEAL N.

INTERNAL
JUGULAR V.

ACCESSORY
N.

Figure 137   The parotid gland: (a) surface view; (b) as seen in a horizontal section between the skull and atlas.

The Structure of the Scalp

The scalp consists of five layers. The outermost layer is hairy skin, the second layer is connective tissue and the third the aponeurotic layer in which are the occipitalis and frontalis muscles. The third layer is called the *galea aponeurotica* or *epicranial aponeurosis* (*galea = helmet*, Latin) and the muscles form its anterior and posterior parts. The skin is attached to the third layer by fibrous septa so that all three layers move together. The epicranial aponeurosis is attached behind to the occipital bone by the occipitalis muscle. Laterally it is attached to the bone above the mastoid process and to the zygomatic arch and anteriorly it fuses with the fascia in the eyelids.

The blood vessels and nerves of the scalp lie in the second layer and the walls of the vessels are attached to the fibrous septa. A wound of the scalp bleeds profusely because the vessels' walls cannot contract and retract and because the scalp has a rich blood supply. This vascularity makes it possible for an avulsed scalp to be sewn back again. If this is done within a reasonable time the replaced tissue will survive. A wound which goes through the three layers gapes but the edges of a wound which does not penetrate the third layer remain together.

The fourth layer of the scalp is loose connective tissue and the fifth layer is the periosteum (pericranium) of the skull bones. Blood due to trauma or fluid due to infection spreads backwards in the fourth layer as far as the occiput, laterally as far as the zygomatic arches and anteriorly into the eyelids or even into the orbit. Fluid deep to the pericranium remains confined to the bone over which it lies because the pericranium on the outer surface of the bone is continuous with that of the inner surface at the fibrous tissue of the sutures.

The Parotid Gland

The Form, Position and Main Relations (figure 137)

The parotid gland (*para = beside, otis = of the ear*, Greek) is the largest of the salivary glands and lies between the ramus of the mandible and the mast-

oid process. It is described as wedge-shaped with the base of the wedge lying superficially and the two sides passing medially so that there are antero-medial and posteromedial surfaces. The gland also extends superficially over the masseter and sterno-cleidomastoid muscles. The gland has also been described as being shaped like a collar stud with the large part of the stud superficial. The facial nerve passes forwards on either side of the neck of the stud.

Most of the relations of the parotid gland are easily remembered if the fingers are placed point-ing medially between the ramus of the mandible and the mastoid process. Anteriorly it is related to the angle of the mandible and the muscles attached to it, the masseter to its outer surface, and the medial pterygoid to its medial surface. Posteriorly the gland is related to the mastoid process and the sternocleidomastoid which is attached to it. Super-iorly are the external auditory meatus and in front of the meatus the temporomandibular joint. By looking at a skull one can see that the medial edge of the gland reaches the styloid process and is therefore related to the muscles and ligaments attached to it. Deep to the styloid process the gland reaches the carotid sheath, containing the internal jugular vein, internal carotid artery and vagus nerve.

There are three important structures passing through the parotid gland. The most superficial is the facial nerve which passes forwards from behind and divides within the gland into its terminal branches appearing above, in front of and below the edge of the gland. Deep to the nerve the retro-mandibular vein is formed in the upper part of the gland (p. 194). In the lower part of the gland the vein divides and joins the external jugular vein and the facial vein. Deep to the veins the external car-otid artery runs upwards in the gland and at the level of the neck of the mandible divides into the superficial temporal and maxillary arteries. The superficial temporal artery passes behind the temporomandibular joint, emerges from the upper part of the gland and runs upwards over the post-erior end of the zygomatic arch. The maxillary artery runs forwards medial to the neck of the mandible.

The Capsule and Duct

The parotid gland has a fibrous capsule which is formed by a splitting of the deep cervical fascia. Superficially the capsule is attached to the zygomatic arch. The deep part of the capsule is attached to the styloid process and the mandible and a thickening of fascia forms the *stylomandibular ligament*. Several lymph nodes are related to the more superficial part of the gland and some of these lie outside and some inside the capsule.

The *parotid duct* is about 5 cm long and emerges from the anterior border of the gland. It runs forwards over the masseter at the anterior edge of which it turns medially at a right angle, pierces the buccinator and after running obliquely forwards for about 1 cm opens on a papilla on the inside of the cheek opposite the upper second molar tooth. The papilla is inflamed in the early stages of *mumps*, a virus infection of the parotid gland (*epidemic parotiditis*). A separate accessory part of the gland lies on the masseter above the duct. *With the teeth clenched the duct can be palpated as it crosses the anterior border of the masseter about 2 cm below the zygomatic arch. The duct is represented by the middle third of a line between the antitragus of the auricle (the projection below and behind the external meatus) and the middle of the junction of the nostril to the cheek and the angle of the mouth.*

The Blood Vessels and Nerves

The arteries are derived from the superficial temporal and facial arteries. The veins from the gland end in the external jugular vein. The secretomotor nerve supply comes from the parasympathetic part of the glossopharyngeal nerve. The preganglionic fibres come from the cells of the inferior salivary nucleus. The branch from the glossopharyngeal nerve runs a complicated course through the petrous temporal and ends in the otic ganglion which lies on the tensor veli palatini muscle (p. 207). The postganglionic fibres join the auriculotemporal nerve which enters the upper part of the gland before turning upwards over the posterior end of the zygomatic arch.

15

The Temporomandibular Joint and Related Structures

The region which is described in this chapter includes not only the joint but the muscles of mastication and their blood and nerve supply. These structures lie in the temporal and infratemporal fossae (figure 138). The former is deep to the zygomatic arch and the latter is in the base of the skull. In front of the infratemporal fossa, the pterygopalatine fossa lies between the pterygoid process of the sphenoid and the posterior surface of the maxilla (figure 138). Most of the structures described lie deep to the ramus of the mandible.

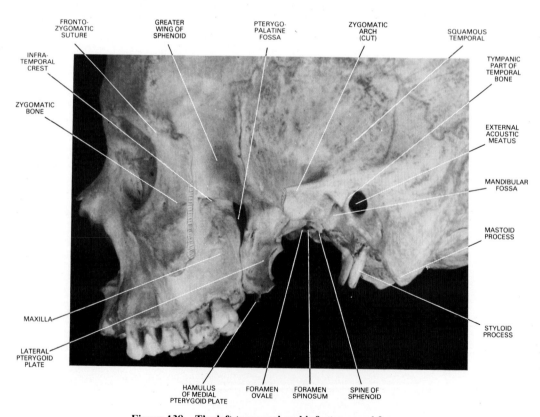

Figure 138   The left temporal and infratemporal fossae.

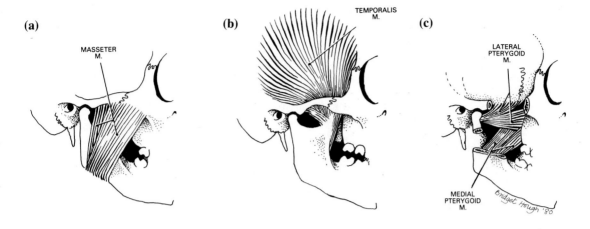

(a)   MASSETER M.

(b)   TEMPORALIS M.

(c)   LATERAL PTERYGOID M.

MEDIAL PTERYGOID M.

Bridget Hough '80

Figure 139   The muscles of mastication: (a) the masseter; (b) the temporalis; (c) the lateral and medial pterygoid muscles.

The Muscles of Mastication

This term is used to describe the main muscles which move the mandible rather than all the muscles involved in chewing. The *masseter muscle* (*maseter = a chewer*, Greek) is attached superiorly to the lower border and deep surface of the zygomatic arch and inferiorly to the outer surface of the ramus and the angle of the mandible (figure 139). Its anterior fibres slope somewhat backwards, are more superficial and may extend as far forwards as the maxilla. The attachment of the posterior deep fibres to the mandible reach as high as the coronoid process. The transverse facial artery, the parotid duct and branches of the facial nerve pass forwards superficial to the masseter, and the parotid gland overlaps the muscle from behind (figure 137). There is a considerable quantity of fat deep to the masseter, between it and the buccinator. This is called the *buccal* or *suctorial pad of fat*. It is comparatively large in an infant and together with the shape of the mandible gives the infant's face its charateristic roundness. It is unlikely that it has any effect on sucking. The masseter elevates the lower jaw and also tends to pull it forwards. *When the teeth are clenched the muscle is easily palpable and is used for finding the facial artery which crosses the lower border of the mandible just anterior to the masseter, and also the*

parotid duct which turns medially at its anterior border. The masseter is supplied by a branch of the mandibular nerve which enters its deep surface by passing through the mandibular notch.

The *temporalis muscle* (figure 139) is attached to the inferior of the two temporal lines and the bone on the side of the skull. These lines form an arch from the frontal bone in front, over the parietal bone, to the temporal bone behind. The *temporalis fascia* is attached to the superior of the two lines. The muscle fibres have an attachment to the deep surface of the fascia. Inferiorly the temporalis passes deep to the zygomatic arch, is attached to the coronoid process and anterior borders of the ramus of the mandible and extends on to its medial surface. The temporalis fascia is attached to the zygomatic arch.

The temporalis muscle pulls the mandible upwards as in closing the jaws. The muscle has posterior horizontal fibres which pull the mandible backwards. *When the teeth are clenched the anterior fibres can be felt above and posterior to the orbit.* The muscle is supplied by branches of the mandibular nerve. The superficial temporal vessels and the cutaneous nerves to the scalp run upwards on the muscle. The maxillary artery is deep to it.

The *lateral* and *medial pterygoid muscles* (figures 139, 140) are deep to the temporalis muscle. The lateral pterygoid is attached to the

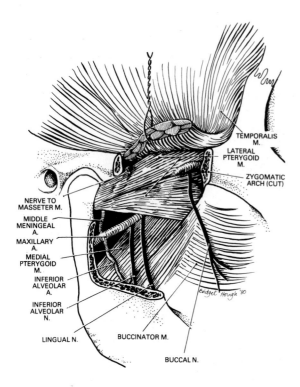

Figure 140   The structures related to the lateral and medial pterygoid muscles.

lateral surface of the lateral pterygoid plate and extends upwards on to the inferior surface of the greater wing of the sphenoid as far laterally as the vertical part of the greater wing. This junction of the horizontal part of the greater wing with the vertical part is marked by the *infratemporal crest*. The fibres of the lateral pterygoid muscle are horizontal and pass backwards to a pit on the anteromedial part of the neck of the mandible. The muscle is also attached to the capsule of the temporomandibular joint and passes through the capsule to be inserted into the disc within the joint. The lateral pterygoid thus pulls the jaw forwards and as it does so it pulls the disc forwards. The muscle is supplied by the mandibular nerve which lies deep to it.

The medial pterygoid muscle is attached to the medial side of the lateral pterygoid plate, the back of the maxilla and the part of the palatine bone which lies in the gap between the lower parts of the pterygoid plates (*the pyramidal process*). The

muscle passes downwards, backwards and laterally to become attached to the inner surface of the ramus of the mandible. In the gap between the muscle and the ramus the lingual and inferior alveolar nerves run forwards. The maxillary artery lies in this gap before passing deep to the lateral pterygoid muscle. The superior constrictor muscle of the pharynx is deep to the medial pterygoid which is supplied by the mandibular nerve. The medial pterygoid pulls the jaw upwards. It may pull the jaw to the opposite side because of its outward obliquity.

These muscles and their upper bony attachments lie in layers (figure 141). The most superficial layer is the masseter and zygomatic arch and the next is the temporalis and coronoid process. The third layer is the lateral pterygoid and the condylar process of the mandible, and the fourth layer more anteriorly is the medial pterygoid. The pharynx lies deep to the medial pterygoid in front and the lateral pterygoid posteriorly. The mandibular nerve is deep to the lateral pterygoid muscle and posterior to the medial pterygoid.

Other muscles are involved in mastication. The role of the *buccinator* (figure 136) has already

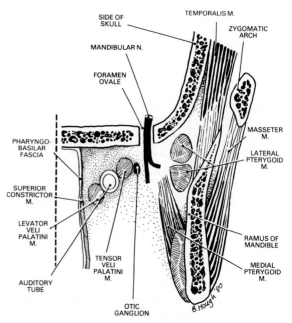

Figure 141   A diagram of the layers of the muscles of mastication in a coronal section of the skull.

been mentioned. In addition some of the muscles attached to the inside of the mandible are involved in opening the mouth – the *mylohyoid*, the *anterior belly of the digastric* and the *geniohyoid*.

The Temporomandibular Joint (figure 142)

In describing this joint as a condyloid synovial joint it should be appreciated that both joints are included. A *condyloid joint* by definition has two projections (condyles) and the two condyles of the mandible are regarded as parts of one joint. Normal functioning of the lower jaw always involves the two joints. On each side the joint is formed superiorly by the concave mandibular fossa extending forwards on to the convex articular

tubercle (eminence) of the temporal bone. The articular surface is limited posteriorly by the petrotympanic part of the temporal bone. The inferior surface of the joint is formed by the convex head of the condylar process of the mandible. The head is cylindrical in outline and is directed backwards as well as medially.

The capsule of the joint is attached superiorly to the temporal bone anterior to the petrotympanic fissure, round the articular area formed by the fossa and articular tubercle, and inferiorly to the neck of the condylar process. The lateral pterygoid muscle is attached to the capsule. The *ligaments* associated with the joint are the *lateral*, the *stylomandibular* and the *sphenomandibular*. The lateral ligament passes downwards and backwards from the posterior end of the zygomatic arch to the lateral and posterior surfaces of the neck of the

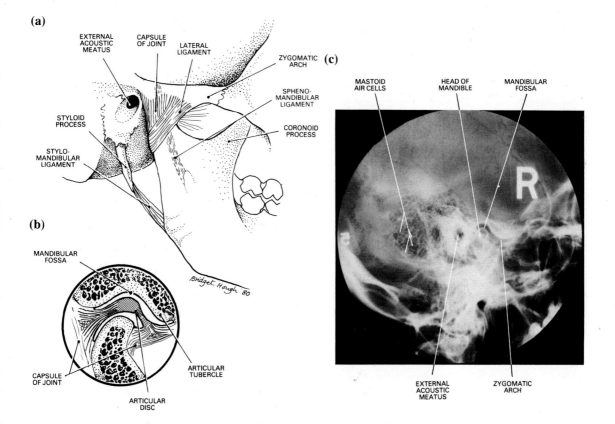

Figure 142   The temporomandibular joint: (a) the ligaments; (b) the articular disc; (c) an X-ray of the right joint.

mandible. The stylomandibular ligament is a thickening of the deep fascia extending from the styloid process to the angle of the mandible. The sphenomandibular ligament is attached superiorly to the spine of the sphenoid bone and inferiorly to the lingula of the mandible.

As in all synovial joints the capsule is lined by synovial membrane which in this joint extends upwards over the neck of the mandible as far as the articular cartilage. Unlike other synovial joints the articulating surfaces are covered by fibrocartilage.

The articular disc within the joint separates the cavity completely into two compartments. The disc is concavoconvex superiorly and concave inferiorly. It therefore fits the joint surfaces. It is attached anteriorly and posteriorly to the capsule and laterally and medially to the inferior surface of the head of the condylar process. The disc is thickest anteriorly where it is attached to the articular eminence, and thin or even perforated where it is related to the anterior wall of the mandibular fossa. Posteriorly the disc has an upper part which is elastic in structure, a lower part which is fibrous and an intervening region which consists of loose vascular tissue. Three different parts have been distinguished in the intermediate region (figure 142).

The neighbouring arteries and nerves supply the joint — the superficial temporal and maxillary arteries and the auriculotemporal and masseteric nerves.

The Movements at the Joint. The movements of the mandible can be described as lowering and raising the lower jaw, protrusion (protraction) and retraction, and side-to-side movements. Chewing involves all these movements to some extent. At the joint itself the movements may be either sliding (translation or gliding) or rotatory. In sliding the disc is pulled forwards together with the head, that is the movement takes place in the upper compartment, and in rotation the head rotates on the inferior surface of the disc, that is in the lower compartment.

Normal *opening of the mouth* begins with slight rotation which is followed by combined rotation and gliding until maximum opening is attained. The axis of movement is approximately through

the lingulae of the mandible, the lower attachment of the sphenomandibular ligaments. The forward movement of the mandibular head can be easily felt by placing a finger in front of or in the external acoustic meatus. The main muscle involved is the lateral pterygoid which is attached to the neck of the mandible, the capsule and the disc, and pulls the mandible and disc forwards. At the same time the digastric and geniohyoid muscles attached to the mandible near the midline anteriorly and the hyoid bone below, pull the jaw downwards so that it rotates. This movement is assisted by gravity and the relaxation of the muscles which close the jaw. The falling open of the jaw during sleep illustrates the effect of gravity. It is possible to pull the jaw backwards from the resting position and then lower the jaw without the normal forward gliding, but the opening of the mouth is much more limited. Opening the jaw against resistance involves the mylohyoid muscles.

When *closing the mouth* from the fully opened position there is initially a slight backward movement. This is followed by combined rotatory and gliding movements until the position of rest is reached. The muscles involved are the masseters, temporales, and medial pterygoids. These six muscles can produce a force varying between 25 and 50 kg. This is insufficient to support the body weight but it is possible for circus performers to hang by their teeth at the top of the tent by biting on a specially made bite-block which enables the forces involved to be applied to their teeth at right angles to their long axis. They are safe so long as they keep their mouth closed. Considerable pain and laceration can result from accidentally biting one's cheek or tongue.

Protrusion of the lower jaw requires slight opening of the mouth in most individuals since the lower front teeth are normally behind the upper front teeth in the position of rest. The mandible is pulled forwards by the lateral pterygoid muscles. *Retraction* is largely the restoration of the protruded jaw to the resting position and is due to relaxation of the lateral pterygoid muscles. The mandible can be pulled backwards for about 3 mm from the position of rest by the posterior horizontal fibres of the temporalis muscles.

Side-to-side movements of the lower jaw are

best described in the following way. When the jaw is moved to the left it rotates about the left condyle as the right condyle is pulled forwards by the right lateral pterygoid and possibly the right medial pterygoid. When the jaw is moved to the right it rotates about the right condyle and the left condyle is pulled forwards by the left pterygoid muscles.

The temporomandibular joint is not infrequently dislocated, usually on one side, often as the result of opening the mouth too widely. This may occur when yawning. The condylar process on the dislocated side becomes lodged in front of the articular tubercle and spasm of the lateral pterygoid muscles keeps it there. Reduction of the dislocation usually requires an anaesthetic to relax the muscles. The dislocation may be reduced by placing a thumb on each side between the back teeth and pushing downwards. This releases the condylar process and the jaw springs back into place. It is important to remove the thumbs quickly or take the preliminary precaution of wrapping something protective round them. Unfortunately in some cases the dislocation tends to recur on yawning, but it is inadvisable to attempt to avoid calls at night by teaching the patient or a relative how to reduce the dislocation.

The Temporal Fossa

This is the space between the zygomatic arch and the lateral wall of the skull (figures 126, 138). The main structure in the space is the temporalis muscle covered by the temporalis fascia. The muscle passes deep to the zygomatic arch to the coronoid process and ramus of the mandible. The fascia is attached to the arch. The parietal, frontal and temporal bones meet the greater wing of the sphenoid at the *pterion* (p. 175). The vessels and nerves to the temporalis lie between it and the skull. Anteriorly the *zygomaticotemporal nerve*, a branch of the maxillary nerve, emerges from the deep surface of the zygomatic bone and passes upwards to the scalp.

The Infratemporal Fossa

This fossa is medial to the anterior part of the temporal fossa and lies below the horizontal part of the greater wing of the sphenoid bone in the base of the skull (figure 138). The medial limit of the fossa is the lateral pterygoid plate and its anterior limit is the posterior surface of the maxilla. In this region there are the lateral and medial pterygoid muscles, the maxillary artery and vein, the pterygoid plexus of veins and the mandibular nerve which is deep to the lateral pterygoid muscle.

The Pterygopalatine Fossa (figure 138)

This is the narrow space between the posterior wall of the maxilla anteriorly and the pterygoid process of the sphenoid bone posteriorly. Medially the fossa is limited by the perpendicular plate of the palatine bone. The lateral opening into the fossa is called the *pterygomaxillary fissure*, through which the maxillary artery enters and the vein leaves the fossa. The fossa also contains the maxillary nerve and the pterygopalatine ganglion which is attached to the nerve.

The Mandibular and Maxillary Nerves and the Maxillary Vessels

The mandibular nerve and otic ganglion

It is convenient to include a description of these structures with the fossae. The *mandibular nerve*, the third division of the trigeminal nerve, emerges from the skull through the foramen ovale in the greater wing of the sphenoid bone. It is deep to the lateral pterygoid muscle and lateral to the pharynx immediately below the skull. The pharynx in this region consists of fascia through which pass two muscles and the *auditory (Eustachian) tube*. The *levator veli palatini* is inferior and medial to the tube and the *tensor veli palatini* is superior and lateral (figure 141). It should be appreciated that the upper border of the superior constrictor of the pharynx, as it passes backwards and then medially from the pterygoid hamulus at the lower end of the medial pterygoid plate to the pharyngeal tubercle on the occipital bone, leaves, inferior to the base of the skull, a triangular space in which lie the two muscles and the auditory tube (figures 194, 195). The mandibular nerve is lateral to the tensor veli palatini and the otic ganglion lies between the nerve and muscle.

The mandibular nerve is about 1.5 cm long and divides into its two main branches, anterior and posterior (figure 143). There are two branches from the main trunk, the *nervous spinosus*, which passes back into the skull through the foramen spinosum and is sensory to the dura mater, and the *nerve to the medial pterygoid muscle*. All the branches of the anterior division are motor except for its continuation, the *buccal nerve*. The *motor branches* are to the *temporalis* and *masseter muscles*, which pass laterally above the lateral pterygoid muscle,

and to the *lateral pterygoid* itself. The buccal nerve passes forwards between the two heads of the lateral pterygoid muscle on to the buccinator and is sensory to the skin and mucous membrane of the lower part of the cheek (figure 140).

The posterior division divides into three large almost entirely sensory branches – the *auriculo-temporal*, *inferior alveolar* and *lingual nerves*; the inferior alveolar has a motor branch. The *auriculo-temporal nerve* is usually described as arising by two roots which embrace the middle meningeal artery. The nerve then passes laterally behind the temporomandibular joint and turns upwards over the posterior end of the zygomatic arch behind the superficial temporal artery. The nerve is distributed mainly to the scalp over the temporal region and also supplies a small part of the skin of the outer surface of the auricle. It is one of the nerves supplying the external acoustic meatus, tympanic membrane and temporomandibular joint. The auriculo-temporal nerve conveys the secretomotor fibres to the parotid gland. These fibres are postganglionic parasympathetic with their cell bodies in the otic ganglion.

The *lingual* and *inferior alveolar nerves* pass downwards deep to the lateral pterygoid muscle and emerge from its lower border to pass forwards between the medial pterygoid muscle and the ramus of the mandible (figure 140). The lingual nerve is anterior and above the inferior alveolar (this is easily remembered by placing the tongue above the lower teeth). The further course of the nerves is outside the region being considered but will be described here and referred to again (p. 222). The lingual nerve then lies under the mucous membrane of the mouth in a groove on the medial side of the body of the mandible at the level of the roots of the third molar tooth. *It can be palpated in this part of its course.* The nerve then passes on to the hyoglossus muscle deep to the mylohyoid muscle and runs forwards into the tongue (figure 144). While lying in this position, the deep part of the submandibular gland is inferior to it, the submandibular ganglion is attached to it, and the hypoglossal nerve is inferior. While on the hyoglossus the nerve crosses lateral to, then below and then medial to the submandibular duct.

The lingual nerve while it is deep to the lateral

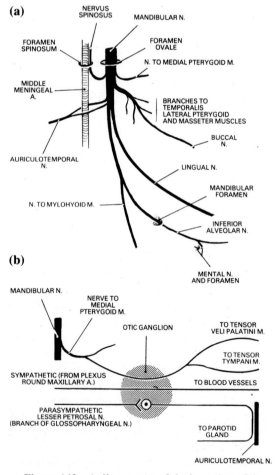

Figure 143   A diagram (a) of the branches of the mandibular nerve, (b) of the connections of the otic ganglion.

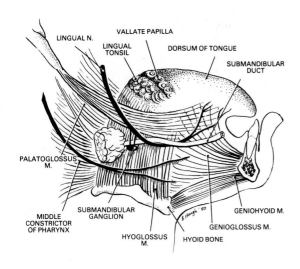

LINGUAL N.
VALLATE PAPILLA
LINGUAL TONSIL
DORSUM OF TONGUE
SUBMANDIBULAR DUCT
PALATOGLOSSUS M.
MIDDLE CONSTRICTOR OF PHARYNX
SUBMANDIBULAR GANGLION
HYOGLOSSUS M.
HYOID BONE
GENIOGLOSSUS M.
GENIOHYOID M.

Figure 144   The relations of the lingual nerve as it lies on the hyoglossus muscle.

pterygoid muscle is joined by a branch of the facial nerve, the *chorda tympani*. The lingual nerve itself is a nerve of general sensation and is distributed to the mucous membrane of the anterior part of the tongue (the part in front of the sulcus terminalis), the floor of the mouth and the lingual surface of the gingiva. The chorda tympani conveys taste fibres from the anterior part of the tongue and preganglionic parasympathetic fibres to the submandibular ganglion. The postganglionic fibres from the ganglion are secretomotor to the sublingual and submandibular salivary glands.

The inferior alveolar nerve passes between the sphenomandibular ligament and the ramus of the mandible and after entering the mandibular foramen runs forwards in the mandibular canal towards the mental symphysis. Before entering the mandibular foramen the inferior alveolar nerve gives off the *nerve to the mylohyoid muscle* which runs downwards in a groove on the mandible inferior to the muscle and supplies the muscle and the anterior belly of the digastric. While in the mandibular canal the nerve supplies the teeth and gives off its *mental branch* which emerges from the mental foramen and is distributed to the skin and mucous membrane of the lower lip and chin from the angle of the mouth to the midline.

It is convenient to describe the *otic ganglion* which is medial to the mandibular nerve and lateral to the tensor veli palatini (figure 141). It is one of the parasympathetic ganglia of the head and neck. Although all these ganglia are associated with branches of the trigeminal nerve, their parasympathetic component comes from a different cranial nerve. In the case of the otic ganglion its parasympathetic fibres come from the glossopharyngeal (ninth cranial) nerve. All the ganglia receive three types of fibre, sympathetic, somatic motor or sensory, and parasympathetic. The first two types of fibre pass through the ganglia and the parasympathetic fibres synapse in the ganglia. The otic ganglion receives postganglionic sympathetic fibres from the plexus round the maxillary artery and they leave the ganglion to go to the blood vessels of the parotid gland. The motor fibres come from the nerve to the medial pterygoid muscle and leave the ganglion to supply the tensor veli palatini and tensor tympani muscles. The parasympathetic fibres reach the ganglion from the glossopharyngeal nerve by a very devious route. A branch of this nerve arises just below the skull, enters the petrous temporal bone and goes to a nerve plexus on the medial wall of the middle ear. From there the fibres leave the middle ear as the *lesser petrosal nerve* which enters the cranial cavity and leaves the skull through or near the foramen ovale to join the otic ganglion. These fibres synapse in the ganglion and the postganglionic fibres join the auriculotemporal nerve and supply the parotid gland with secretomotor and vasodilator fibres.

The *general motor and sensory distribution of the mandibular nerve* is as follows. The motor branches supply the masseter, temporalis, lateral and medial pterygoids, mylohyoid, anterior belly of the digastric, tensor veli palatini and tensor tympani, all derived from the mesoderm of the first pharyngeal (branchial) arch. The sensory branches supply the skin of the side of the scalp, part of the skin of the auricle, external acoustic meatus and cheek, the skin of the lower lip, the mucous membrane of the mandibular gingiva, floor of the mouth and anterior two-thirds of the tongue and all the teeth of one half of the lower jaw and possibly the lower central incisor of the other side. It also supplies the dura mater of the middle cranial fossa.

Disease affecting one part of the distribution of the nerve may produce pain referred to the distribution of another branch; for example, caries in a lower tooth can produce pain referred to the ear. In certain conditions affecting the mandibular nerve characterised by spontaneous pain from the areas supplied by its branches, it may be necessary to attempt to destroy the fibres of the nerve by injecting alcohol into the nerve. The nerve is reached by passing a needle through the masseter, mandibular notch and lateral pterygoid muscle and thus injecting the main trunk below the foramen ovale (figure 141). In cancer of the tongue associated with intractable pain the lingual nerve may be cut as it lies next to the mandible. When a dentist injects an anaesthetic around the inferior alveolar nerve the lingual nerve is also affected. Although almost inevitable it is also necessary in order to anaesthetise the labial gingiva.

The maxillary nerve and pterygopalatine ganglion

Only a small part of this nerve is seen in this region, that is in the pterygopalatine fossa, but because

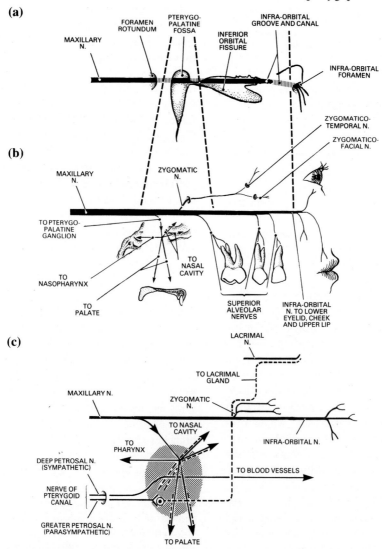

Figure 145   The maxillary nerve: a diagram of (a) its course, (b) its branches, (c) the pterygopalatine (sphenopalatine) ganglion. (The interrupted lines indicate postganglionic parasympathetic fibres.)

so many of the branches of the nerve arise in the fossa the nerve is described here. The maxillary nerve, the second division of the trigeminal nerve, leaves the skull through the foramen rotundum in the greater wing of the sphenoid bone (figure 145). (This foramen can be seen only from the inside of the skull.) The nerve passes forwards into the pterygopalatine fossa and continues into the orbit through the medial part of the inferior orbital fissure. The nerve runs forwards on the floor of the orbit into the infra-orbital groove which becomes the infra-orbital canal and opens on to the face at the infra-orbital foramen. It is possible to pass a flexible wire from the foramen rotundum through everything which has been named so that the tip of the wire appears on the face. The maxillary nerve is called the *infra-orbital nerve* after it enters the orbit.

In the pterygopalatine fossa the maxillary nerve gives off (1) the *zygomatic nerve*, which enters the orbit through the inferior orbital fissure; (2) *branches to the pterygopalatine ganglion*; (3) the *posterior superior alveolar nerve*, which enters the posterior wall of the maxilla and supplies the molar teeth (figure 145(b)). The zygomatic nerve divides near the front of the orbit into two branches which pass through the zygomatic bone. One branch, the *zygomaticofacial*, ends in the skin over the zygomatic bone and the other, the *zygomaticotemporal*, ends in the scalp in the temporal region. The branches to the ganglion continue uninterruptedly through the ganglion and emerge as five branches: (1) the *nasopalatine nerve*, which enters the nasal cavity through the sphenopalatine foramen and mainly supplies the septum of the nose and the palate; (2) the *lateral posterior superior nasal nerves*, which enter the nasal cavity through the same foramen and supply part of the lateral wall of the nose; (3) the *greater* and (4) the *lesser palatine branches*, which pass downwards to the posterolateral angle of the hard palate and supply the palate and palatine tonsil; (5) the *pharyngeal branch*, which passes backwards in the roof of the pterygopalatine fossa to the nasopharynx.

The infra-orbital nerve in the orbit gives off the *middle* and *anterior superior alveolar nerves* which run in the lateral wall of the maxilla to the pre-molar, canine and incisor teeth. The infra-orbital nerve on the face is distributed to the lower eyelid, anterior part of the cheek, the upper lip and the edge of the anterior nasal aperture.

The *pterygopalatine (sphenopalatine) ganglion* is attached to the maxillary nerve and lies near the medial wall of the fossa (figure 145(c)). It receives a large sensory branch from the maxillary nerve which leaves the ganglion as the branches already referred to. In addition the *nerve of the pterygoid canal* joins the ganglion. This nerve, which comes from the middle cranial fossa, contains postganglionic sympathetic fibres from the plexus surrounding the internal carotid artery (*deep petrosal nerve*) and preganglionic parasympathetic fibres from the facial nerve (*greater petrosal nerve*). The parasympathetic fibres synapse in the ganglion and the postganglionic fibres either return to the maxillary nerve and travel with the zygomatic branch into the orbit and supply secretomotor fibres to the lacrimal gland, or go independently into the orbit to the gland. In the orbit the fibres usually join the lacrimal nerve before supplying the gland. Mucous glands in the palate, nasal cavity and nasopharynx may receive a parasympathetic secretomotor innervation through branches of the ganglion travelling in the sensory nerves already mentioned. The sympathetic fibres pass through the gland and supply blood vessels.

The general distribution of the maxillary nerve is as follows. It gives off a meningeal branch before it leaves the skull. Outside the skull it supplies the skin of the side of the scalp, the front of the cheek, the lower eyelid, the upper lip and a small part of the edge of the nostril. It also supplies most of the mucous membrane of the nasal cavity, the roof of the mouth (both surfaces of the soft and hard palate), the upper teeth and gingiva and the lining of the maxillary air sinus. Disease involving any part supplied by the maxillary nerve may result in pain being referred to another site. Intractable pain from the area of distribution of the maxillary nerve may be treated by injection of alcohol into the nerve as it lies in the pterygopalatine fossa. The needle is inserted below the middle of the zygomatic arch and directed medially in front of the lateral pterygoid plate to a depth of 6–7 cm.

(a)

(b)

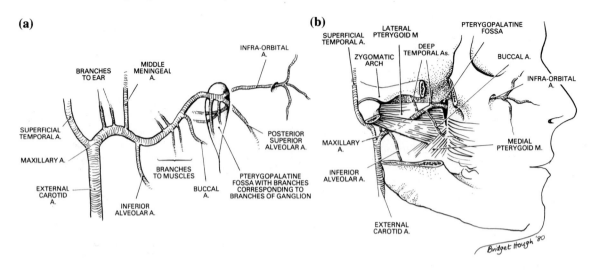

Figure 146   The maxillary artery: (a) its branches; (b) its main relations.

The maxillary artery and vein (figure 146)

This artery is one of the terminal branches of the external carotid which divides behind the neck of the mandible in the parotid gland. The maxillary artery passes deep to the neck of the mandible between it and the sphenomandibular ligament. It then runs forwards and medially deep to the temporalis muscle and passes either medial to the lower head of the lateral pterygoid muscle or between its two heads and enters the pterygopalatine fossa where it lies anterior to the ganglion.

The branches of the artery correspond to a large extent with the branches of the mandibular and maxillary nerves. There are branches to the external acoustic meatus (corresponding with the auricular part of the auriculotemporal nerve) and the middle ear (running a similar course to that of the chorda tympani branch of the facial nerve). The *middle meningeal artery* enters the cranial cavity through the foramen spinosum and the *accessory meningeal* through the foramen ovale. The middle meningeal artery is an important branch. It runs upwards between the sphenomandibular ligament and lateral pterygoid muscle and then between the roots of the auriculotemporal nerve before entering the foramen spinosum. Inside the skull it runs laterally and forwards on the squamous part of the temporal bone for about 1–2 cm and divides into an *anterior (frontal)* and *posterior (parietal) branch*.

The anterior branch runs more or less upwards on to the greater wing of the sphenoid towards the antero-inferior angle of the parietal bone. In this part of its course the anterior branch lies in a groove or canal and is near the pterion. The anterior branch continues on the parietal bone about 1 cm behind the coronal suture and then divides into branches which pass upwards and also backwards. The posterior branch curves backwards on the squamous temporal and parietal bones. The middle meningeal artery supplies the trigeminal ganglion and the roots of the trigeminal nerve and the middle ear as well as the dura mater and the diploe of the bones of the vault of the skull. The surface markings of the intracranial course of the middle meningeal artery is as follows. *Its entry through the foramen spinosum is marked by the posterior end of the zygomatic arch. It divides 2 cm above the middle of the arch. The anterior branch crosses the pterion which is 4 cm above the middle of the arch and continues towards the vertex of the skull to a point midway between the nasion and glabella.* It lies lateral to the motor area of the cerebral cortex in this part of its course.

The importance of the middle meningeal artery lies in the possibility of its being torn in linear fractures of the temporal region due to blows on the side of the skull. Its anterior branch is particularly liable to be damaged as it lies in the groove or canal on the parietal bone near the pterion. This results in an *extradural haemorrhage* which develops rapidly and produces compression effects on the brain. These effects become increasingly obvious within 24 h following injury and the possibility of such a complication after a blow on the side of the head must be kept in mind. Death will ensue unless the skull is opened, usually by trephining, the blood or clot removed and the torn artery tied. This life-saving procedure usually results in complete recovery.

The *inferior alveolar artery* runs with the nerve of the same name and gives off similar branches, namely the mylohyoid and mental.

The next group of branches go to the muscles of mastication — the *masseteric*, *temporal* and *pterygoid*. There is a *buccal branch* which accompanies the buccal nerve to the surface of the buccinator.

The maxillary artery gives off a number of branches in the pterygopalatine fossa — the *posterior superior alveolar*, the *greater palatine* (which gives off lesser palatine branches), the *artery of the pterygoid canal*, the *pharyngeal*, and the *sphenopalatine*. The sphenopalatine artery enters the nasal cavity and supplies both the lateral wall and the septum. The maxillary artery ends as the *infra-orbital artery* which has a similar course and distribution as the infra-orbital nerve.

The *maxillary vein* is a short vessel which drains the pterygoid plexus of veins lying between the temporalis and lateral pterygoid muscles. This plexus receives many of the veins corresponding with the muscular branches of the artery and the branches which arise in the pterygopalatine fossa. The plexus communicates with the intracranial venous sinuses, particularly the cavernous sinus through the adjacent foramina and also with the facial vein. The maxillary vein passes backwards between the sphenomandibular ligament and the neck of the mandible and joins the superficial

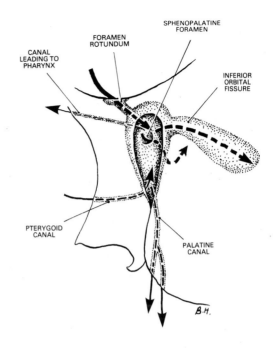

Figure 147   The pterygopalatine fossa.

temporal vein to form the retromandibular vein (p. 194).

The pterygopalatine fossa presents some difficulties which may be alleviated by a description of the foramina, etc., which enter and leave it (figure 147). Laterally the *pterygomaxillary fissure* leads into the fossa from the infratemporal region. Medially the *sphenopalatine foramen* opens into the nasal cavity at the posterior end of the middle concha. Posteriorly the canal for the pharyngeal branch of the maxillary nerve and artery, the *foramen rotundum* and the *pterygoid canal* open into the fossa. Anteriorly the fossa opens into the orbit through the *inferior orbital fissure*. The *palatine canal* passes downwards to the posterolateral angle of the hard palate.

16

The Neck I

The skeleton of the neck is formed by the seven cervical vertebrae (p. 186). The upper three or four vertebrae lie above the level of the lower border of the mandible so that the neck may be said to extend upwards towards the base of the skull behind the mandible. The length of the neck is variable and a graceful, long neck is apparently necessary for success as a ballet dancer. It is unlikely, however, that the ability to dance even classical ballet depends on the length of one's neck. Among some tribes lengthening of the neck by wearing metal rings is more apparent than real, and is achieved by pushing down the ribs and clavicle (figure 148). The result is that the neck muscles atrophy and if the rings are removed the head falls over and suffocation ensues, unless a brace is used and the muscles are exercised. Removal of the rings was used as a punishment for adultery.

The neck contains in the midline the downward continuations of the alimentary and respiratory tracts, blood vessels and their branches, lymph nodes and lymphatic vessels, several groups of muscles (prevertebral, infra- and suprahyoid, and long superficial muscles, the sternocleidomastoid and trapezius), the last cranial nerves, the cervical spinal nerves forming the cervical plexus, the beginning of the brachial plexus and the cervical part of the sympathetic trunk.

The Skin and Surface Markings

Anteriorly the skin of the neck usually shows a

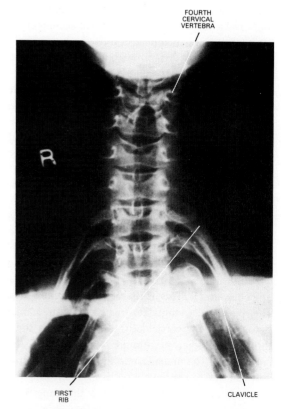

FOURTH
CERVICAL
VERTEBRA

R

FIRST
RIB

CLAVICLE

Figure 148 **An anteroposterior X-ray of the neck of a Padaung tribeswoman of Burma after the removal of the metal rings worn round her neck (reproduced by kind permission of John M. Kershishian, Washington, D.C.). Compare with figure 132(d).**

number of transverse creases, the number of which is determined to some extent by the amount of fat. On the back of the neck the skin is bound down to the underlying fascia. Frequently in old age vertical folds appear in the front of the neck due to the loss of elastic tissue in the deeper layers of the skin.

The ventral rami of the second, third and fourth cervical nerves supply the skin of the neck except for a strip of skin supplied by their dorsal rami on either side of the midline at the back. The second and third cervical nerves supply the skin behind the auricle by the *lesser occipital nerve*, the skin of and below the auricle by the *great auricular nerve*, and the skin below the mandible by the *transverse cervical nerve*. The skin inferior to this area, extending to the clavicle, is supplied by the *supraclavicular nerves* (from the third and fourth cervical nerves) (figure 135). The dorsal rami of the second and third cervical nerves (the *greater occipital* and *third occipital nerves* respectively) and the *dorsal ramus of the fourth cervical nerve* supply the skin at the back of the neck.

The lower border of the mandible, *its angle and the posterior border of the ramus can be palpated. The* mastoid process *is easily felt behind the ear and midway between the mastoid process and angle of the mandible the* transverse process of the atlas *can be palpated. The* body of the hyoid bone, *the* laryngeal prominence *(Adam's apple), the* cricoid cartilage *and the* rings of the trachea *are palpable in the midline in the front of the neck.*

Inferiorly passing from the midline laterally, the jugular notch, *the projecting* medial end of the clavicle, *the* sternoclavicular joint, *the* clavicle *and the* acromioclavicular joint *mark the lower limit of the neck. Above the medial third of the clavicle, the* first rib *can be pressed upon especially if the head is inclined to the same side. The lateral sloping line from the neck to the shoulder is formed by the underlying* trapezius muscle *which can be followed downwards to the clavicle and acromion. In the midline at the back if the head is bent forwards the* spinous processes of the sixth and seventh cervical *and* first thoracic vertebrae *are visible. The most prominent is usually that of the first thoracic vertebra. The upper cervical vertebrae cannot be palpated posteriorly. The* external occipital protuberance *can be felt in the midline superiorly.*

Anteriorly in the midline the body of the hyoid bone *can be felt and followed laterally to its* greater cornua (horns) *which are more easily palpable than the body especially if the thumb and index finger are applied to the sides of the neck. The* laryngeal prominence *of the* thyroid cartilage *and the* cricoid cartilage *can be followed laterally although the lower part of the thyroid cartilage is obscured by overlying structures. The hyoid bone is only slightly inferior to the lower edge of the mandible unless the head is tilted backwards and is at the level of the third or fourth cervical vertebra. The cricoid cartilage is at the level of the sixth cervical vertebra and the jugular notch at the level of the second thoracic vertebra.*

The hyoid bone (figure 149)

This bone is shaped like the letter U and has a central *body* which is about 1 cm in height and 3 cm wide. (The Greek letter U becomes a Y in English; aspirate the Y, that is add the letter H, and add the suffix *oid = like* and the result is the word *hyoid*.) The lower part of the body on each side continues backwards and somewhat upwards as the *greater cornua* which are about 3 cm long. The

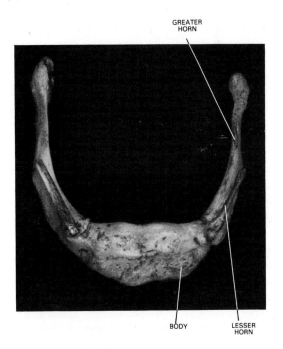

GREATER
HORN

BODY

LESSER
HORN

Figure 149   The hyoid bone.

lesser cornua project backwards from the upper lateral angle of the body and are about 1 cm long. The upper part of the body of the hyoid bone and the lesser cornua develop from the second pharyngeal arch and the lower part of the body and the greater cornua from the third pharyngeal arch. The bone ossifies in cartilage from six centres, two for the body and one for each horn. Ossification begins late in fetal life and shortly after birth. The lesser cornua frequently remain attached by fibrous tissue to the body. The hyoid bone has a large number of muscles attached to it. They can be grouped as those superior to the bone, *suprahyoid*, and those inferior to the bone, *infrahyoid*. The hyoid bone is attached to the thyroid cartilage by the thyrohyoid membrane and to the styloid process of the temporal bone by the stylohyoid ligament. On the whole, the infrahyoid muscles fix the hyoid bone so that the suprahyoid muscles can move the tongue or mandible or act on the pharyngeal wall.

The Superficial Fascia

The superficial fascia contains anteriorly the *platysma muscle* which forms a sheet extending downwards beyond the clavicle and upwards over the mandible to which it is attached (figure 136). The muscle reaches the angle of the mouth (p. 195). It is supplied by the cervical branch of the facial nerve. The muscle can be demonstrated by jerking the angle of the mouth downwards — the muscle appears as vertical folds in the neck.

In the superficial fascia the *cutaneous nerves* run to the skin, the great auricular and lesser occipital upwards behind the ear, the transverse cervical anteriorly across the neck and the supraclavicular downwards over the clavicle. All the nerves appear from beneath the sternocleidomastoid muscle at about the middle of its posterior border. The *external jugular vein* (figure 134(b)) runs downwards and backwards from the anterior to the posterior border of the sternocleidomastoid muscle. Superiorly it emerges from the parotid gland and is formed by the union of the posterior branch of the retromandibular vein and the posterior auricular vein. The external jugular vein pierces the deep fascia at the posterior border of the sternocleidomastoid muscle above the clavicle and receives the anterior jugular vein before joining the subclavian vein. The external jugular vein is important in so far as its distension is visible in raised venous pressure due to heart failure. The height of the column of blood above the clavicle is a rough guide to the increase in the venous pressure.

Anteriorly the *anterior jugular veins* pass downwards on either side of the midline from the chin to the jugular notch. The two veins have numerous cross-anastomoses. Each vein pierces the deep fascia above the jugular notch and passes laterally deep to the sternocleidomastoid muscle to join the external jugular vein.

Posteriorly the subcutaneous fat is loculated by septa joining the skin with the deep fascia. Infection of the subcutaneous region, forming a *carbuncle*, is very painful due to the non-distensible nature of the tissue.

The Deep Fascia (figure 150)

Functionally the arrangement of the deep fascia provides smooth surfaces over which structures or organs can move, for example when turning the head and neck or when swallowing. Clinically the fascia creates planes along which infection can spread. It must be said that the existence of the definite layers of fascia usually described may depend to some extent on the way in which the tissues are fixed. It is customary to describe (1) a *superficial (investing) layer*, (2) a *prevertebral layer*, (3) a *pretracheal layer*, (4) the *carotid sheath*.

The Superficial (Investing) Layer. This layer extends round the whole circumference of the neck. Posteriorly it is attached in the midline to the external occipital protuberance and the spinous processes of the cervical vertebrae. Passing laterally the fascia encloses the trapezius. At the oblique lateral edge of the muscle the two layers fuse and continue round the side of the neck covering the area between the trapezius and sternocleidomastoid muscles (this area is called the posterior triangle). The fascia splits to enclose the sternocleidomastoid and at its anterior edge the two layers fuse and

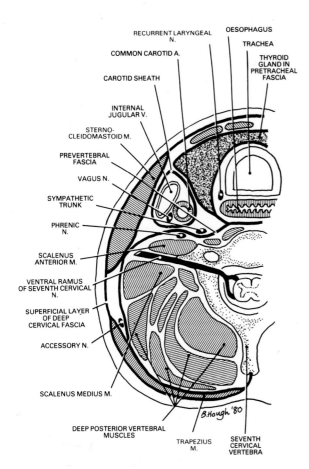

RECURRENT LARYNGEAL N.
OESOPHAGUS
TRACHEA
COMMON CAROTID A.
THYROID GLAND IN PRETRACHEAL FASCIA
CAROTID SHEATH
INTERNAL JUGULAR V.
STERNO-CLEIDOMASTOID M.
PREVERTEBRAL FASCIA
VAGUS N.
SYMPATHETIC TRUNK
PHRENIC N.
SCALENUS ANTERIOR M.
VENTRAL RAMUS OF SEVENTH CERVICAL N.
SUPERFICIAL LAYER OF DEEP CERVICAL FASCIA
ACCESSORY N.
SCALENUS MEDIUS M.
B.Hough '80
DEEP POSTERIOR VERTEBRAL MUSCLES
TRAPEZIUS M.
SEVENTH CERVICAL VERTEBRA

Figure 150   A transverse section of the neck at the level of the seventh cervical vertebra to show the arrangement of the deep fascia.

cover the area between the muscle and the midline anteriorly (this is called the anterior triangle). In the midline the fascia is attached to the mandible and the hyoid bone.

Superiorly the fascia is attached to the lower border of the body of the mandible and splits to enclose the submandibular gland. At the posterior border of the ramus of the mandible the fascia splits to enclose the parotid gland and passing over the masseter muscle is attached to the zygomatic arch. At the upper pole of the parotid gland the fascia becomes attached to the lateral surface of the mastoid process and from there it passes back-

wards along the superior nuchal line. Deep to the parotid gland a thickening of the fascia forms the stylomandibular ligament. Inferiorly on the front of the neck the fascia is attached to the clavicle. Above the manubrium the fascia splits into two layers which enclose the *suprasternal space* containing the lower ends of the anterior jugular veins and the sternal heads of the two sternocleidomastoid muscles.

The Prevertebral Layer. This is a transverse lamina of fascia lying in front of the prevertebral muscles of the neck. This lamina is attached to the transverse processes of the cervical vertebrae and extends laterally over the muscles forming the floor of the posterior triangle. The fascia then continues round the posterior vertebral muscles deep to the upper part of the trapezius. Superiorly the prevertebral fascia is attached to the base of the skull and inferiorly is continuous with the anterior longitudinal ligament of the vertebral column. The posterior triangle is covered by two layers of the cervical fascia and the spinal accessory nerve lies between the two layers. The branches of the spinal nerves are deep to the prevertebral fascia, as is the subclavian artery. As the subclavian artery enters the axilla (armpit) it takes with it a sheath of the prevertebral fascia (the *axillary fascia*). In front of the bodies of the vertebrae the prevertebral fascia is separated from the pharynx by loose connective tissue (the *retropharyngeal space*).

The Pretracheal Layer. As the name implies, this layer lies in front of the trachea. Its upper part splits, encloses the thyroid gland and is attached above the thyroid gland to the thyroid cartilage. It is attached to the cricoid cartilage and can be followed downwards into the mediastinum where it fuses with the fibrous pericardium. The pretracheal fascia extends laterally and fuses with the carotid sheath. It also extends round the trachea and oesophagus and passes behind them so that infection can spread downwards into the mediastinum from behind the oesophagus as well as from in front of the trachea. If followed upwards this posterior part becomes continuous with the fascia round the constrictor muscles of the pharynx.

A further layer of fascia between the posterior part of the pretracheal layer and prevertebral fascia called the *alar fascia* has been described. It is attached to the transverse processes of the cervical vertebrae.

The Carotid Sheath. This is the name given to the tubular fascia surrounding the common and internal carotid arteries, the internal jugular vein and the vagus nerve. The sheath extends from the base of the skull to the thorax and is thinner on its lateral side to allow distension of the internal jugular vein. Because of the sheath, the vagus nerve accompanies the large vessels if they are moved. The sympathetic trunk, lying behind and medial to the sheath, does not move because it remains embedded in the prevertebral fascia.

The Trapezius and Sternocleidomastoid Muscles

These two large muscles on each side are comparatively superficial and, since they are innervated by the spinal accessory nerve, they are regarded as being derived from the same embryonic mass of muscle, which is part of the branchial musculature.

The Trapezius Muscle (figure 14). This muscle has an extensive origin from the midline of the back extending from the external occipital protuberance to the twelfth thoracic vertebra. The *ligamentum nuchae* is a mass of fibro-elastic tissue attached to the atlas and the spinous processes of the second to the sixth cervical vertebrae. The trapezius is attached to the ligamentum nuchae and the spinous processes of the vertebrae from the sixth cervical to the twelfth thoracic. The fibres of the muscle pass laterally — the upper fibres, which are also attached to the medial part of the superior nuchal line, downwards, the middle transversely and the lower upwards, and are attached to the lateral third of the posterior border of the clavicle, the medial border of the acromion and the upper border of the spine of the scapula. Because of its attachment to the pectoral girdle the trapezius is regarded as a muscle of the upper limb. One trapezius can, however, turn the head to the oppo-

site side and both muscles can extend the head. In addition the trapezius braces back and elevates the shoulder, and rotates the scapula so that its inferior angle moves outwards. These movements are considered more fully with the shoulder region of the upper limb (p. 359). Besides its motor nerve supply from the spinal accessory nerve the trapezius receives a sensory (proprioceptive) innervation from the third and fourth cervical spinal nerves.

The Sternocleidomastoid Muscle (figures 150, 151, 152). The lower end of the sternocleidomastoid muscle (*kleis = key*, Greek; the clavicle is shaped like a key) is attached by a rounded tendon 2 cm in diameter to the upper border of the manubrium and by flat muscular fibres, 5–6 cm wide, to the medial third of the upper surface of the clavicle (figure 151). Superiorly the muscle is attached to the outer surface of the mastoid process, and the lateral part of the superior nuchal line (*nucha = nape of neck*, Latin; *cervix* and *collum*, Latin, are also used).

The sternocleidomastoid has a large number of structures related to it, some of which are superficial to it and have already been mentioned — the platysma, the external jugular vein, some of the cutaneous branches of the cervical plexus, the parotid gland (figures 134–136). The muscle covers the large vessels of the neck, the last four cranial nerves, the cervical spinal nerves forming the cervical and brachial plexuses and many muscles.

The right sternocleidomastoid muscle turns the head to the left and tilts the head so that it approaches the shoulder of the same side. The left muscle produces the opposite effect. This is the position of the head in *torticollis* (*wry-neck*), which may be congenital or due to spasm or shortening of the muscle. Infection of the lymph nodes in the neck may produce reflex spasm of the muscle. Both muscles flex the head and neck in the recumbent position or against resistance when standing. They do not extend the head, as is sometimes stated. The muscles can also be used as accessory muscles of respiration. Their attachment to the manubrium enables them to lift the rib cage upwards, an action similar to that of the scalene muscles attached to the first rib. This upward movement of the superior part of the cage results in the whole cage moving

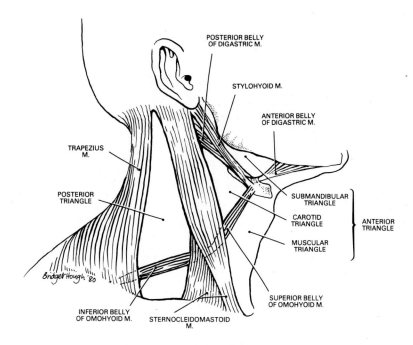

POSTERIOR BELLY
OF DIGASTRIC M.

STYLOHYOID M.

ANTERIOR BELLY
OF DIGASTRIC M.

TRAPEZIUS
M.

POSTERIOR
TRIANGLE

SUBMANDIBULAR
TRIANGLE

CAROTID
TRIANGLE

ANTERIOR
TRIANGLE

MUSCULAR
TRIANGLE

Bridget Hough '80

SUPERIOR BELLY
OF OMOHYOID M.

INFERIOR BELLY
OF OMOHYOID M.

STERNOCLEIDOMASTOID
M.

Figure 151   The triangles of the neck, lateral view.

so that its anteroposterior and transverse diameters are increased.

The sternocleidomastoid muscle, in addition to its motor nerve supply from the spinal accessory nerve, also receives a sensory (proprioceptive) nerve supply from the second and third cervical spinal nerves.

The Triangles of the Neck (figure 151)

The neck is divided into two large triangles. The *anterior triangle* is bounded laterally by the anterior border of the sternocleidomastoid, medially by the midline and superiorly by the lower border of the mandible. The *posterior triangle* is bounded anteriorly by the posterior border of the sternocleidomastoid, posteriorly by the anterior border of the trapezius and inferiorly by the clavicle between the attachments of these two muscles. The posterior triangle presents a problem of description because its apex at the occipital bone is posterior and the rest of the triangle winds round the lateral side of the neck so that its base at the clavicle is anterior. It is suggested that the triangle be called the *lateral*

region of the neck which is a better name but does not overcome the fact that its apex is posterior and base is anterior.

The anterior triangle

This triangle is conveniently subdivided by small muscles into (1) the *muscular triangle*, (2) the *carotid triangle*, (3) the *submandibular triangle*. In addition the single *submental triangle*, below and behind the chin, lies on both sides of the midline.

The Muscular Triangle (figure 152)

This triangle is bounded above and laterally by the superior belly of the omohyoid muscle, below and laterally by the lower part of the anterior border of the sternocleidomastoid and medially by the midline. Its name refers to the muscles which it contains, the *sternohyoid*, *sternothyroid* and *thyrohyoid* (figure 152). The important structure in this triangle, deep to the muscles, is the *thyroid gland* which lies lateral to the larynx and trachea.

(a)

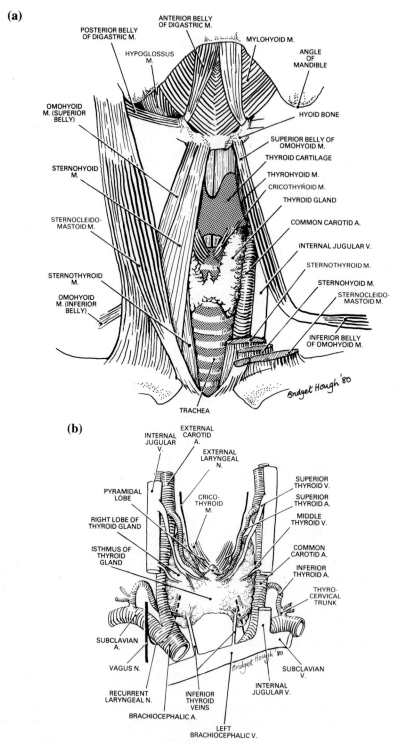

Figure 152   (a) The muscular and submental triangles, anterior view. (b) The arteries and veins of the thyroid gland.

The *omohyoid muscle* has two bellies joined by the intermediate tendon. The inferior belly is attached to the upper border of the scapula near its scapular notch (*omos = shoulder*, Greek) and passes forwards and upwards across the lower part of the posterior triangle to lie deep to the sternocleidomastoid. The intermediate tendon lies here and is attached by a band of deep fascia to the region of the sternoclavicular joint. The muscle is angled at the tendon so that the superior belly has a more upward direction as it crosses the carotid sheath to become attached to the body of the hyoid bone.

The *sternohyoid* is attached to the deep surface of the upper part of the manubrium and passes upwards to the body of the hyoid bone. The *sternothyroid* is also attached to the manubrium and passes upwards deep to the sternohyoid to the lamina of the thyroid cartilage. The *thyrohyoid* is attached to the lamina of the thyroid cartilage and extends upwards to the body of the hyoid bone.

All these muscles are collectively known as the *infrahyoid muscles* and also, apart from the omohyoid, as the *strap muscles*. They are innervated by the ventral rami of the first, second and third cervical nerves and are involved in chewing, swallowing and phonation. In all these activities they fix the hyoid bone to enable other muscles, mainly the suprahyoid, to act from a fixed point.

The Thyroid Gland (figure 152). This is the largest of the endocrine glands. It consists of two pear-shaped *lateral lobes*, about 5–6 cm in height and 2–3 cm wide and anteroposteriorly. The lobes are joined by a narrow band called the *isthmus*, about 1 cm in height. The upper limit of the lateral lobe is the attachment of the sternothyroid muscle to the lamina of the thyroid cartilage (*thyreos = shield*, Greek). The wider lower part extends downwards as far as the sixth tracheal ring. The lobes extend sufficiently far back to lie lateral to the pharynx and oesophagus which lie behind the larynx and trachea. The carotid sheath and its contents lie behind the lobe lateral to the pharynx and oesophagus. The thyroid gland is covered by the sternothyroid and sternohyoid muscles.

The isthmus lies anterior to the second, third and fourth tracheal rings. There may be an upward extension of the isthmus near the midline (the *pyramidal lobe*). The pyramidal lobe may be connected to the hyoid bone by a fibrous or fibro-muscular band. There may be small pieces of thyroid tissue in the midline of the neck between the floor of the wall and the pyramidal lobe. These develop in relation to the thyroglossal duct which extends in the fetus from the tongue to the isthmus and usually disappears. Remains of the thyroglossal duct may form cysts in the midline of the neck.

In addition to the sheath formed by the pretracheal fascia there is a capsule surrounding the gland. The venous plexus around the gland lies within the capsule.

The arteries supplying the gland (figure 152(b)) are the *superior thyroid* from the external carotid and the *inferior thyroid* from the thyrocervical trunk, a branch of the subclavian artery. The superior thyroid artery accompanied by the external laryngeal nerve passes downwards and supplies the upper pole and anterior part of the gland. The inferior thyroid artery accompanied by the recurrent laryngeal nerve passes upwards and supplies the lower pole and posterior part of the gland. The parathyroid glands, two on each side, are embedded in the posterior surface of the gland, and are supplied by the inferior thyroid arteries. There are anastomoses between the superior thyroid arteries along the upper border of the isthmus and between the superior and inferior thyroid arteries. There may be an ascending artery, the *thyroidea ima* (*ima = lowest*, Latin), from the arch of the aorta or one of its larger branches passing to the isthmus.

The veins from the gland are differently arranged. The venous plexus within the capsule of the gland is drained on each side by *superior* and *middle thyroid veins* which pass laterally and join the internal jugular vein. (This arrangement is somewhat variable.) The *inferior thyroid veins*, one on each side, pass downwards and join the left brachiocephalic vein.

The *lymphatic vessels* from the thyroid gland go to prelaryngeal, pretracheal, and paratracheal nodes. Some vessels pass downwards to nodes in the superior mediastinum. Other vessels from the gland pass laterally to the deep cervical nodes which lie along the internal jugular vein and some on the left side pass directly to the thoracic duct.

Enlargement of the thyroid gland may occur during menstruation and pregnancy. A pathological enlargement is called a *goitre* which produces a bulging in the neck. The gland can enlarge backwards, or downwards towards or into the thorax, but it cannot enlarge upwards because of the attachment of its fascial sheath and the sternothyroid muscles to the thyroid cartilage. An enlarged gland can press on the trachea and interfere with respiration. Pressure on one of the nerves related to the thyroid arteries resulting in changes in the voice usually indicates a malignant growth of the gland. One or more of these laryngeal nerves may be cut in the operation of removal of the gland (*thyroidectomy*). The posterior part of each lobe of the gland is usually left behind in order to prevent *myxoedema*, a condition which would develop due to the complete absence of the gland, and to ensure that the parathyroid glands are not removed.

The Parathyroid Glands. There are usually four of these glands, two superior and two inferior, each about 3 mm wide, 1 mm anteroposteriorly and 6 mm in length. The glands lie posterior to the thyroid lobes inside the capsule, the superior about the middle of the posterior surface and the inferior nearer the inferior pole of the lobe. The four parathyroid glands are supplied by the inferior thyroid arteries, although it has been observed that tying both arteries does not lead to necrosis of the four glands.

The Carotid Triangle (figure 153)

This triangle is bounded laterally by the anterior border of the sternocleidomastoid, superiorly by the posterior belly of the digastric and inferiorly by the superior belly of the omohyoid. It contains the common carotid artery and the beginning of its two divisions, the internal and external carotid

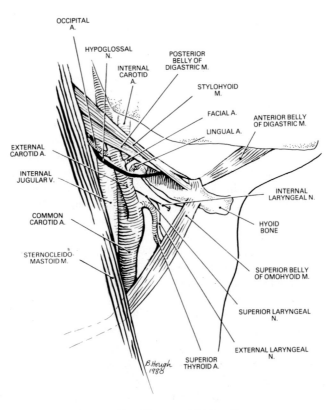

Figure 153   The carotid triangle.

arteries. It also contains part of the internal jugular vein and some of its tributaries, some branches of the external carotid artery, parts of the vagus and hypoglossal nerves and some of the muscles attached to the hyoid bone (the hyoglossus and middle constrictor of the pharynx). Most of these structures are overlapped from behind by the sternocleidomastoid muscle, but more anteriorly the greater cornu of the hyoid bone and the thyroid cartilage are covered by only the skin and the platysma.

Almost all of these structures, for example the blood vessels and nerves and their branches, are best described as complete entities, and the muscles with the tongue and pharynx.

The Submandibular (Digastric) Triangle

This triangle is bounded above by the lower border of the body of the mandible and below by the two bellies of the digastric diverging from its intermediate tendon which is attached to the hyoid bone. The floor of the triangle is formed by the mylohyoid muscle on which lie the facial artery and submandibular salivary gland. The facial vein is superficial to the gland. The internal and external carotid arteries, internal jugular vein and hypoglossal and accessory nerves lie deep to the posterior belly of the digastric.

The Digastric, Stylohyoid, Mylohyoid and Geniohyoid Muscles. The *digastric muscle*, as the name implies, has two bellies, a posterior which is attached to the mastoid notch medial to the mastoid process and an anterior which is attached to a depression at the side of the mental symphysis (figure 153). The two bellies are joined at an angle to each other by an intermediate tendon which is attached to the body of the hyoid bone. The *stylohyoid muscle* is attached to the styloid process of the temporal bone, runs downwards and forwards with the posterior belly of the digastric and is attached to the hyoid bone where it splits to enclose the intermediate tendon of the digastric (figure 153). The stylohyoid and posterior belly of the digastric are innervated by the facial nerve. The anterior belly receives its nerve supply from the mylohyoid nerve,

a branch of the inferior alveolar nerve which is a branch of the mandibular nerve (p. 206). The stylohyoid muscle and the posterior belly of the digastric help to keep the hyoid bone steady when the anterior belly pulls the mandible downwards against resistance. The internal and external carotid arteries and some of the branches of the latter, the hypoglossal and accessory nerves and the internal jugular vein are deep to the posterior belly of the digastric and the stylohyoid muscle which are deep to the sternocleidomastoid.

The *mylohyoid muscle* is attached to the mylohyoid line on the inner surface of the body of the mandible (figures 152, 154, 186). The posterior fibres pass backwards and slightly downwards to the hyoid bone and the middle and anterior fibres from each side meet in a midline raphe extending from the mental symphysis to the hyoid bone. The two muscles together form the floor of the mouth. The inferior surface is mainly in the submandibular triangle and is therefore related to the digastric muscle, the superficial part of the submandibular gland, the facial artery and the mylohyoid nerve and vessels. The superior (oral) surface is related to the deep part of the submandibular gland and its duct and its neighbouring structures – the hyoglossus muscle, the hypoglossal and lingual nerves and the submandibular ganglion (figure 144).

The mylohyoid muscle is supplied by the mylohyoid nerve, a branch of the inferior alveolar nerve. The muscle pulls the mandible downwards especially against resistance and also pushes the tongue upwards in the first (oral) stage of swallowing.

The *geniohyoid muscles* (figure 184) lie on the superior surface of the mylohyoid on either side of the mandible. They are attached to the lower of the tubercles on each side of the inner surface of the mandible lateral to the symphysis. The geniohyoid passes backwards and is attached to the hyoid bone. The ventral ramus of the first cervical nerve which joins the hypoglossal nerve supplies this muscle through a branch of the hypoglossal nerve. The geniohyoid depresses the mandible in opening the mouth.

The Submandibular Gland (figures 137, 144, 154).

This gland has two parts, a superficial and a deep. The superficial part lies in the submandibular tri-

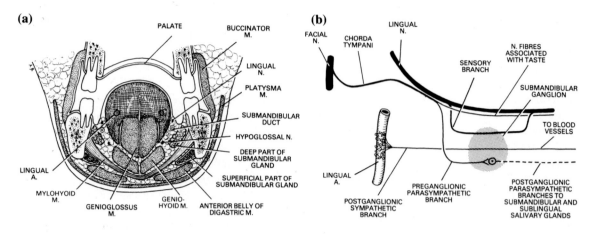

Figure 154 (a) A coronal section through the mouth at the level of the second/third molar teeth. (b) A diagram of the connections of the submandibular ganglion.

angle and is continuous with the deep part round the posterior edge of the mylohyoid muscle. The deep part therefore lies inside the mouth since the mylohyoid muscles form its floor. The superficial part is enclosed in a capsule formed by deep cervical fascia attached to the mandible, and is 3 cm in its greatest diameter and about 2 cm in its other dimensions. *Its position is indicated by placing the thumb deep to the ramus or posterior part of the body of the mandible in front of the angle.* In this situation the submandibular fossa of the mandible is lateral, the mylohyoid muscle is superior and medial and the skin and platysma with the facial vein are inferior (superficial) to the gland. The facial artery lies in a groove in the superior part of the gland and then becomes more superficial as it passes to the lower border of the mandible where it can be felt pulsating. The mylohyoid nerve and vessels lie between the gland and the mylohyoid muscle. The superficial part of the gland extends posteriorly beyond the mylohyoid and becomes related to the hyoglossus and the lateral wall of the pharynx. The submandibular lymph nodes are closely related to the superficial part of the gland and some nodes may be embedded in it.

The deep part of the gland (figure 154) lies between the hyoglossus muscle and the upper surface of the mylohyoid with the lingual nerve superior and the hypoglossal nerve inferior. The submandibular ganglion, suspended from the lingual nerve, lies between the gland and the hyoglossus muscle. The submandibular duct passes forwards from the deep part of the gland and lies between the sublingual gland and the tongue in the floor of the mouth. The lingual nerve becomes lateral to the duct and then passes under it to become medial. The duct opens on a papilla lateral to the frenulum of the tongue in the floor of the mouth (figure 185).

The secretomotor and vasodilator nerve supply of the submandibular gland is from the chorda tympani, a branch of the facial nerve. The chorda tympani leaves the facial nerve while it runs in the facial canal which is in the medial wall of the middle ear. The chorda tympani leaves the temporal bone through the petrotympanic fissure, which is posterior to the temporomandibular joint, and joins the lingual nerve (p. 207). The secretomotor fibres go to the submandibular ganglion and synapse there. The postganglionic fibres return to the lingual nerve and supply the sublingual gland and possibly the submandibular gland. It appears that most of the preganglionic fibres supplying the submandibular gland synapse in the gland itself.

The submandibular gland can be palpated between a finger of one hand placed in the floor of the mouth and a finger of the other hand placed deep to the posterior half of the body of the mandible. A stone in the duct of the gland can be palpated in a similar manner. The obstruction by the stone can produce a swelling of the gland seen in the floor of the mouth and/or neck deep to the mandible.

The Submandibular Ganglion (figure 154(b)). This is one of the parasympathetic ganglia of the head and neck. It is attached to the lingual nerve by two nerve filaments and lies on the hyoglossus muscle near the deep part of the submandibular gland. It receives three types of nerve fibres: (1) sensory from the lingual nerve; (2) sympathetic from the plexus round the facial artery; (3) parasympathetic from the chorda tympani, which travels via the lingual nerve. Only the parasympathetic fibres synapse in the ganglion. The sympathetic are postganglionic fibres with their cell bodies in the superior cervical ganglion and pass through the ganglion to supply blood vessels in the submandibular and sublingual glands. The sensory fibres rejoin the lingual nerve and are distributed with it. The postganglionic parasympathetic nerve fibres supply the sublingual gland and some small glands in the floor of the mouth. The submandibular gland is innervated by parasympathetic fibres which synapse in the gland itself.

The Submental Triangle

This triangle is formed by the two anterior bellies of the digastric muscles and the body of the hyoid bone (figure (152(a)). It is covered by the skin, platysma and deep fascia. The anterior jugular veins begin in the superficial fascia deep to the platysma. In the triangle there are one or two lymph nodes which receive lymphatic vessels from the tip of the tongue, the floor of the mouth and the incisor teeth. These vessels pass through the mylohyoid muscle. Infection of these structures can present as painful enlarged nodes in the neck below the mandible. The nodes drain to the submandibular nodes.

The posterior triangle (the lateral region of the neck) (figure 155)

This triangle, bounded posteriorly by the lateral border of the trapezius, anteriorly by the posterior border of the sternocleidomastoid and inferiorly by the middle third of the clavicle, has its apex at the superior nuchal line of the occipital bone, and its base at the clavicle. Because of this it is difficult to follow the arrangement of the structures in it and one has to recall that the triangle winds round the side of the neck. The floor is therefore formed superiorly by posterior muscles and inferiorly by anterior muscles. The splenius capitis is the most superior muscle although some of the vertical fibres of the *semispinalis capitis* may appear above its upper border. The *splenius capitis* passes upwards and laterally from the lower cervical and upper thoracic spinous processes to the mastoid process deep to the sternocleidomastoid. Inferior to the splenius capitis the levator scapulae passes downwards and backwards from the transverse processes of the upper four cervical vertebrae to the upper part of the medial border of the scapula. The next two muscles are prevertebral and are the *scalenus medius* and a small part of the *scalenus anterior*, most of which is covered by the lower part of the sternocleidomastoid. The scalene muscles are attached to the transverse processes of the cervical vertebrae, the medius to the posterior tubercles and the anterior to the anterior tubercles.

The *inferior belly of the omohyoid* passes upwards and forwards across the lower part of the posterior triangle and lies deep to both the trapezius and sternocleidomastoid. The whole triangle is covered by two layers of deep fascia. The more superficial is part of the investing layer and the deeper layer is part of the prevertebral fascia. Between these two layers the spinal accessory nerve passes downwards and backwards on the levator scapulae round the side of the neck, *from about the middle of the posterior border of the sternocleidomastoid to the anterior border of the trapezius, 5–6 cm above the clavicle. These two points can be used as the surface marking of the nerve.* At about the same point on the posterior border of the sternocleidomastoid cutaneous branches of the cervical plexus appear, the great auricular and the lesser occipital, passing upwards, the transverse cervical, passing forwards, and the supraclavicular, passing downwards (figure 155). Their segmental origins and distribution are described on p. 213 (figure 135).

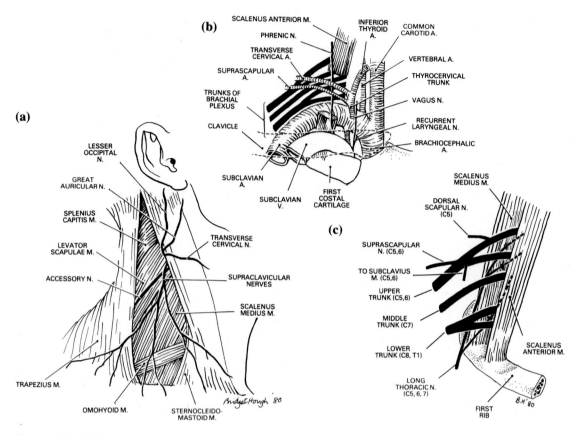

Figure 155   (a) The posterior triangle. (b) The omoclavicular (subclavian) triangle. (c) The roots and trunks of the brachial plexus.

The triangle above the inferior belly of the omo-hyoid (the *occipital triangle*) requires no further description. Inferior to the omohyoid there are important structures — part of the subclavian artery and vein and part of the brachial plexus. This region is now known as the *omoclavicular triangle*, was called the *supraclavicular* or *sub-clavian triangle* and corresponds with the *greater supraclavicular fossa* (the *lesser supraclavicular fossa* is the hollow between the two heads of the sternocleidomastoid). Although one can describe the structures in the omoclavicular triangle it is more desirable to look at this region with the sternocleidomastoid detached from the clavicle and sternum and turned upwards. This reveals the scalenus anterior muscle lying in front of the sub-clavian artery and behind the subclavian vein, as these vessels pass laterally from the neck into the upper limb.

The Subclavian Artery. On the right this artery arises from the brachiocephalic artery where it divides behind the sternoclavicular joint into the subclavian and common carotid arteries (figure 155(b)). On the left the subclavian artery arises from the arch of the aorta and passes upwards to enter the neck at the level of the sternoclavicular joint. The subclavian artery grooves the upper sur-face of the first rib and ends at its outer border where is becomes the axillary artery. It is custom-ary to divide the artery into three parts, relative to the scalenus anterior the first, second and third parts being medial to, behind and lateral to the muscle respectively. It is simpler to consider the relations of the whole of the subclavian artery rather than those of each part.

The subclavian vein is anterior and inferior to the artery and is separated from its middle part by the scalenus anterior. The subclavian artery is anterior to and grooves the apex of the lung, the dome of the pleura and the suprapleural membrane. The scalenus medius muscle is attached to the first rib behind the artery with the lower trunk of the brachial plexus intervening. The middle and upper trunks of the plexus lie above the artery. The internal jugular vein passes in front of the medial part of the artery and joins the subclavian vein to form the brachiocephalic vein. On the left the terminal part of the thoracic duct passes in front of the artery to join the beginning of the brachiocephalic vein.

On the right the phrenic nerve while lying on the scalenus anterior enters the thorax. On the left the nerve crosses the medial part of the artery. The vagus nerve passes anterior to the first part of the subclavian artery and on the right gives off the right recurrent laryngeal nerve which passes upwards and medially behind the artery. The sympathetic trunk is posterior to the artery. The ansa subclavia (*ansa = loop*, Latin) passes from the middle cervical ganglion downwards in front of and then upwards behind the subclavian artery to the inferior cervical ganglion lying posteriorly (figure 161).

The external jugular vein and some of its tributaries are anterior to the artery where it lies on the first rib lateral to the scalenus anterior. *The artery is relatively superficial here and can be pressed on to the first rib lateral to the lower end of the sternocleidomastoid.* This is a pressure point well known to first-aid personnel for decreasing or stopping haemorrhage from the arteries of the upper limb. The manoeuvre is easier if the head is bent to the same side. More medially the sternocleidomastoid lies in front of the artery separated from it by the scalenus anterior and subclavian vein.

The subclavian artery can be indicated in the living by an arching band about 1 cm wide beginning at the sternoclavicular joint and ending medial to the middle of the clavicle. The highest level of the arch is about 3 cm above the level of the clavicle.

The Subclavian Vein. This vein begins at the outer border of the first rib as a continuation of the axillary vein from the upper limb. It ends at the medial border of the scalenus anterior by joining the internal jugular vein to form the brachiocephalic vein. The subclavian vein lies in front of and inferior to the subclavian artery, from which it is separated by the scalenus anterior. On the right the phrenic nerve lies between the vein and the muscle. On the left the nerve is more medial and lies between the vein and the artery. The vein is separated from the apex of the lung by the artery. The clavicle is anterior to the vein.

Its main tributary is the external jugular vein, which receives most of the superficial veins of the head and neck. Apart from a vein from the lower part of the back of the neck (the dorsal scapular) the subclavian vein does not receive the veins corresponding with the branches of the artery.

The Branches of the Subclavian Artery. (1) The *vertebral artery* arises from the most medial part of the subclavian artery, passes upwards and enters the foramen transversarium of the sixth cervical vertebra. In this part of its course the vertebral artery lies in a triangle formed laterally by the scalenus anterior, medially by the longus colli and inferiorly by the transverse process of the seventh cervical vertebra (figure 161). The artery is anterior to the ventral rami of the seventh and eighth cervical spinal nerves and the sympathetic trunk and posterior to the common carotid and inferior thyroid arteries (in front of nerves and behind arteries).

The vertebral artery runs almost vertically upwards through the foramen transversarium of the cervical vertebrae anterior to the ventral rami of the cervical spinal nerves to the foramen of the axis (figure 156). The artery then passes laterally to enter the foramen transversarium of the atlas. It runs medially behind the lateral mass of the atlas lateral to the ventral ramus of the first cervical nerve and then forwards over the lateral end of the posterior arch of the atlas, inferior to the posterior atlanto-occipital membrane. The dorsal ramus of the first cervical nerve lies between the artery and the arch. The artery enters the skull through the foramen magnum. After piercing the dura mater and arachnoid the vertebral arteries join and form the basilar artery.

The vertebral artery is surrounded by a plexus of veins as it runs through the foramina transversaria and also by a postganglionic plexus of nerve

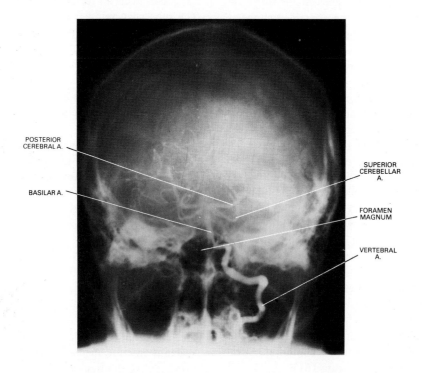

POSTERIOR
CEREBRAL A.

BASILAR A.

SUPERIOR
CEREBELLAR
A.

FORAMEN
MAGNUM

VERTEBRAL
A.

Figure 156   An arteriogram of the vertebral artery.

fibres whose cell bodies are in the inferior cervical and first thoracic ganglia (usually combined to form one ganglion). In the region of the lower cervical vertebrae the plexus of veins forms a single vertebral vein which joins the brachiocephalic vein.

The vertebral artery gives off spinal branches which enter the vertebral canal through the intervertebral foramina and supply the spinal cord, the spinal nerve roots and meninges and also the vertebrae. In the region of the posterior arch of the atlas (the suboccipital triangle, p. 332) the vertebral artery gives off muscular branches. Within the skull the artery supplies the meninges, the spinal cord by means of long descending spinal arteries, and the cerebellum.

(2) *The internal thoracic (mammary) artery* arises medial to the scalenus anterior and passes downwards into the thorax. Its course and distribution are described on p. 16.

(3) *The thyrocervical trunk* arises from the subclavian artery at the same level as the internal thoracic artery and runs upwards in the same triangle in which the vertebral artery lies. After a short course of about 1 cm it divides into the inferior thyroid, superficial cervical and suprascapular arteries. The *inferior thyroid artery* runs upwards in front of the vertebral artery and behind the carotid sheath to the lower pole of the thyroid gland. As it approaches the gland the artery is closely related to the recurrent laryngeal nerve.

The inferior thyroid artery gives branches not only to the thyroid and parathyroid glands but also to the neighbouring muscles, and the larynx, trachea, pharynx and oesophagus. The inferior laryngeal artery accompanies the recurrent laryngeal nerve into the larynx.

The *transverse cervical* and the *suprascapular arteries* pass laterally and backwards superficial to the scalenus anterior and phrenic nerve then across the trunks of the brachial plexus and finally deep to the trapezius. (The cervical artery is superior to the scapular — the neck is superior to the scapula). The transverse cervical artery passes upwards deep to the trapezius. The suprascapular artery runs laterally with the suprascapular nerve deep to the clavicle and the inferior belly of the omohyoid to the suprascapular notch on the superior border of the scapula. The nerve and artery enter the supraspinous fossa of the scapula separated by the ligament bridging the notch. The nerve is below the ligament. The artery is widely distributed and supplies the muscles, bones and joints related to the scapula and clavicle. Its branches form part of the anastomosis round the shoulder joint and also the anastomosis round the scapula.

(4) *The costocervical trunk* arises from the posterior aspect of the subclavian artery as it lies behind the scalenus anterior. The costocervical trunk arches backwards over the cervical pleura and, on the neck of the first rib, divides into the *deep cervical* and *superior intercostal arteries*. The deep cervical artery passes upwards and then backwards below the transverse process of the seventh cervical vertebra into the deep postvertebral muscles among which it ascends towards the occiput. The artery is distributed mainly to these muscles.

The superior intercostal artery passes downwards on the necks of the first and second ribs. On the neck of the first rib the artery lies between the sympathetic nerve trunk (medial) and the branch of the ventral ramus of the first thoracic nerve (lateral) as it passes upwards to join the brachial plexus (figure 158). The superior intercostal artery gives off the posterior intercostal artery of the first and second intercostal spaces.

(5) *The dorsal scapular artery* arises from the subclavian artery lateral to the scalenus anterior and passes laterally and backwards over the brachial plexus and deep to the levator scapulae. It is accompanied by the dorsal scapular nerve (formerly the nerve to the rhomboid muscles) and passes downwards deep to the muscles attached to the medial border of the scapula. The artery supplies the muscles and takes part in the scapular anastomosis.

The preceding description of the branches of the subclavian artery may be the single commonest arrangement but frequently the origin of the branches and the way in which they divide are different from the arrangement described. One of the commonest is for the dorsal scapular artery to arise from the transverse cervical. Frequently the transverse cervical and suprascapular arteries arise by a common trunk from the thyrocervical trunk or separately from the subclavian artery.

In addition to the subclavian artery becoming the main artery of the upper limb, it is important to appreciate that the vertebral artery supplies the spinal cord, hindbrain, midbrain and the posterior part of the forebrain, that the internal thoracic artery passes through the thorax and into the abdominal wall and by means of its branches provides anastomotic channels with the thoracic and abdominal aortae, that one of the branches supplies the thyroid gland and that several of the branches form anastomotic connections with arteries in the back of the neck, in the region of the shoulder joint and around the scapula.

The Trunks of the Brachial Plexus. The brachial plexus which innervates the upper limb is formed by the ventral rami of the fifth, sixth, seventh and eighth cervical and first thoracic spinal nerves. (These are usually called the *roots* of the plexus, a somewhat misleading term because *roots* also refers to the origin of the spinal nerves from the spinal cord.) The cervical spinal nerves emerge from the vertebral canal through the intervertebral foramina. The first is above the atlas, the eighth is below the seventh cervical vertebra. The spinal nerves divide almost immediately into a small dorsal and a large ventral ramus. The dorsal rami pass backwards and in general terms are distributed to the deep muscles of the back and the skin at the side of the midline (p. 12). The ventral rami pass laterally behind the vertebral artery and lie in the groove between the tubercles of the transverse processes. The ventral ramus of the first cervical nerve passes forwards medial to the vertebral artery and lateral to the lateral mass of the atlas and that of the eighth cervical nerve passes above the first rib. The ventral rami emerge from between the scalenus anterior which is attached to the anterior tubercles, and the scalenus medius which is attached to the posterior tubercles. Those of the upper four cervical spinal nerves form the cervical plexus (p. 235) and the lower four take part in the formation of the brachial plexus. In the lower part of the posterior triangle above the subclavian artery, the trunks of the brachial plexus pass downwards and laterally. The fifth and sixth ventral rami form the *upper trunk*, the seventh continues as the *middle trunk* and the eighth cervical and first thoracic form the *lower trunk* (figure 155(b), (c)). The trunks pass downwards and laterally behind the clavicle where each divides into *anterior* and *posterior divisions*. Their further course is considered with the upper limb (p. 354).

In the posterior triangle the trunks are superficial, being covered by the skin, platysma and deep fascia. The lower trunk is posterosuperior to the subclavian artery. *They can be palpated above the artery and feel like tense cords.* The external jugular vein and the scapular and cervical branches of the thyrocervical trunk are superficial to the nerve trunks.

There is a contribution to the phrenic nerve from the ventral ramus of the fifth cervical nerve, and muscular branches to the scalene muscles and longus colli from most of the ventral rami. There are in addition branches from this part of the brachial plexus to the upper limb. Two nerves are important, the *suprascapular* and the *long thoracic*. Two are unimportant — the *nerve to the subclavius muscle* from the upper trunk (the fifth and sixth cervical nerves) and the *dorsal scapular nerve* (from the fifth cervical) which supplies the rhomboid muscles. The *suprascapular nerve* arises from the upper trunk and passes laterally with the suprascapular artery deep to the trapezius and the omohyoid. It enters the supraspinous fossa deep to the ligament bridging the scapular notch, and supplies the supraspinatus and infraspinatus muscles.

The *long thoracic nerve* is formed by separate branches from the fifth, sixth and seventh ventral rami. The branches pass downwards deep to the rest of the brachial plexus and the axillary artery, and join on the upper part of the external surface of the serratus anterior, which is supplied by the nerve.

In a baby the upper trunk may be injured during delivery due to the head and neck being pulled downwards and backwards to release the shoulder from under the symphysis pubis. It is also caused by accidents, such as falling off a motorcycle, in which the point of the shoulder is thrust downwards and the head is pushed sideways. This produces a condition called *Erb–Duchenne paralysis* or *palsy* (W.H. Erb, 1840–1921, German neurologist; G.B.A. Duchenne, 1806–1875, French neurologist). The ventral rami of the fifth and sixth cervical nerves are torn and the muscles supplied by these nerves are paralysed. Briefly, the patient cannot abduct and laterally rotate the upper limb at the shoulder, cannot flex and supinate the forearm and cannot extend the hand at the wrist. This will be more fully understood after studying the anatomy of the upper limb. A commoner condition affecting this part of the brachial plexus is due to pressure on the contribution of the first thoracic nerve to the brachial plexus. This nerve has to pass upwards and laterally over the first rib to join the ventral ramus of the seventh cervical nerve. The possible causes of pressure on this nerve are a cervical rib (p. 189) because the nerve has to ascend further to join the seventh cervical nerve, spasm of the scalenus anterior which elevates the first rib, or excessive fatigue associated with a sliding downwards of the upper limb girdle on the chest wall. Pressure on this branch of the first thoracic nerve results in weakness and later paralysis of the small muscles of the hand which are supplied by this nerve.

17

The Neck II

The larynx and trachea, and pharynx and oesophagus, lie in the midline and are dealt with in later chapters. The remaining structures in the neck are the prevertebral muscles, the carotid arteries and their branches, the internal jugular vein and its tributaries, the sympathetic ganglionated trunk and the last four cranial nerves, the glossopharyngeal, vagus, accessory and hypoglossal. Since almost all the lymph nodes are in the neck these are also described in this chapter.

The Prevertebral Muscles and the First Rib (figures 157, 158)

The Longus Colli. This muscle has a vertical part attached to the front of the bodies of the cervical vertebrae, a superior oblique part attached to the transverse processes of the middle cervical vertebrae and passing upwards and medially to the anterior tubercle of the atlas, and an inferior oblique part which is attached to the front of the bodies of the upper three thoracic vertebrae and passes upwards and laterally to the transverse processes of the middle cervical vertebrae.

The Longus Capitis. Its inferior attachment is to the transverse processes of the lower cervical vertebrae. The muscle passes upwards and medially to the occipital bone in front of the foramen magnum.

The Rectus Capitis Anterior and *Rectus Capitis Lateralis.* These small muscles are attached to the

front of the anterior arch and lateral mass of the atlas respectively and pass vertically upwards to the occipital bone in front of the condyle and foramen magnum.

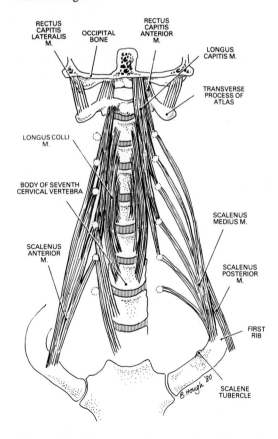

Figure 157   The prevertebral muscles of the neck.

(a)

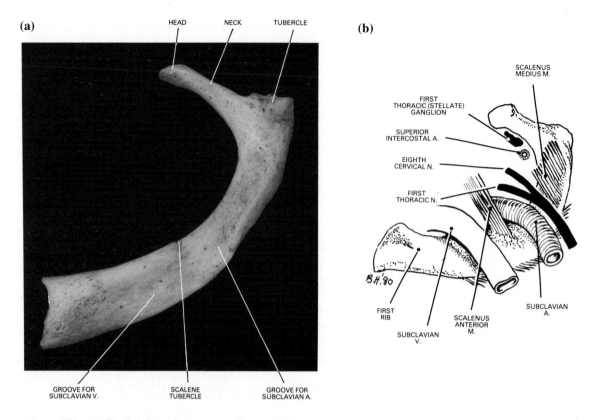

(b)

Figure 158   (a) The left first rib (upper surface). (b) The structures related to the upper surface of the first rib.

All these muscles are supplied by the ventral rami of cervical nerves, the small muscles by that of the first and the two larger muscles by several. If the muscles of both sides contract at the same time, they flex the head and neck. Acting on one side, the muscles produce lateral bending of the cervical part of the vertebral column. Oblique fibres on one side produce rotation. The two small muscles between the atlas and occipital bone are part of a group of muscles most of which are posterior (suboccipital). They mainly function for the fine adjustment of the position of the head and thus indirectly of the eyes.

The Scalenus Anterior. This muscle is an important landmark in the neck. It is attached to the anterior tubercles of the transverse processes of the third to sixth cervical vertebrae. The fibres pass downwards and slightly laterally and are attached to the scalene tubercle on the medial border of the first rib and also to the adjacent area on its upper surface. Many of its relations have been referred to. The sterno-cleidomastoid almost completely covers the scalenus anterior. The inferior belly of the omohyoid passes upwards and forwards between the two muscles. The phrenic nerve passes vertically downwards on its anterior surface, and branches of the subclavian artery (transverse cervical and supra-scapular) pass backwards on the surface of the scalenus anterior superficial to the phrenic nerve. The subclavian artery is behind and the subclavian vein in front of the muscle. The ventral rami of the cervical nerves pass laterally and emerge between the scalenus anterior and medius. Medial to the scalenus anterior is the triangle containing the vertebral artery, the inferior thyroid artery, the sympathetic trunk and the transverse process of the seventh cervical vertebra (figure 161). On the left side the termination of the thoracic duct is also in this triangle.

The Scalenus Medius. The upper attachment of this muscle is to the posterior tubercles of the transverse processes of all the cervical vertebrae except that of the first. The fibres pass downwards and are attached to the upper surface of the first rib behind the subclavian artery.

The Scalenus Posterior. This is the smallest of the scalene muscles and is attached to the posterior tubercles of the lower cervical vertebrae. The muscle passes downwards and slightly laterally and is attached to the outer surface of the second rib.

All the scalene muscles are innervated by the ventral rami of several of the cervical spinal nerves. They can act on the vertebral column. If the muscles of both sides contract, flexion is produced. The muscles of one side produce lateral bending. The scalene muscles are important accessory muscles of respiration. By pulling upwards on the first and second ribs the whole thoracic cage is pulled upwards and the result is an increase in the diameters of the thorax. These muscles contract in deep and forced inspiration. In some subjects they contract in quiet inspiration.

The First Rib (figure 158). This rib has some special features. Unlike the third to the twelfth ribs it has upper and lower surfaces and medial and lateral borders. The angle and tubercle at the back of the lateral border coincide. The side to which a first rib belongs is determined by finding the grooves on the anterior half of its upper surface. It is obvious that the concave border is medial and that the posterior end has a head for articulation with the body of the first thoracic vertebra. The *scalene tubercle*, not always as obvious as one is led to believe, is on the medial border and is nearer its anterior end.

The anterior groove in the upper surface is for the subclavian vein and the posterior groove, usually deeper than the anterior, is for the subclavian artery and the lower trunk of the brachial plexus. The scalenus anterior is attached to the scalene tubercle and the adjacent area of the upper surface between the two grooves. The scalenus medius is attached to the area behind the posterior groove. The sympathetic trunk, usually the fused inferior cervical and first thoracic ganglia, is anterior to the neck of

the rib. The superior intercostal artery crosses the medial border between the sympathetic trunk and the lower trunk of the brachial plexus.

The first digitation of the serratus anterior muscle is attached to the middle of the outer border and the subclavius muscle and costoclavicular ligament are attached to the anterior end of the upper surface. The suprapleural membrane is attached to the medial border.

The Common Carotid Artery (figures 150, 152, 153)

The common carotid artery enters the neck at the level of the sternoclavicular joint at the side of the trachea. On the right the artery is one of the two branches of the brachiocephalic artery. On the left the common carotid is a direct branch of the arch of the aorta. The artery as it passes upwards in the neck becomes deeper and lies anterior to the transverse processes of the cervical vertebrae. At the level of the upper border of the thyroid cartilage the artery divides into the external and internal carotid arteries. The internal carotid artery continues upwards in the line of the common carotid to the base of the skull. The internal jugular vein is lateral to the common carotid artery but at the sternoclavicular joint the vein is anterior to the artery. The vagus nerve lies posterior and between the vein and artery. All three structures are in the carotid sheath.

The lower part of the artery is covered by the sternocleidomastoid but at the level of the transverse process of the sixth cervical vertebra the artery is comparatively superficial and can be pressed against the transverse process on which there is a small projection called the *carotid tubercle*. The inferior belly of the omohyoid is anterior to the artery at the same level.

The prevertebral fascia is posterior to the carotid sheath and the sympathetic ganglionated trunk lies in or on the prevertebral fascia. As the artery lies on the cervical transverse processes the scalenus anterior is lateral and the longus colli medial. The trachea with the oesophagus behind it and the larynx with the pharynx behind it are medial to the artery. On the right, the recurrent laryngeal nerve passes medially behind the common carotid and then runs upwards between the trachea and oesophagus. On the left the nerve is in this latter position at a lower level.

The nerve loop called the *ansa cervicalis (hypoglossi)* formed by the union of its *superior root* (from the hypoglossal nerve) and *inferior root* (from the cervical plexus) lies anterior to the carotid sheath (figure 160). The remaining structures related to the common carotid artery have already been referred to – the vertebral artery is posterior, the superior and middle thyroid veins are anterior as they join the internal jugular vein and the lateral lobe of the thyroid gland usually extends posteriorly as far as the carotid sheath.

At the division of the internal carotid artery there is a dilatation called the *carotid sinus*, where there is a thickening of the outer coat and a thinning of the middle coat of the artery. In the adventitia, the outer coat, there are sensory nerve endings which come from the *sinus nerve*, a branch of the glossopharyngeal nerve. These react to changes in blood pressure, that is they are baroreceptors. Behind the division of the common carotid artery there is a small structure called the *carotid body*. This has sensory nerve endings from the glossopharyngeal and vagus nerves which respond to changes in the oxygen and carbon dioxide content of the blood, that is they are chemoreceptors.

Normally there are no branches from the common carotid artery apart from its two terminal divisions.

The common carotid can be marked in the neck by a vertical line drawn from the sternoclavicular joint to a point 1 cm below the tip of the greater horn of the hyoid bone.

The Internal Carotid Artery (figures 153, 159, 168)

This artery continues upwards to the base of the skull in a line continuous with that of the common carotid artery. The external carotid artery is at first medial to the internal and then becomes lateral and more superficial. The internal carotid lies anterior to the transverse processes of the third second and first cervical vertebrae in the carotid

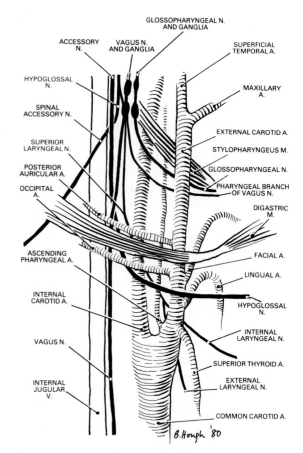

Figure 159   Some of the relations of the carotid arteries, the internal jugular vein and the glossopharyngeal, vagus, accessory and hypoglossal nerves.

sheath with the internal jugular vein lateral to it and the vagus nerve posterior and between the vein and the artery. At the base of the skull the vein is posterior to the artery. The pharynx is medial to the carotid sheath. The sternocleidomastoid is anterior with the posterior belly of the digastric and stylohyoid muscles passing downwards deep to the sternocleidomastoid and superficial to the artery.

The pharyngeal branch of the vagus nerve and the glossopharyngeal nerve with the stylopharyngeus muscle pass forwards between the internal and external carotid artery. The superior laryngeal nerve is deep and the hypoglossal nerve is superficial to both arteries. A long styloid process and a part of the parotid lie between the two arteries. At the base of the skull, the last four cranial nerves lie between the internal jugular vein and the internal carotid artery.

There are no branches of the internal carotid artery in the neck. *The position of the internal carotid artery in the neck can be indicated by a line which begins inferiorly 1 cm below the tip of the greater horn of the hyoid bone and ends above at the neck of the mandible.*

The internal carotid artery enters the skull vertically through the carotid canal in the petrous temporal bone accompanied by the *internal carotid nerve*, an upward continuation of the superior cervical sympathetic ganglion. The artery almost immediately turns medially and forwards in front of the middle and internal parts of the ear, from which it is separated by a thin plate of bone. The artery lies above the fibrocartilage in the foramen lacerum and then turns forwards into the cavernous venous sinus. This part of its course is described in the section on the inside of the skull (p. 258).

The External Carotid Artery and its Branches (figures 152, 153, 159)

The external carotid artery, one of the two divisions of the common carotid artery, is at first medial and anterior to the internal carotid artery. As it runs upwards the external carotid passes lateral to the internal and enters the parotid gland, in which it is deep to the retromandibular vein, which in turn is deep to the facial nerve. Within the gland and at the level of the neck of the mandible the external carotid artery divides into its terminal branches, the *superficial temporal* and *maxillary arteries*.

The main structures related to the internal carotid artery are also related to the external. The sternocleidomastoid and deep to it the posterior belly of the digastric and stylohyoid muscles are superficial to the artery. The structures passing deep to, between and superficial to the internal and external carotid arteries have been given on p. 232. *The position of the external carotid artery is indicated by a line passing upwards from a point 1 cm below the tip of the greater horn of the hyoid bone to a point just behind the neck of the*

mandible; the line passes behind the angle of the mandible.

The external carotid artery is distributed mainly to the structures of the neck and on the outside of the skull. These are conveniently grouped as (1) a small but long branch to the base of the skull, the *ascending pharyngeal*; (2) a descending, the *superior thyroid*; (3) and (4) two branches passing backwards, the *occipital* and the *posterior auricular*; (5) and (6) branches passing forwards, the *lingual* and the *facial*; and (7) and (8) the terminal branches.

The Ascending Pharyngeal Artery. This artery is a slender branch which arises from the origin of the external carotid artery and runs upwards between the pharynx and carotid sheath. It supplies the pharyngeal muscles and gives off a branch to the palate. At the base of the skull the artery ends as a number of branches which enter the cranial cavity through various foramina and supply the meninges.

The Superior Thyroid Artery (figure 152). Arising from the external carotid artery just above its origin, the superior thyroid artery runs downwards and medially deep to the infrahyoid muscles and lateral to the pharynx. It is accompanied by the external laryngeal nerve. This close association endangers the nerve in the operation of thyroidectomy. One of its branches is the *superior laryngeal artery* which enters the larynx with the internal laryngeal nerve through the thyrohyoid membrane. The superior thyroid artery supplies the upper pole and anterior part of the thyroid gland, the external aspect of the larynx and the sternocleidomastoid and infrahyoid muscles.

The Lingual Artery (figure 153). This artery often arises by a common trunk with the facial artery. *If they arise separately the origin of the lingual artery is just below the hyoid bone and that of the facial just above it.* The lingual artery loops upwards on the middle constrictor of the pharynx where it is crossed superficially by the hypoglossal nerve. Further forwards the artery lies deep to the hyoglossus muscle and the nerve superficial. The artery continues its course beyond the hyoglossus, to the tip of the tongue lateral to the genioglossus, and is accompanied by the lingual nerve. As the artery lies deep to the hyoglossus it gives off the *dorsal lingual arteries* which supply the back of the tongue and the neighbouring palatoglossal fold, the tonsil and the soft palate. The main artery supplies the rest of the tongue and also the sublingual salivary gland and floor of the mouth.

The Facial Artery (figures 134(a), 153). From its origin just above the level of the hyoid bone the facial artery loops upwards on the middle constrictor of the pharynx and descends towards the lower border of the mandible. The artery then passes between the mandible and the submandibular gland, winds round the lower border of the mandible 4 cm anterior to the angle where it can be felt pulsating. It has a tortuous course upwards on the face in which it lies in a plane between several of the muscles (p. 191).

The facial artery as it lies on the pharynx gives off the *ascending palatine artery* which passes upwards on the superior constrictor to the palate and gives off tonsillar branches. The main *tonsillar artery* is a branch of the facial artery. The tonsillar arteries pierce the superior constrictor and enter the palatine tonsil. The facial artery also supplies the submandibular gland and before entering the face gives off the *submental artery* which runs medially inferior to the mylohyoid muscle. This artery and the branches of the facial artery on the face have a rich anastomosis with branches of the lingual, maxillary, and ophthalmic arteries.

The facial artery may loop upwards on to the superior constrictor of the pharynx and become a lateral relation of the palatine tonsil where it may be inadvertently cut in tonsillectomy.

The Occipital and Posterior Auricular Arteries (figures 134(a), 159). Their origins are at the level of the lower and upper borders of the posterior belly of the digastric respectively and they run backwards superficial to the internal carotid artery, internal jugular vein and last three cranial nerves. The hypoglossal nerve hooks round the origin of the *occipital artery* before becoming superficial to the carotid arteries. The occipital artery continues backwards

and lies in a groove medial to the mastoid notch to which the posterior belly of the digastric is attached. In this position the artery is deep to the muscles attached to the mastoid process. The artery ends in the superficial fascia (second layer) of the scalp. Along its course the occipital artery gives off branches to the sternocleidomastoid and other muscles, the auricle and scalp. A long descending branch passes downwards deep to the trapezius and anastomoses with the superficial cervical and deep cervical arteries, branches of the subclavian artery. Meningeal branches enter the cranial cavity through several foramina including the mastoid and jugular.

The *posterior auricular artery* leaves the digastric muscle and turns upwards between the auricle and the mastoid process. It supplies branches to the parotid gland, auricle and scalp. An important branch is the *stylomastoid artery* which enters the stylomastoid foramen and supplies the facial nerve, middle ear, antrum, mastoid air cells and semicircular canals which are also supplied by the labyrinthine artery.

The Superficial Temporal Artery (figure 134(a)). Being one of the terminal branches of the external carotid artery it begins behind the neck of the mandible in the parotid gland. The artery passes laterally and then upwards over the posterior end of the zygomatic arch where it is anterior to the auriculotemporal nerve and can be felt pulsating. Its branches supply the parotid gland, external acoustic meatus, temporalis muscle and fascia and scalp. While in the parotid gland it gives off the *transverse facial artery* which passes forwards on the face between the zygomatic arch and parotid duct.

The Maxillary Artery (figure 146). This artery has been described with the region in which it lies (p. 210). Briefly the artery passes forwards from its origin posteromedial to the neck of the mandible to become medial to the lateral pterygoid muscle by passing inferior to the whole muscle or between its two heads. The artery then enters the pterygopalatine fossa through the pterygomaxillary fissure. Its branches correspond with the branches of both the mandibular and maxillary nerves. The branches from the artery lateral to the lateral pterygoid muscle enter bony foramina. The most important of these is the inferior alveolar. Deep to the lateral pterygoid the branches are mainly muscular with one important branch passing through a foramen (the middle meningeal artery) and in the pterygopalatine fossa the branches again enter foramina and supply part of the nasal cavity, palate and orbit, as well as the upper teeth.

The Internal Jugular Vein (figures (134(b), 150, 153, 159)

Almost all the blood from the cranial cavity enters the internal jugular vein and it also receives a number of veins in the neck. There is, however, a considerable venous return from the neck and extracranial part of the head to the subclavian vein via the external jugular vein, and the vertebral, inferior thyroid and deep cervical veins end in the brachiocephalic veins.

The internal jugular vein begins at the jugular foramen as a continuation of the sigmoid venous sinus which is inside the skull (p. 261). The vein runs vertically downwards in the carotid sheath lateral to the internal and then the common carotid arteries with the vagus nerve posterior and between the vein and artery. At the base of the skull the vein is posterior to the artery with the last four cranial nerves between them. At its entry to the thorax the vein is anterior as well as lateral to the artery before joining the subclavian vein to form the brachiocephalic vein.

The main relations of the internal jugular vein are the same as those of the internal and common carotid arteries with minor differences. Posteriorly the vein lies on the transverse processes of the cervical vertebrae but being somewhat more lateral than the internal carotid artery the vein lies on the cervical plexus and origin of the phrenic nerve. Inferiorly the internal jugular vein is in front of the medial part of the subclavian artery. The sternocleidomastoid muscle covers the vein. Superiorly the posterior belly of the digastric with the occipital and posterior auricular arteries and the stylohyoid muscle and inferiorly the omohyoid cross superficial to the vein. The parotid gland and

styloid process are anterolateral to the vein and lower down the accessory nerve passes backwards superficial to it.

Dilatations at the beginning and end of the vein are called the *superior* and *inferior jugular bulbs*. Above the inferior bulb there is a valve. The inferior petrosal sinus leaves the skull through the jugular foramen and joins the superior bulb.

In addition to the blood from the brain, the tributaries to the vein are veins from the tongue and pharynx and the facial vein. The vein from the front of the tongue and sublingual gland is superficial to the hyoglossus muscle and because it runs with the hypoglossal nerve it is called the *vena comitans of the hypoglossal nerve* (*comitans = accompanying*, Latin). The veins from the back of the tongue are deep to the hyoglossus muscle and form the *lingual vein*. The superior and middle thyroid veins cross anterior to the common carotid artery and join the internal jugular vein. The facial vein corresponds approximately with the facial artery to which it is posterior on the face. The facial vein is superficial in the submandibular triangle and joins the internal jugular vein near the greater cornu of the hyoid bone.

Along the whole length of the internal jugular vein there are lymph nodes which receive afferent vessels from other lymph nodes in the neck. The nodes along the vein drain downwards into a single vessel called the jugular lymph trunk which on the right joins the subclavian lymph trunk to form the right lymph duct or on the left opens separately into the thoracic duct. On the right the right lymph duct enters the beginning of the right brachiocephalic vein.

The Cervical Plexus

The ventral rami of the first four cervical spinal nerves form this plexus, which is in the form of a series of loops on the transverse processes of the upper cervical vertebrae deep to the internal jugular vein. The branches of the plexus may be grouped as follows.

(1) There are *communicating branches* with the hypoglossal, accessory and vagus nerves and the sympathetic trunk. The branch to the hypoglossal

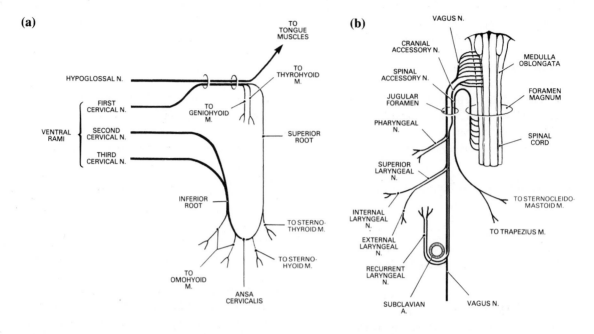

Figure 160   (a) The formation of the ansa cervicalis. (b) The distribution of the accessory nerve.

nerve comes from the first cervical nerve (figure 160) and leaves as branches to the geniohyoid and thyrohyoid muscles and the *superior root of the ansa cervicalis* (formerly called the *descendens hypoglossi* and *ansa hypoglossi*). The sympathetic branches are grey rami communicantes (postganglionic fibres) from the superior cervical ganglion.

(2) *Muscular branches* supply prevertebral muscles — the rectus capitis lateralis and anterior (from the first cervical nerve) and the longus colli and capitis, and scalene muscles. A branch of the second and third cervical nerves forms the *inferior root of the ansa cervicalis* (formerly the *descendens cervicalis*). The roots and ansa lie on the carotid sheath and give off branches to the omohyoid, sternothyroid and sternohyoid muscles.

(3) *Sensory branches* supply the trapezius and sternocleidomastoid muscles and also form the cutaneous nerves which have already been described (p. 213) — the great auricular, lesser occipital, transverse cervical and supraclavicular nerves (figures 135, 155(a)).

(4) The *phrenic nerve* (figures 46, 150) comes from the third and fourth cervical nerves and receives a branch from the fifth cervical nerve. The phrenic nerve, the most important branch of the plexus, passes downwards on the scalenus anterior from its lateral to its medial border and enters the thorax behind the subclavian vein. Its further course is described on p.   . The phrenic nerve is a mixed nerve (approximately one-third of its fibres are sensory) and is motor to the diaphragm and sensory to the mediastinal and diaphragmatic pleura, the fibrous and parietal serous pericardium and the diaphragmatic peritoneum. Irritation of any of these serous membranes may produce referred pain to the tip of the shoulder, a region which is supplied by the fourth cervical spinal nerve.

The Glossopharyngeal Nerve (figure 159)

The *ninth cranial nerve*, the *glossopharyngeal*, leaves the skull through the jugular foramen with the vagus and accessory nerves. They all lie between the internal jugular vein and internal carotid artery which is anterior. The glossopharyngeal nerve has a superior and inferior ganglion in the jugular foramen. Together with the stylopharyngeus the nerve passes downwards and forwards between the internal and external carotid arteries. The nerve passes superficial to the stylopharyngeus and ends in the back of the tongue.

The glossopharyngeal nerve contains (1) fibres of general sensation which come from the *posterior third of the tongue* (that is posterior to and including the sulcus terminalis), and from most of the *lining of the pharynx* including the fauces and tonsil; (2) fibres of *taste* from the posterior third of the tongue and also the vallate papillae; (3) sensory fibres from the *carotid body and sinus*; (4) sensory fibres from the lining of the *middle ear and auditory tube*. The cell bodies of all these fibres are in the inferior ganglion. A branch of the glossopharyngeal nerve is *motor to the stylopharyngeus*. The nerve also contains preganglionic *parasympathetic fibres* which pursue a complicated course. A branch of the glossopharyngeal nerve, the *tympanic nerve*, goes to the tympanic plexus on the medial wall of the middle ear and contains parasympathetic fibres. In the middle ear the *lesser petrosal nerve* is formed, enters the cranial cavity and leaves it usually through the foramen ovale to join the otic ganglion (p. 207). The parasympathetic fibres synapse in the ganglion and the postganglionic fibres join the auriculotemporal nerve and supply the secretomotor fibres to the parotid gland.

The Vagus Nerve in the Neck
(figures 150, 159)

The *vagus*, the *tenth cranial nerve*, leaves the skull through the jugular foramen and passes downwards inside the carotid sheath between and posterior to the internal and common carotid arteries and the internal jugular vein. There are two *ganglia* on the vagus nerve as it leaves the skull, a smaller *superior* (about 3 mm long) which lies in the jugular foramen and larger *inferior* (about 25 mm long) lying just below the foramen. Below the superior ganglion the vagus is joined by the cranial accessory nerve which is distributed with the laryngeal and pharyngeal branches of the vagus (figure 160).

While in the jugular foramen sensory branches arise from the superior ganglion, a *meningeal branch*

which re-enters the skull and an *auricular branch* which supplies part of the lining of the external acoustic meatus and part of the outer surface of the tympanic membrane. It also supplies part of the skin of the cranial surface of the auricle. It is thought that stimulation of this nerve while the ear is being syringed may cause slowing of the heart and fainting because of reflex stimulation of the vagal nerve supply to the heart. Wax in the ear or syringing can also cause reflex coughing due to irritation of the auricular branch reflexly stimulating the internal laryngeal nerve, a branch of the vagus supplying the mucous membrane of the larynx above the vocal folds. The auricular branch is also known as the *alderman's nerve* because traditionally an alderman during a gargantuan aldermen's dinner stroked the back of his ear or stimulated the external acoustic meatus with his finger to increase reflexly his gastric secretions in order to cope with the very large meal.

The *pharyngeal branch* of the vagus nerve from the inferior ganglion passes forwards between the internal and external carotid arteries to the pharyngeal plexus of nerves (figures 159, 160). The branch is mainly motor and derived from the cranial accessory nerve. It supplies all the muscles of the pharynx except the stylopharyngeus and all the muscles of the palate except the tensor veli palatini.

The *superior laryngeal nerve* also arises from the inferior ganglion and passes downwards posterior and then medial to the internal carotid artery. The nerve divides into the *external* and *internal laryngeal nerves* (figures 159, 160, 194). The external laryngeal nerve accompanies the superior thyroid artery and supplies the cricothyroid muscle. The nerve may be cut during the operation of thyroidectomy. The internal laryngeal nerve pierces the thyrohyoid membrane with the superior laryngeal artery and is distributed mainly as sensory fibres to the lining of the larynx above the vocal folds, and the mucous membrane adjacent to the laryngeal opening. This nerve is the sensory part of the cough reflex which is initiated if anything solid or liquid enters the larynx.

On the right side the *recurrent laryngeal nerve* is given off from the vagus as it crosses the subclavian artery before entering the thorax (figure 155(b)). The recurrent laryngeal nerve passes below and then behind the subclavian artery and then medially and upwards behind the common carotid artery and reaches the interval between the oesophagus and trachea. The nerve passes upwards deep to the inferior constrictor and supplies all the muscles of the larynx except the cricothyroid and is sensory to the larynx below the level of the vocal folds. The nerve also supplies the inferior constrictor of the pharynx, and motor and sensory fibres to the trachea and the upper part of the oesophagus.

On the left side the recurrent laryngeal nerve arises in the thorax as the vagus crosses to the left of the arch of the aorta (p. 50). The left recurrent laryngeal nerve passes upwards and enters the neck in the groove between the trachea and oesophagus. On both sides of the neck the recurrent laryngeal nerve accompanies the inferior thyroid artery (the exact relationship is variable and may be different on the two sides of the neck). The nerve may be involved in the operation of thyroidectomy. The motor fibres in both the external and recurrent laryngeal nerves are mainly from the cranial accessory nerve.

Each vagus nerve gives off in the neck two or three *cardiac branches* which descend into the thorax and end in the deep cardiac plexus of nerves except for the lowest branch on the left side which joins the superficial cardiac plexus. These nerves are largely motor parasympathetic.

The Accessory Nerve

The *accessory, the eleventh cranial nerve*, is formed by the union of a *spinal part* which comes from the upper five cervical segments of the spinal cord and a *cranial part* which comes from the medulla oblongata of the hindbrain (figure 106(b)). The roots of the spinal part emerge from the spinal cord between the dorsal and ventral roots of the spinal nerves and run upwards. They unite and form a nerve trunk which enters the skull through the foramen magnum, posterior to the vertebral artery. The cranial part emerges as a series of rootlets which join and pass laterally towards the jugular foramen. The spinal and cranial parts unite and form the accessory nerve which leaves the

skull through the jugular foramen within the same sheath of dura mater as the vagus nerve. (The name *accessory nerve* refers to the cranial part, being an accessory nerve to the vagus.) Immediately below the jugular foramen the cranial part joins the vagus nerve and the spinal part passes backwards between the internal carotid artery and internal jugular vein and crosses the internal jugular vein anteriorly and also the transverse process of the atlas. The spinal part pierces the sternocleidomastoid, continues downwards and backwards deep to the muscle and appears at about the middle of its posterior border in the posterior triangle. The nerve runs downwards and backwards across the posterior triangle to pass deep to the lateral border of the trapezius 5 cm above the clavicle (figure 155(a)).

The spinal accessory nerve is motor to the sternocleidomastoid and trapezius muscles. Both receive proprioceptive fibres from the cervical spinal nerves, the sternocleidomastoid from the second and third and the trapezius from the third and fourth. *The surface marking of the upper part of the nerve is from in front of the external acoustic meatus to the transverse process of the atlas which can be palpated midway between the angle of the jaw and the mastoid process. The rest of the nerve is indicated by a line drawn from the transverse process of the atlas to the anterior border of the trapezius 5 cm above the clavicle. This line crosses the posterior border of the sternocleidomastoid about its middle.*

In an operation involving removal of all the lymph nodes of the neck, the spinal accessory nerve, especially where it is superficial in the posterior triangle, is liable to be damaged. The trapezius is paralysed and the patient cannot shrug and brace back his shoulder. The nerve may be damaged in a fracture of the skull involving the jugular foramen. This would affect the sternocleidomastoid as well. Irritation of the nerve due to inflamed lymph nodes in the neck is common in children. Spasm of the sternocleidomastoid muscle causes torticollis — the head is turned to the opposite side and tilted to the same side.

The cranial accessory nerve is distributed through the laryngeal and pharyngeal branches of the vagus — the superior and recurrent laryngeal and the pharyngeal nerves. The cell bodies of these motor fibres form the major part of the *nucleus ambiguus* of the hindbrain. Some of the fibres from this nucleus join the glossopharyngeal and vagus nerves. Those in the glossopharyngeal nerve supply the stylopharyngeus. The nucleus ambiguus supplies all the muscles of the larynx, pharynx and palate except the tensor veli palatini which is supplied by the mandibular nerve. The nucleus ambiguus may be affected by a vascular lesion with the result that the muscles of the palate, pharynx and larynx are involved and swallowing and speech are affected. This is marked if both nuclei are affected — swallowing is difficult, speech is weak and nasal and there is considerable danger of food passing into the larynx.

The effects of lesions of the individual nerves of the larynx are discussed with that organ (p. 317).

The Hypoglossal Nerve

The *hypoglossal, twelfth cranial, nerve* leaves the skull through the hypoglossal (anterior condylar) canal of the occipital bone medial to the jugular foramen. The nerve passes laterally behind the vagus and glossopharyngeal nerves and internal carotid artery, and runs downwards between the internal jugular vein and internal carotid artery in front of the vagus nerve (figures 153, 159). The hypoglossal nerve becomes more superficial and hooks round the occipital artery to pass forwards superficial to the internal and external carotid arteries. The nerve is superficial to the loop of the lingual artery and is crossed by the facial vein. In this part of its course the nerve is deep to the posterior belly of the digastric and stylohyoid muscles. It enters the mouth by passing superficial to the hyoglossus and deep to the mylohyoid. While on the hyoglossus the hypoglossal nerve is inferior to the lingual nerve, and the submandibular gland and duct and the submandibular ganglion lie between the nerves (figure 144). The hypoglossal nerve runs forwards to the tip of the tongue.

The hypoglossal nerve receives branches from the first cervical and vagus nerves. Sensory fibres in these branches are distributed to the dura mater of the posterior cranial fossa. The motor fibres in the first cervical nerve leave the hypoglossal nerve as branches to the geniohyoid and thyrohyoid muscles and as the upper root to the ansa cervicalis (p. 236). The hypoglossal nerve is motor to the intrinsic and extrinsic muscles of the tongue, except the palatoglossus, which is supplied by the pharyngeal branch of the vagus through the pharyngeal plexus of nerves.

If the hypoglossal nerve on one side is injured the muscles of the tongue of that side waste and the tongue, if protruded, is pushed to the affected side. Speech and swallowing are not markedly affected. If both nerves are affected the whole tongue wastes and lies motionless on the floor of the mouth. The initiating (oral part) of swallowing is almost impossible and speech is slow and indistinct.

The Cervical Part of the Sympathetic System

The sympathetic ganglionated trunk extends from the base of the skull to the hollow of the sacrum in the pelvis (p. 50). The cervical part of the trunk consists of three *ganglia, inferior, middle* and *superior*, and is continuous inferiorly with the thoracic part of the trunk (figure 161). The superior ganglion continues upwards as the internal carotid nerve which accompanies the internal carotid artery into the temporal bone and forms a plexus round that artery. The cervical sympathetic trunk lies behind and slightly medial to the carotid sheath on or in the prevertebral fascia. The preganglionic fibres come from the upper four or five thoracic spinal segments via the white rami communicantes of the upper four or five intercostal nerves and the thoracic part of the sympathetic trunk (p. 50). These preganglionic fibres synapse in the cervical ganglia and postganglionic grey fibres leave the ganglia to be distributed to the structures in the head and neck.

The *superior cervical ganglion*, thought to be formed by the fusion of four cervical ganglia, is about 2.5 cm long and lies in front of the transverse processes of the second and third cervical vertebrae behind the internal carotid artery. Most of the preganglionic fibres which synapse in the superior ganglion are derived from the first thoracic

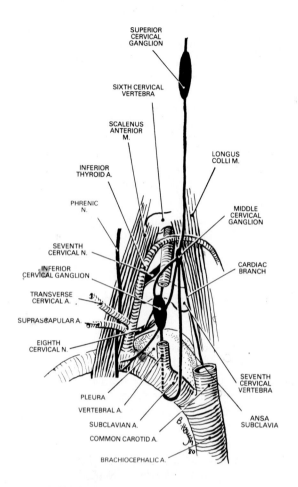

Figure 161   The cervical sympathetic ganglia.

The *middle cervical ganglion* is smaller than the superior and lies at the level of the transverse process of the sixth cervical vertebra. It is probably formed by the fusion of two ganglia. Postganglionic fibres from the middle ganglion (1) go to the fifth and sixth cervical spinal nerves; (2) go to the thyroid and parathyroid glands as a plexus round the inferior thyroid artery which lies near the ganglion; (3) form a cardiac branch which descends into the thorax and joins the deep cardiac plexus. A loop called the *ansa subclavia* connects the middle ganglion with the inferior and passes downwards in front of the medial part of the subclavian artery and below and then upwards behind the artery to join the inferior ganglion.

The *inferior cervical ganglion* is usually fused with the first thoracic to form the *cervicothoracic (stellate) ganglion* and lies on the transverse process of the seventh cervical vertebra and neck of the first rib behind the vertebral artery. Postganglionic fibres from the ganglion (1) join the seventh and eighth cervical and first thoracic spinal nerves; (2) form a plexus round the subclavian artery and its branches; (3) form a cardiac branch which goes to the deep cardiac plexus. The plexus on the vertebral artery accompanies that vessel into the cranial cavity and is regarded by some authorities as more important in relation to the cerebral vessels than the internal carotid plexus.

The preganglionic sympathetic fibres supplying the head and neck and also the upper limb are derived from the upper five thoracic spinal segments, mainly the upper three. Most of the sympathetic fibres for the upper limb are derived from the second and third thoracic segments and in order to denervate the upper limb of its sympathetic supply removal of the second and third thoracic ganglia is adequate. The operation is carried out for conditions involving spasm of the blood vessels of the hand and also for excessive palmar sweating.

Since all the preganglionic fibres of the cervical sympathetic trunk pass through the cervicothoracic ganglion, pressure on this ganglion, which lies in the thoracic inlet behind the suprapleural membrane and cervical pleura, can result in a loss of sweating in the neck, face and scalp on the affected side. In addition the postganglionic fibres which accompany the internal carotid artery cease to

spinal cord segment. Postganglionic fibres from the superior ganglion (1) join the upper four cervical spinal nerves and the glossopharyngeal, vagus and hypoglossal nerves; (2) continue upwards as the internal carotid nerve into the skull; (3) join the pharyngeal plexus of nerves; (4) form a plexus round the external carotid artery and its branches (these may leave the artery and travel with branches of the trigeminal nerve); (5) form a cardiac branch, which on the right descends behind the common carotid and subclavian arteries and arch of the aorta and joins the deep cardiac plexus, and on the left lies in front of the common carotid artery then to the left of the aortic arch and usually joins the superficial cardiac plexus.

function. These supply the dilatator pupillae muscle and the smooth muscle of the elevator of the upper eyelid. This would also follow removal of the cervicothoracic ganglion in the operation referred to above. *Horner's syndrome* is the name given to the condition in which the pupil is small, *meiosis* (= *a state of being smaller*, Greek), the upper lid droops, *ptosis* (= *a falling*, Greek), the eyeball is sunken (*enophthalmos*) and there is loss of sweating (*anhydrosis*) of the skin of the head and neck (J.H. Horner, 1831–86, Swiss ophthalmologist). This condition most frequently results from pressure on the cervicothoracic ganglion at the inlet of the thorax.

The Lymph Nodes of the Neck (figure 162)

These are arranged in two groups, *superficial* and *deep*. Most of the superficial nodes form a ring at the junction of the head and neck and are sub-divided as follows. Posteriorly there are *occipital nodes* along the superior nuchal line of the occipital bone and *retro-auricular nodes* behind the auricle. Their afferent vessels go to the deep cervical nodes. For some obscure reason the occipital nodes are enlarged in the early stage of German measles.

The *parotid* and *preauricular nodes* are in front of the external acoustic meatus and are usually superficial to the parotid gland. One or two nodes may be embedded in the gland itself. The afferent vessels to these nodes come from the side of the scalp, the anterior parts of the external ear (pinna and meatus), the middle ear and the lateral halves of the eyelids.

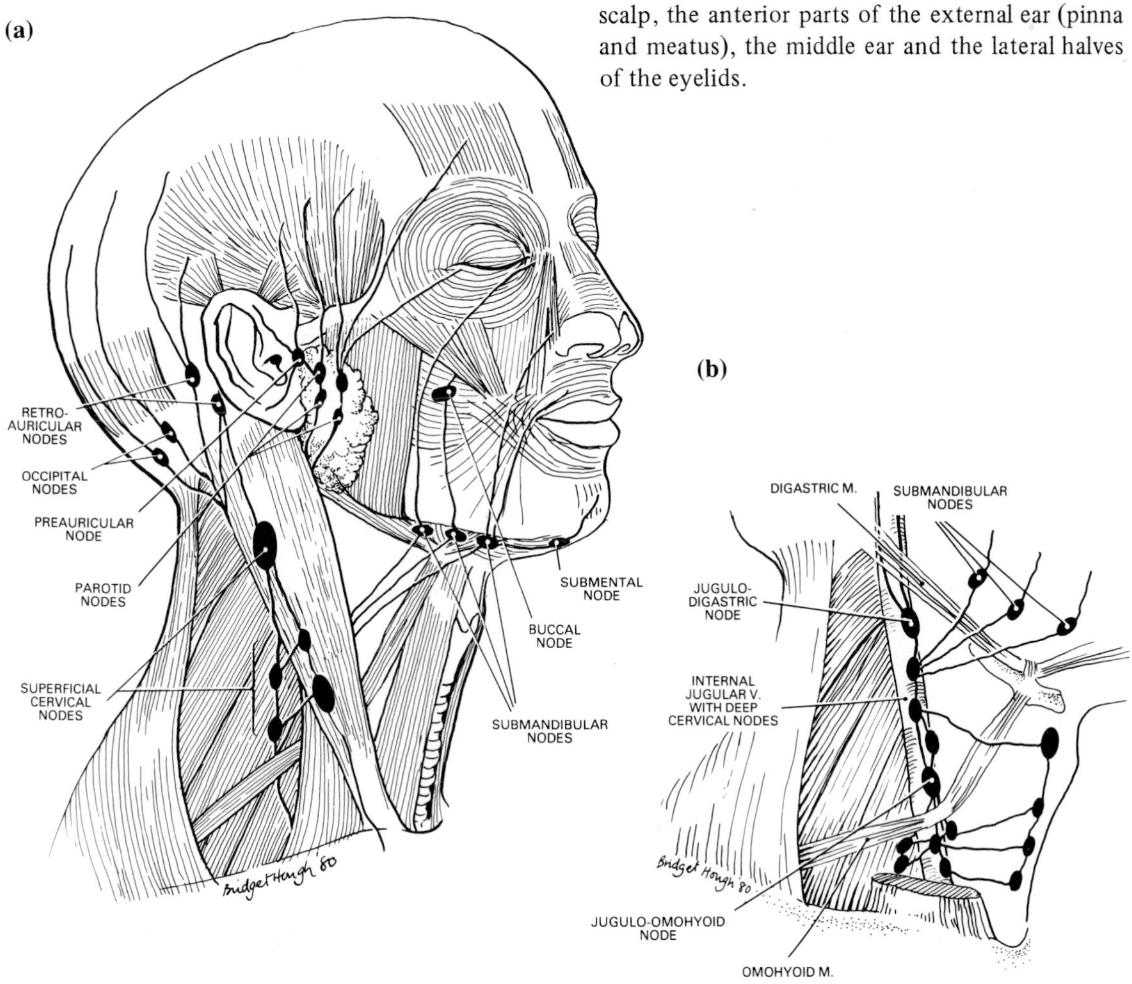

(a)

(b)

Figure 162   The lymph nodes of the head and neck: (a) superficial; (b) deep.

The *submandibular nodes* lie near or in the submandibular gland, between the mandible and mylohyoid muscle. Their afferent vessels come from an extensive area including most of the lips and cheek, the anterior part of the scalp, the medial halves of the eyelids, the upper and lower teeth and gingivae, the side of the tongue, the posterior part of the floor of the mouth and the vestibule and anterior part of the nasal cavity. Painful enlargement of these nodes is common because infection of the regions they drain (mouth, teeth, inner parts of the eyelids, vestibule of the nasal cavity) is common. It is surprising how often the enlarged painful nodes produce the first or main complaint from the patient. The *source* of the infection must be traced. The submandibular nodes also receive the efferent vessels from the submental nodes. The efferent vessels from the submandibular nodes go to the deep cervical.

The *submental nodes* are posterior to the lower border of the mandible and inferior to the mylohyoid muscle. They receive vessels from the tip of the tongue and the anterior part of the mouth which pierce the mylohyoid muscle, and vessels from the central part of the lower lip. The afferent vessels go mainly to the submandibular nodes but some pass directly to the deep cervical nodes.

There are superficial nodes (1) on the surface of the sternocleidomastoid muscle along the external jugular vein; (2) vertically near the midline of the neck along the anterior jugular vein; (3) diagonally along the accessory nerve in the posterior triangle. The afferent vessels to these nodes come from the skin and their efferent vessels go to the deep cervical nodes.

The *deep cervical nodes* are arranged longitudinally along the internal jugular vein and are divided into *superior* and *inferior*. The efferent vessels from all the superficial nodes drain directly or indirectly into the deep nodes. The lymph from some of the deeper tissues of the neck, the upper part of the larynx, lower part of the pharynx and beginning of the oesophagus drains directly into the deep cervical nodes. The vessels from the deep nodes drain downwards and eventually form the *jugular lymph trunk*, which on the right side joins the *subclavian lymph trunk* from the axillary nodes to form the *right lymph duct*, which usually joins the beginning of the right brachiocephalic vein. On the left the jugular and subclavian lymph ducts usually join the thoracic duct.

There are some deep lymph nodes in front of and at the sides of the larynx and trachea. Vessels from the larynx, trachea and thyroid gland drain into these nodes from which efferent vessels go to the lower deep cervical nodes. The deep cervical nodes which lie where the posterior belly of the digastric crosses the internal jugular vein are called the *jugulodigastric nodes*. These nodes receive lymphatic vessels from the tonsil. The node where the omohyoid muscle crosses the vein is called the *jugulo-omohyoid* and receives lymph from the tongue which also drains into the jugulodigastric node.

There are also some lymph nodes behind the nasopharynx in front of the vertebral column (*retropharyngeal*). The pharyngeal tonsil (p. 309) drains into these nodes which drain into the deep cervical nodes. Infection of the retropharyngeal nodes may lead to a *retropharyngeal abscess* which is difficult to incise because of its position. Even if incised there is the danger of the inhalation of the pus from the abscess.

A summary of the lymphatic drainage of the different parts and organs of the head and neck is given in table 5 on p. 322.

18

The Cranial Cavity

The cranial cavity contains the brain with its meninges and blood vessels and the cranial nerves which enter and emerge from the brain. The cerebrospinal fluid is produced inside the brain and leaves it to enter the subarachnoid space between two of the meninges. It is re-absorbed mainly into the veins in the cranial cavity.

The Bony Features

The bones of the inside of the skull can be examined by means of a horizontal cut which passes through the skull about 4 cm above the nasion and external occipital protuberance.

The *skull cap* (figure 163(a)) consists of a triangular piece of the occipital bone posteriorly, almost the whole of the parietal bones and part of the frontal bone anteriorly. The anteroposterior *sagittal suture* between the parietal bones, and the transverse *coronal suture* between the parietal and frontal bones are present, although internally they may not be very obvious in the skull of a subject over 40 years old. A part of the *lambdoid suture* between the parietal and occipital bones is present.

In the skull cap anteriorly the cavities in the frontal bone on either side of the midline (the *frontal sinuses*) may be cut through. Internally above the frontal sinuses there is the midline *frontal crest*. Passing backwards from the crest the *sagittal sulcus*, which widens posteriorly, reaches the *internal occipital protuberance* below the level of the cut. On either side of the sulcus there are depressions of varying size. The bone related to these depressions is often very thin. On the parietal bone grooves for the middle meningeal vessels pass horizontally backwards and almost vertically upwards behind the coronal suture. The vertical groove may be quite deep or even form a canal. Reference has already been made to the possibility of these vessels being torn due to injury (p. 210).

The interior of the base of the skull is divided for descriptive purposes into the anterior, middle and posterior cranial fossae.

The Anterior Cranial Fossa (figure 163(b))

This is defined as the anterior part of the inside of the floor of the cranial cavity limited posteriorly by the *lesser wings* of the sphenoid bone. When followed medially the posterior edge of the lesser wing curves backwards and ends as the *anterior clinoid process* (*kline = bed*, Greek, *clinoid = like a bedpost*). Most of the anterior cranial fossa is formed by the *orbital plates* of the frontal bone which form the major part of the roof of the orbits. The ridges on the plates correspond with the sulci of the frontal lobes. Between the orbital plates there is a gap which is filled by the *cribriform plate* (*cribrum = sieve*, Latin) and a vertical midline projection called the *crista galli* (*cock's comb*, Latin). Both are parts of the ethmoid bone. Anterior to the crista galli the *foramen caecum*

(a)

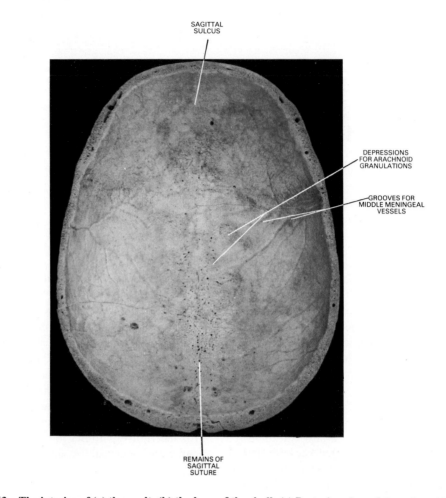

SAGITTAL
SULCUS

DEPRESSIONS
FOR ARACHNOID
GRANULATIONS

GROOVES FOR
MIDDLE MENINGEAL
VESSELS

REMAINS OF
SAGITTAL
SUTURE

Figure 163   The interior of (a) the vault, (b) the base of the skull. (c) Posterior view of the sphenoid bone.

(*caecum = blind*, Latin) occasionally communicates with the nasal cavity. Immediately behind the cribriform plates a part of the body of the sphenoid bone forms the *jugum sphenoidale* (*jugum = yoke*, Latin), and behind the jugum there is a groove. Lateral to the groove, the *optic canal* leads into the orbit.

The Middle Cranial Fossa (figure 163(b), (c))

This is limited anteriorly by the lesser wings of the sphenoid bone and posteriorly on each side by the upper border of the petrous temporal bone. This fossa is described as having a central part and a lateral part on each side. The central part consists mainly of the upper surface of the body of the

sphenoid bone and is hollowed out to form the *sella turcica* (*Turkish saddle*, Latin) the deepest part of which is called the *hypophyseal fossa*. The hypophysis cerebri lies in this fossa. A transverse bony projection called the *dorsum sellae* limits the sella posteriorly. The *posterior clinoid processes* form the lateral limits of the dorsum sellae. The *carotid sulcus* is an anteroposterior groove on each side of the sella turcica. The posterior end of the groove turns laterally and passes above the *foramen lacerum* between the petrous temporal and sphenoid bones.

The lateral part of the middle cranial fossa is formed mainly by the *greater wing* of the sphenoid bone. Anteriorly and medially the greater wing is separated from the lesser wing by the *superior*

(b)

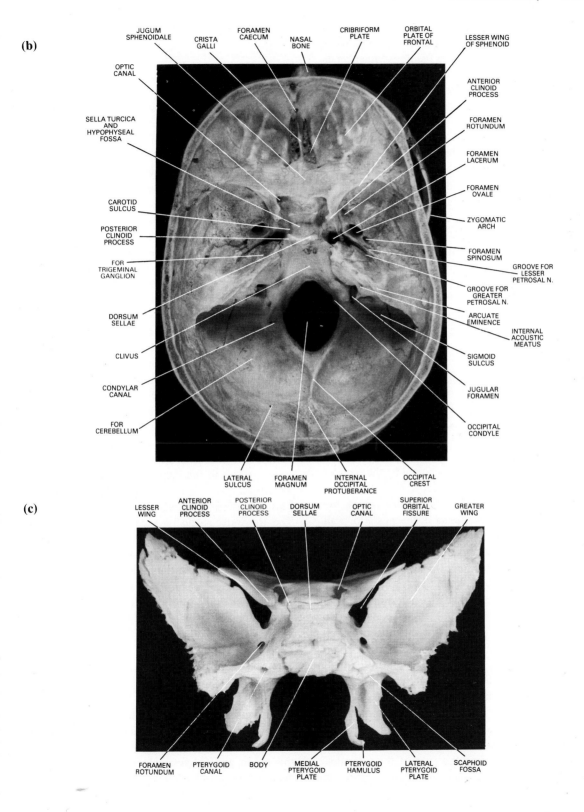

JUGUM SPHENOIDALE

CRISTA GALLI

FORAMEN CAECUM

NASAL BONE

CRIBRIFORM PLATE

ORBITAL PLATE OF FRONTAL

LESSER WING OF SPHENOID

OPTIC CANAL

ANTERIOR CLINOID PROCESS

FORAMEN ROTUNDUM

SELLA TURCICA AND HYPOPHYSEAL FOSSA

FORAMEN LACERUM

FORAMEN OVALE

CAROTID SULCUS

ZYGOMATIC ARCH

POSTERIOR CLINOID PROCESS

FORAMEN SPINOSUM

GROOVE FOR LESSER PETROSAL N.

FOR TRIGEMINAL GANGLION

GROOVE FOR GREATER PETROSAL N.

DORSUM SELLAE

ARCUATE EMINENCE

INTERNAL ACOUSTIC MEATUS

CLIVUS

SIGMOID SULCUS

CONDYLAR CANAL

JUGULAR FORAMEN

FOR CEREBELLUM

OCCIPITAL CONDYLE

LATERAL SULCUS

FORAMEN MAGNUM

INTERNAL OCCIPITAL PROTUBERANCE

OCCIPITAL CREST

(c)

LESSER WING

ANTERIOR CLINOID PROCESS

POSTERIOR CLINOID PROCESS

DORSUM SELLAE

OPTIC CANAL

SUPERIOR ORBITAL FISSURE

GREATER WING

FORAMEN ROTUNDUM

PTERYGOID CANAL

BODY

MEDIAL PTERYGOID PLATE

PTERYGOID HAMULUS

LATERAL PTERYGOID PLATE

SCAPHOID FOSSA

orbital fissure which leads into the orbit and is directed laterally, upwards and forwards when looked at from behind. The fissure is wider medially than laterally. Immediately behind its medial end the *foramen rotundum* leads into the pterygopalatine fossa. About 1 cm posterior and slightly lateral to the foramen rotundum the *foramen ovale* leads downwards into the infratemporal fossa. The *foramen spinosum* is posterolateral to the foramen ovale. From the foramen spinosum a groove passes laterally and forwards and then turns upwards on to the squamous temporal bone which forms the lateral part of the middle cranial fossa. The greater wing of the sphenoid passes anteriorly as well as laterally and turns upwards to meet the frontal, parietal and temporal bones at the *pterion*.

The posterior wall of the lateral part of the middle fossa is formed by the anterosuperior surface of the petrous temporal bone. Its medial end forms part of the boundary of the foramen lacerum. The *carotid canal* which runs vertically and then medially and forwards in the petrous temporal bone opens on to the upper part of the foramen lacerum, the lower part of which in the living is closed by fibrocartilage. There are two grooves on this surface of the petrous temporal bone, a lateral which leads to the foramen ovale and contains the lesser petrosal nerve and a medial which leads to the foramen lacerum and contains the greater petrosal nerve. The medial groove leads to a canal on the anterior wall of the foramen lacerum, the *pterygoid canal*, which ends in the posterior wall of the pterygopalatine fossa. The greater petrosal nerve joins the deep petrosal nerve from the internal carotid sympathetic plexus and forms the nerve of the pterygoid canal which passes through the canal to the pterygopalatine ganglion (p. 209).

The upper border of the petrous temporal bone is grooved. The medial end of the upper border, where the trigeminal nerve lies, is flat. The nerve passes forwards to the trigeminal ganglion which lies in a hollow area at the medial end of the antero-superior wall of the petrous bone. Posterolateral to the grooves for the petrosal nerves there is the *arcuate eminence* due to the underlying anterior (superior) semicircular canal. Lateral to the eminence the bone forming the roof of the tympanic cavity (the middle ear) and the mastoid antrum is

called the *tegmen tympani* (*tegmen = roof*, Latin).

The Posterior Cranial Fossa (figure 163(b))

The occipital bone forms the major part of the posterior cranial fossa. Anteriorly in front of the foramen magnum the basilar part of the occipital bone is continuous with the body of the sphenoid. This sloping surface is called the *clivus* (*clivus = hill*, Latin) and ends superiorly as the dorsum sellae and posterior clinoid processes.

On each side the postero-superior surface of the petrous temporal forms the anterolateral wall of the posterior fossa. The medial end of the petrous temporal bone articulates with the sphenoid and occipital bones at the *petro-occipital suture*. The jugular foramen lies between the petrous temporal and the occipital bones. Almost directly above the jugular foramen, on the petrous temporal bone, there is the *internal acoustic meatus*.

The *foramen magnum* is narrowed antero-laterally by the encroachment of the *occipital condyles*. The opening of the *hypoglossal canal* lies above the middle of the edge of the condyle. More superiorly and just behind the condyle the opening of the *condylar canal* may be present. Behind the foramen magnum the *occipital crest* runs upwards in the midline to the *internal occipital protuberance*. The edges of the *sagittal sulcus* pass upwards in the midline from the protuberance. The transverse sulcus on each side passes laterally from the protuberance, curves anteriorly and grooves the postero-inferior angle of the parietal bone. The groove continues downwards, medially and forwards as the *sigmoid sulcus* which lies on the internal aspect of the mastoid process and then on the occipital bone to end at the jugular foramen.

The External Features of the Brain (figure 164)

It is necessary to describe briefly the main parts of the brain in order to follow the description of its coverings (meninges) and large blood vessels and the origin and intracranial course of the cranial nerves. Most of the human brain consists of the

(a)

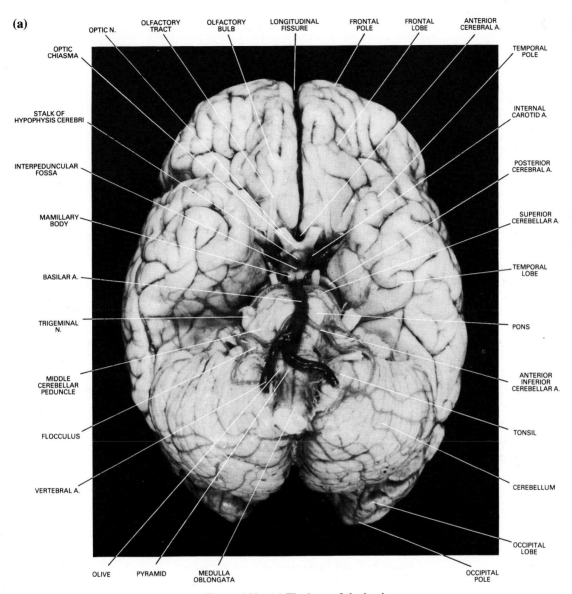

Figure 164 **(a) The base of the brain.**

cerebral hemispheres which are part of the *fore-brain*. These overgrow the rest of the brain so that its different parts can most easily be seen only from its inferior surface. Because the brain is bent forwards its inferior surface was originally anterior. The *hindbrain* lies posteriorly and consists of the *medulla oblongata*, the upward continuation of the spinal cord through the foramen magnum, the *pons*, which on the surface appears as a transverse bridge whose lower border marks the upper limit

of the medulla oblongata, and the *cerebellum* into which the pons can be followed laterally.

The medulla oblongata is about 2.5 cm long and about 1 cm wide. On its anterior surface it has a vertical midline groove. The *pyramid* lies on each side of the groove and is enlarged near the pons. The *olive* is a vertical structure, about 1 cm long, at the side of the pyramid immediately inferior to the pons. The olive is separated from the pyramid by a groove which extends towards the spinal cord.

(b)

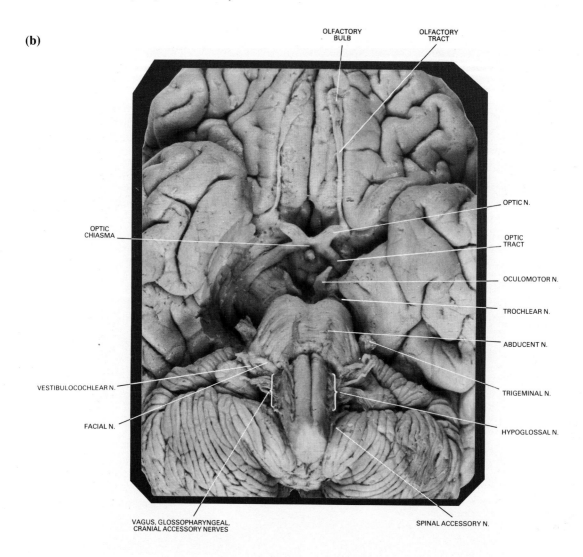

OLFACTORY BULB

OLFACTORY TRACT

OPTIC N.

OPTIC CHIASMA

OPTIC TRACT

OCULOMOTOR N.

TROCHLEAR N.

ABDUCENT N.

VESTIBULOCOCHLEAR N.

TRIGEMINAL N.

FACIAL N.

HYPOGLOSSAL N.

VAGUS, GLOSSOPHARYNGEAL, CRANIAL ACCESSORY NERVES

SPINAL ACCESSORY N.

Figure 164   (b) The origin of the cranial nerves.

Lateral to the olive near the pons on the postero-lateral aspect of the medulla the *inferior cerebellar peduncle* passes upwards into the cerebellum. The groove between the olive and the inferior peduncle extends downwards to the spinal cord.

The pons is about 3.5 cm wide and 3 cm long. It has transverse fibres on its surface and narrows laterally to form the *middle cerebellar peduncle*. The pons on its anterior surface has a longitudinal midline groove about 3 mm wide. The medulla and most of the pons lie in a wide groove between the cerebellar hemispheres and conceal the middle part

of the cerebellum (the *vermis*). The surface of the cerebellum has a large number of fissures. The part of the hemisphere adjacent to the medulla and just above the foramen magnum is called the *tonsil*. The *flocculus* of the cerebellum lies immediately below the lateral part of the pons. The cerebellum is about 10 cm wide, 5 cm long and 4 cm thick.

The *midbrain* is the smallest of the subsections of the brain and is about 1.5 cm long, 2.5 cm wide and 2 cm thick. Little of the midbrain can be seen from the inferior surface, but the *cerebral ped-uncles* which are part of the midbrain can be

(c)

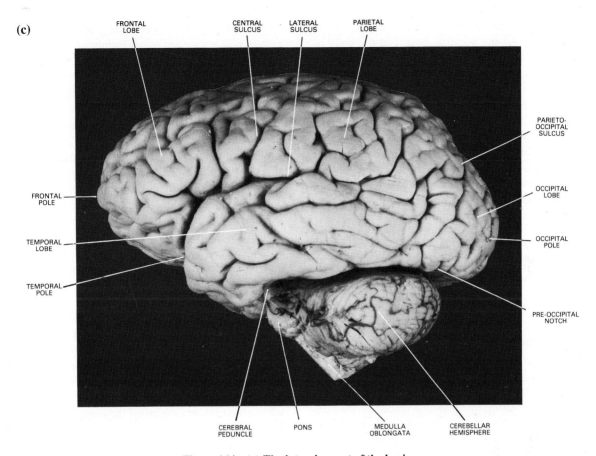

Figure 164 (c) The lateral aspect of the brain.

identified passing upwards and laterally from the upper border of the pons. Each peduncle enters a cerebral hemisphere. Between the diverging peduncles there is a space called the *interpeduncular fossa* in which there are from behind forwards the paired *corpora mamillaria*, the attachment of the *stalk of the hypophysis cerebri* and the *optic chiasma (chiasma = two lines placed crosswise*, Greek). The region between the corpora mamillaria and the optic chiasma is called the *hypothalamus* and is part of the forebrain. The optic chiasma is formed by the union of the *optic nerves* as they pass backwards and medially from the optic canals. The chiasma divides into the diverging *optic tracts*. Each tract winds round a cerebral peduncle and disappears from view.

The forebrain is divided into two parts, the cerebral hemispheres (the *telencephalon*) and a much smaller part which lies above the midbrain, the *diencephalon (di = between, tele = end, encephalon = brain*, all Greek: the *between brain* is between the midbrain and the main part of the forebrain). On the inferior aspect of the brain the *temporal lobes* lie lateral to the cerebral penduncles and extend forwards beyond the optic chiasma. In front of the optic chiasma the midline *longitudinal fissure* separates the *frontal lobes*. The *olfactory bulb* continuing backwards as the *olfactory tract* to the side of the optic chiasma lies in a sulcus lateral to the longitudinal fissure. The frontal lobes are separated from the temporal lobes by a deep sulcus which extends on to the lateral surface of the hemisphere.

The relation of the inferior surface of the brain to the inside of the base of the skull is as follows. The cerebellar hemispheres lie in the posterior cranial fossa. The medulla oblongata, pons and midbrain lie on the sloping clivus formed by the basilar part of the occipital bone and the body of the sphenoid. The interpeduncular fossa lies above the sella turcica with the hypophysis cerebri in its fossa. The optic chiasma lies *behind* the sulcus which is between the optic canals. The temporal lobes lie in the lateral parts of the middle cranial fossa and extend as far forwards as the lesser wings of the sphenoid bone. The frontal lobes lies on the orbital plates of the frontal bone and the olfactory bulb on the cribriform plate of the ethmoid.

In a lateral view of the brain the cerebral and cerebellar hemispheres of one side are the main structures visible. The hemispheres are covered by grey matter called the *cortex* which is deeply grooved in what may appear to be an unpatterned manner. Many of the grooves (*sulci*), although somewhat variable as between different brains, are easily identifiable and are used for dividing the brain into lobes. (An area of the cerebral cortex between two sulci is called a *gyrus.*)

The *lateral sulcus (of Sylvius)* passes backwards and slightly upwards on the lateral surface about two-thirds below its upper border (Jacques Dubois = Sylvius, a Latin, more learned version of Dubois, 1478–1555, French anatomist). Anteriorly the sulcus extends through the whole thickness of the hemisphere and separates the frontal lobe from the temporal lobe. The lesser wing of the sphenoid bone lies in this part of the sulcus. *The surface marking of the lateral sulcus is indicated by a line beginning at the pterion (4 cm above the middle of the zygomatic arch) and extending backwards and slightly upwards for about 7 cm. Posteriorly the line turns upwards and ends at the parietal eminence.*

The *central sulcus (of Rolando)* passes downwards, forwards and laterally for about 10 cm from just behind the middle of the upper border of the hemisphere at an angle of about 70° and ends above the lateral sulcus (L. Rolando, 1773–1831), Italian anatomist). *The central sulcus can be indicated on the surface by a line beginning superiorly about 1 cm behind the vertex of the skull (the highest point of its sagittal plane) and passing downwards and forwards for about 10 cm towards the midpoint of the zygomatic arch.*

The pre-occipital notch is on the lower lateral border of the cerebral hemisphere about 5 cm in front of its posterior end. The parieto-occipital sulcus, which is a deep sulcus mainly on the medial surface, extends on to the superolateral surface almost vertically above the pre-occipital notch.

The frontal lobe lies anterior to the central sulcus and above the lateral sulcus. Its anterior end is called the *frontal pole*. The *temporal lobe* lies below the lateral sulcus and in front of an imaginary line between the parieto-occipital sulcus and the pre-occipital notch. Its anterior end is called the *temporal pole*. The *parietal lobe* is bounded anteriorly by the central sulcus, posteriorly by the line between the parieto-occipital sulcus and the pre-occipital notch and inferiorly by the lateral sulcus extended backwards to meet this line. The *occipital lobe* lies behind the line joining the parieto-occipital sulcus to the pre-occipital notch. Its posterior end is the *occipital pole*.

From behind only the posterior parts of the cerebral and cerebellar hemispheres are visible, separated by a horizontal fissure. The longitudinal fissure of the cerebrum separates the cerebral hemispheres. Centrally in the depth of the fissure the hemispheres are joined by a large transverse band of fibres about 10 cm long called the *corpus callosum*. In a superior view the only parts of the brain which can be seen are the cerebral hemispheres separated by the longitudinal cerebral fissure.

The Meninges

The brain (and spinal cord) are covered by three meninges (*meninx = membrane*, Greek), an outer *dura mater*, a middle *arachnoid (mater)* and an inner *pia mater* (*mater = mother*, Latin; a curious use of the word *mother*; it was thought that all the membranes in the body were derived from the meninges, which therefore may be regarded as the *mother* of all membranes).

The Dura Mater

Within the skull the dura mater has two layers, an outer which is the endosteum of the skull bones (*endosteal layer*) and an inner or *meningeal layer*

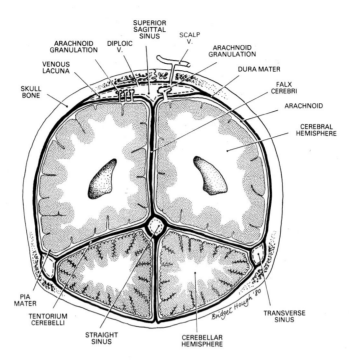

Figure 165 **The meninges of the brain as shown by a coronal section through the posterior parts of the cerebral and cerebellar hemispheres.**

(figure 165). Over most of the brain the layers are united, but along certain lines they separate and form spaces (*sinuses*) which contain the venous blood from the brain. The endosteal layer is continuous with the pericranium through the sutures and foramina, and is adherent to the bone at these sites and to the base of the skull. The meningeal (inner) layer is continuous with the spinal dura mater through the foramen magnum where the endosteal layer fuses with the periosteum of the edge of the foramen. The meningeal layer also ensheaths the cranial nerves as they pass through the foramina of the skull.

The meningeal layer of dura mater forms septa between parts of the brain (figure 166). The *falx cerebri* (*falx* = *sickle*, Latin) lies in the longitudinal fissure between the cerebral hemispheres. It is narrow in front where it is attached to the crista galli and becomes deeper posteriorly where it has a straight inferior edge attached to the upper surface of the tentorium cerebelli. The upper edge of the falx extends from the crista galli to the internal occipital protuberance and contains the superior

sagittal sinus. The shorter, free, inferior, curved edge contains the inferior sagittal sinus which continues into the straight sinus lying between the falx cerebri and the tentorium cerebelli.

The *tentorium cerebelli* (*tentorium* = *tent*, Latin) is an arched crescentic fold of dura mater between the cerebellum inferiorly and the occipital lobes of the cerebral hemispheres superiorly (figures 166, 167). The anterior free edge bounds a notch (the *tentorial incisure*) in which lie the midbrain and the middle narrow part of the cerebellum (vermis). The free edge passes forwards round the midbrain and is attached on each side to the anterior clinoid process. The outer convex edge of the tentorium is attached to the internal occipital protuberance and laterally to the edges of the groove on the occipital and parietal bones. This attached edge of the tentorium contains the transverse venous sinus and continues on to the upper border of the petrous temporal to the posterior clinoid process. The free edge passes superior to the attached edge on each side in the region of the clinoid processes. The superior petrosal sinus lies in

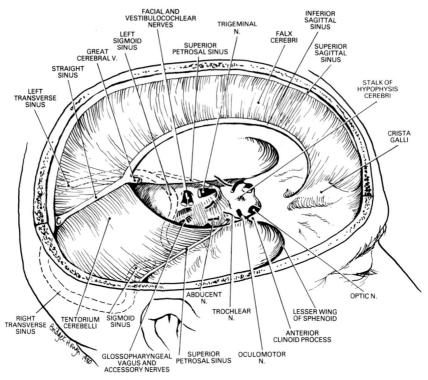

Figure 166   A lateral view of the falx cerebri and tentorium cerebelli.

the tentorium where it is attached to the petrous temporal bone.

Just lateral to the apex of the petrous temporal there is an extension forwards of the dura below the superior petrosal sinus into the middle cranial fossa. This extension, the *cavum trigeminale*, passes between the endosteal and meningeal layers of the dura mater and contains the motor and sensory roots of the trigeminal nerve, as they pass over the petrous temporal, and also the posterior part of the trigeminal ganglion. The walls of the cave fuse with the anterior part of the ganglion. The cavum trigeminale is more easily understood if one thinks of its being produced by the trigeminal nerve and ganglion pushing the meningeal dura forwards over the medial end of the petrous temporal bone into the middle cranial fossa at the side of the sella turcica.

There is a vertical fold of meningeal dura between the two cerebellar hemispheres, the *falx cerebelli*. It is attached to the internal occipital crest and the inferior surface of the tentorium cerebelli.

The *diaphragma sellae* is a horizontal fold of dura mater roofing over the sella turcica and covering the hypophysis cerebri (pituitary gland). It has a central hole through which passes the infundibulum (stalk) of the hypophysis. The diaphragma is attached to the clinoid processes.

The dura mater has a number of *meningeal vessels* which lie outside it in the so-called *extradural space*. In the anterior cranial fossa the arteries are derived from the internal carotid or its branches. The main artery of the middle fossa is the middle meningeal (p.   ). In the posterior fossa the meningeal arteries come from the vertebral and occipital arteries.

The *nerve supply* of the dura mater in the anterior and middle fossae is mainly from the three divisions of the trigeminal nerve. In the posterior cranial fossa the nerves are derived from the upper three cervical spinal nerves. The meningeal branches from the hypoglossal and vagus nerves are thought to be derived from the same spinal nerves.

The Arachnoid (Mater)

As its name suggests (*arachne = spider, spider's web*, Greek) the arachnoid is a thin, delicate membrane. It is related closely to the dura mater but there is a *subdural space* into which haemorrhage can occur. The arachnoid is separated from the underlying pia mater by the *subarachnoid space*, which contains the cerebrospinal fluid and larger blood vessels. Fine strands of tissue cross the space and connect the arachnoid with the pia mater. The cranial nerves, as they leave the brain, carry a sheath of arachnoid with them, but this extends only as far as the foramina through which they pass.

Since the pia mater dips into the sulci of the cerebral cortex and the arachnoid bridges these gaps, the subarachnoid space extends into the sulci of the brain. In some sites the space between the arachnoid and pia mater is enlarged and forms *cisternae*. The largest is between the inferior surface of the cerebellum and the upper posterior surface of the medulla oblongata, the *cerebello-medullary cisterna* (*cisterna magna*). There is also a *pontine cisterna* on the ventral surface of the pons and an *interpeduncular cisterna* between the cerebral peduncles. Both these cisternae contain large arteries supplying the brain. The cerebello-medullary cistern can be entered by a hollow needle pushed accurately and slowly through the tissues in the midline between the occipital bone and the atlas to the appropriate depth. By means of this procedure (*cisternal puncture*) a specimen of cerebrospinal fluid can be obtained. Cisternal puncture is not usually attempted unless a lumbar puncture (p. 336) has failed to obtain some fluid.

The arachnoid projects into the venous sinuses in the form of small structures called *villi* (*villus = tuft of hair*, Latin) which usually form clusters called *arachnoid granulations*. These lie in the hollows at the side of the superior sagittal sinus and less frequently of the other venous sinuses. The villus pushes the dura mater into the venous sinus but at the top of the villus the dura mater is absent and the arachnoid fuses with the endothelial lining of the venous sinus. The arachnoid granulations are the main means whereby cerebrospinal fluid returns to the circulation.

The Pia Mater

The pia mater (*pius = tender, kind*, hence *delicate*, Latin) consists of very fine connective tissue containing a plexus of small blood vessels. This membrane is closely adherent to the surface of the brain and dips into the sulci of both the cerebral and cerebellar hemispheres. The pia extends as a sheath round the small blood vessels as they enter the brain substance. Together with the lining cells (ependyma) of the cavities (ventricles) of the brain the pia mater forms the roof of the third and fourth ventricles. Invaginations of pia mater covered by ependyma into all the ventricles form the choroid plexuses which produce the cerebrospinal fluid.

The arachnoid and pia mater are regarded to some extent as a single structure and form the *leptomeninges* (*leptos = thin*, Greek). They develop together and become separated by cerebrospinal fluid, and it has been suggested that the outer layer of the pia mater is really an inner part of the arachnoid. The dura mater consisting of much denser connective tissue is referred to as the *pachymeninx* (*pachus = thick*, Greek). Functionally the dura mater with its partitions separates the cranial cavity into compartments and limits the extent to which the whole brain moves. Anteroposterior movement tends to be greater than side-to-side movement and in head injuries severe lacerations of the brain can occur where the midbrain meets the free edge of the tentorium cerebelli and the temporal lobe meets the posterior border of the lesser wing of the sphenoid bone. The main function of the arachnoid is related to the re-absorption of the cerebrospinal fluid by the villi. The pia mater is intimately linked with the blood supply of the brain and the production of cerebrospinal fluid through the choroid plexuses. The perivascular extensions of the pia mater, subarachnoid space and arachnoid into the brain are not regarded as a means whereby an exchange of substances or fluid can take place between the nervous tissue and the cerebrospinal fluid. The cerebrospinal fluid, which is under low pressure, is easily displaced and one of its main functions is to allow for the normal changes in the intracranial volume which result from changes in the blood supply.

Infection of the meninges, *meningitis*, may be bacterial or viral or may be due to the spread of an infection from outside the skull. In addition to the general signs and symptoms due to the central nervous system being affected, the cerebrospinal fluid shows changes of pressure, colour and content. The fluid can be withdrawn and examined by lumbar or cisternal puncture. Because the subarachnoid space extends along the nerves for a short distance, the cranial nerves may be affected. This particularly applies to the optic nerve which is surrounded by the meninges along its whole length to where it emerges from the eyeball. Infection may spread towards the eyeball. The infection can also spread into the brain along the extensions of the subarachnoid space which accompany the arteries.

Sometimes adhesions form in the region of the tentorium and the midbrain (*basal meningitis*), so that the cerebrospinal fluid which is produced mainly inside the forebrain and leaves through holes in the roof of the hindbrain below the tentorium, cannot pass upwards into the subarachnoid space round the forebrain. Since most of the fluid is absorbed through the arachnoid granulations projecting into the superior sagittal sinus and the choroid plexuses continue to produce cerebrospinal fluid, *hydrocephalus* (*water on the brain*) results.

Fractures of the anterior cranial fossa in the region of the cribriform plate may be associated with tearing of the meninges and loss of cerebrospinal fluid, usually bloodstained, through the nose. Fractures of the middle cranial fossa involving the ear and tearing of the meninges may result in loss of cerebrospinal fluid from the external acoustic meatus. Usually there is also bleeding from the nose or the external meatus in these fractures.

Fractures of the posterior cranial fossa may involve the basilar part of the occipital bone and the meninges lying on it. Inferior to the basilar part is the nasopharynx and there may be bleeding and escape of cerebrospinal fluid into the nasopharynx. The nerves in the jugular foramen may be involved. To test the integrity of the glossopharyngeal nerve taste sensations of the posterior third of the tongue are investigated (p. 290). Interruption of the vagus may produce cardiac and respiratory effects (palpitation, rapid pulse, slow breathing). If the vagus nerve is involved below where the cranial accessory joins it, the palate on the affected side does not move upwards and backwards on saying '*Ah*'. To test the spinal part of the accessory nerve shrugging the shoulder (one of the actions of the trapezius) and turning the head to the opposite side (one of the actions of the sternocleidomastoid) are attempted. These movements cannot be carried out if the spinal accessory nerve is not functioning.

The Intracranial Course of the Cranial Nerves

The Olfactory (First Cranial) Nerve. The cell bodies of the fibres which form the olfactory nerve bundles are in the olfactory mucous membrane in the roof of the nasal cavity and adjacent areas of the septum and lateral walls. The nerve bundles pass through the holes of the cribriform plate in the anterior cranial fossa and synapse with neurons whose cell bodies are in the olfactory bulb (figure 164). The axons of these neurons form the olfactory tract. Fractures of the anterior cranial fossa may separate partly or completely the bulb from the olfactory nerves so that partial or complete loss of smell results on one or both sides of the nasal cavity.

The Optic (Second Cranial) Nerve. It is estimated that there are over one million fibres in the optic nerve. These fibres are the central processes of the ganglion cells of the retina. In the eyeball they converge on to the area of the retina called the optic disc and leave the posterior pole of the eyeball to pass backwards in the orbit and enter the cranial cavity through the optic canal in the lesser wing of the sphenoid bone (figures 166, 167). The ophthalmic artery going from the cranial cavity into the orbit lies inferior to the optic nerve in the optic canal. The optic nerves join to form the *optic chiasma* which lies over the hypophysis cerebri. The chiasma divides and forms the optic tracts which wind round the cerebral peduncles (figure 164). Most of the fibres end in the lateral geniculate body. The internal carotid artery lies lateral to the optic chiasma and the anterior cerebral

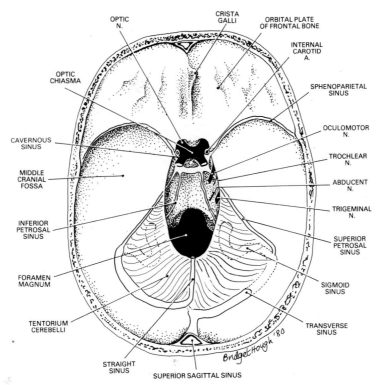

OPTIC N.

CRISTA GALLI

ORBITAL PLATE OF FRONTAL BONE

OPTIC CHIASMA

INTERNAL CAROTID A.

SPHENOPARIETAL SINUS

OCULOMOTOR N.

CAVERNOUS SINUS

TROCHLEAR N.

MIDDLE CRANIAL FOSSA

ABDUCENT N.

TRIGEMINAL N.

INFERIOR PETROSAL SINUS

SUPERIOR PETROSAL SINUS

FORAMEN MAGNUM

SIGMOID SINUS

TENTORIUM CEREBELLI

TRANSVERSE SINUS

STRAIGHT SINUS

SUPERIOR SAGITTAL SINUS

Figure 167   A superior view of the tentorium cerebelli and some of the intracranial venous sinuses.

artery, one of the terminal branches of the internal carotid artery, passes forwards above the optic nerve into the longitudinal cerebral fissure.

Within the chiasma the fibres from the outer temporal halves of the retina remain on the same side and the fibres from the inner nasal halves cross over. Because of this arrangement a tumour of the hypophysis cerebri which grows upwards can press on the central part of the chiasma. This affects the crossed fibres and therefore the fibres from the inner halves of the retina. Since the outer halves of the fields of vision are projected on to the inner halves of the retina, there is a bitemporal loss of vision. Calcification of the internal carotid arteries may occur in the region of the optic chiasma and cause pressure on the outer halves of the chiasma. The result is that the fibres from the outer halves of the retinae are affected and there is a binasal loss of the fields of vision.

The Oculomotor (Third Cranial) Nerve. The oculomotor nerve arises from the midbrain and emerges medial to the cerebral peduncle between the posterior cerebral and superior cerebellar arteries. The nerve passes forwards lateral to the posterior clinoid process into the cavernous sinus between the free and attached edges of the tentorium cerebelli (figure 167). The oculomotor nerve lies in the upper part of the lateral wall of the cavernous sinus above the trochlear nerve (figure 171) and divides into superior and inferior branches. These enter the orbit through the superior orbital fissure within the fibrous ring which in the orbit encircles the optic canal and medial end of the fissure. While in the cavernous sinus the oculomotor nerve receives branches from the sympathetic plexus round the internal carotid artery and branches from the ophthalmic nerve.

The oculomotor nerve supplies all the extrinsic muscles in the orbit except the superior oblique and the lateral rectus. The nerve also contains preganglionic parasympathetic fibres which synapse in the ciliary ganglion. The postganglionic fibres supply the sphincter pupillae and the ciliary muscle.

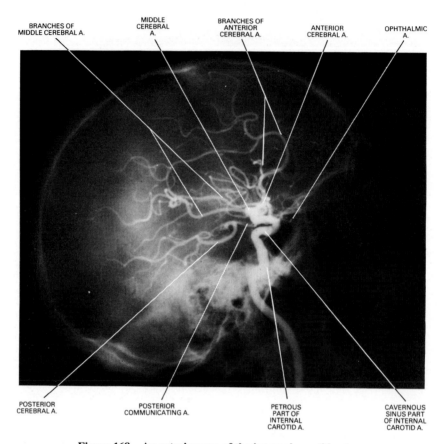

BRANCHES OF
MIDDLE CEREBRAL A.

MIDDLE
CEREBRAL
A.

BRANCHES OF
ANTERIOR
CEREBRAL A.

ANTERIOR
CEREBRAL A.

OPHTHALMIC
A.

POSTERIOR
CEREBRAL A.

POSTERIOR
COMMUNICATING A.

PETROUS
PART OF
INTERNAL
CAROTID A.

CAVERNOUS
SINUS PART
OF INTERNAL
CAROTID A.

Figure 168   An arteriogram of the internal carotid artery.

The Trochlear (Fourth Cranial) Nerve. This thread-like nerve is much smaller than the oculomotor (3000 as compared with 24 000 fibres). The trochlear nerve (*trochlea = pulley*, Latin; the nerve supplies the superior oblique muscle which winds round a bony pulley in the orbit) is the only cranial nerve which emerges from the brain on its posterior surface at the junction of the hindbrain with the midbrain.

The nerve winds round the lateral side of the cerebral peduncle and enters the cavernous sinus below the free edge of the tentorium cerebelli (figure 167). In the sinus the nerve lies on its lateral wall inferior to the oculomotor and superior to the ophthalmic nerves. The trochlear nerve enters the orbit through the superior orbital fissure outside the fibrous ring, crosses to the medial side of the orbit superior to the muscles, and supplies the superior oblique muscle.

The Trigeminal (Fifth Cranial) Nerve. This nerve has a large sensory and small motor root. The motor root is medial to the sensory at about the middle of the lateral part of the pons where the motor root emerges and the sensory root enters the hindbrain (figure 164). The sensory root, about 8 mm wide, passes forwards over the medial end of the upper border of the petrous temporal bone with the motor root inferior to it. It contains about 140 000 fibres (compare this with the number of optic nerve fibres). The sensory root joins the crescentic *trigeminal ganglion* which lies in the cavum trigeminale of dura mater in a hollow on the medial part of the anterosuperior surface of the petrous temporal bone, lateral to and above the foramen lacerum. The internal carotid artery is medial to the ganglion and the cavernous sinus is anterosuperior.

From the convex anterior border of the ganglion

the three divisions of the trigeminal nerve emerge. The *ophthalmic nerve* passes forwards in the lateral wall of the cavernous sinus inferior to the trochlear nerve and divides into its three branches, the *lacrimal*, *frontal* and *nasociliary nerves* which enter the orbit through the superior orbital fissure. The lacrimal and frontal nerves are outside the fibrous ring.

The *maxillary nerve* passes forwards from the ganglion inferior to the cavernous sinus and leaves the cranial cavity through the foramen rotundum to enter the pterygopalatine fossa. Its further course and distribution are described on p. 209.

The *mandibular nerve* emerges from the lateral part of the ganglion and leaves the skull almost immediately by passing downwards through the foramen ovale. The motor root of the trigeminal nerve, which is inferior to the ganglion, accompanies the mandibular nerve and joins it just below the foramen. The branches of the mandibular nerve are described on p. 206.

In intractable pain involving all the divisions of the trigeminal nerve alcohol may be injected into the ganglion by a needle inserted into the foramen ovale (p. 208). Treatment may take the form of cutting the sensory root where it joins the ganglion.

The Abducent (Sixth Cranial) Nerve. This nerve containing about 6000 fibres emerges from the hindbrain at the lower border of the pons near the midline. It runs forwards and upwards to the apex of the petrous temporal bone next to the dorsum sellae. The nerve bends downwards acutely over the apex and enters the cavernous sinus in which it lies lateral and then inferior to the internal carotid artery. The abducent nerve enters the orbit through the superior orbital fissure within the fibrous ring. It is inferior to the oculomotor and nasociliary nerves as it passes laterally to supply the lateral rectus muscle.

The Facial (Seventh Cranial) Nerve. The facial nerve has a large medial motor root and a smaller lateral root (the *nervus intermedius*) which is both sensory and motor parasympathetic. The two roots emerge laterally at the lower border of the pons and are medial to the vestibulocochlear nerve. They pass laterally with the vestibulocochlear

nerve and usually join before entering the internal acoustic meatus in which the facial nerve is anterosuperior to the vestibulocochlear nerve. The further course of the nerve in the temporal bone is described with the ear (p. 282) and its course and distribution after emerging from the stylomastoid foramen on p. 196.

The Vestibulocochlear (Eighth Cranial) Nerve. As the name suggests this nerve consists of two parts, the nerve associated with the sense of balance (*vestibular*) and the nerve of hearing (*cochlear*). Both nerves come from the internal ear and emerge from the internal acoustic meatus to enter the hindbrain at the lateral end of the lower border of the pons. The vestibular nerve is medial to the cochlear. Within the internal meatus and at the lower border of the pons the eighth nerve is closely related to the facial nerve. In both positions these nerves may be affected, for example, by a tumour of the eighth nerve, by a tumour of the cerebellum or by a fracture involving the internal meatus. Disturbances of balance and hearing and weakness and paralysis of the facial muscles occur.

The Glossopharyngeal, Vagus and Accessory (Ninth, Tenth and Eleventh Cranial) Nerves. The glossopharyngeal, vagus and cranial accessory nerves emerge as a series of rootlets from the groove lateral to the olive and its continuation inferiorly, and leave the cranial cavity in the middle compartment of the jugular foramen in which the inferior petrosal sinus is anteromedial and the sigmoid sinus is posterolateral. The glossopharyngeal nerve, formed by three or four rootlets, crosses the flocculus of the cerebellum (figure 164) and enters the jugular foramen anterior to the vagus nerve and separated from it by fibrous tissue which may ossify. The vagus nerve, formed by about 10 rootlets, passes through the jugular foramen in the same sheath of dura mater and arachnoid as the accessory nerve. The cranial part of the accessory nerve is formed by three or four rootlets from the medulla oblongata and joins the spinal part which arises from the upper five cervical segments. The spinal accessory nerve enters the skull through the foramen magnum, and passes laterally to join the cranial accessory nerve which leaves the skull through the jugular foramen. The course and distribution of these nerves in the neck are described on pp. 236–239.

The Hypoglossal (Twelfth Cranial) Nerve. This nerve arises from the medulla oblongata as a series of rootlets between the pyramid and the olive. The rootlets join and enter the hypoglossal canal from which the nerve emerges medial to the jugular foramen. The course and distribution of the hypoglossal nerve are described on p. 239.

In head injuries, movements of the brain inside the skull may result in the tearing of a nerve because of the attachment of the dural sheath of the nerve to the edge of the foramen through which the nerve goes.

The Arteries in the Cranial Cavity

These include the internal carotid and vertebral arteries and the arteries to the meninges. The most important of the *meningeal arteries* is the branch of the maxillary artery, the middle meningeal, which enters the cranial cavity through the foramen spinosum (p. 210). The internal carotid, vertebral and ophthalmic arteries also give off meningeal branches. In the posterior cranial fossa there are meningeal branches from the occipital artery.

The Internal Carotid Artery
(figures 168, 169, 170, 171)

The course of the internal carotid artery in the neck from its origin from the common carotid artery at the level of the upper border of the thyroid cartilage and its passage through the carotid canal in the petrous temporal bone are described on p. 232. The artery comes to lie on the fibrocartilage in the foramen lacerum where it turns forwards and enters the cavernous sinus. In the sinus the artery continues to run forwards and lies in a groove at the side of the sella turcica. It then turns upwards to lie medial to the anterior clinoid process where it pierces the dura mater. While in the cavernous sinus the artery is covered by lining endothelium and is superior and medial to the abducent nerve

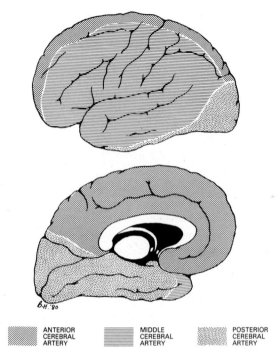

ANTERIOR CEREBRAL ARTERY   MIDDLE CEREBRAL ARTERY   POSTERIOR CEREBRAL ARTERY

Figure 169   The cortical distribution of the cerebral arteries.

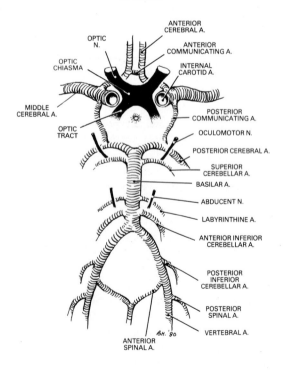

Figure 170   The cerebral arterial circle.

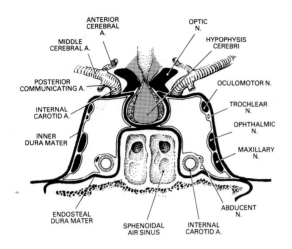

Figure 171   A coronal section through the cavernous sinus, viewed posteriorly.

(figure 171). The oculomotor, trochlear and oph-thalmic nerves on the lateral wall of the sinus are lateral to the artery. In the subarachnoid space the artery turns backwards below the optic nerve to lie lateral to the optic chiasma. It ascends again and at the medial end of the lateral sulcus divides into its terminal branches, the *anterior* and *middle cerebral arteries*.

The internal carotid artery while in the petrous temporal bone gives off a small branch to the middle ear. Small branches are also given off in the cavernous sinus to the trigeminal ganglion, the walls of the sinus, the meninges and the hypo-physis cerebri. The arteries to the hypophysis are important (p. 263). The internal carotid artery, as it lies medial to the anterior clinoid process, gives off the *ophthalmic artery* which enters the orbit by passing through the optic canal where it lies inferior to the optic nerve. Its course and distribu-tion are described with the orbit (p. 263).

Before dividing into its terminal branches the internal carotid artery gives off the *posterior communicating artery* which passes backwards and anastomoses with the posterior cerebral artery. It forms part of the circular anastomosis between the two internal carotid and two vertebral arteries (p. 260). Near the origin of the posterior communi-cating artery the *anterior choroidal artery* arises and passes backwards over the cerebral peduncle

to enter the cerebral hemisphere on its medial sur-face and end in the choroid plexus of the lateral ventricle.

The *anterior cerebral artery* passes forwards and medially above the optic nerve and enters the longitudinal cerebral fissure. The two anterior cerebral arteries are joined by the *anterior communicating artery* and lying almost next to each other pass upwards and then backwards in the fissure round the anterior end of the corpus cal-losum. They continue backwards over its upper surface to its posterior end and anastomose with branches of the posterior cerebral arteries. The anterior cerebral arteries give off *cortical branches* which supply most of the medial surface and a strip of the lateral surface of the cerebral hemi-sphere along its upper border (figure 169). Near their origin the anterior cerebral arteries give off *central branches* which enter the adjacent part of the hemisphere.

The *middle cerebral artery*, usually larger than the anterior, passes laterally into the lateral sulcus and then backwards and divides into a number of branches. The middle cerebral artery by its *cortical branches* supplies most of the superolateral surface of the cerebral hemispheres (figure 169). Its *central branches* supply the inner part of the hemisphere. One of the central branches was labelled by Charcot as the *artery of cerebral haemorrhage* because of the frequency with which it ruptures (J.M. Charcot, 1825–93, French neurologist).

The Vertebral Arteries (figures 156, 161, 170)

Each artery arises from the medial end of the sub-clavian artery and its course in the neck is described on p. 225. It passes upwards through the transverse processes of the upper six cervical vertebrae and having reached the atlas turns backwards behind its lateral mass and then medially over its posterior arch. The vertebral arteries pass upwards through the foramen magnum anterior to the spinal acces-sory nerves and after piercing the dura mater and arachnoid run medially in front of the medulla oblongata. The arteries unite at the lower border of the pons and form the basilar artery.

The vertebral artery in the cranial cavity gives

off (1) a *posterior spinal artery* which descends in relation to the dorsal spinal roots; (2) an *anterior spinal artery* which supplies the anterior part of the medulla before descending in the anterior median fissure of the spinal cord (the two anterior spinal arteries unite to form one artery); (3) the *posterior inferior cerebellar artery* which often gives origin to the posterior spinal artery and supplies the posterior and inferior parts of the cerebellum, the lateral part of the medulla oblongata and the choroid plexus of the fourth ventricle.

The Basilar Artery and the Circulus Arteriosus Cerebri (figure 170)

The basilar artery is formed by the union of the two vertebral arteries at the lower border of the pons. It passes upwards and forwards in a groove in the midline of the pons and lies on the basilar part of the occipital bone and body of the sphenoid. At the upper border of the pons the artery divides into the *posterior cerebral arteries*. The basilar artery gives off branches to the pons, a branch to the internal ear (*labyrinthine* or *internal auditory artery*) which enters the internal acoustic meatus, and two cerebellar arteries, the *anterior inferior* and *superior cerebellar arteries*. The anterior inferior cerebellar arises near the beginning of the basilar artery and is closely related to the facial and vestibulocochlear nerves. The superior cerebellar artery arises near the division of the basilar artery and is posterior to the oculomotor nerve.

The *posterior cerebral artery* passes laterally round the cerebral peduncle of the midbrain and then above the tentorium cerebelli to supply the whole of the occipital lobe (figure 169). On the inferior surface the posterior cerebral artery extends further forwards than on the medial and superolateral surfaces and supplies the temporal lobe. The branches are *cortical* and *central*. There are also *choroidal branches* to the choroid plexuses of the third and lateral ventricles.

The *circulus arteriosus (of Willis)* (figure 170) is formed by the three cerebral arteries on each side and one anterior and two posterior communicating arteries (T. Willis, 1621–75, English anatomist and physician). The anterior communicating artery joins the two anterior cerebral arteries and a posterior communicating artery on each side joins the internal carotid artery to the posterior cerebral. The arterial circle lies in the interpeduncular cisterna and surrounds the optic chiasma, the stalk of the hypophysis cerebri and the mamillary bodies. It is thought that normally the arterial circle does not provide anastomotic channels between the internal carotid and vertebral arteries. Arteriograms of the vertebral artery and the internal carotid artery confirm this. Movements of the head, however, open up the connections between the arteries forming the circle because the movements of the head narrow or occlude temporarily one of the branches. If there is obstruction to one branch of the arterial circle, the other branches may be able to provide alternative channels for a blood supply to the affected part. This depends to a large extent on whether the obstruction is rapid or slow. If rapid, a cerebral artery and its branches behave like end-arteries and the part supplied necroses.

The effects of blocking one of the large cerebral arteries or one of their branches depend on the functions of the part of the brain supplied by the artery. Only some examples are given. The posterior cerebral artery supplies the visual area of the cerebral cortex and some form of loss of vision results from blocking of that artery. (This also applies to the vertebral artery.) The middle cerebral artery supplies most of the main motor and general sensory areas and, on the left side in right-handed people, the speech areas of the cerebral cortex. Motor and sensory disturbances on the opposite side of the body and speech defects result from thrombosis (clotting) of the left middle cerebral artery. The anterior cerebral artery, however, supplies the motor area for the opposite *lower* limb. Thrombosis of the anterior cerebral artery produces a paralysis of the lower limb of the opposite side.

The Intracranial Veins and Venous Sinuses

The Veins of the Brain

The veins of the brain have thin non-muscular walls and no valves and their arrangement is different from that of the arteries. Most of the *cortical veins* on the superolateral and medial surfaces pass upwards to the superior sagittal sinus. The anterior of these veins are at right angles to the sinus but the posterior pass forwards so that the blood in them is flowing in the opposite direction to that of the blood in the sinus. A large vein on the lateral surface of the hemisphere in the lateral sulcus, the *middle cerebral vein*, joins the cavernous sinus. The middle cerebral vein is connected above to the superior sagittal sinus and below to the transverse sinus by anastomotic veins. The veins on the inferior surface of the hemisphere are joined by veins from inside the hemisphere and form the *basal vein* which passes backwards and joins the great cerebral vein. The *internal cerebral vein* is formed by veins from the interior of the hemisphere and runs backwards below the corpus callosum. The two internal cerebral veins join and form the *great cerebral vein* below the posterior end of the corpus callosum in the transverse fissure which lies between the posterior end of the corpus callosum and the upper surface of the midbrain. The great cerebral vein joins the *straight sinus* which runs in the junction of the falx cerebri with the tentorium cerebelli.

In head injuries, because the brain may move inside the skull, the veins from the brain may be torn at their entry into the sinuses. This results in a *subdural haemorrhage* which tends to show signs and symptoms several days after the injury. This lucid interval has to be kept in mind following any head injury which resulted in loss of consciousness.

The Venous Sinuses

The large channels for the venous blood from the cranial cavity take the form of venous sinuses whose walls are formed by the two layers of the dura mater (figures 165, 166, 167). The walls are devoid of muscle and the sinuses have an endothelial lining which is continuous with that of the veins connected with the sinuses. *The superior sagittal sinus* lies in the upper border of the falx cerebri and begins at the crista galli (figure 166). It runs backwards, grooving the frontal, parietal and occipital bones as far as the internal occipital protuberance, where it usually turns to the right

and forms the *right transverse sinus*. It receives the blood from the superior cerebral veins and communicates with the veins of the scalp through the parietal emissary veins which are near the posterior end of the sagittal suture. There may be an emissary vein in the foramen caecum in front of the crista galli connecting the superior sagittal sinus with the nasal veins. The arachnoid granulations project into the sinus (figure 165).

Venous lacunae (spaces) in the dura mater at the side of the sinus receive blood from meningeal and diploic veins (figure 165). These lacunae have several openings into the sinus and arachnoid granulations project into them from below.

The *straight sinus* passes backwards in the junction between the falx cerebri and the tentorium cerebelli to the internal occipital protuberance where it usually turns to the left and forms the *left transverse sinus*. The straight sinus is formed by the union of the *great cerebral vein* with the *inferior sagittal sinus* which runs in the inferior concave free border of the falx cerebri. The straight sinus also receives veins from the cerebellum. At the internal occipital protuberance the superior sagittal sinus and straight sinus usually form connections (the *confluence of the sinuses*) which vary from a common pool of blood from which the right and left transverse sinuses arise, to a small anastomotic vein connecting the two transverse sinuses. The *occipital sinus* passes upwards in the midline from the posterior edge of the foramen magnum to the confluence of the sinuses. (The confluence of the sinuses was called the *torcula Herophili*, the *winepress of Herophilus*, a Greek physician and anatomist who worked in Alexandria in about 300 BC. He wrote about the brain, duodenum and genitalia and distinguished between nerves and blood vessels. Because of his work he was called the *father of anatomy*.)

The transverse sinus curves laterally, forwards and slightly upwards in the attached edge of the tentorium. When it reaches the petrous temporal bone the transverse sinus turns downwards and becomes the *sigmoid sinus* (figures 166, 167). Where the sinus turns downwards it is joined by the *superior petrosal sinus* which runs along the upper border of the petrous temporal bone. Veins from the inferior parts of the cerebral and cerebellar hemispheres also join the transverse sinus.

The *sigmoid sinus* passes downwards and then medially and forwards on the mastoid part of the temporal bone and the jugular process of the occipital bone to the jugular foramen through which it passes to become the superior bulb of the internal jugular vein. In the foramen the sinus is posterolateral to the glossopharyngeal, vagus and accessory nerves. The upper part of the sigmoid sinus is medial to the mastoid antrum and air cells. Mastoid and condylar emissary veins join the sigmoid sinus. *The surface marking of the transverse sinus is a band slightly convex upwards about 1 cm wide extending from the external occipital protuberance to a point 4 cm behind and 2 cm above the external acoustic meatus. (It can be confirmed on a skull that this marks the postero-inferior angle of the parietal bone.) The sigmoid sinus is indicated by continuing the band downwards and forwards to the attachment of the auricle and then following the attachment to a point 1 cm above the tip of the mastoid process.*

The *cavernous sinus*, about 2 cm long and 1 cm wide, lies at the side of the body of the sphenoid bone and extends anteriorly from the superior orbital fissure to the medial end of the petrous temporal bone behind. Its roof and lateral wall consist of the inner layer of dura mater and its floor and medial wall of endosteal dura (figure 171). The anterior border of the free edge of the tentorium as it passes to the anterior clinoid process indicates the junction of the roof and lateral wall of the sinus. The interior of the sinus is apparently crossed by fibrous trabeculae forming a number of spaces or channels, but it has been suggested that there are few trabeculae in the adult and they are seen in the cadaver because of the collapse of the walls of the sinus.

On the lateral wall of the sinus from above downwards the oculomotor, trochlear and ophthalmic nerves pass forwards to the superior orbital fissure. The internal carotid artery surrounded by a plexus of sympathetic nerves runs forwards on the medial wall with the abducent nerve inferior and lateral to it. These structures are separated from the blood in the sinus by a covering of endothelium. The maxillary nerve runs forwards to the foramen rotundum embedded in the dura of the lateral wall. The trigeminal ganglion in its cave of dura mater lies posterolateral to the sinus and the wall of the cave fuses with the lateral wall of the sinus. The hypophysis cerebri and sphenoidal air sinus lie medially.

The tributaries of the cavernous sinus are the two ophthalmic veins from the orbit, the middle cerebral vein from the lateral surface of the hemisphere, some inferior cerebral veins, and the sphenoparietal sinus which runs on the parietal bone and the edge of the lesser wing of the sphenoid. Through the ophthalmic veins the cavernous sinus communicates with the facial vein. Infection may spread from the face to the sinus along these channels and may cause thrombosis. The nerves passing through the sinus may be affected. Emissary veins passing through the foramen ovale or foramen lacerum connect the cavernous sinus with the pterygoid plexus of veins. The cavernous sinuses communicate with each other through the *anterior* and *posterior intercavernous sinuses* which lie in the anterior and posterior borders of the diaphragma sellae.

Most of the blood in the cavernous sinus drains into the *superior* and *inferior petrosal sinuses*. The superior petrosal sinus passes laterally along the upper border of the petrous temporal to the transverse sinus and the inferior petrosal sinus passes downwards and then laterally in the petro-occipital suture to the medial end of the jugular foramen through which it passes to join the superior bulb of the internal jugular vein.

Diploic, Emissary and Meningeal Veins

These veins form communications between the veins inside and outside the skull. The *diploic veins* between the two layers of bone of the cranium have relatively wide channels (2–3 mm), are thin-walled and have no valves. Because of their beaded appearance and the thinning of the bone adjacent to them diploic veins can be recognised in an X-ray of the skull. *Meningeal veins*, corresponding with the meningeal arteries, drain blood from the dura mainly into the lacunae of the superior sagittal sinus. They also communicate with the diploic veins. *Emissary veins* connect the veins of the scalp, face and pterygoid region with the intracranial sinuses. They are important because of the possibility of the spread of infection from the face or scalp to the sinuses.

The Hypophysis Cerebri (Pituitary Gland)

This endocrine gland, resembling a pea and about 1 cm in diameter, lies in the hypophyseal fossa of the body of the sphenoid and is attached by the infundibulum to the base of the brain in the interpeduncular fossa between the optic chiasma anteriorly and the corpora mamillaria posteriorly (figure 164). As it lies in the fossa it is roofed over by the diaphragma sellae, which is attached to the clinoid processes and has a hole for the passage of the infundibulum. The optic chiasma lies above the anterior part of the gland. On each side there is the cavernous sinus and between the hypophysis and the floor of the fossa there is a venous sinus which joins the cavernous sinuses. The sphenoidal air sinus is inferior to the hypophysis (figure 171). The gland has a capsule which fuses with the meninges.

The terminology of the subdivisions of the hypophysis is confusing. It is therefore suggested that the part that grows upwards from the roof of the mouth be called the *adenohypophysis* and the part that grows downwards from the diencephalon the *neurohypophysis*. The neurohypophysis has three parts, the median eminence where the infundibulum is attached to the brain, the central part of the infundibulum and the posterior part of the hypophysis (figure 172). The adenohypophysis consists of the anterior part of the gland and its extension upwards round the central part of the infundibulum.

The arteries supplying the hypophysis come from the internal carotid arteries. The *superior hypophyseal artery* supplies the upper and lower parts of the infundibulum in which they form tufts of capillaries from which vessels pass downwards into the anterior part of the gland where they form sinusoids related to the cells of this part of the gland (figure 172). The hormone releasing and inhibiting factors produced by the hypothalamus use this portal system of vessels to reach the anterior part of the gland.

The *inferior hypophyseal arteries* supply the posterior (neural) part of the hypophysis. The neurohypophysis receives a nerve supply from some of the hypothalamic nuclei. The fibres of these cells convey their neurosecretions to the posterior part of the hypophysis from where they pass into the blood stream.

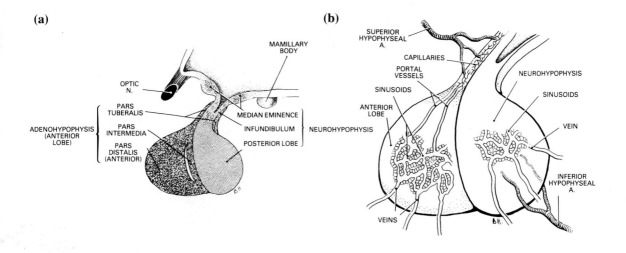

Figure 172   (a) The hypophysis cerebri (pituitary gland). (b) The blood supply of the hypophysis cerebri.

19

The Orbit and Ear

The Orbit

The orbit contains the peripheral organ of vision, the eyeball, and its muscles, nerves and blood vessels. Anteriorly, various parts of the lacrimal apparatus lie within the orbit and eyelids which with the tears protect the front of the eyeball and keep its anterior surface moist.

The bony walls of the orbit (figure 173)

The orbit has a roof, floor, medial wall and lateral wall. The medial wall is in the sagittal plane and the lateral wall slopes medially as it passes backwards. The narrow posterior part of the orbit is often called the *apex*. At the apex the *superior orbital fissure* between the lesser and greater wings

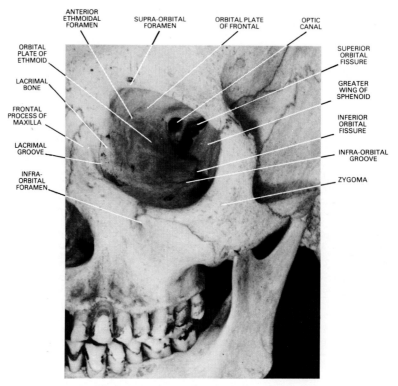

Figure 173   The walls of the left orbit.

of the sphenoid bone is the main communication between the orbit and cranial cavity. The *optic canal* lies above the medial end of the superior fissure. The *roof* is formed mainly by the orbital plate of the frontal bone with the lesser wing of the sphenoid bone posteriorly. The *floor* is formed mainly by the roof of the maxillary sinus. The orbital process of the palatine bone forms a small part of the floor posteriorly. The *lateral wall* is formed anteriorly by the zygomatic bone and posteriorly by the greater wing of the sphenoid. The *inferior orbital fissure*, leading to the infratemporal fossa laterally and the pterygopalatine fossa medially, lies posteriorly between the lateral wall and floor.

The *medial wall* is formed from in front backwards by the frontal process of the maxilla, the lacrimal bone, the orbital plate of the ethmoid bone (the largest part of the wall) and the body of the sphenoid. On the anterior part of the medial wall the *lacrimal groove* is formed by the lacrimal bone and maxilla. The groove is limited anteriorly by the lacrimal crest of the maxilla and posteriorly by the lacrimal crest of the lacrimal bone. Both crests at their lower ends pass laterally and fuse together to form a foramen.

The eyelids and lacrimal apparatus

The Eyelids (figure 174(a))

The eyelids consist of an outer layer of thin skin continuous at the edge of the lid with an inner layer of modified skin called the *conjunctiva*, fibres of the orbicularis oculi muscle, a plate of dense connective tissue and prominent glands perpendicular to the edge of the lid between the conjunctiva and connective tissue.

The skin is freely movable over the underlying muscle since it is separated from it by loose connective tissue in which fluid readily collects. The connective tissue deep to the muscle is continuous with the connective tissue of the fourth layer of the scalp and fluid or blood in this layer may pass into the eyelids. The plate of dense connective tissue, the *tarsus* (formerly the *tarsal plate*, a term regarded as tautological because *tarsus* means *plate*, although it also means *eyelid*), is about 2.5 cm wide. In the upper eyelid it is about 1 cm in height and in the lower about 0.5 cm. The elevator of the upper eyelid, *levator palpebrae superioris*, which comes from within the orbit is attached to the upper border of the plate (*palpebra = eyelid*, Latin). Some fibres of the inferior rectus muscle may be attached to the lower plate. The *orbital septum* is a layer of connective tissue which is attached to the edges of the orbit and extends into the eyelids to become continuous with the tarsal plates. The levator palpebrae superioris has to pass through this septum to become attached to the anterior surface of the upper tarsal plate. The orbital septum is thickened laterally and medially to form the *lateral* and *medial palpebral ligaments* which are attached to the zygomatic bone and maxilla respectively.

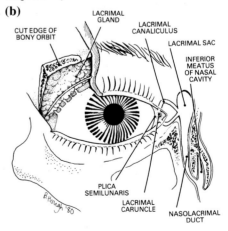

Figure 174 (a) A vertical section through an upper eyelid. (b) The right lacrimal apparatus.

The *tarsal (Meibomian) glands* lie in grooves on the deep surface of the tarsal plates parallel to each other in a single row perpendicular to the edge of the eyelids (H. Meibom, 1638–1700, German physician). They are modified sebaceous glands. Their secretion spreads over the margins of the lids and due to its surface tension is thought to be one factor in preventing the tears overflowing on to the cheek and reducing their evaporation. At the edge of the eyelids the eyelashes curl away from the eyeball. *Styes* are infections of modified sweat glands which open at the side of the eyelashes.

The *conjunctiva* consists of non-keratinised stratified squamous epithelium and a very thin transparent layer of connective tissue containing a large number of small blood vessels. The conjunctiva is reflected on to the sclera (white) of the eyeball on all sides, forming the *conjunctival sac*, and becomes further modified in front of the clear part of the eyeball, the cornea. Infection with resultant engorgement of the blood vessels is seen in *conjunctivitis*. If the lower eyelid is pulled downwards and the eyeball turned upwards the reflection of the conjunctiva can be easily seen. It is impossible to see this reflection from the upper eyelid on to the eyeball because of the much larger upper eyelid and tarsal plate. It is important to be able to evert the upper eyelid in order to inspect its deep surface should there be a foreign body adherent to it. If the patient looks downwards the upper eyelid can be turned upwards round the upper edge of the tarsal plate. One should do this by holding the edge of the eyelid and not pulling on the eyelashes.

At the medial angle between the edges of the eyelids there is a small red body called the *lacrimal caruncle (caruncle = small piece of flesh, Latin)* which consists of modified skin and usually has a few fine hairs projecting from it. Lateral to the caruncle the *plica semilunaris* is a semicircular fold of thickened conjunctiva which is more easily seen if the eyeball is turned outwards. It may be homologous with the *nictitating membrane* of some reptiles and mammals.

The *sensory nerve supply* of the upper eyelid is from the ophthalmic nerve (lacrimal, supratrochlear and infratrochlear branches) and that of the lower eyelid is from the maxillary nerve (infra-orbital

branch). The *arterial blood supply* is from the ophthalmic and facial arteries. The *veins* from the eyelids drain to the facial vein and the ophthalmic veins and form an important communication between the veins of the face and those of the orbit and cranium. The region of the outer angle of the eyelids has *lymphatic vessels* which go to the lymph nodes related to the parotid gland. The region of the inner angle drains to the submandibular nodes.

In lesions of the facial nerve the patient cannot close the eye completely because the orbicularis oculi supplied by the facial nerve is paralysed. The levator of the upper eyelid functions because its nerve supply, the oculomotor nerve, is intact. If the oculomotor nerve is affected, *ptosis*, a drooping of the upper eyelid results.

The Lacrimal Apparatus (figure 174(b))

The *lacrimal gland* lies in a hollow in the upper lateral part of the front of the orbit and extends into the lateral region of the upper eyelid. The orbital part (2.5 cm x 1 cm) is the larger and is continuous with the palpebral part round the lateral edge of the levator palpebrae superioris. The ducts of the gland open into the conjunctival sac. Removal of the palpebral part results in the loss of tears because the ducts of the orbital part do not open independently into the sac. The tears consist almost entirely of water and contain very small quantities of inorganic salts and a bacterial enzyme. The secretomotor nerve supply of the gland is from the greater petrosal branch of the facial nerve. The branch is preganglionic parasympathetic and synapses in the pterygopalatine ganglion (figure 145). The postganglionic fibres enter the orbit through the inferior orbital fissure either separately or with the zygomatic branch of the maxillary nerve. In the orbit the fibres pass either directly or via the lacrimal nerve to the gland.

The tears pass across from the lateral side of the conjunctival sac to its medial side due to capillary attraction and the blinking of the eyelids. This movement of tears requires eyelids lying close to the eyeball. If they become everted, especially the lower eyelid, a possible consequence of old age or wearing a monocle, the tears flow down the cheek. Most of the tears have evaporated before they reach the *lacrimal canaliculi*, one in each eyelid. On the edge of the eyelid there is a small *lacrimal papilla* about 5 mm lateral to the inner angle. A small aperture, the *lacrimal punctum*, opens on to the papilla and leads into the lacrimal canaliculus. The superior canaliculus passes upwards and the inferior downwards for about 3 mm and both bend sharply medially for about 5 mm before joining the lacrimal sac. The *lacrimal sac* is the upper part of a structure which lies in the fossa formed by the maxilla and lacrimal bone on the anterior part of the medial wall of the orbit and continues downwards and laterally in the lateral wall of the nose as the *nasolacrimal duct*. The lacrimal bone and the inferior concha form its medial wall. The duct opens into the anterior part of the inferior meatus of the nasal cavity. The lacrimal sac is behind the medial paplebral ligament and in front of the lacrimal part of the orbicularis oculi.

Normally little of the tears reach the inferior meatus. Slight excess results in sniffing and a greater excess leads to tears flowing down the cheeks. The production of tears is a carefully balanced process and requires repeated closure of the eyelids to prevent excessive evaporation.

Holding the eyelids open for 20–30 min can cause drying of the cornea with serious damage to its surface cells.

It is important to examine in a mirror the eyelids and anterior part of the eyeball and identify many of the features described.

The eyeball (figure 175)

The eyeball is an almost spherical structure, in the adult about 2.5 cm in diameter, with a wall which consists of three coats. The interior of the eyeball contains fluid under pressure and is divided into two compartments by a vertical partition. The posterior compartment is much larger than the anterior.

The Outer Coat. This is called the *sclera* (*skleros = hard*, Greek) and is commonly referred to as the *white of the eye*. The anterior transparent part of the sclera is the *cornea* (*corneus = horny*, Latin) which forms about one-sixth of the circumference and is of a different radius from that of the sclera. The cornea and sclera are continuous at the *corneosclerotic junction* or *limbus* (*limbus = edge*, Latin). Near the inner aspect of this junction there is a circular space called the *sinus venosus sclerae* in

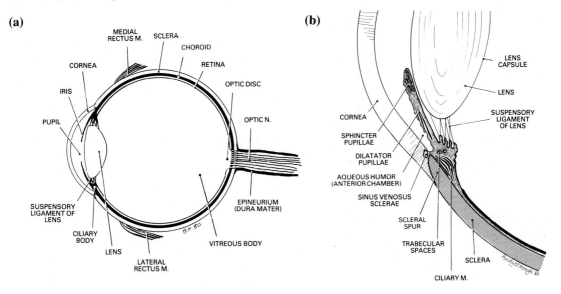

(a)

(b)

Figure 175 (a) A horizontal section through the eyeball. (b) An enlargement of the corneosclerotic junction and ciliary body.

front of which there is loose tissue. The *iris*, the coloured part of the eye (*iris = rainbow*, Greek) and ciliary body are attached to the *scleral spur* which is formed by the scleral edge projecting forwards where it is continuous with the cornea (figure 175(b)).

The sclera is about 1 mm thick posteriorly and about 5 mm thick anteriorly and consists of dense white fibrous tissue. It is surrounded by the fascial sheath of the eyeball and the muscles which are attached to the sclera take a sheath of fascia with them as they pass backwards from the eyeball. The sclera is pierced posteriorly by the fibres of the optic nerve, the sheath of which fuses with the sclera. The anterior part of the sclera is covered by the conjunctiva.

The cornea, in addition to transmitting light, is the major refractive medium of the eyeball. *Astigmatism* is usually due to an error in the curvature of the cornea which should be the section of an almost perfect sphere. Nine-tenths of the thickness of the cornea consists of layers of transparent connective tissue fibres whose external surface is covered by a modified conjunctiva consisting of several layers of cells similar to non-keratinised stratified squamous epithelium. Injury to the surface cells can heal without an opacity but infection and trauma affecting the deeper layers often result in corneal opacities which can be treated by corneal grafts. These are among the more successful of grafting operations because of the structure of the cornea, although even in the cornea the results are much improved if the donor's and host's tissues are well matched.

The cornea is avascular and richly innervated by the ophthalmic nerve. Abrasions of the cornea are very painful and the sensitivity of the cornea to touch is the basis of the *corneal reflex* in which touching the cornea results in reflex contraction of the orbicularis oculi.

The Middle Coat. This coat is called the *uveal tract* or *vascular coat* (*uva = grape*, Latin) and consists of the *choroid* which lines the sclera as far as the corneosclerotic junction (*chorion = skin*, Greek) where it is called the *ciliary body* (figure 175(b)). The ciliary body becomes the *iris*, the coloured part of the eye which is a circular structure separated

from the cornea, with a hole in its centre called the *pupil*. The choroid consists of an outer layer of pigmented cells which prevent light passing through the sclera and the scattering of the light which enters the interior of the eye through the pupil. It has been compared with the blackening of the inside of a camera. The vascular layer has nutritive functions in relation to the outer parts of the retina.

The ciliary body contains smooth muscle fibres (the *ciliary muscle*) which make it more bulky than the adjacent choroid and iris. The *suspensory ligament of the lens* is attached to the posterior surface of the ciliary body. When the ciliary muscle contracts it pulls the suspensory ligament inwards so that it is relaxed. The *capsule of the lens* to which the suspensory ligament is attached slackens and the *lens* becomes more biconvex. By this means the eye can focus on near objects. The ciliary muscle is innervated by postganglionic parasympathetic fibres whose cell bodies are in the ciliary ganglion. The preganglionic fibres are branches of the oculomotor nerve.

The ciliary body also contains loose, vascular tissue continuous with a number of radiating *processes* which produce the fluid circulating in the anterior part of the eyeball. The fluid passes through the pupil into the space between the iris and the cornea and is reabsorbed into the sinus venosus sclerae (p. 267).

The iris contains smooth muscle arranged as an inner circular *sphincter pupillae* and outer radially arranged *dilatator pupillae*. The sphincter is supplied by postganglionic parasympathetic fibres whose cell bodies are in the ciliary ganglion. The preganglionic fibres come from the oculomotor nerve. The dilatator is supplied by postganglionic sympathetic fibres whose cell bodies are in the superior cervical ganglion. The preganglionic fibres have their cell bodies in the first thoracic segment of the spinal cord.

The colour of the iris is due to pigment cells. In the newborn of some groups of people there are practically no pigment cells and because of the way the other elements of the iris absorb and reflect the light the eyes are pale blue. If pigment cells develop the colour of the iris darkens and can become dark brown.

The Inner Coat. This coat is called the *retina* which is the light sensitive layer. It extends on to the ciliary body and iris but in this site contains no nerve elements and is therefore non-functioning. The retina is thickest posteriorly (0.5 mm) and thins anteriorly (0.1 mm), although both the optic disc and fovea at the back are much thinner areas. The *optic disc*, slightly medial to the posterior pole of the eyeball, is the region where the fibres forming the optic nerve converge and pass backwards through the choroid and sclera. The disc is paler than the rest of the retina, has a sharp medial border and has no visual elements in it. It is therefore known as the *blind spot*. In the centre of the disc the branches of the central artery and vein of the retina divide and go to the four retinal quadrants. About 3 mm lateral to the optic disc

there is a small yellowish area, the *macula lutea* (= *yellow spot*, Latin), with a central depressed area, the *fovea centralis*, where vision is most acute (figure 176 (b)).

With reference to the traditional 10 layers of the retina, seven of these are formed by the three basic elements responsible for reacting to the stimulus of light and transducing the stimulus into action potentials which pass along the optic nerve (figure 176(a)). The layer of rods and cones is peripheral, that is nearer the choroid than the centre of the eyeball, so that the light has to pass through eight of the layers of the retina before reaching the rods and cones. Besides the *rods and cones*, *bipolar cells* and *ganglion cells*, the three basic elements, there are additional cells in the retina and most of their cell bodies are in the sixth layer which is formed by the cell bodies of the bipolar cells.

The *cones* are used in bright light and for colour discrimination. There are only cones at the macula lutea and when looking at an object it is always focused on to the maculae. The number of cones in the retina falls rapidly as one passes from the macula. The *rods* increase in density as one passes from the macula and are used in dim light. The pigments which they contain are bleached out in bright light and re-form in dim light so that objects

(a)

PIGMENTED CELL LAYER   CONE   ROD

LAYER OF RODS AND CONES

OUTER NUCLEAR LAYER

OUTER PLEXIFORM LAYER

INNER NUCLEAR LAYER

INNER PLEXIFORM LAYER

LAYER OF GANGLION CELLS

OPTIC FIBRE LAYER

LIGHT

LIGHT

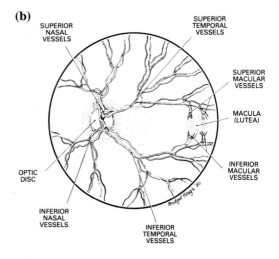

(b)

SUPERIOR NASAL VESSELS

SUPERIOR TEMPORAL VESSELS

SUPERIOR MACULAR VESSELS

MACULA (LUTEA)

INFERIOR MACULAR VESSELS

OPTIC DISC

INFERIOR NASAL VESSELS

INFERIOR TEMPORAL VESSELS

Figure 176 **(a) A diagram of the basic structure of the retina. (b) The optic disc and macula lutea of the left eye. (Reproduced from** *Hamilton's Textbook of Human Anatomy* **by courtesy of the Editors and the Macmillan Press.)**

previously not visible are seen. The process is called *dark adaptation*. There are about six times as many rods as cones in the retina.

The retina receives a *blood supply* from two sources. The central artery of the retina (a branch of the ophthalmic artery) has already divided into four branches when it enters the optic disc (figure 176(b)). Each branch supplies a quadrant. The central artery and its branches are end-arteries and blockage of any of them results in loss of function of the appropriate part of the retina. The outer layers of the retina as far as the layer of the bipolar cells are supplied by arteries of the choroid. The veins of the retina correspond with the arteries.

Detachment of the retina is a condition which occurs either spontaneously or due to a blow on the eye. A tear in the retina allows fluid to pass outside the layer of the rods and cones, and vision is lost to the extent that the retina is separated. The condition is usually progressive and the objective of treatment is to re-attach the retina in order to prevent further separation.

The Contents of the Eyeball. These consist of the *aqueous humour* anteriorly and the *vitreous body* posteriorly, separated by the lens and its suspensory ligament (figure 175). The aqueous humour (*humor = fluid*, Latin) is a clear watery fluid produced by the ciliary processes of the ciliary body which are in a plane posterior to the iris. The fluid passes through the pupil and is absorbed at the iridocorneal angle into connective tissue spaces which communicate with the venous sinus of the sclera (figure 175(b)). From there the fluid re-enters the circulation. The aqueous humour nourishes the avascular cornea and lens, and is continuously produced. It is under pressure and if its circulation and/or absorption are interfered with the intra-ocular pressure rises, a condition called *glaucoma* (*glaukos = green*, Greek; the colour refers to the reflection seen through the cornea). The effect is the loss of the peripheral part of the fields of vision due to pressure on the retina. This is progressive and glaucoma is one of the commonest causes of blindness in Britain.

The *lens* consists largely of concentric laminae of lens fibres surrounded by a capsule which is elastic and transparent, as is the rest of the lens.

The capsule is attached round its circumference to the suspensory ligament which peripherally is attached to the ciliary body beyond the ciliary processes. Up to the age of about 40 years the lens is the means whereby near objects are focused on to the retina. This is called *accommodation*. Contraction of the ciliary muscle relaxes the suspensory ligament and the capsule, so that the lens becomes more biconvex. Accommodation is always accompanied by convergence of the eyes so that only one image is seen. The reflex involved in focusing on near objects is usually called the *accommodation–convergence reflex*. The pupil also constricts. After about 40–45 years of age the lens becomes less elastic and the ability to accommodate is gradually lost and lenses are required for close work. This condition is called *presbyopia* (*presbus = old man*, Greek; an unkind word to people aged 40 years and possibly resented by feminists since presbyopia also occurs in women). Progressive loss of transparency frequently occurs in old age and is called *cataract*, a condition which may also be traumatic or congenital.

The *vitreous body* occupies about four-fifths of the interior of the eyeball and lies behind the lens and suspensory ligaments (*vitreus = glassy*, Latin). It is transparent, colourless and jelly-like, consisting of water (99 per cent), with a small amount of mucoprotein. The vitreous body is under pressure and a penetrating wound of the eyeball results in its loss. Since it is irreplaceable the eyeball shrinks and vision is lost.

Refraction. The cornea, aqueous humour, lens and vitreous body constitute the refractive media of the eye. The cornea is responsible for about three-quarters of refraction and the lens for the remaining quarter. If the eyeball is too large the image falls in front of the retina, a condition called *myopia* (*short sightedness*). If the eyeball is too small the image falls behind the retina, a condition called *hypermetropia* (*long sightedness*). These conditions can be corrected by appropriate lenses.

The muscles, fascia and ligaments (figure 177)

The muscles which move the eyeball are called the

(a)

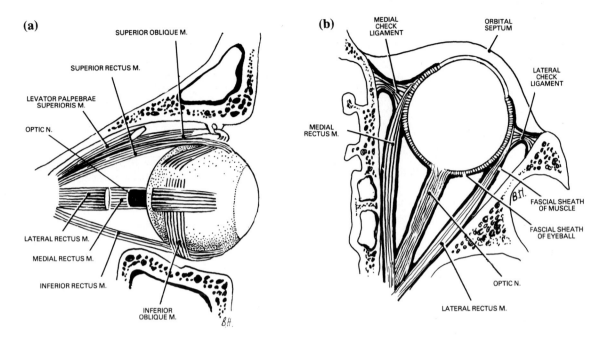

(b)

Figure 177   (a) The extrinsic muscles of the right eyeball (the lateral wall of the orbit has been removed). (b) The fascia of the right eyeball seen from above.

extrinsic muscles. These include the elevator of the upper eyelid (levator palpebrae superioris). The *intrinsic muscles* are the ciliary muscle and the sphincter and dilatator pupillae. The *levator palpebrae superioris* is attached to the roof of the orbit above the optic canal, passes forwards inferior to the roof and spreads out as an aponeurosis to become attached to the upper edge of the tarsal plate and skin of the upper eyelid. The levator contains some smooth muscle fibres which are supplied by sympathetic fibres whose cell bodies are in the superior cervical ganglion. The rest of the muscle is supplied by the oculomotor nerve.

The muscles moving the eyeball are the four recti and two obliques. The *recti (superior, inferior, lateral* and *medial)* are attached posteriorly to the appropriate part of the fibrous ring surrounding the optic canal and the medial end of the superior orbital fissure. They run forwards and each is attached by a tendon to the corresponding part of the sclera about 6 mm behind the edge of the cornea. The *superior oblique* is attached to the sphenoid bone above and medial to the optic canal,

runs forwards above the medial rectus and, just within the superomedial edge of the orbital margin, hooks round the *trochlea*, a fibrocartilaginous pulley on the frontal bone. The tendon passes backwards and laterally inferior to the superior rectus and is attached to the upper surface of the sclera behind the equator of the eyeball. The *inferior oblique*, unlike the rest of the muscles, lies entirely in the front of the orbit. It is attached medially to the maxilla in front of the nasolacrimal canal, passes laterally and backwards below the inferior rectus and is attached to the sclera behind the equator of the eyeball.

The lateral rectus is supplied by the abducent nerve, the superior oblique by the trochlear nerve and the remaining muscles by the oculomotor nerve.

The following, an over-simplification, are the actions of extrinsic muscles. The lateral rectus pulls the eyeball outwards and the medial rectus pulls it inwards. The superior rectus pulls the eyeball upwards and inwards, and the inferior rectus downwards and inwards. The superior oblique pulls the eyeball downwards and outwards and together with the inferior rectus pulls the eyeball downwards. The inferior oblique pulls the eyeball upwards and outwards, and in conjunction with the superior rectus pulls it upwards. All the movements are described in terms of movements about either a transverse axis (the eyeball moves upwards and downwards) or a vertical axis (the eyeball moves outwards and inwards). The eyeball, however, can also rotate about an anteroposterior axis (clockwise and counterclockwise movements). For example, the inferior oblique of the left eyeball produces a clockwise rotation. It is accepted that almost any movement of the eyeball involves at least three muscles.

The eyeball is surrounded by a fascial sheath which is fused anteriorly to the sclera at the cornea and posteriorly to the sheath of the optic nerve (figure 177(b)). The extrinsic muscles as they pass from the sclera take a fascial covering with them. The sheath of the lateral rectus is attached to the zygomatic bone and that of the medial rectus to the lacrimal bone. These are called the *lateral* and *medial check ligaments* respectively. The *suspensory ligament of the eyeball* is a thickening of the fascia of the inferior rectus attached on each side to a check ligament. The sheaths of the superior and inferior recti extend forwards and become attached to the superior and inferior tarsal plates respectively.

All the structures in the orbit are embedded in fatty tissue in which variable amounts of smooth muscle fibres are found. A decrease in the amount of fat leads to the characteristic sunken-eye appearance of the starving. An increase in the amount of fat may be the cause of the protrusion of the eyeball (*exophthalmos*) in exophthalmic goitre.

The nerves of the orbit (figure 178)

The intracranial parts of these nerves have been described on pp. 255–257. The optic nerve leaves the orbit through the optic canal; the oculomotor, the trochlear, the branches of the ophthalmic and the abducent nerves enter through the superior orbital fissure; the maxillary nerve enters through the inferior orbital fissure. The relation of the entrance of the nerves through the superior orbital fissure to the fibrous ring at the medial end of the fissure appears to be important and the simplest way to recall this is to remember that the lacrimal, frontal and trochlear nerves from the lateral to the medial side enter outside the ring (L, F, T outside the ring).

The Optic Nerve. The optic nerve emerges from the eyeball slightly medial to the posterior pole and is formed by the central processes of the ganglion cells of the retina. As it passes backwards within the cone formed by the recti muscles, the optic nerve is crossed superiorly from the lateral to the medial side by the ophthalmic artery and nasociliary nerve. At the same point the ciliary ganglion, attached to the nasociliary nerve, is lateral. The optic nerve is tortuous to allow for movements of the eyeball.

The nerve leaves the orbit through the optic canal in which the ophthalmic artery lies inferolateral to the nerve. Nearer the eyeball the central artery of the retina is inferior to the optic nerve and just behind the eyeball the artery sinks into the centre of the nerve. The optic nerve which develops as an outgrowth from the brain is surrounded by extensions of the meninges which fuse with the sclera and fascia of the eyeball. Increased intracranial pressure results in increased pressure of the fluid in the subarachnoid space. This produces a protrusion at the optic disc, called *papilloedema*, which can be seen with an ophthalmoscope.

The Oculomotor Nerve. Before entering the orbit the nerve has already divided into superior and inferior branches. The superior supplies the levator palpebrae superioris and superior rectus; the inferior supplies the medial and inferior recti and inferior oblique and a preganglionic parasympathetic branch to the ciliary ganglion.

Division of the oculomotor nerve results in a marked loss of movements of the eyeball (only downward and outward movements are possible), drooping of the upper eyelid (ptosis), loss of accommodation due to paralysis of the ciliary muscle and a dilated pupil due to paralysis of the sphincter pupillae.

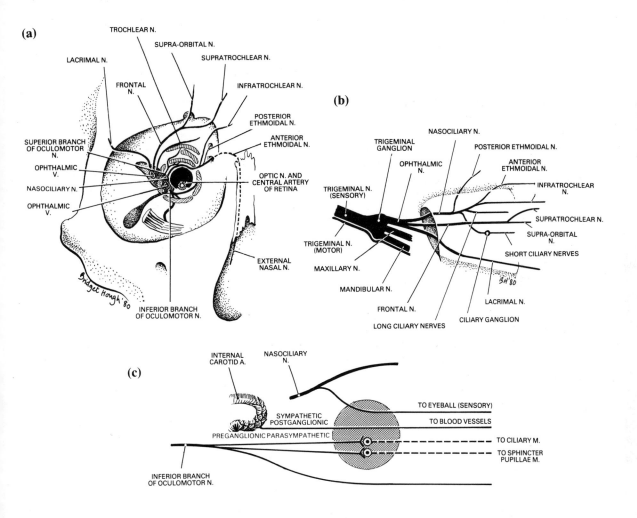

Figure 178 **(a) The nerves of the orbit. (b) The branches of the ophthalmic nerve. (c) The ciliary ganglion.**

The Trochlear Nerve. After entering the orbit it passes medially above the levator of the upper eyelid to supply the superior oblique muscle. If the nerve is injured, downward and outward movements of the eyeball are affected.

The Abducent Nerve. After entering the orbit, it supplies the lateral rectus muscle. This nerve is not infrequently affected and this is said to be due to its angulation both when it passes through the dura and over the apex of the petrous temporal bone. Paralysis of the lateral rectus muscle results in occasional double vision (*diplopia*). It only occurs when attempting to look laterally with the affected eye. At the same time an observer will notice a squint.

The Lacrimal, Frontal and Nasociliary Nerves (figure 178(b)). The *lacrimal nerve* runs forwards along the upper border of the lateral rectus, traverses the lacrimal gland which it supplies and is distributed to the lateral part of the skin of the upper eyelid. The postganglionic parasympathetic nerves from the pterygopalatine ganglion to the lacrimal gland may join the lacrimal nerve to supply the gland.

The *frontal nerve* passes forwards on the upper surface of the levator palpebrae superioris and divides at the level of the back of the eyeball into the larger lateral supra-orbital nerve and more medial supratrochlear nerve. The *supra-orbital nerve* continues forwards and after entering the supra-orbital notch or foramen is distributed to the skin of the upper eyelid, forehead and scalp as far as the vertex. The *supratrochlear nerve* passes forwards above the trochlea and is distributed to the skin of the upper eyelid and medial part of the forehead.

The *nasociliary nerve* runs forwards lateral to the optic nerve and then passes medially above the nerve with the ophthalmic artery. It continues inferior to the medial rectus as the *anterior ethmoidal nerve* in the anterior ethmoidal canal between the roof and medial wall of the orbit. The nerve then lies within the skull on the cribriform plate of the ethmoid bone and enters the nasal cavity at the side of the crista galli. It grooves the deep surface of the nasal bone and supplies the skin of the external nose by passing between the nasal bone and cartilage as the *external nasal nerve*. The anterior ethmoidal nerve is distributed to the ethmoidal, sphenoidal and frontal air sinuses and a small part of the lining of the nasal cavity. Within the orbit the nasociliary nerve supplies sensory fibres to the ciliary body, iris and cornea through the *long ciliary nerves* which come off where the nasociliary nerve crosses the optic nerve and usually contain postganglionic sympathetic fibres which supply the dilatator pupillae. The branches of the nasociliary nerve to the ciliary ganglion continue through the ganglion and emerge as some of the *short ciliary nerves* which are sensory to the back of the eyeball. The *infratrochlear nerve* passes forwards between the superior oblique and medial rectus and supplies the medial part of the skin of the upper eyelid and adjacent part of the external nose. The *posterior ethmoidal nerve* enters the posterior ethmoidal canal and supplies some of the ethmoidal air sinuses.

In general terms the ophthalmic division of the trigeminal nerve, a wholly sensory nerve, is distributed to (1) the anterior part of the meninges; (2) the contents of the orbit; (3) the skin of the forehead, anterior part of the scalp, upper eyelid and

side of the external nose, except for the edge of the external nasal aperture; (4) the lining of all the paranasal air sinuses except that of the maxillary sinus; (5) a small part of the lining of the nasal cavity. Conditions affecting the nerve or its branches result in pain radiating along the distribution of the nerve or its branches. The supra-orbital nerve shows this most frequently. *The surface marking of the* supra-orbital notch *which can be felt and where the nerve may be injected is the supra-orbital margin about 2.5 cm from the midline.*

The Maxillary Nerve. This nerve enters the orbit through the inferior orbital fissure from the pterygopalatine fossa and is accompanied by its zygomatic branch which usually contains the postganglionic parasympathetic motor fibres to the lacrimal gland. The latter supply the gland. The zygomatic nerve enters the orbital surface of the zygomatic bone usually as two branches and the maxillary nerve passes forwards on the floor of the orbit to enter the infra-orbital groove where it continues as the infra-orbital nerve. The infra-orbital nerve continues into the infra-orbital canal and *emerges on the face at the* infra-orbital foramen *0.5 cm below the lower margin of the orbit about 2.5 cm from the midline (p. 209).*

The Autonomic Nerves of the Orbit. Postganglionic sympathetic fibres reach the orbit either as a plexus round the ophthalmic artery or as a branch of the carotid plexus which comes off in the cavernous sinus and enters the orbit through the superior orbital fissure either separately or as part of the nasociliary nerve. In the orbit the sympathetic fibres supply the blood vessels, the dilatator pupillae and any smooth muscle in the orbit, including that of the levator palpebrae superioris. The effects of interruption of the sympathetic nerve supply to the orbit (Horner's syndrome) are described on p. 241.

The *ciliary ganglion* (figure 178(c)) is connected to the oculomotor and nasociliary nerves and lies lateral to the optic nerve. It is a parasympathetic ganglion in that only the parasympathetic fibres from the oculomotor nerve synapse in it. The sensory and sympathetic components pass through the ganglion. The former are branches of the naso-ciliary nerve and the latter may be the independent branch referred to above or travel in the nasociliary nerve. All the branches which come from the gang-lion are called the *short ciliary nerves* and may be sensory, sympathetic or parasympathetic. The sensory fibres supply part of the eyeball, the sympathetic supply the blood vessels, and the para-sympathetic the ciliary muscle and the sphincter pupillae. (The sympathetic supply of the dilatator pupillae enters the eyeball without passing through the ganglion.) The accommodation—convergence reflex (p. 270) involving the parasympathetic is accompanied by constriction of the pupil. Shining a light into the eye also produces constriction of the pupil (the *light reflex*) but this reflex follows a different neuronal pathway from that of accom-modation.

The ophthalmic artery and veins (figure 179)

The internal carotid artery before dividing into its terminal branches within the cranium gives off the *ophthalmic artery* which enters the orbit through the optic canal where it lies inferolateral to the optic nerve. The artery within the cone of muscles becomes lateral to the nerve and then crosses it superiorly to become medial and continue forwards between the superior oblique and medial rectus muscles. At the front of the orbit the artery divides into its terminal branches, the *supratrochlear* and the *dorsal nasal* which are distributed to the skin of the forehead and adjacent skin of the external nose.

Before the ophthalmic artery becomes lateral to the optic nerve it gives off the *central artery of the retina* which continues forwards inferior to the optic nerve and sinks into it 1 cm behind the eyeball. Just behind the retina the central artery divides into two branches each of which divides again so that superior, inferior, lateral and medial branches are visible at the optic disc (p. 270). The central artery of the retina is an end-artery. Block-age of this artery results in complete blindness of the affected eye.

The remaining branches of the ophthalmic artery are related to the branches of the ophthal-

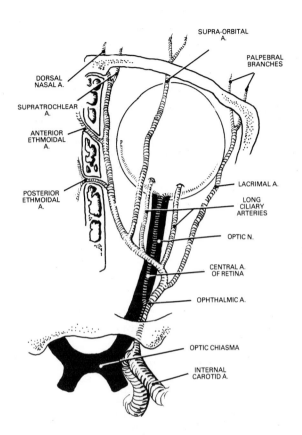

Figure 179   The ophthalmic artery.

mic nerve. Laterally the *lacrimal artery* goes to the lacrimal gland and upper eyelid. More medially the *supra-orbital artery* passes above the levator palpe-brae superioris and continues forwards with the supra-orbital nerve. The *posterior* and *anterior ethmoidal arteries* accompany the nerves of the same names and are distributed to the walls of the ethmoidal and frontal air sinuses and nasal cavity. The anterior ethmoidal artery ends on the skin of the side of the nose. The *posterior ciliary arteries* enter the eyeball posteriorly round the optic nerve. The *anterior ciliary arteries* come from the muscu-lar branches of the ophthalmic artery and enter the eyeball near the attachments of the muscles.

The ophthalmic artery constitutes an important anastomosis between the internal and external carotid arteries through the arteries of the face and scalp.

There are two *ophthalmic veins*, a *superior*

which begins near the anteromedial part of the orbit near the upper eyelid and runs backwards along the course of the ophthalmic artery, and an *inferior* which runs backwards along the inferior rectus muscle. Both veins end in the cavernous sinus by passing through the superior orbital fissure. Usually one vein lies inside and the other outside the fibrous ring. The *central vein of the retina*, which, just behind the eyeball, is in the middle of the optic nerve, leaves the nerve and ends in the cavernous sinus. There are important communications between the veins of the orbit and the veins of the scalp and face and infection may spread to the cavernous sinus from the face via the veins of the orbit.

The Ear

All parts of the ear (external, middle and internal) lie in the temporal bone except for the pinna or auricle which is attached to the tympanic part of the bone (figure 180(c)). The internal ear contains

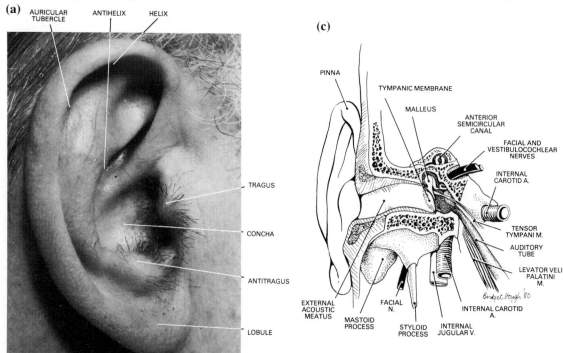

Figure 180   The right auricle (a) of an elderly male, (b) of a young woman. (c) A coronal section through the right external, middle and internal ears seen from the front.

both the peripheral organ of hearing and the vestibular apparatus which provides information about the position of the head in space and its movements, linear, angular and rotatory. Sounds are conducted by the external ear to the tympanic membrane which lies between it and the middle ear. The vibrations of the membrane are transmitted across the middle ear by a chain of small bones, the auditory ossicles, to the internal ear. The cochlear nerve is stimulated by fluid waves in the internal ear set up by the movements of the ossicles.

The external ear

The Pinna or Auricle. This structure, consisting largely of elastic cartilage and covered by skin, projects backwards and to a variable extent laterally from the side of the head. The skin on the outer surface is firmly adherent to the cartilage but on the inner surface is slightly mobile. The outer surface of the pinna has a number of ridges, elevations, hollows and grooves indicated in figure 180(a). Of these the *helix, antihelix, tragus, antitragus* and *lobule* are often referred to (*tragus = goat*, Latin and may refer to the thick hairs attached to it; this type of hair surrounds the external acoustic orifice and there are finer hairs over the rest of the outer surface). Near the upper end of the helix there is a tubercle of variable size (*Darwin's tubercle*, probably erroneously thought to be the remains of the pointed part of the quadruped ear). The lobule consists of fibrofatty tissue and does not contain cartilage. There is considerable variation in the depth of the groove between the lobule and the adjacent skin of the face.

The cartilage of the pinna extends inwards as a short cylinder deficient posterosuperiorly. It is attached to the lateral edge of the bony part of the external meatus. Small ligaments and muscles attach the auricle to the neighbouring areas of the skull. The muscles are supplied by the facial nerve. The outer surface of the auricle has a sensory nerve supply mainly from the auriculotemporal nerve and the inner surface is supplied mainly by the great auricular nerve which also supplies the helix, antihelix and outer surface of the lobule. The facial nerve may give a sensory branch to the concha which is behind the opening of the meatus. Evidence of this sensory innervation is seen in facial herpes zoster in which blisters appear in the skin of the meatus due to a virus infection of the cell bodies of the nerve fibres. The superficial temporal and posterior auricular arteries supply the auricle. The lymphatic vessels of the anterior part of the auricle go to the parotid lymph nodes and those from the inner surface to the mastoid nodes.

The External Acoustic (Auditory) Meatus. This canal, about 2.5 cm long from the concha to the tympanic membrane is cartilaginous in its outer third and bony in its inner two-thirds (figure 180(c)). The bony part is formed by the tympanic part of the temporal bone and is deficient in its upper posterior part which is completed by the squamous temporal bone. As the meatus passes medially it curves upwards and backwards. The tympanic membrane lies obliquely in a groove at the medial end of the meatus so that the lower part of the membrane is more medial than its upper part. The meatus is oval with the longer axis lying horizontally and narrowed at the junction of the cartilaginous with the bony part. Young children have a habit of pushing small objects into their orifices (mouth, nose or ear) and a small bead once pushed beyond this narrow part becomes lodged and very difficult to remove.

The meatus is lined by skin firmly adherent to the underlying bone and as a result any infection is very painful. The skin of the cartilaginous part is hairy and contains special wax (ceruminous) glands which look like sweat glands. The hairs and the wax are considered to be obstacles to the entry of foreign bodies, dead or alive. The wax lining the canal may make it impervious to water. Excess wax may block the meatus and cause partial deafness or may lodge on the membrane and interfere with its function. When syringing the meatus, its vagal nerve supply has to be kept in mind because of the possibility of reflex vagal slowing of the heart. Reference has already been made to this branch of the vagus nerve being called the *alderman's nerve* (p. 237).

By means of an aural speculum and light it is possible to examine the external surface of the

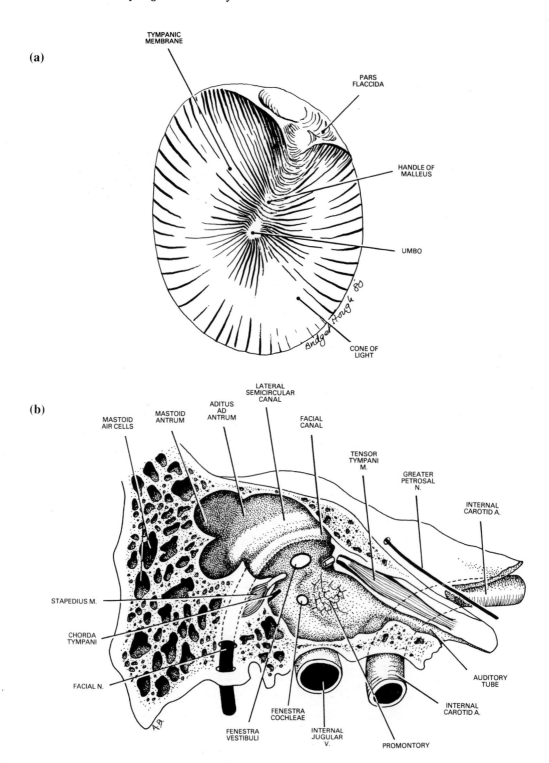

Figure 181   (a) The outer surface of the right tympanic membrane. (b) The medial wall of the right middle ear.

(c)

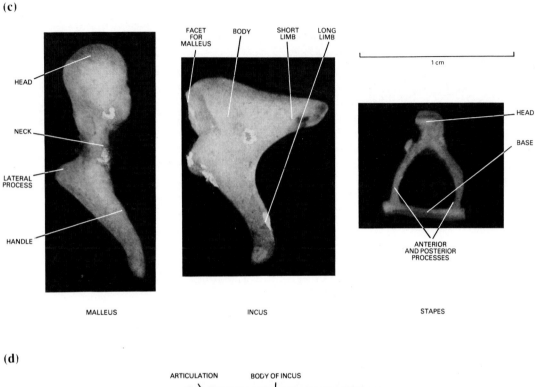

MALLEUS   INCUS   STAPES

(d)

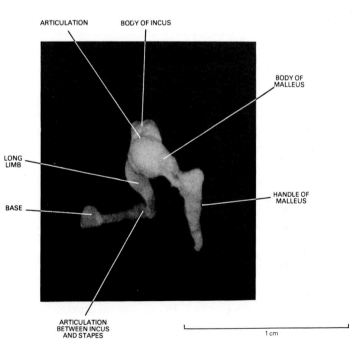

(c) The auditory ossicles. (d) The left auditory ossicles seen from the front.

tympanic membrane (figure 181(a)). The pinna is pulled upwards and backwards to straighten the meatus and it is important to remember that the meatus is short in a young child. The tympanic membrane appears pinkish and slightly glistening. The centre of the membrane, the *umbo*, is depressed where the handle of the malleus is attached (*umbo = boss of a shield*, Latin). The handle passing upwards and forwards can be seen through the membrane which presents a *flaccid part* above, anterior to the handle and a bright area, *the cone of light*, below and anterior to it. In infections of the middle ear the membrane usually bulges into the meatus and loses its glistening appearance.

The middle ear (tympanic cavity) (figures 180(c), 181(b))

This cavity in the petrous temporal bone is rectangular. The space is about 1.5 cm high and anteroposteriorly but only about 0.5 cm from its lateral to medial side. Where the tympanic membrane bulges medially at the umbo this measurement is reduced to about 0.2 cm. The *epitympanic recess* is that part of the cavity extending above the level of the upper border of the tympanic membrane. It is convenient to describe the six sides of the space as the roof, the floor and the anterior, posterior, medial and lateral walls.

The *roof* is formed by a thin plate of bone, the *tegmen tympani* (*tegmen = covering*, Latin) which extends posteriorly over the mastoid antrum and anteriorly over the canal for the auditory (Eustachian) tube. The meninges and temporal lobe of the brain lie on the tegmen tympani. The *floor* of the tympanic cavity is formed by bone separating the cavity from the superior bulb of the internal jugular vein.

The *anterior wall* has two openings in its upper part, a superior through which the tendon of the tensor tympani enters the middle ear and an inferior which is the lateral (posterior) end of the auditory tube. The openings are separated by bone projecting into the cavity. The tendon hooks round this projection and passes to the handle of the malleus. The middle ear is lined by ciliated mucous columnar epithelium continuous with that of the nasopharynx through the auditory tube. The tube, described with the pharynx (p. 310), is the means whereby the pressure on the two sides of the tympanic membrane is equalised and is opened during swallowing. The lower part of the anterior wall is separated by bone from the internal carotid artery.

The *posterior wall* of the cavity separates it from the air spaces in the petrous temporal bone, the largest of which is the *mastoid antrum* lying immediately posterior to the middle ear (*antron = cave*, Greek). The opening into the antrum (*aditus to the antrum*) lies on the posterior wall near the medial wall and the roof. Below the aditus there is a projection of bone called the *pyramid* out of which comes the *stapedius muscle* which is attached to the stapes. Medial to the aditus the *lateral semicircular canal* produces a bulge. The *facial nerve* runs downwards in a canal between the posterior and medial walls, medial to the aditus.

The *medial wall* is lateral to the internal ear and has two openings. The upper, which is oval, is called the *fenestra vestibuli* and has the footpiece of the stapes lodged in it. The lower which is round is called the *fenestra cochleae* and is closed by a membrane. The *promontory* is a projection on the medial wall anterior to these openings. The promontory lies over the basal turn of the cochlea (*cochlea = snail's shell*, Latin). There is a plexus of nerves on the promontory. The *facial nerve* runs backwards in a bony canal in the upper border of the medial wall from its *ganglion* which lies in the upper anterior angle of the wall.

The *lateral wall* contains the *tympanic membrane* and extends above the level of the membrane. The *chorda tympani*, a branch of the facial nerve, emerges posteriorly from a small canal at the level of the upper border of the tympanic membrane and runs forwards on its medial surface between the handle of the malleus and long process of the incus. The nerve leaves the tympanic cavity through a small canal at the junction of the lateral wall and floor of the cavity. It emerges from the skull through the petrotympanic fissure and joins the lingual nerve (p. 207 and p. 222).

The Tympanic Membrane. This structure separating the external from the middle ear lies at an angle of about 50° to the external meatus. It is more or less circular and about 1 cm in diameter. Its outer surface is modified epidermis supplied by the auriculotemporal and vagus nerves. Its inner surface consists of mucous columnar cells and is supplied by the glossopharyngeal nerve. Between these two layers there are fibres of a special composition unlike collagen or elastin arranged circularly and radially. The appearance of the membrane as viewed with an aural speculum is described on p. 280.

The Mastoid Antrum and Air Cells. The *antrum* is a cavity behind the middle ear and communicates with it by the aditus to the antrum. The tegmen tympani covers the antrum, the sigmoid sinus is posterior and the lateral semicircular canal is medial. The facial nerve is anterior and then inferior to the antrum. *The surface marking of the mastoid antrum is the* suprameatal triangle *(of MacEwan) (Sir William MacEwan, 1848–1924, Glasgow surgeon) which lies above and behind the tympanic part of the temporal bone. The triangle is indicated by a horizontal line along the upper edge of the external acoustic meatus, a vertical line along its posterior edge and an oblique line along its posterosuperior edge. If the auricle is pulled forwards the triangle can be felt as a depression.* As already stated there is in the infant less than 5 mm of bone between the antrum and the surface as compared with about 15 mm in the adult.

The *mastoid air cells* are extensions of the antrum but unlike the antrum, which is present at birth, the air cells develop mainly after the second year when the mastoid process develops. The number and extent of these cells vary a great deal so that the mastoid process may be almost solid dense bone or the air cells may fill the mastoid process and extend into the squamous and petrous parts of the temporal bone.

Infection of the antrum and air cells may occur as an extension of infection from the middle ear, which in children is readily infected via the auditory tube from the nasopharynx. Not only is infection of bone difficult to eradicate, but the infection may spread to the temporal lobe of the brain through the tegmen tympani, to the internal ear, to the sigmoid sinus or to the cerebellum. Apart from these possible complications, infection of the middle ear (*otitis media*) often interferes with hearing and may result in a conduction deafness.

The Auditory Ossicles. These are three small bones extending from the lateral to the medial wall (figure 181(c), (d)). The lateral bone, the *malleus (malleus = hammer*, Latin) has a *head* which lies in the epitympanic recess and a *handle* which passes downwards and backwards to the middle of the tympanic membrane to which it is attached at the umbo. The posterior surface of the head of the malleus articulates with the body of the incus by means of a synovial joint. The malleus has an *anterior process* attached to the floor of the tympanic cavity and a *lateral process* attached to the edge of the flaccid part of the tympanic membrane. The tensor tympani is attached to the handle near the head. The chorda tympani passes forwards medial to the handle.

The middle ossicle, the *incus (incus = anvil*, Latin) has a *body* which lies in the epitympanic recess and articulates anteriorly with the head of the malleus. The body has two widely diverging processes. The *long process* passes downwards and backwards behind and parallel to the handle of the malleus. Its lower end turns medially and articulates with the stapes. The *short process* projects backwards and is attached to the posterior wall near the roof. The chorda tympani passes forwards lateral to the long process.

The medial ossicle, the *stapes (stapes = stirrup*, Latin), is about half the length of the malleus and has a head, two limbs and a base. The *head* points laterally and articulates by a synovial joint with the long process of the incus. The *limbs, anterior* and *posterior*, pass medially from the head and are joined by the oval *base* (footpiece of the stirrup) which lies in the fenestra vestibuli. The base is attached to the edges of the fenestra by a ligament. The stapedius muscle supplied by the facial nerve is attached to the head of the stapes near its limbs.

Sound waves passing along the external meatus cause the tympanic membrane to vibrate. These vibrations are transmitted across the middle ear by the ossicles to the fenestra vestibuli and thence to the internal ear. When the footpiece of the stapes moves, it rocks about its long axis. It does not move inwards and outwards. The waves are amplified about 50 times since the tympanic membrane is about 20 times the area of the footpiece and the lever action of the ossicles increases the movements by a factor of two or three. The tensor tympani and stapedius muscles contract reflexly to dampen down excessive movements of the ossicles due to sounds of high intensity.

The Nerves Related to the Middle Ear. The *tympanic branch of the glossopharyngeal nerve* and *sympathetic fibres* from the continuation of the carotid plexus which surrounds the branches of the internal carotid artery form a plexus on the promontory of the medial wall. The glossopharyngeal part of the plexus supplies sensory fibres to the lining of the middle ear, antrum and auditory tube. It also gives off the preganglionic parasympathetic *lesser petrosal nerve* which leaves the petrous temporal bone in the middle cranial fossa and eventually ends in the otic ganglion (p. 206).

The *facial nerve* runs in a bony canal along the upper and then the posterior border of the medial wall. The *geniculate ganglion* lies at the anterior end of the upper border where the facial nerve having passed laterally across the vestibule of the internal ear bends backwards (*genu = knee*, Latin). About 5 mm above the stylomastoid foramen the *chorda tympani* leaves the facial nerve and runs upwards and laterally in the posterior wall from which it emerges to pass forwards between the middle and inner layers of the tympanic membrane. (The nerves, muscles and ossicles lie outside the lining of the middle ear.) The chorda tympani contains taste fibres whose cell bodies are in the geniculate ganglion and preganglionic parasympathetic fibres which end in the submandibular ganglion (p. 207). The facial nerve also supplies the stapedius and gives off the *greater petrosal nerve* which is a preganglionic parasympathetic nerve and leaves the petrous temporal bone in the middle cranial fossa. This nerve passes towards the foramen lacerum and eventually ends in the pterygopalatine ganglion (p. 208). The postganglionic fibres from the ganglion supply the lacrimal gland and nasal and palatine mucous glands.

The Blood Vessels and Lymphatics. The blood supply to the middle ear comes from the posterior auricular, maxillary and internal carotid arteries. The veins form a communication between the intracranial venous sinuses and the extracranial pterygoid venous plexus. The lymphatic vessels go to either the parotid or deep cervical nodes.

The internal ear

The internal ear consists of the *osseous labyrinth*, which is a series of cavities in the petrous temporal bone, and a *membranous labyrinth* which lies in these cavities. A fluid called *endolymph* lies within the membranous labyrinth which in turn is surrounded by *perilymph*. The osseous labyrinth consists of the three *semicircular canals* which are posterior, the bony *cochlea* which is anterior and the *vestibule* which lies between the canals and cochlea (figures 182, 183).

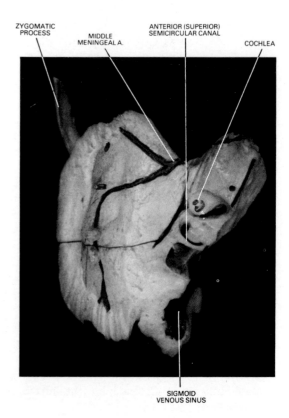

ZYGOMATIC PROCESS   MIDDLE MENINGEAL A.   ANTERIOR (SUPERIOR) SEMICIRCULAR CANAL   COCHLEA

SIGMOID VENOUS SINUS

Figure 182   A superior view of the left temporal bone to show the position of the labyrinth.

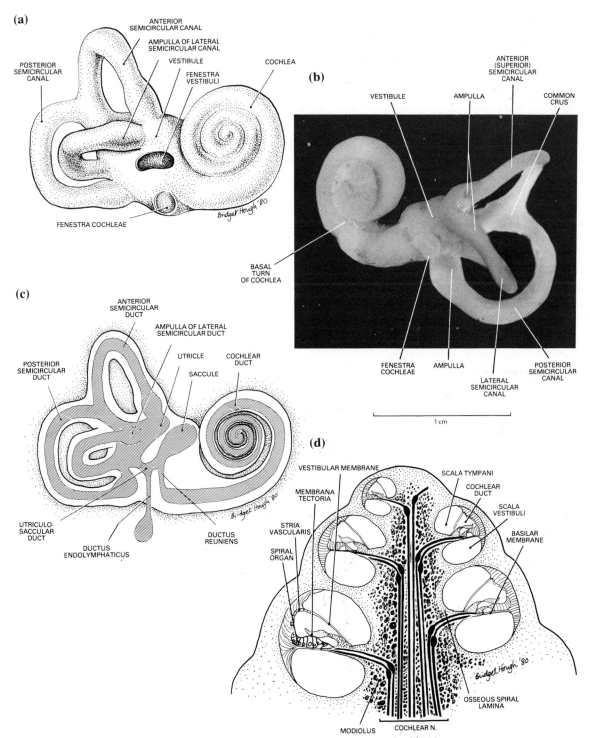

Figure 183 (a) The right osseous labyrinth. (b) A lateral view of a cast of a left human labyrinth.
(c) The membranous labyrinth placed inside the bony labyrinth (the cochlea has been opened out).
(d) A vertical section through the cochlea.

The Osseous Labyrinth

The Semicircular Canals. The three *canals*, about 1 mm in diameter, are *anterior* (superior), *posterior* and *lateral*. The anterior and posterior have a common opening into the medial wall of the vestibule. Their opposite ends are dilated to form *ampullae* about 2 mm in diameter (*ampulla = jar*, Latin) and open separately into the vestibule. The anterior and posterior canals are at right angles to each other and are at an angle of 45° to the sagittal plane, the anterior being anterior and lateral, and the posterior, posterior and lateral. The lateral canal is horizontal and its ampulla opens into the lateral wall of the vestibule (figure 183(a)).

The Cochlea. The bony cochlea has about two and three-quarter turns and lies on its side so that the basal turn is inferior and produces the promontory on the medial wall of the middle ear. The apex is directed laterally. The cochlea if unravelled is about 30 mm long. Its base is about 10 mm wide and its height (base to apex) is about 5 mm. The cochlea has a central pillar of bone, the *modiolus* (*modiolus = hub*, Latin) which has a perforated base for the cochlear nerve adjacent to the lateral end of the internal acoustic meatus. A shelf of bone, the *osseous spiral lamina*, winding round the modiolus like the thread of a screw, projects outwards. A lower basilar and upper vestibular membrane pass from the edge of the lamina to the outer wall of the bony cochlea so that it is divided into three channels, an upper *scala vestibuli*, a middle *cochlear duct* and a lower *scala tympani* (*scala = staircase*, Latin). In the base of the coil the scala vestibuli begins at the fenestra vestibuli. The scala vestibuli is continuous with the scala tympani at the apex of the coil through an opening called the *helicotrema* (*trema = hole*, Latin) and the scala tympani ends at the fenestra cochleae. The cochlear nerve and ganglion lie in the modiolus and the peripheral processes of the bipolar ganglion cells pass into the spiral lamina and basilar membrane (figure 183(d)).

The Vestibule. This lies medial to the middle ear, is ovoid in shape and about 5 mm in diameter. The five openings of the semicircular canals open on to the vestibule more or less posteriorly and the fenestra vestibuli and fenestra cochleae open on to its lateral wall. Its medial wall is at the lateral end of the internal acoustic meatus and has perforations for the peripheral processes of the vestibular nerve whose ganglion lies in the internal meatus. The scala vestibuli and scala tympani open on to its anterior wall, the former near the fenestra vestibuli and the latter near the fenestra cochleae.

The Membranous Labyrinth

The Semicircular Ducts. Their arrangement is similar to that of the canals and they have a dilated *ampulla* at one end. It is important to appreciate that parts of the membranous labyrinth are attached to the wall of the osseous labyrinth and are not floating in perilymph. In the ampulla of each duct, where it is attached to the bony wall, there is a thickening called the *ampullary crest*. This thickening is the end-organ in which some of the fibres of the vestibular nerve end. The three ducts open into the utricle which is the posterior part of the membranous labyrinth in the vestibule.

The Utricle and Saccule (figure 183(c)). These two parts of the membranous labyrinth communicate with each other by a narrow channel. The utricle is posterior and the saccule anterior and the saccule communicates with the cochlear duct by the *ductus reuniens*. From the posterior part of the saccule a diverticulum (the *ductus endolymphaticus*) extends towards and lies behind the internal acoustic meatus. A part of the wall of both the utricle and saccule is thickened to form the *maculae*. Each macula is an end-organ in which fibres of the vestibular nerve end. The histological structure of the ampullary crests and the maculae is similar (there are otoliths on the maculae and not on the crests) and they are stimulated by movement of the endolymph. This results in stimulation of the vestibular nerve. It is thought that the ampullary crests of the semicircular canals convey information about rotatory and angular movements of the head and that the maculae are associated with linear and tilting movements. Disease of the semicircular ducts, utricle and saccule results in attacks of giddiness of varying severity.

The Cochlear Duct (figure 183(c), (d)). This is a spiral tube which lies in the bony cochlea between the scala vestibuli above and the scala tympani below. The floor of the duct is formed by the basilar membrane and the roof by the vestibular membrane. In section the duct appears triangular and is attached medially to the osseous spiral lamina. Laterally its wall is formed by the thickened endosteum of the bony canal lined by thin vascular tissue (*stria vascularis*). The upper end of the cochlear duct is closed and its lower end communicates with the saccule. The end-organ of hearing (*the spiral organ*) lies on the basilar membrane. The fibres of the cochlear nerve pass from the osseous spiral lamina into the basilar membrane and make contact with the end-organ. Movements of the basilar membrane due to waves in the perilymph result in stimulation of the cells of the end-organ which in turn stimulate the cochlear nerve.

The Perilymph and Endolymph. The *perilymph* is the fluid within the osseous labyrinth outside the membranous labyrinth. It is similar to cerebrospinal fluid and the space within which it lies communicates with the subarachnoid space through a small canal which opens on to the petrous temporal bone forming the anterior wall of the jugular foramen. Movements of the stapes produce pressure waves in the perilymph and these waves pass through the perilymph in the scala vestibuli and scala tympani. This results in movements of the basilar membrane.

The *endolymph* in the membranous labyrinth is different in composition from that of the perilymph (for example, it contains a larger number of potassium ions) and is probably produced by the stria vascularis of the wall of the cochlear duct and the lining cells of the semicircular ducts. The fluid is thought to be absorbed at the dilated end of the ductus endolymphaticus.

Hearing defects are usually classified as *conduction deafness* and *sensory* or *neuronal deafness*. In the former there is some interference with the conduction of sounds from the external to the internal ear, for example wax in the external meatus or disease affecting the tympanic membrane, auditory ossicles or auditory tube. In sensory deafness sounds, having reached the internal ear in the normal way without interference, fail to stimulate the cochlear nerve in the appropriate manner. For example, the deafness of old age is due to a progressive degeneration of the basilar membrane beginning at the base of the cochlear coil and thus affecting sounds of high pitch so that the condition begins with a high tone deafness. Since sounds can be conducted through the temporal bone to the internal ear, conduction deafness is more easily treated than neuronal deafness by means of a hearing aid.

20

The Oral Cavity and Palate

The Lips, Cheeks and Vestibule of the Mouth

The *oral cavity* or *mouth* is the space bounded anteriorly by the lips, laterally by the cheeks and superiorly by the palate. The floor is muscular with the tongue lying posteriorly and the two mylo-hyoid muscles joined in the midline anteriorly. The mouth opens posteriorly into the oropharynx through the *isthmus of the fauces (fauces = throat*, Latin) which is bounded laterally by the palato-glossal folds. The space between the cheeks extern-ally and the teeth and alveolar processes of the maxilla and mandible internally, is called the *vesti-bule of the mouth*. When the teeth are together the vestibule communicates behind the last molar teeth with the oral cavity proper, the part of the mouth within the alveolar processes.

The Lips. These are two fleshy folds consisting largely of muscles covered by skin externally and mucous membrane internally. Both are firmly bound down to the underlying tissue. Laterally the lips meet at the *angle of the mouth*. The *naso-labial groove* which deepens with age runs down-wards and laterally from the ala of the nose at the cheek towards the angle of the mouth and ends about 1 cm lateral to it. The *labiomarginal groove* running downwards and slightly inwards from the angle of the mouth towards the lower border of the mandible makes its appearance only with advancing age.

The *philtrum* of the upper lips is the vertical, midline, shallow groove between the nose and the edge of the lips (p. 191). There is considerable variation in the vertical height of the upper lip. This influences its mobility and it is said that the male has a less mobile upper lip than the female.

The *red margin* of the lips indicates the change from the keratinised, hairy skin on the outside to the non-keratinised epithelium of a transitional zone between the skin and the mucous membrane. There is considerable variation in the colour, visible width of the red zone and its shape, and cosmetic efforts are made to alter or improve these.

There are numerous serous, mucous and salivary glands in the mucous membrane of the lips (*labial glands*). Both lips have a *frenulum* which is a mid-line, vertical fold of mucous membrane between their deep surface and the gum. The upper is much larger than the lower (*frenum = bridle*, Latin).

The lips consist largely of the *orbicularis oris muscle* (p. 195) and have a rich blood and nerve supply (figures 134, 135). The main arteries come from the *facial artery* and the veins go to the *facial vein*. The nerve supply to the muscles is the *facial nerve*. The sensory nerves of the upper lip come from the *maxillary nerve (infra-orbital branch)* and those of the lower lip from the *mandibular nerve (mental branch of the inferior alveolar nerve)*. There is a specially rich sensory innervation of the lips. This, together with the large area of represent-ation for the lips on both the motor and sensory cortex of the cerebral hemispheres, is related to their functions in speech.

The lips are usually closed when chewing and

almost invariably closed when swallowing. Their closure is essential for suckling in an infant so that the lips can form a seal round the nipple or teat. A common congenital defect which may be uni- or bilateral is a *cleft (hare) lip* in which the upper lip has failed to develop properly. The result is an inability to effect this closure and consequent difficulty in feeding. Usually an immediate temporary closure of the defect is made and subsequently the defect is permanently repaired.

The Cheeks. Their structure is similar to that of the lips — a layer of muscle, mainly the *buccinator*, covered externally by skin and internally by mucous membrane. The posterior limit of the outside of the cheek extends further than that of the inside which is marked by a palpable fold between the maxilla and mandible containing the *pterygomandibular raphe*.

External to the posterior part of the buccinator there is a pad of fat which extends backwards between the buccinator and masseter muscles and the other muscles of mastication. This pad of fat is relatively much larger in the newborn and infant and although there is some doubt about its having a specific function in suckling it is called the *buccal* or *suctorial pad*. Its presence is one of the reasons why a healthy baby's face invariably appears round. The other factors are the size and shape of the upper and lower jaws.

The *parotid duct* runs forwards in the cheek over the masseter, pierces the fat and the buccinator and opens on to the inside of the cheek at the *parotid papilla* opposite the second upper molar tooth.

The *facial artery*, the *infra-orbital branch* of the *maxillary artery* and the *transverse facial branch* of the *superficial temporal artery* supply the cheek, which has a sensory innervation from the *maxillary* and *mandibular nerves*.

The Vestibule of the Mouth. Defined as that part of the mouth between the lips and cheeks, and teeth and gums, the vestibule has the *parotid ducts* opening into it, one on each side, and contains the *frenula of the lips*.

The Tongue

The tongue is a muscular organ which has a free, mobile, anterior part, horizontal at rest, and a more fixed, posterior, vertical part (the *root*) (figure 184). The anterior part is in the mouth and the posterior part in the pharynx.

The Surfaces of the Tongue (figure 185). The upper surface of the anterior part and the posterior surface of the posterior part are called the *dorsum*, a confusing term unless one thinks of the whole tongue pointing upwards. The *sulcus terminalis*, a V-shaped groove with its apex pointing backwards, divides the dorsum of the tongue into an anterior two-thirds and a posterior third. The part of the tongue behind the sulcus terminalis differs in development, innervation and structure from that in front of it. Immediately behind the apex of the sulcus there is a small depression, the *foramen caecum*, which marks the site of origin of the thyroid diverticulum.

The dorsal surface of the tongue is covered by a fairly thick, non-keratinised, stratified epithelium covered with different types of papillae. The largest of these, the *vallate*, form a single row in front of the sulcus terminalis and are about 2–4 mm in diameter. They consist of a circular central elevation surrounded by a groove which in turn is surrounded by a narrow wall (*vallum = rampart* or *ditch*, Latin). There are taste buds in the walls of the groove. The *fungiform papillae*, as their name suggests, resemble toadstools. They are about 1 mm in diameter, contain taste buds and are found at the apex and edges of the tongue. The *filiform papillae (filum = thread*, Latin) are the most numerous and are like threads with a pointed tip. They are found over the whole of the anterior part of the tongue and do not contain taste buds. Other types of papillae varying in their shape are also described (*foliate, lentiform, conical*).

The posterior third of the dorsum of the tongue has an irregular surface due to nodules of lymphatic tissue (the *lingual tonsil*). There are serous and mucous glands in the submucosa. Behind this part of the tongue, between it and the epiglottis, there

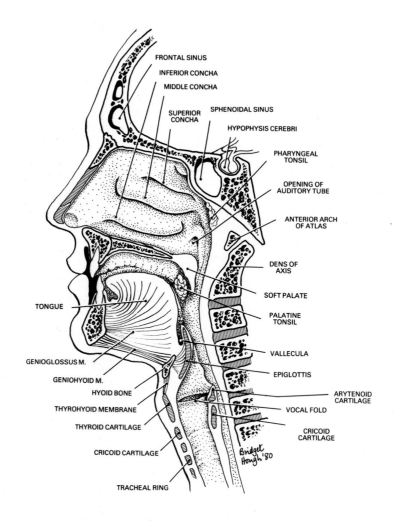

Figure 184   A sagittal section through the nasal cavity, mouth, pharynx and larynx.

is a space in which there are a sagittal midline fold of mucous membrane, the *median glosso-epiglottic fold*, and a fold on each side, the *lateral glosso-epiglottic folds*. These folds bound two hollows called the *valleculae* (*vallecula = little valley*, Latin).

The inferior surface of the anterior part of the tongue (figure 185(b)) is covered by a much thinner mucous membrane than that on the dorsum, with the result that the *deep lingual (ranine) vein* can be seen passing towards the apex (*rana = frog*, Latin; the appearance of the region below the tongue is thought to resemble the undersurface of a frog). Running parallel and lateral to the vein there is a fimbriated fold (*fimbria = fringe*, Latin).

The *lingual frenulum* is a vertical midline between the tongue and the floor of the mouth. The *sublingual fold* due to the underlying sublingual salivary gland passes laterally from the frenulum between the inferior surface of the tongue and the floor of the mouth. On each side of the frenulum there is a small papilla on to which the submandibular duct opens.

The Muscles of the Tongue (figure 186). The muscles are divided into intrinsic and extrinsic. The *intrinsic fibres* are confined to the tongue itself, are mainly in the anterior part and are arranged in vertical, horizontal and longitudinal

(a)

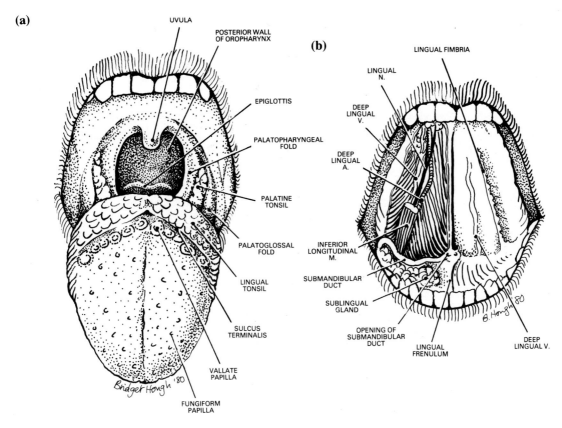

(b)

Figure 185   (a) The upper (dorsal) surface of the tongue. (b) The inferior surface of the tongue and the floor of the mouth.

groups. The *vertical* are at the sides of the tongue, the *transverse* are attached to a sagittal fibrous partition and the *longitudinal* (*superior* and *inferior*) are only found immediately deep to the surfaces of the tongue. The vertical fibres flatten and broaden the tongue, the transverse produce a narrowing and lengthening and the longitudinal turn the tip upwards (superior fibres) or downwards (inferior fibres).

The *extrinsic muscles* have an attachment to structures outside the tongue. The *hyoglossus muscle* is attached to the greater cornu and part of the body of the hyoid bone and passes vertically upwards into the tongue. It forms the most lateral part of the tongue except superiorly where the styloglossus mingles with it. The hyoglossus has a number of important relations (figure 144). The posterior belly of the digastric and stylohyoid

muscles are superficial to it posteriorly and the mylohyoid muscle overlaps it anteriorly. The lingual and hypoglossal nerves pass downwards and forwards on its superficial surface with the submandibular ganglion suspended from the lingual nerve between them. The deep part of the submandibular gland, its duct and sublingual gland are on the superficial surface of the muscle and the lingual artery and glossopharyngeal nerve pass forwards deep to it. The hyoglossus pulls the tongue downwards if the hyoid bone is fixed by the infrahyoid muscles.

The *styloglossus muscle* is attached to the styloid process of the temporal bone and passes downwards and forwards into the tongue where it mingles with the fibres of the hyoglossus. The styloglossus pulls the tongue upwards and backwards. The *genioglossus* is attached to the upper

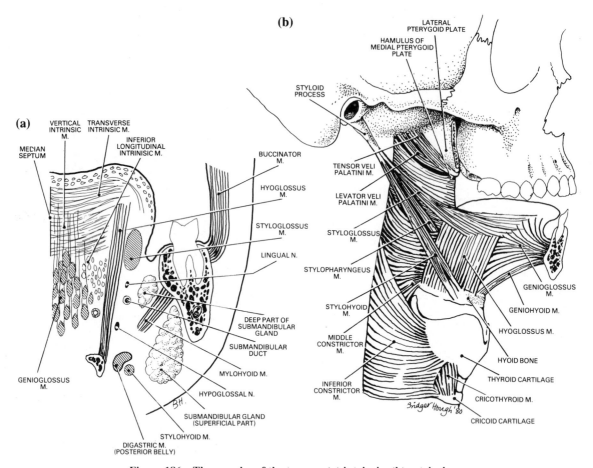

Figure 186   The muscles of the tongue: (a) intrinsic; (b) extrinsic.

part of the mental spine (formerly the superior genial tubercle). It is a fan-shaped muscle lying in the sagittal plane near the midline, and its fibres spread out into the tongue from the tip to the base. Most of its fibres, however, pass backwards so that its main effect is to pull the tongue forwards. The lowest fibres are attached to the body of the hyoid bone. The fibres going to the tip pull it downwards. If both genioglossi contract they produce a sagittal midline furrow in the tongue.

The *palatoglossus* arises from the soft palate, passes laterally into the palatoglossal fold and descends to enter the tongue and mingle with the fibres of the styloglossus. Besides pulling the tongue upwards it is an important muscle in swallowing in which action it closes the isthmus of the fauces both before and after the food passes from the mouth into the oropharynx.

The Nerve and Blood Supply of the Tongue. The muscles are supplied by the hypoglossal nerve. The exception is the palatoglossus which is supplied by the pharyngeal plexus. The motor nerve of this plexus is the pharyngeal branch of the vagus. The sensory innervation is both general and special (taste) and the innervation of the anterior two-thirds is different from that of the posterior third (pre- and postsulcal parts). The lingual nerve, a branch of the mandibular, is the nerve of general sensation of the anterior two-thirds of the tongue. The chorda tympani (p. 222), a branch of the facial nerve, joins the lingual nerve and supplies taste fibres to the anterior two-thirds. The glossopharyngeal nerve supplies both fibres of general sensation and taste to the posterior third of the tongue. The taste buds of the vallate papillae, although anterior to the sulcus terminalis, are supplied by the glossopharyngeal nerve. The vagus nerve through the internal laryngeal nerve supplies taste buds in the region of the epiglottis.

The lingual artery (p. 233), a branch of the external carotid, is the main *artery* supplying the tongue. It enters the tongue deep to the hyoglossus muscle. The *veins* draining the tongue either accompany the artery or run superficial to the hyoglossus near the hypoglossal nerve. The veins end in the facial or internal jugular vein.

The *lymphatic drainage* of the tongue (p. 322) is very important because carcinoma of the tongue spreads early and rapidly via the lymphatic vessels.

The Functions of the Tongue. The tongue is used in sucking, chewing and swallowing and is especially important for sucking in an infant. In chewing it pushes the food between the teeth and in swallowing it pushes the food backwards towards the oropharynx between it and the palate. The tongue is of paramount importance in speech and it is the organ of taste. If paralysed all the motor functions are difficult or impossible. If one side is paralysed, on protrusion the tongue deviates to the affected side.

The Teeth

Only the gross structure, the main differences between the types of teeth and some indication of their time of eruption are given.

The Gross Structure of a Tooth (figure 187(a)). A tooth consists of a core of *pulp* lying in the *pulp cavity* and surrounded by *dentine* which is covered in its upper part by *enamel* and in its lower part by *cement*. The *crown* of the tooth is the part covered by enamel which extends for a short distance below the edge of the gingiva. The surfaces of the crowns which meet when the teeth are brought together (*occlusal surface*) have one or more projections called *cusps*. The *root* is the part covered by cement and the *neck* of the tooth is between the root and the crown. If a tooth has more than one root the pulp and pulp cavity extend into each root. The tip of each root is open (*apical foramen*) and blood and lymphatic vessels and nerves enter

and leave the tooth through this opening. Each tooth lies in a *dental alveolus* (*alveolus = hollow*, Latin) in the alveolar arches of the mandible and maxilla. The alveolus is lined by a thin layer of dense bone to which the cement of the tooth is attached by the fibrous *periodontal membrane*. The term *periodontium* may be used to include the dense bone, odontal ligament, cement and the part of the gum below the level of the visible crown.

The Different Types of Teeth. Teeth are classified as *incisor*, *canine*, *premolar* and *molar*. There are two sets of teeth, *deciduous* (*milk*) and *permanent*. The deciduous teeth in each quadrant from in front backwards are two incisors (*central* and *lateral*), one canine and two molars. The permanent teeth in each quadrant (figure 187(b)) are two incisors, one canine, two premolars and three molars (there may be only two molars). The *incisor teeth* are flattened with a chisel-like edge and as their name implies they are used for cutting. The *canine teeth* also used for cutting or tearing food have a pointed extremity. They derive their name from their prominence in dogs. Their roots are the longest of the roots of the teeth and bulge sufficiently to produce a palpable elevation on the face. The *premolar* (*bicuspid*) *teeth* have two cusps and the upper premolars may have two roots. The *molar teeth* have three, four or five cusps. The upper molars usually have three roots and the lower two, although the third molars frequently have only one root. The premolar and molar teeth are used for grinding the food.

The Time of Eruption of the Teeth. The first of the deciduous teeth to erupt is the lower central incisor at about 6 months. This is followed by the eruption of the upper central incisors and the lateral incisors so that the eight incisor teeth are usually present at the end of the first year. The first molars, followed by the canines and finally the second molars, erupt during the next year or 18 months and a baby may be expected to have all its 20 deciduous teeth by the age of 30 months.

Although it is usually said that the first permanent tooth to erupt is the first molar behind the deciduous teeth at about 6 years (*6-year molar*), not infrequently the deciduous lower central

(a)

(b)

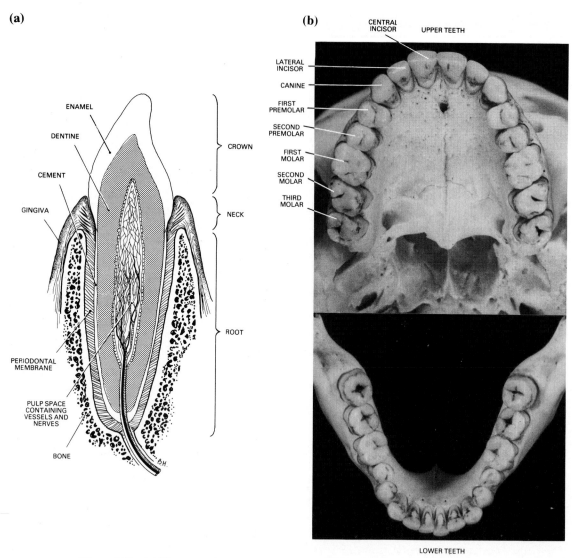

Figure 187 (a) The general structure of a tooth. (b) The upper and lower teeth.

incisor falls out and is replaced by the permanent lower central incisor before the eruption of the 6-year molar. From 7 years to 12 years the deciduous teeth fall out due to resorption of their roots and are replaced by the erupting permanent teeth. The eight incisor teeth are present by the age of 8 years and by the age of 12 years there are usually seven teeth in each quadrant. The third molar erupts after the age of 17 years and usually before 25 years. It is not uncommon for one or more of the third molars to remain unerupted. (In different populations the incidence varies from less than 1

per cent to 25 per cent.) Because of the direction of the eruption of the lower third molar (it is directed forwards as well as upwards) it is much more commonly impacted against the second molar than the upper third molar which erupts posteriorly as well as downwards. An impacted third molar (*wisdom tooth*) can be a problem which requires surgical intervention.

Considerable changes in the maxilla and mandible and especially in their alveolar processes occur during the eruption of the teeth. While the deciduous teeth are erupting the main growth is in an

(a)

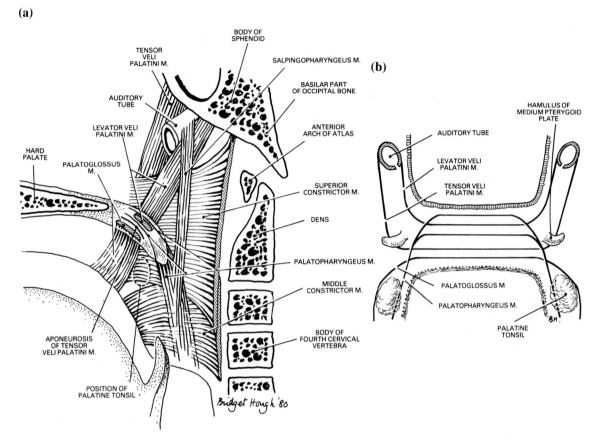

Figure 188   (a) **The muscles of the right side of the palate viewed from the inside of the mouth. (b) A diagram of the structure of the soft palate.**

anteroposterior direction, but during the eruption of the permanent teeth there is also a considerable increase in growth from side to side and vertically and in the size of the maxillary sinus.

The arch formed by the upper teeth is different from that formed by the lower. The upper arch is described as elliptical and the lower as parabolic. When the teeth are brought together the upper incisors normally lie in front of the lower. Because of the width of the upper incisors, especially the central, an upper tooth occludes with its corresponding lower tooth and also part of the next tooth; for example, the upper canine meets the lower canine and the lower first premolar. Although the posterior part of the lower arch is wider than that of the lower, the outer surface of the upper molars lies outside that of the lower molars because the latter slope inwards.

The Palate

The palate forms the roof of the mouth and the floor of the nasal cavity and is divided into the larger anterior *hard (bony) palate* and posterior *soft (muscular) palate*.

The Hard Palate (figure 187(b)). This is arched transversely and is formed anteriorly by the palatine processes of the maxilla, and posteriorly (about one-quarter) by the horizontal processes of the palatine bones. It is bounded anteriorly and laterally by the alveolar processes of the maxillae covered by the gingivae. The soft palate is attached to its posterior edge. Anteriorly the mucous membrane on both its surfaces is firmly bound down to the underlying periosteum, forming a mucoperiosteum which on its oral surface is transversely ridged.

The mucous membrane posteriorly is less firmly attached and contains a number of mucous glands. There is a small midline papilla overlying the incisive fossa just behind the incisive teeth.

The Soft Palate (figure 188). This hangs downwards from the posterior edge of the hard palate so that it has an anterior (inferior or oral) surface and a posterior (superior or pharyngeal) surface. The soft palate consists mainly of muscles attached to an aponeurosis and is covered by a mucous membrane on both its surfaces. In the midline the conical *uvula* (*uvula = little grape*, Latin) hangs downwards from the posterior free edge. It is of varied length, 5–15 mm. Laterally the posterior edge divides into an anterior *palatoglossal arch* (*anterior pillar of the fauces*) and a posterior *palatopharyngeal arch* (*posterior pillar of the fauces*). The *palatal aponeurosis*, which is the expanded tendon of the tensor veli palatini muscle, is attached to the posterior edge of the hard palate. The other muscles are attached mainly to the anterior thicker part of the aponeurosis.

Two muscles enter the soft palate from above. The *tensor veli palatini* (figures 141, 186(b), 188, 194, 196) which is outside the pharynx, is attached to the base of the skull (the scaphoid fossa of the pterygoid process of the sphenoid bone) and the lateral surface of the auditory tube and passes downwards. Its tendon hooks round the hamulus at the lower end of the medial pterygoid plate and passes medially above the buccinator to become internal to the pharynx and enter the soft palate in which it forms the palatal aponeurosis. The *levator veli palatini* (figures 186(b), 188), which is inside the pharynx, is attached to the medial surface of the auditory tube and the adjacent part of the petrous temporal anteromedial to the carotid canal. The muscle passes downwards and enters the soft palate in which it lies between the two layers of the palatopharyngeus muscle.

Two muscles leave the soft palate and pass downwards. The *palatopharyngeus* attached to the aponeurosis and posterior edge of the hard palate has two layers which laterally join and pass downwards in the palatopharyngeal arch behind the palatine tonsil (figure 188). The muscle enters the pharynx in which it forms part of a layer of muscle

deep to the pharyngeal constrictors (p. 306). Part of the muscle is attached to the posterior border of the thyroid cartilage. The *palatoglossus* (figure 188) is attached to the inferior surface of the palatal aponeurosis and passes laterally and then downwards into the palatoglossal arch anterior to the palatine tonsil. The muscle enters the upper lateral part of the tongue.

There are slips of muscle (the *musculus uvulae*) running anteroposteriorly in the aponeurosis from the posterior edge of the hard palate near the midline into the uvula.

The Nerve and Blood Supply of the Palate. The tensor veli palatini is innervated by the mandibular nerve. The remaining muscles are innervated by the pharyngeal plexus whose motor branch is the pharyngeal branch of the vagus nerve. The cells of origin of these fibres are in the nucleus ambiguus in the hindbrain and most of the fibres leave in the cranial accessory nerve which joins the vagus. The sensory innervation of both surfaces of the whole palate is almost entirely from the maxillary nerve (the greater and lesser palatine and nasopalatine branches). The glossopharyngeal nerve innervates a small part of the soft palate laterally. The facial nerve via some of the fibres of its greater petrosal branch which pass through the pterygopalatine ganglion into the lesser palatine nerve supplies taste fibres to the soft palate.

The arteries to the palate come from the facial, maxillary and ascending pharyngeal arteries. The veins go mainly to the pterygoid plexus of veins.

The Functions of the Soft Palate. The soft palate is pulled upwards and backwards mainly by the levator veli palatini muscles so that the nasopharynx is closed off from the oropharynx. This occurs in swallowing and phonation except in the production of the nasal consonants. The closure is assisted by the formation of a horizontal ridge on the posterior wall of the pharynx produced mainly by the superior constrictor of the pharynx. The palatoglossal muscles close off the oral cavity from the oropharynx and the palatopharyngeal muscles shorten the pharynx and elevate the larynx in swallowing.

During development the two lateral halves of

the palate may fail (partially or completely) to fuse with each other and with the nasal septum so that varying degrees of *cleft palate* are produced. The severer forms which extend into the hard palate are often associated with unilateral or bilateral cleft lip. These conditions present considerable problems in feeding and later in speech. Repair of a cleft palate is usually postponed to the time when the child is about 18 months old. The repair, however, is complicated by a lack of tissue both transversely and anteroposteriorly so that it is difficult to bring the edges together and also to produce a soft palate long enough for an adequate closure of the oropharynx from the nasopharynx.

The Oral Cavity Proper

This part of the mouth is bounded laterally and anteriorly by the *alveolar processes* of the maxillae and mandible. The *tongue* occupies most of the floor which, below the free part of the tongue, is formed by the *mylohyoid muscles* with the *geniohyoid muscles* on either side of the midline. The roof is formed by the *palate*. Posteriorly the oral cavity opens into the oropharynx through the *oropharyngeal isthmus* (the isthmus of the fauces) bounded laterally by the palatoglossal folds.

Most of the other features of the oral cavity have been described. On the roof there are the *incisive papilla* and *transverse ridges* (*rugae*) passing laterally from the midline *palatine raphe* as far back as the level of the first molar teeth. The mucous membrane over the soft palate appears darker because it is thinner than that over the hard palate and contains muscles.

The *tongue* lies in the floor. On its *dorsal surface* (figure 185(a)) there are the papillae, sulcus terminalis, foramen caecum and lingual tonsil (p. 287). If the anterior part of the tongue is elevated its *inferior surface* with the lingual frenulum, fimbriated fold and deep lingual vein are visible (figure 185(b)). In the floor of the mouth inferior to the tongue the sublingual salivary gland forms the sublingual fold. On each side of the frenulum there is a papilla on to which the submandibular duct opens.

The *sublingual gland* (figure 185(b)) is almond-shaped and is about 3 cm long and 1 cm wide. It lies between the tongue and mandible in the sublingual fossa of the mandible above the mylohyoid line and therefore lies on the mylohyoid muscle. The genioglossus muscle is medial to the gland. The ducts of the lateral posterior part of the gland open separately into the floor of the mouth. A duct from the medial anterior part opens into the submandibular duct. The gland is supplied by postganglionic, parasympathetic, secretomotor nerve fibres whose cell bodies are in the submandibular ganglion. The preganglionic fibres are in the chorda tympani, a branch of the facial nerve.

In the mouth posteriorly, the soft palate with its uvula hangs downwards. Laterally the posterior margin of the soft palate divides into the anterior *palatoglossal arch* and posterior *palatopharyngeal arch* (p. 294). On each side the *palatine tonsil* lies between the two folds. (This structure is in the lateral wall of the oropharynx and is described on p. 309). There are pits (crypts) on the medial surface of the tonsil. The *supratonsillar fossa* lies above the tonsil between the folds. The lower pole of the tonsil is covered by the *triangular fold* of mucous membrane.

When the oral cavity is examined with a good light and a tongue depressor all the above features of the roof, floor and posterior part can be seen. The posterior wall of the nasopharynx is visible through the isthmus of the fauces. The teeth and gingivae can be inspected and the papilla on to which the parotid duct opens is seen on the inside of the cheek opposite the upper second molar tooth. If the subject makes the sound 'Ah' the soft palate should rise. In addition a clearer view of the oropharynx is obtained.

When the mouth is opened widely the pterygomandibular fold is seen. It passes downwards and somewhat laterally from behind the posterior end of the maxillary alveolar process. The fold contains the pterygomandibular raphe, the upper end of which is attached to the hamulus of the medial pterygoid plate. The hamulus may produce a visible small elevation. Both the palpable hamulus and raphe are used by dentists as landmarks for anaesthetising the inferior alveolar nerve lying lateral to the raphe.

21

The External Nose, Nasal Cavity and Paranasal Air Sinuses

The upper respiratory passages include the nasal cavity, pharynx, larynx and trachea. Since part of the pharynx is common to both the alimentary and respiratory passages, there must be a mechanism which can prevent food entering the air passages. This mechanism is provided by the upper part of the larynx. The larynx is also closed in strong muscular effort in which the chest is fixed, a manoeuvre which is also used when increasing intra-abdominal pressure in order to cough or to assist the evacuation of hollow abdominal organs in a downward direction.

The upper respiratory passages cleanse, warm and moisten the air but only within certain limits, as is evidenced by the deposition of carbon particles in the interstices of the lungs. The typical respiratory epithelium (ciliated, mucous, columnar) performs these functions. In addition the air passages must be so constructed that they do not collapse if the external air pressure is greater than that of the air in the respiratory passages. To some extent part of the passages can enlarge their diameter mainly by relaxing the smooth muscle in their walls in order to increase the intake of air.

Air can be breathed through the mouth but the loss of the functions of the nasal epithelium and also smell is a considerable disadvantage. The mouth plays an important role in thermoregulation in some animals and in these mouth breathing has a special significance.

The Maxilla, Palatine and Ethmoid Bones and Inferior Concha

It is necessary to describe some of the bones which form the lateral wall of the nasal cavity, especially the maxilla, ethmoid and palatine.

The Maxilla (figure 189). The two maxillae form the upper jaw. The main part of each maxilla is called the *body* which is hollow. The body has four surfaces. The *upper surface* forms most of the floor of the orbit. The *anterior surface* is on the face, is also directed downwards and laterally and is palpable below the zygomatic bone. The *posterior surface* forms the anterior wall of the infratemporal and pterygopalatine fossae. Between the anterior and posterior surfaces a thickened ridge of bone, resisting the stresses of biting and chewing, passes upwards from the first molar tooth. The *nasal surface* is medial and forms most of the lateral part of the wall of the nasal cavity. In the disarticulated bone this surface has a large opening about 2 cm in diameter which is very much reduced in the living by the encroachment of neighbouring bones. The *lacrimal groove* on the anterosuperior part of the surface leads upwards into the orbit. Behind the opening into the maxillary sinus there is a vertical groove which is converted into a canal by the perpendicular plate of the palatine bone which articulates with this part of the maxilla and

(a)   **(b)**

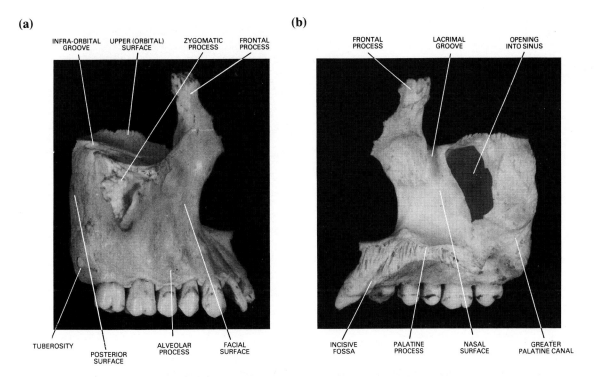

Figure 189   The right maxilla: (a) lateral view; (b) medial view.

overlaps the opening into the sinus.

The maxilla has four processes. The *alveolar process* is inferior, forms half an arch and has sockets for the teeth. The *palatine process* projects medially from the upper part of the alveolar process and forms with the opposite maxillary palatine process the major part of the hard palate. The *incisive fossa* just behind the incisive teeth in the midline is formed when the two palatine processes articulate with each other. The *frontal process* projects upwards from the anteromedial part of the body, articulates with the frontal bone and forms the anterior limit of the medial wall of the orbit where it articulates posteriorly with the lacrimal bone and forms a hollow for the lacrimal sac. The *zygomatic process* is on the superolateral part of the body and has a flattened, roughened area which articulates with the zygomatic bone.

The Ethmoid Bone (figure 190(a)). This bone (*ethmos = sieve*, Greek) has a midline *perpendicular plate*. The *cribriform plate* projects horizontally and laterally about 1 cm below its upper end and

forms most of the roof of the nasal cavity. The *crista galli* is the part of the perpendicular plate above the level of the cribriform plate and is in the anterior cranial fossa. The *ethmoidal labyrinth* is suspended from the lateral edge of the cribriform plate. The lateral surface of the labyrinth is formed by the *orbital plate of the ethmoid* and is in the medial wall of the orbit. Most of the labyrinth consists of small air cells, some of which open on to the surface and are completed by articulation with the frontal, lacrimal, sphenoidal and palatine bones and maxilla.

The medial surface of the labyrinth forms part of the lateral wall of the nasal cavity. The *superior* and *middle conchae* project medially and then downwards from the medial surface. The spaces between the conchae and the medial wall are called *meatuses*, *superior* and *middle*. Some of the ethmoidal air cells form a projection in the middle meatus, the *bulla ethmoidalis*. The *uncinate process* projects downwards and backwards below the bulla (*uncus = hook*, Latin). The *hiatus semilunaris* is the groove between the uncinate process and the

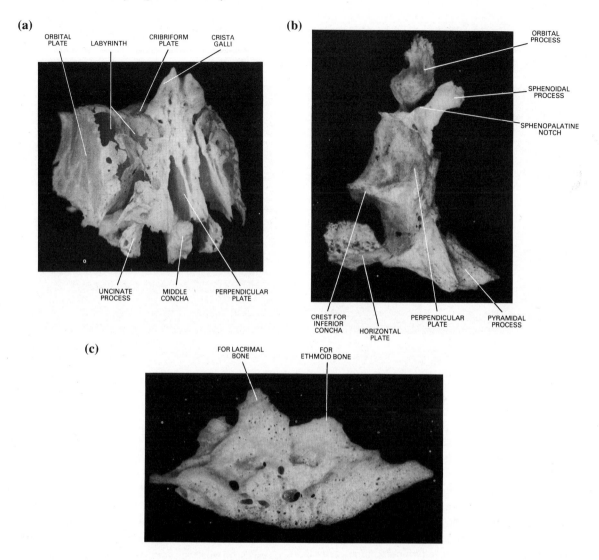

(a)

ORBITAL PLATE   LABYRINTH   CRIBRIFORM PLATE   CRISTA GALLI

UNCINATE PROCESS   MIDDLE CONCHA   PERPENDICULAR PLATE

(b)

ORBITAL PROCESS

SPHENOIDAL PROCESS

SPHENOPALATINE NOTCH

CREST FOR INFERIOR CONCHA   HORIZONTAL PLATE   PERPENDICULAR PLATE   PYRAMIDAL PROCESS

(c)

FOR LACRIMAL BONE   FOR ETHMOID BONE

Figure 190   **(a) An anterolateral view of the ethmoid bone. (b) A posteromedial view of the right palatine bone. (c) The medial surface of the right inferior concha.**

bulla and leads upwards into a canal in the laby-rinth called the *infundibulum* (figure 192). This leads upwards into the frontal air sinus.

The Palatine Bone (figure 190(b)). This consists largely of a *horizontal plate*, which forms part of the hard palate, and a *perpendicular plate* which forms part of the lateral wall of the nasal cavity where it covers the posterior part of the opening into the maxillary sinus. On the lateral side of the perpendicular plate there is a vertical groove which

completes with a similar groove on the maxilla the vertical *greater palatine canal*. Inferiorly this canal opens on to the hard palate at the lateral end of the horizontal plate and has branches, the *lesser palatine canals*, which open behind the greater canal.

The upper end of the perpendicular plate divides into a lateral *orbital process*, which forms a small posterior part of the floor of the orbit, and a medial *sphenoidal process* which articulates with the inferior surface of the body of the sphenoid bone. The notch between the processes is converted into a foramen by the sphenoid bone, the *sphenopalatine foramen*, which forms a communication between the pterygopalatine fossa and the nasal cavity. The lower end of the perpendicular plate projects backwards forming the *pyramidal process* and filling the space between the medial and lateral pterygoid plates.

The Inferior Concha (figure 190(c)). This is an elongated, thin, curved plate of bone on the lower part of the lateral wall of the nasal cavity. It extends forwards and articulates with the maxilla, and backwards and articulates with the perpendicular plate of the palatine bone. Anteriorly between these articulations an upward projection meets a downward projection of the lacrimal bone. These two projections lie over the anterior part of the maxillary hiatus. They also exclude the nasolacrimal duct from the middle meatus so that the duct opens into the inferior meatus, the space between the inferior concha and the lateral wall of the nose. A projection upwards from about the middle of the concha and a posterior projection further reduce the size of the maxillary opening.

The External Nose (figure 191(a), (b))

The external nose is bony superiorly, where it is formed by the two nasal bones articulating with each other in the midline, and cartilaginous inferiorly. A number of nasal cartilages is described and the largest of these forms part of the external openings of the nasal cavity, the *nares* or *anterior nasal apertures*. This cartilage passes inferior to the septal cartilage in the midline and forms the mobile part of the septum which can easily be moved from side to side. Inferiorly and posteriorly some fibrofatty tissue completes the external nose.

The skin of the nose is supplied mainly by the ophthalmic nerve. The lateral edge of the nares is supplied by the maxillary nerve. There are external nasal muscles which produce twitching of the nose and can enlarge or reduce the size of the openings. Active dilatation of the nostrils can be achieved by some people and is seen in conditions which cause difficulty in breathing. These muscles are supplied

by the facial nerve. The skin over the prominent part of the nose is unusual in that it contains sebaceous glands opening independently on to the surface and not into hair follicles. The stratified squamous epithelium of the skin of the nose extends for a short distance into the lowest part of the nasal cavity (the *vestibule*). In addition to normal hairs, longer, thicker hairs, called *vibrissae*, are seen in the vestibule.

The Nasal Cavity (figures 191(c), 192)

The nasal cavity lies above the oral cavity, below the cranial cavity and inferomedial to the orbits. There is *one* nasal cavity divided into two by a vertical nasal septum, usually deviated to one side of the midline and each half of the nasal cavity has four walls — a roof, a floor, an outwardly sloping lateral wall and a medial wall common to the two halves. The anterior openings to the exterior are usually horizontal and are called the *nares* and the posterior vertical openings into the nasopharynx are called the *choanae* (*posterior nasal apertures*; *choana = funnel*, Latin).

The Walls of the Nasal Cavity. The main part of the *roof* is horizontal and is formed by the cribriform plate of the ethmoid bone. Posteriorly the roof slopes downwards and backwards and is formed by the body of the sphenoid and anteriorly it slopes downwards and forwards inferior to the frontal and nasal bones. The *floor* is much wider than the roof and is formed by the hard and soft palates.

The *nasal septum* (figure 191(c)) is partly bony, partly cartilaginous. The bony part is posterior and is formed by the perpendicular plate of the ethmoid bone superiorly and the vomer inferiorly. Superiorly the perpendicular plate extends from the body of the sphenoid bone behind to the nasal bones in front. The vomer is posterior to the perpendicular plate as well as inferior and lies below the body of the sphenoid bone. Its lower border fuses with the ridge formed in the midline by the two halves of the hard palate. The septal cartilage lies in the anterior angle formed by the perpendicular plate and the vomer and extends forwards to

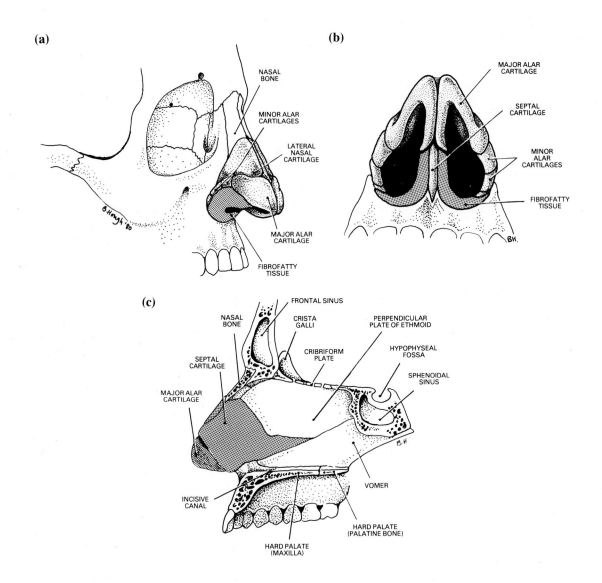

(a)

NASAL
BONE

MINOR ALAR
CARTILAGES

LATERAL
NASAL
CARTILAGE

MAJOR ALAR
CARTILAGE

FIBROFATTY
TISSUE

(b)

MAJOR ALAR
CARTILAGE

SEPTAL
CARTILAGE

MINOR
ALAR
CARTILAGES

FIBROFATTY
TISSUE

(c)

FRONTAL SINUS

NASAL
BONE

CRISTA
GALLI

CRIBRIFORM
PLATE

SEPTAL
CARTILAGE

PERPENDICULAR
PLATE OF ETHMOID

HYPOPHYSEAL
FOSSA

SPHENOIDAL
SINUS

MAJOR ALAR
CARTILAGE

VOMER

INCISIVE
CANAL

HARD PALATE
(PALATINE BONE)

HARD PALATE
(MAXILLA)

Figure 191   (a) The external nose. (b) The nares (external nasal apertures). (c) The nasal septum.

become attached to the external nasal cartilages superiorly and anteriorly but not inferiorly. The *vomeronasal organ* is a blind recess extending backwards along the lower edge of the septal cartilage and has an opening behind the incisive canal. It is the remnant of an organ associated with olfaction in reptiles.

The *lateral wall* of the nasal cavity slopes downwards and laterally and is irregular because of the *superior*, *middle* and *inferior conchae* (*turbinate*

bones) projecting medially and then downwards into the cavity (*concha = shell*, Latin; *turbinatus = like a scroll*, Latin). The inferior is a separate bone and the other two are part of the ethmoid bone. The space between a concha and the lateral wall of the nose is called a *meatus* (*meatus = passage*, Latin; plural *meatus* not *meati*, but *meatuses* is an accepted Anglicised plural). There are therefore three meatuses, inferior, middle and superior. The narrow space above the superior concha is called the *spheno-ethmoidal recess* because it lies between the ethmoid bone laterally and the sphenoid bone posteriorly.

The nasolacrimal duct opens into the anterior part of the inferior meatus and the maxillary and frontal sinuses and anterior and middle ethmoidal air cells into the middle meatus. The posterior ethmoidal air cells open into the superior meatus and the sphenoidal sinus opens into the posterior wall of the spheno-ethmoidal recess.

The *choanae* are the vertical posterior openings of the nasal cavity on either side of the midline. They are about 2.5 cm high and 1 cm wide. The posterior edge of the vomer separates the openings. Laterally they are bounded by the medial ptery-goid plate which is continuous anteriorly with the perpendicular plate of the palatine bone. The lower edge of the choanae is formed by the posterior border of the hard palate to which the soft palate is attached. The body of the sphenoid bone and extensions of the palatine bone and vomer form the upper boundary.

The Lining of the Nasal Cavity. The stratified squamous epithelium of the vestibule just within the nares has already been referred to. The rest of the cavity is lined by respiratory epithelium except for the thicker, yellowish, olfactory epithelium on the roof and adjacent parts of the lateral walls and septum. The nerve fibres from the olfactory receptor cells in this epithelium form bundles which pass through the holes in the cribriform plate to the olfactory bulb.

The respiratory epithelium is ciliated, mucous, columnar, and deep to it there are mucous and serous glands. The lining is thickest over the conchae, especially the inferior, and septum and is thinnest in the floor of the cavity and meatuses. The amount of subepithelial cavernous tissue, consisting of dilated thin-walled capillaries with arteriovenous anastomoses, determines the thickness.

The functions of the nasal cavity are olfaction and changing the inspired air. The serous and mucous glands make the air moist and produce a sticky surface to which particles in the air adhere. (Breathing industrial fog demonstrates this function.) The special vascular cavernous tissue warms the air and the cilia bend backwards and convey the mucus towards the nasopharynx whence it passes downwards and is swallowed. It has been suggested that the conchae cause turbulence of the inspired air. The old name, turbinate bones, apparently had a functional as well as a structural significance. In infection of the nasal cavity swelling of the thick lining together with increased mucous secretion may block the nasal cavity and the openings into the sinuses, especially that of the maxillary sinus. The lining of the nasal cavity is continuous with that of the paranasal sinuses, the nasolacrimal duct and the nasopharynx, and indirectly with that of the auditory tube and middle ear, so that infection can spread to any of these structures.

The Blood and Nerve Supply of the Nasal Cavity. The *arteries* to the nasal cavity are derived from the ophthalmic, maxillary and facial. The vestibular area of the septum receives a particularly rich blood supply and is frequently the site of *epistaxis* (nose-bleeding). It is called *Little's* or *Kiesselbach's area*, depending to some extent on which country one belongs to (James Little, 1836–85, American surgeon; Wilhelm Kiesselbach, 1839–1902, German laryngologist). The *veins* correspond with the arteries. There are venous communications between the nasal cavity and the veins on the inferior surface of the frontal lobe through the foramen caecum and cribriform plate.

The *nerves of general sensation* are derived mainly from the maxillary nerve except for an area, anteriorly and superiorly, which is supplied by the ophthalmic nerve. The maxillary branches include the infra-orbital nerve to the vestibule, the anterior superior dental nerve and the nasopalatine and lateral nasal nerves which enter the nasal cavity from the pterygopalatine fossa through the spheno-palatine foramen situated near the posterior end of the middle concha. There are also important sympathetic vasomotor fibres to the blood vessels and parasympathetic secretomotor and vasodilator fibres to the glands. These run in the sensory nerves. The preganglionic parasympathetic fibres are from the facial nerve which synapse in the pterygo-palatine ganglion (p. 208).

The *olfactory nerves* have been described.

The Paranasal Air Sinuses

The word *sinus* means a *space* and has no specific meaning, hence the addition of the word *air* to indicate the contents. *Paranasal* refers to the position of these sinuses. They are found in the frontal, maxillary, ethmoid and sphenoid bones.

The Frontal Sinuses (figure 193). These lie above the nasal cavity on either side of the midline posterior to the superciliary arches, the thickened bone above the medial part of the orbit. Each sinus is pyramidal in shape and is about 2–3 cm in height, depth and width. The septum separating the sinuses is rarely in the midline and a sinus can extend laterally and backwards over most of the roof of the orbit. The sinus is related inferolaterally to the orbit, inferiorly to the nasal cavity and laterally to the meninges and frontal lobe of the brain. It opens into the middle meatus by the frontonasal duct or the infundibulum (figure 192).

The Maxillary Sinus (figure 193(a)). This is the cavity in the body of the maxilla. It may be said to have five walls. The *facial wall* is antero-infero-lateral and can be felt through the cheek below the zygomatic bone. In this wall there are branches of the anterior and middle superior alveolar nerves. The *posterior wall* is related medially to the pterygo-palatine fossa in which lie part of the maxillary artery, the pterygopalatine ganglion and the maxillary nerve. More laterally is the infratemporal fossa containing part of the maxillary artery, the pterygoid muscles and branches of the mandibular nerve (p. 205). In the posterior wall there are branches of the posterior superior alveolar nerve.

The *roof* of the sinus forms most of the floor of the orbit in which run the infra-orbital vessels and nerve. The *floor* of the sinus is related to the roots of the first and second molar teeth. The roots of the second and first premolars may also project into the floor.

The *medial* or *nasal wall* forms a large part of the lateral wall of the nose. In the disarticulated bone it has a large opening (figure 189(b)). This, however, is reduced in size by the encroachment of neighbouring bones, the palatine posteriorly, the ethmoidal superiorly, and the inferior concha inferiorly, so that there remains an opening about

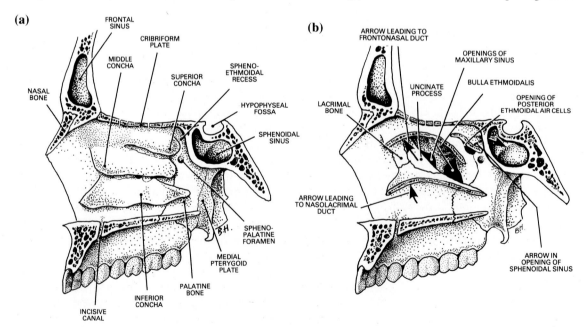

Figure 192   The lateral wall of the nasal cavity: (a) to show the conchae; (b) to show the meatuses (the conchae have been partially removed).

(a)

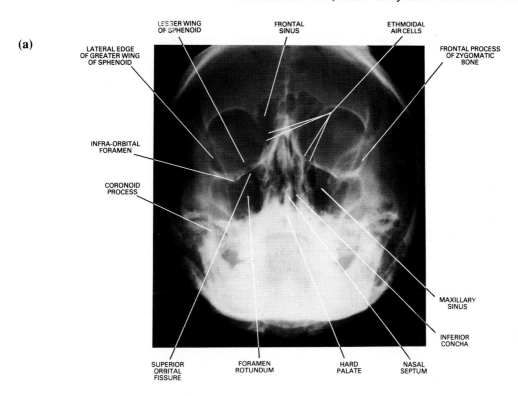

LESSER WING
OF SPHENOID

FRONTAL
SINUS

ETHMOIDAL
AIR CELLS

LATERAL EDGE
OF GREATER WING
OF SPHENOID

FRONTAL PROCESS
OF ZYGOMATIC
BONE

INFRA-ORBITAL
FORAMEN

CORONOID
PROCESS

MAXILLARY
SINUS

INFERIOR
CONCHA

SUPERIOR
ORBITAL
FISSURE

FORAMEN
ROTUNDUM

HARD
PALATE

NASAL
SEPTUM

(b)

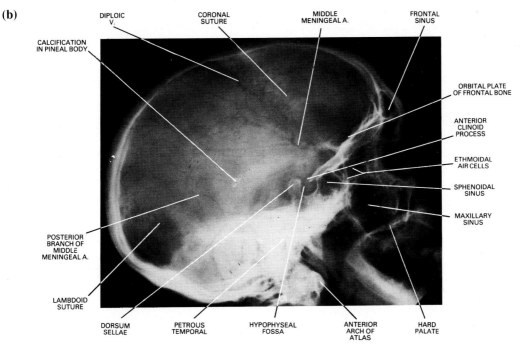

DIPLOIC
V.

CORONAL
SUTURE

MIDDLE
MENINGEAL A.

FRONTAL
SINUS

CALCIFICATION
IN PINEAL BODY

ORBITAL PLATE
OF FRONTAL BONE

ANTERIOR
CLINOID
PROCESS

ETHMOIDAL
AIR CELLS

SPHENOIDAL
SINUS

MAXILLARY
SINUS

POSTERIOR
BRANCH OF
MIDDLE
MENINGEAL A.

LAMBDOID
SUTURE

DORSUM
SELLAE

PETROUS
TEMPORAL

HYPOPHYSEAL
FOSSA

ANTERIOR
ARCH OF
ATLAS

HARD
PALATE

Figure 193   **(a) An X-ray of the skull to show the frontal and maxillary sinuses and ethmoid air sinuses (cells).
(b) A lateral X-ray of the skull.**

3–4 mm in diameter into the hiatus semilunaris of the middle meatus. There may be a second opening inferior to the hiatus. Anteromedial to the sinus is the nasolacrimal duct (figure 192(b)).

The possible signs and symptoms of a growth in the maxillary sinus form a good example of applied anatomy. There may be bloodstained discharge from the nose, pain from the region supplied by the infra-orbital nerve or the superior alveolar nerves (toothache), a swelling on the hard palate, proptosis of the eye (the eye is pushed forwards due to the upward growth of the tumour; *proptosis = a falling forwards*, Greek), a swelling on the face, and epiphora (tears passing downwards on the cheek due to blocking of the nasolacrimal duct; *epiphora = a sudden burst, as of tears*, Greek). It should be emphasised that some of the symptoms, for example blood-stained nasal discharge and toothache, have much commoner causes than malignant tumours of the maxillary sinus. It has been said that students die many times before they qualify.

The Sphenoidal Sinus (figures 192, 193). This is a cavity in the body of the sphenoid bone usually divided into two sinuses by a thin septum which is seldom in the midline. The hypophysis cerebri and the optic chiasma are superior and the cavernous sinus and internal carotid artery are superolateral. The size of the sinuses varies but they are about 2 cm in height, depth and width. By extension the sinus can become closely related to the optic or ophthalmic nerves or the nerve of the pterygoid canal. The sinuses lie behind the superior part of the nasal cavity and open into the spheno-ethmoidal recess. The anterior wall of the sinus is formed by a thin plate of bone with an opening in its upper half.

The Ethmoidal Air Cells (Sinuses) (figures 173, 193). These lie in the labyrinth of the ethmoid. Their number and size vary inversely to each other. There are usually between 10 and 15 and they are divided into *anterior, middle* and *posterior*. The anterior open into the infundibulum of the ethmoid, the middle on to the bulla ethmoidalis (both open into the middle meatus) and the posterior into the superior meatus. Many of the ethmoidal cells are completed by neighbouring bones, the frontal, lacrimal, maxilla and palatine. The plate of bone separating the cells from the orbit is very thin.

All the sinuses are lined by ciliated, mucous, columnar epithelium continuous with that of the nasal cavity. The epithelium, however, is thin, except at the openings of the sinuses. They are all supplied by the ophthalmic nerve and artery except the maxillary sinus which is supplied by the maxillary nerve and artery. The sinuses make the head lighter and add resonance to the voice but comparative anatomy suggests that they have temperature regulating and olfactory functions in other animals. These functions have been lost in man but the sinuses have persisted. There is no evidence that air enters and leaves them during respiration.

Clinically they are important because of the ease with which infection can spread to them from the nasal cavity. The commonest to be infected is the maxillary sinus and is usually referred to as *sinusitis* or an *antrum* by the layman (the maxillary sinus was called the *antrum of Highmore* – Nathaniel Highmore, 1613–85, English anatomist). Because the opening is small and is situated well above the floor, drainage from the maxillary sinus, in the upright position, is poor.

The paranasal sinuses can be investigated by means of X-rays (figure 193(b)). In addition fluid in the maxillary sinus can be seen by *transillumination* (if fluid is present the sinus or sinuses are opaque when a light is shone into the mouth of the patient in a dark room) and detected by aspiration through the inferior meatus (usually called *antral puncture*).

All the sinuses are small or absent at birth. They grow slowly to the age of 7 or 8 years and then rapidly during the second dentition.

22

The Pharynx and Cervical Oesophagus

The Pharynx

Although the pharynx, which extends from the base of the skull to the sixth cervical vertebra, is usually regarded as part of the alimentary tract, the part behind the nasal cavity (the *nasopharynx*) is entirely respiratory, and the part behind the mouth (the *oropharynx*) and behind the larynx (the *laryngopharynx*) is both respiratory and alimentary.

The pharynx is a muscular tube about 12 cm long, wider above (about 4 cm) than below (about 1.5 cm) where it becomes continuous with the oesophagus. Its anterior wall is largely deficient and opens into the nasal and oral cavities and inferiorly into the larynx. The pharynx lies anterior to the cervical vertebrae (figure 184).

The posterior and lateral muscular walls are formed mainly by the three constrictors. Three muscles pass into the pharyngeal wall from above, the *stylopharyngeus*, *palatopharyngeus* and *salpingopharyngeus* (*salpinx = tube*, Greek).

The Constrictor Muscles (figures 194, 195)

The *superior constrictor* is attached to the pterygomandibular raphe which extends from the hamulus of the medial pterygoid plate to the posterior end of the mylohyoid line on the inner surface of the mandible. At its upper end the muscle extends on to the medial pterygoid plate and at its lower end on to the mucous membrane adjacent to the mylo-hyoid line. From their origin the highest fibres arch backwards and upwards and are attached to the pharyngeal tubercle on the basilar part of the occipital bone. Since the hamulus is at a lower level than the tubercle there is a space between the upper border of the muscle and the base of the skull. This is filled by the membranous *pharyngobasilar fascia* passing, as its name suggests, between the pharynx and the base of the skull. The auditory tube with the levator veli palatini on its medial side, and the tensor veli palatini on its lateral side, lie in this space. The rest of the fibres of the superior constrictor fan out and, passing backwards and medially, enter the fibrous pharyngeal raphe running longitudinally in the middle of the posterior wall of the pharynx. Some of the superior fibres are joined by muscle fibres from the soft palate and, on movement of the palate, form a ridge on the posterior wall of the nasopharynx, the *ridge of Passavant* (P.G. Passavant, 1815–93, German physician).

The *middle constrictor* is attached to the greater and lesser horns of the hyoid bone and the lower end of the stylohyoid ligament. It fans out as it passes backwards and then medially into the posterior raphe. It is external to the superior but internal to the inferior constrictor.

The part of the *inferior constrictor* attached to the oblique line on the lamina of the thyroid cartilage and to a fibrous arch over the cricothyroid muscle is called the *thyropharyngeus*, and the part attached to the lateral surface of the arch of the cricoid cartilage is called the *cricopharyngeus*. Its

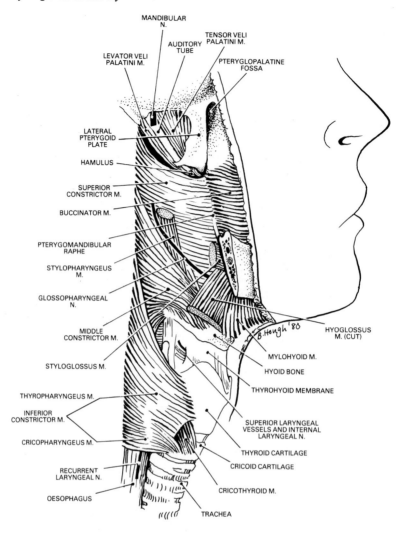

Figure 194   A lateral view of the constrictor muscles of the pharynx.

lowest part is horizontal, is continuous with the circular fibres of the oesophagus and acts like a sphincter. The inferior constrictor passes backwards and medially and is inserted into the posterior raphe.

The Stylopharyngeus, Palatopharyngeus and Salpingopharyngeus Muscles

The *stylopharyngeus* is attached to the medial side of the base of the styloid process and passes downwards superficial to the superior constrictor and deep to the middle constrictor (figure 194). It is attached to the posterior border of the thyroid cartilage and its fibres mingle with those of the middle constrictor. The *salpingopharyngeus* (figure 195) is attached to the lower border of the cartilaginous part of the auditory tube, passes downwards on the inner surface of the constrictors and mingles with the fibres of the palatopharyngeus. The *palatopharyngeus* (figure 188) has two layers of muscle in the soft palate. The upper is immediately deep to the mucous membrane of the pharyngeal surface and the lower is deep to the levator veli palatini. The two layers pass laterally, join and continue downwards in the palatopharyngeal fold behind the palatine tonsil. In the pharyngeal wall

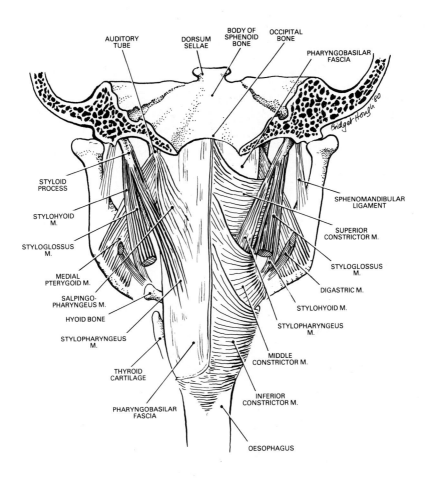

AUDITORY
TUBE

DORSUM
SELLAE

BODY OF
SPHENOID
BONE

OCCIPITAL
BONE

PHARYNGOBASILAR
FASCIA

STYLOID
PROCESS

STYLOHYOID
M.

STYLOGLOSSUS
M.

MEDIAL
PTERYGOID M.

SALPINGO-
PHARYNGEUS M.

HYOID BONE

STYLOPHARYNGEUS
M.

THYROID
CARTILAGE

PHARYNGOBASILAR
FASCIA

SPHENOMANDIBULAR
LIGAMENT

SUPERIOR
CONSTRICTOR M.

STYLOGLOSSUS
M.

DIGASTRIC M.

STYLOHYOID M.

STYLOPHARYNGEUS
M.

MIDDLE
CONSTRICTOR M.

INFERIOR
CONSTRICTOR M.

OESOPHAGUS

Figure 195   A posterior view of the muscles of the pharynx.

the fibres spread out, and, with the stylopharyngeus, form a longitudinally running layer of muscle internal to the constrictors. Some of the fibres of the palatopharyngeus join the pharyngeal raphe and some are attached to the thyroid cartilage.

The Main Relations of the Pharynx

The bodies of the cervical vertebrae covered by some of the prevertebral muscles and fascia are posterior. The carotid sheath and its contents and the ascending pharyngeal artery as they lie anterior to the transverse processes of the cervical vertebrae

are lateral. Anteriorly there are the posterior openings of the nasal and oral cavities and larynx from above downwards (figure 196). The glossopharyngeal nerve is lateral to the superior constrictor and runs downwards along the posterior border of the stylopharyngeus before crossing superficial to that muscle and entering the tongue deep to the hyoglossus together with the lingual artery. The internal laryngeal nerve and an accompanying artery lie between the middle and inferior constrictors before entering the larynx through the thyrohyoid membrane and the external laryngeal nerve runs downwards on the inferior constrictor and pierces it to supply the cricothyroid muscle.

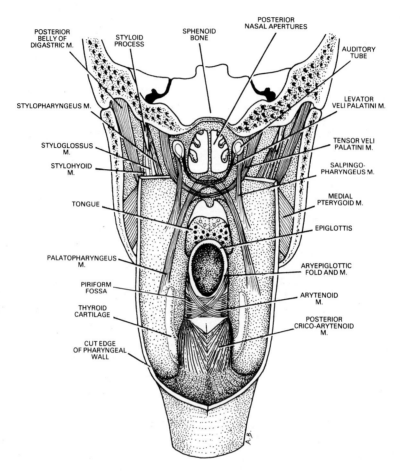

Figure 196   **A posterior view of the naso-, oro- and laryngopharynx after dividing the pharyngeal raphe longitudinally and turning the pharyngeal wall laterally on each side.**

The recurrent laryngeal nerve and a laryngeal artery pass upwards deep to the inferior constrictor on their way to the larynx. The lingual and facial arteries loop upwards on the middle constrictor and the facial artery may reach the lateral surface of the superior constrictor. In this position the artery lies lateral to the palatine tonsil which is medial to the superior constrictor.

The Nerve and Blood Supply of the Pharynx

The *nerve supply* of the stylopharyngeus is from the glossopharyngeal nerve. The remaining five muscles are supplied by the pharyngeal plexus which lies on the external surface of the middle constrictor. The pharyngeal branch of the vagus nerve is the motor nerve of the plexus and is derived mainly from the cranial accessory nerve. The cell bodies of the fibres supplying all the muscles are in the nucleus ambiguus of the hindbrain.

Most of the lining receives its sensory nerve supply from the glossopharyngeal nerve which also partly supplies the tonsillar region and the soft palate. The maxillary nerve supplies the region of the nasopharynx and the recurrent laryngeal nerve supplies the lowest part of the pharynx.

The *arteries* of the pharynx come from the ascending pharyngeal, the facial, the maxillary and the lingual. The *veins* go to the internal jugular and facial veins.

The Nasopharynx (figure 184)

This part of the pharynx lies behind the posterior nasal openings (choanae) of the nasal cavity and in front of the atlas, and is roofed over by the basilar part of the occipital bone and body of the sphenoid. Inferiorly it is continuous with the oropharynx at the level of the soft palate.

On the posterior wall there is a mass of lymphoid tissue called the *pharyngeal tonsil* (*adenoid*) which is much larger in children than in adults. If enlarged, often due to inflammation, it may project forwards, obstruct the choanae and lead to mouth-breathing. This may affect the growth of the jaws, particularly the upper, which are narrowed so that the face looks pinched. The lymphoid tissue may extend into the roof or laterally to the region of the opening of the auditory tube (*tubal tonsil*) whose medial end opens on the lateral wall of the nasopharynx. Lymphatic vessels go from the adenoid to nodes lying behind the pharynx (retropharyngeal) and in front of the atlas.

The opening of the auditory tube projects superiorly and posteriorly and is at the level of and 1 cm behind the inferior meatus of the nasal cavity. A catheter (always referred to as a *Eustachian catheter*) can be passed along the floor of the nasal cavity and inserted into the Eustachian (auditory) tube. This is done to test the patency of the tube and possibly unblock it. (The tube was described by Bartolommeo Eustachio, 1520–74, Italian anatomist.)

The Oropharynx (figure 184)

This part of the pharynx lies behind the oral cavity and in front of the second and third cervical vertebrae. The palatoglossal folds are regarded as the boundary between the oropharynx and the mouth. Superiorly the oropharynx communicates with the nasopharynx and inferiorly with the laryngopharynx.

A mass of lymphoid tissue, the *palatine tonsil* (usually referred to as the *tonsil*), lies in the lateral wall of the oropharynx in a space called the *tonsillar sinus* between the palatoglossal (anterior) and palatopharyngeal (posterior) folds. The tonsil may extend upwards into the soft palate or medially into the tongue or forwards into the palatoglossal fold. This explains why it may be difficult to remove all the lymphoid tissue unless it is carefully dissected out. The tonsil is much larger in the child than in the adult.

Laterally the palatine tonsil is separated from the superior constrictor by a fibrous capsule. The medial surface has a number of pits (*tonsillar crypts*), in which chronic infection can reside, a deep recess, the *intratonsillar cleft*, in its upper part, and a small fold of mucous membrane inferiorly, the *plica triangularis*.

The tonsillar artery from the facial artery enters the lower pole of the tonsil. A large vein from the soft palate passes downwards lateral to the tonsil and then passes laterally to pierce the pharyngeal wall. This vein is at risk when the tonsils are removed. *Tonsillectomy* (removal of the tonsils) is a common operation and one of the main dangers is the inhalation of blood while the patient is unconscious following the operation.

The sensory innervation of this region is from both the maxillary and glossopharyngeal nerves. Since the area innervated by each nerve varies in different people, some individuals gag more readily than others. Gagging is due to touching the area supplied by the glossopharyngeal nerve which supplies the sensory part of the swallowing reflex.

The Laryngopharynx (figures 184, 196)

This part of the pharynx lies behind the opening of the larynx, in front of the fourth, fifth and sixth cervical vertebrae. At the lower border of the cricoid cartilage the pharynx becomes the oesophagus. The laryngeal opening is bounded anteriorly by the epiglottis, laterally by the aryepiglottic folds and posteriorly by the arytenoid cartilages and the tissue between them. Lateral to the opening between it and the lamina of the thyroid cartilage there is a space called the *piriform fossa* (figure 199(b)). The internal laryngeal nerve having pierced the thyrohyoid membrane passes to the larynx deep to the mucous membrane lining the fossa.

The Structure and Functions of the Pharynx

The pharynx consists of three coats — an inner mucous membrane, a middle fibrous coat and an outer muscular layer. The mucous membrane is covered by stratified squamous epithelium in the oro- and laryngopharynx and by ciliated mucous columnar epithelium in the nasopharynx where there are also mucous glands. The fibrous layer is thickened superiorly where it forms the pharyngobasilar fascia between the upper edge of the superior constrictor and the base of the skull.

The functions of the pharynx are respiratory and alimentary. It conducts air from the nasal cavity and mouth to the larynx and food from the mouth to the oesophagus. The walls of the nasopharynx are relatively rigid and its cavity is always patent, unlike that of the oro- and laryngopharynx. The auditory tube leading to the middle ear is opened during swallowing and equalises the pressure on the two sides of the tympanic membrane between the external and middle ear. The salpingopharyngeus, palatopharyngeus and possibly the tensor veli palatini muscles are responsible for this. The stylo- and palatopharyngeus muscles due to their attachment to the thyroid cartilage lift up the larynx in swallowing. The constrictors by a descending wave of contraction propel the food downwards.

Auditory (Pharyngotympanic, Eustachian Tube) (figures 141, 188, 194)

This is a communication between the nasopharynx and the cavity of the middle ear. In the adult it is about 3.5 cm long and is directed laterally, upwards (about 30° from the horizontal) and backwards (about midway between the coronal and sagittal planes) from the nasopharynx. Its lateral third is a bony canal in the petrous part of the temporal bone. The medial two-thirds are cartilaginous and lie between the petrous temporal and greater wing of the sphenoid. The cartilage is a plate folded over so that inferiorly and laterally there is a gap filled by fibrous tissue. Its lateral end is attached to the ragged medial end of the bony part. The projecting medial end in the nasopharynx has

already been described (p. 309) and is the widest part of the tube. It is narrowest at the junction of the bony and cartilaginous parts. The tube is lined by ciliated mucous columnar epithelium continuous with that of the nasopharynx and middle ear.

If one looks at the position of the tube in the skull, the foramen spinosum and foramen ovale are anterior. The middle meningeal artery and the mandibular nerve are therefore anterior to the tube. The tensor veli palatini is attached to the anterolateral surface of the tube and intervenes between the tube and the mandibular nerve. The levator veli palatini is attached to its posteromedial surface (figures 141, 194).

In babies and young children the tube is more horizontal and the bony part wider than in the adult. It is thought that upper respiratory infections in early life spread more readily to the middle ear because of these differences.

As already stated, the function of the tube is to equalise the pressure on the two sides of the tympanic membrane. If the tube is blocked for a long time, the air in the middle ear is absorbed, the auditory ossicles are dislocated and one form of conduction deafness results.

The Cervical Oesophagus

One of the disadvantages of studying anatomy in regions is the division of obviously continuous structures. The oesophagus begins at the level of the cricoid cartilage (the sixth cervical vertebra) and continues into the thorax behind the trachea more or less in the midline. Its thoracic part and abdominal parts are described on p. 51 and p. 82 respectively.

In the neck the vertebral column is posterior and the carotid sheath and lobes of the thyroid gland are lateral to the oesophagus (figure 150). The trachea is anterior to its right border so that the cervical oesophagus is more easily approached from the left. The recurrent laryngeal nerve runs upwards between the trachea and oesophagus. At the thoracic inlet on the left side the thoracic duct lies behind the left border of the oesophagus and almost immediately arches forwards behind the carotid sheath to join the beginning of the left brachiocephalic vein.

The cervical oesophagus is supplied by the inferior thyroid artery and its veins go to the inferior thyroid vein. The muscle of this part of the oesophagus is skeletal and is supplied by the recurrent laryngeal nerve. Its lymphatic vessels drain to the deep cervical nodes.

The beginning of the oesophagus, where it is narrowed partly by the inferior constrictor muscle, is about 15 cm from the incisor teeth. The oesophagus can be investigated by means of a barium swallow (p. 52) and by direct vision by means of an oesophagoscope.

Swallowing (Deglutition)

During chewing the food is pushed between the teeth by the buccinator muscles and the tongue. The food is then formed into a bolus (*bolus = lump*, *morsel*, Latin) which is pressed backwards between the tongue and hard palate. This stage of swallowing is *voluntary*. The tip of the tongue is raised by its intrinsic muscles and the back of the tongue by the styloglossus muscles. The floor of the mouth is also raised by the contraction of the mylohyoid muscles which also elevate the hyoid bone. Other suprahyoid muscles, for example the geniohyoid and anterior belly of the digastric, also contract and produce this elevation. The palatoglossal folds are brought together by the palatoglossal muscles as the bolus passes through the oropharyngeal isthmus and help to push the bolus into the oropharynx. It is said that another effect of their contraction is to prevent the food returning into the mouth.

The second, *involuntary*, stage of swallowing now follows and is initiated by the contact of the food with the wall of the oropharynx activating the *swallowing reflex*. The bolus passes downwards into the oesophagus propelled by waves of contraction by the constrictors. The bolus is prevented from passing upwards into the nasopharynx by the approximation of the soft palate to the posterior pharyngeal wall. The soft palate is raised by the levator veli palatini and kept taut by the tensor veli

palatini. The closure is assisted by the transverse ridge on the posterior pharyngeal wall formed by the upper fibres of the superior constrictor and those fibres of the palatopharyngeus which pass backwards and mingle with the superior constrictor. This band of muscle is the *palatopharyngeal sphincter*.

Food does not pass into the larynx as a rule because the larynx is lifted up by the action of the stylopharyngeus, palatopharyngeus and salpingopharyngeus so that the opening is tucked up behind the tongue and approaches the posterior surface of the epiglottis which helps to close the laryngeal opening. In addition the edges of the opening, the aryepiglottic folds, are pulled together by the aryepiglottic and arytenoideus muscles. If any food enters the larynx the cough reflex, mediated by the internal laryngeal nerve, is set up in an attempt to expel the food. In addition, the vocal folds (p. 317) are approximated and close the larynx lower down. Should anything pass beyond the vocal folds (a favourite example is half a peanut in a child) it is likely to pass down the trachea into the right bronchus and lodge in a lobar or segmental bronchus.

That the larynx rises can be confirmed by placing a finger on the laryngeal prominence formed by the thyroid cartilage and swallowing. The hyoid bone also rises but less than 1 cm as compared with the rise of about 2.5 cm by the larynx. The pharynx is lifted up at the same time and it has been suggested that the resulting bunching up of its mucous membrane in the region of the laryngeal opening remains for a short time after the pharynx is lowered and contributes to the closing of the entrance to the larynx.

Some minor differences are described in relation to swallowing fluids. In the mouth the two genioglossi on both sides of the midline of the tongue form a longitudinal channel along which the fluid is squirted by the intrinsic muscles. In the second stage the fluid is usually divided into two on the two sides of the epiglottis and passes downwards into the oesophagus along the lateral food channels, that is in the piriform fossae at the sides of the laryngeal opening. It is suggested that solid food may also pass downwards in these channels.

23

The Larynx and Cervical Part of the Trachea

The Larynx

The larynx is that part of the air passages between the oropharynx and the trachea. It lies in the middle of the anterior part of the neck opposite the fourth, fifth and sixth cervical vertebrae and is about 5 cm long, 4 cm wide and 3.5 cm in its anteroposterior diameter. It is smaller in the female in all its dimensions, a difference in size which becomes marked at puberty.

The larynx is known as the *voice box* and is the means whereby the egressive air stream resulting in speech is controlled and modified. The larynx also controls the pitch of the voice whether speaking or singing. An egressive air stream, however, can be produced by the pharynx and pharyngeal speech can be developed in an individual who has had his larynx removed and has learned to swallow air and expel it in a reasonably controlled manner. The phrasing may be deficient and the voice have a belching quality, but clearly recognisable speech is produced.

The Skeleton of the Larynx (figure 197). This consists of a number of cartilages connected by membranes. The hyoid bone (p. 213) may also be included (figure 149). The largest of the cartilages is the *thyroid* which consists of two quadrilateral *laminae* joined anteriorly at an angle to form a forward projection called the *laryngeal prominence* (*Adam's apple*). This is much more marked in men than in women. The two laminae meet at an angle of about 90° in men and an angle of about 120° in women. (The angle is measured posteriorly.) The *thyroid notch* is immediately above the prominence and the posterior borders of the laminae project upwards and downwards as the *superior* and *inferior cornua*. On the external surface of the lamina the *oblique line* runs downwards and forwards from the superior cornu towards the lower border.

The *cricoid cartilage* is shaped like a ring with an anterior *arch* and a posterior *lamina* (*cricos = ring*, Greek). The lower border of the arch and lamina is horizontal and the upper border of the arch when followed backwards rises considerably and becomes continuous with the upper border of the lamina. The arch is about 6 mm high and the lamina about 25 mm high. Where the arch becomes the lamina there is a small facet on the middle of the outer surface for articulation with the inferior cornu of the thyroid cartilage at the synovial *cricothyroid joint*. On the upper lateral angle of the lamina there is another facet facing upwards and laterally for articulation with the arytenoid cartilage at the synovial *crico-arytenoid joint*. There is a vertical median ridge on the posterior surface of the lamina to which the longitudinal muscle fibres of the oesophagus are attached.

There are two *arytenoid cartilages* each of which has four triangular surfaces. One of the surfaces is markedly concave hence the name of the cartilage (*arytaina = ladle*, Greek). The base articulates with the cricoid cartilage at the crico-arytenoid joint. The apex curves backwards and medially and is elongated by the *corniculate cartil-*

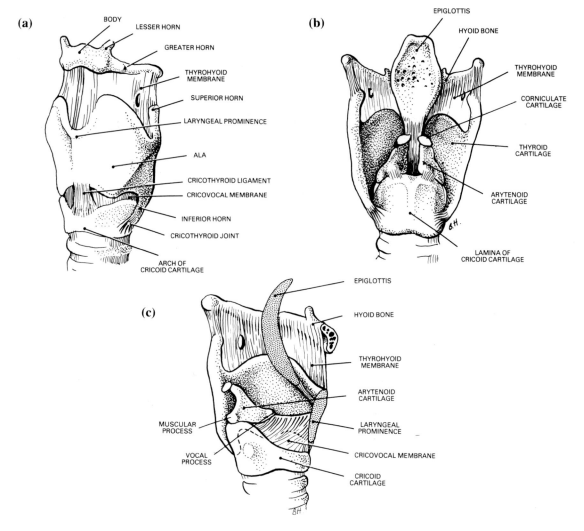

Figure 197   The cartilages, membranes and ligaments of the larynx: (a) anterolateral view; (b) posterior view; (c) lateral view from the right after removal of the right half of the thyroid cartilage, epiglottis and hyoid bone.

age which is attached to it. The inferior border of the medial surface is prolonged forwards as the *vocal process*. The posterior surface of the arytenoid cartilage is flat and its inferior border is prolonged laterally as the *muscular process*. The remaining surface faces anterolaterally.

The *epiglottis* consists largely of a leaflike elastic cartilage which is narrow below where it is attached to the posterior upper part of the angle between the laminae of the thyroid cartilage just below the thyroid notch. The broad upper part of the epiglottis lies behind the tongue and the hyoid

bone to which it is attached by the *hyo-epiglottic ligament*. The lateral borders of the epiglottis are continuous through the *aryepiglottic folds* with the arytenoid cartilages. The *cuneiform cartilage* lies in the aryepiglottic fold anterior to the corniculate cartilage. The posterior surface of the epiglottis has a projection in its lower part called the *tubercle*, and a number of pits in which are mucous glands.

The thyroid cartilage is attached to the hyoid bone by the *thyrohyoid membrane*. This passes upwards behind the body and greater cornua of the hyoid bone and is attached to their upper border. There is a bursa between the membrane and the body. Inferiorly the membrane is attached to the upper border of the laminae and the superior cornua of the thyroid cartilage. The membrane is thickened in the midline anteriorly (*median thyrohyoid ligament*) and its posterior border is called the *lateral thyrohyoid ligament*. The epiglottis and piriform fossa of the pharynx are posterior to the membrane and the infrahyoid muscles are anterior.

The *cricothyroid ligament* has a median thickened part between the upper border of the arch of the cricoid cartilage and the lower border of the lamina of the thyroid cartilage. More laterally it is attached to the upper border of the cricoid arch and passes upwards *deep* to the lamina of the thyroid cartilage (figure 197(c)). This part is also called the *conus elasticus* or *cricovocal membrane* and has a free upper edge attached posteriorly to the vocal process of the arytenoid cartilage and anteriorly to the deep aspect of the laryngeal prominence. This edge is called the *vocal ligament* and forms the skeleton of the vocal fold. There is a structure similar to but much thinner than the conus elasticus in the wall of the larynx above the vestibular fold and extending upwards to the ary-epiglottic fold. It is called the *quadrangular membrane* (figure 199(b)). This, together with the conus elasticus, constitutes the *fibro-elastic membrane of the larynx*.

The epiglottis is attached to the thyroid cartilage by the *thyro-epiglottic ligament*. The anterior surface of the epiglottis is connected to the back of the tongue by a *median glosso-epiglottic fold* and two *lateral glosso-epiglottic* folds, one on each side. The space on either side of the median fold is called the *vallecula*.

The thyroid, cricoid and major part of the arytenoid cartilages may begin to ossify as early as 30 years of age and by 60 years some ossification is usually present in all of them. The elastic cartilages (the epiglottis, the corniculate and cuneiform cartilages and the apices of the arytenoid cartilages) do not ossify.

The Muscles of the Larynx. These are divided into *extrinsic* and *intrinsic*. The former include all the infrahyoid and some of the suprahyoid muscles

(pp. 219, 222), and some of the pharyngeal muscles (for example the stylopharyngeus). Extrinsic muscles are defined as muscles passing between the larynx and other structures.

The intrinsic muscles include the *cricothyroid*, which is attached to the lateral surface of the arch of the cricoid cartilage (figure 198(a)). The fibres pass backwards to the lower border of the thyroid lamina and the inferior cornu. The superior constrictor is attached to a fibrous arch passing over the muscle and the conus elasticus is medial to it. The muscle is supplied by the external laryngeal nerve, a branch of the superior laryngeal. When the cricothyroid contracts the lower part of the thyroid cartilage rotates about the cricothyroid joints and moves downwards and forwards, or alternatively the upper anterior part of the cricoid cartilage moves upwards and backwards. In either case the vocal folds are tensed and may be lengthened.

The *arytenoideus muscle* is unpaired, passes between the posterior surfaces of the arytenoid cartilages, and extends as far laterally as the muscular processes (figure 198(b)). The deep fibres are *transverse* and the more superficial are *oblique*. The latter cross in the midline passing from one muscular process upwards towards the opposite apex and some of them continue into the ary-epiglottic fold to form the *aryepiglottic muscle*. The muscle is supplied by the recurrent laryngeal nerve. When it contracts it pulls the two arytenoid cartilages together at the crico-arytenoid joints and approximates (adducts) the vocal folds. The aryepiglottic muscles close the laryngeal opening by pulling the folds together.

The *posterior crico-arytenoid muscle* (figure 198(b)) is attached to the posterior surface of the lamina of the cricoid cartilage and passes upwards and laterally to the arytenoid muscular process. The lowest fibres are almost vertical. The muscle is supplied by the recurrent laryngeal nerve. Its action is to abduct the vocal fold by rotating the arytenoid cartilage laterally at the crico-arytenoid joint, and its vertical fibres pull the arytenoid cartilage backwards and tense the vocal fold.

The *lateral crico-arytenoid muscle* (figure 198(c)) is attached to the upper border of the cricoid arch and passes upwards and backwards to the muscular process of the arytenoid cartilage.

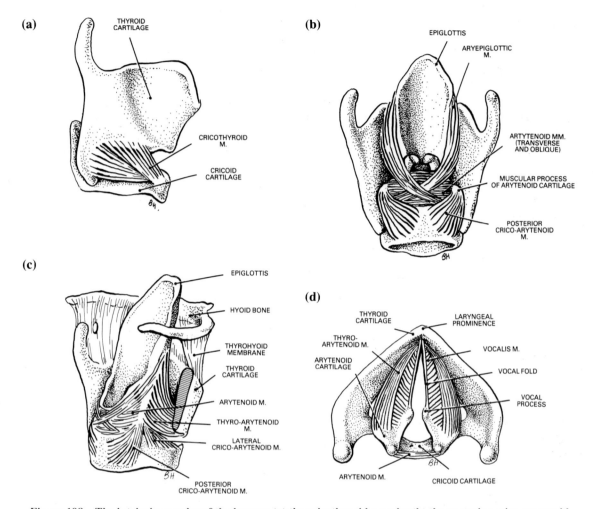

Figure 198   The intrinsic muscles of the larynx: (a) the cricothyroid muscle; (b) the posterior crico-arytenoid, the arytenoid and the aryepiglottic muscles; (c) the right lateral crico-arytenoid, thyro-arytenoid and vocalis muscles after removal of part of the right half of the thyroid cartilage; (d) the thyro-arytenoid and vocalis muscles seen from above.

It is supplied by the recurrent laryngeal nerve. The muscle adducts the vocal fold by rotating the arytenoid cartilage medially at the crico-arytenoid joint.

The *thyro-arytenoid muscle* (figure 198(c), (d)) is attached to the inner surface of the lamina of the thyroid cartilage near the midline and passes backwards to become attached to the anterolateral surface of the arytenoid cartilage. The most medial fibres, lying lateral to the vocal ligament, form the *vocalis muscle* and are attached to the ligament. The superior fibres pass into the aryepiglottic fold and form the *thyro-epiglottic muscle*. The muscle

is supplied by the recurrent laryngeal nerve. The thyro-arytenoids rotate the arytenoid cartilages medially at the crico-arytenoid joints so that the vocal folds are adducted. They also pull the arytenoid cartilages forwards and thus relax the vocal folds. The vocalis is said to alter the functioning length of the vocal folds since its fibres are attached to only the posterior half of the vocal ligament. When they contract they cause relaxation of the posterior half but the anterior half of the fold remains tense. The thyro-epiglottic muscle pulls the ary-epiglottic folds laterally.

(a)

(b)

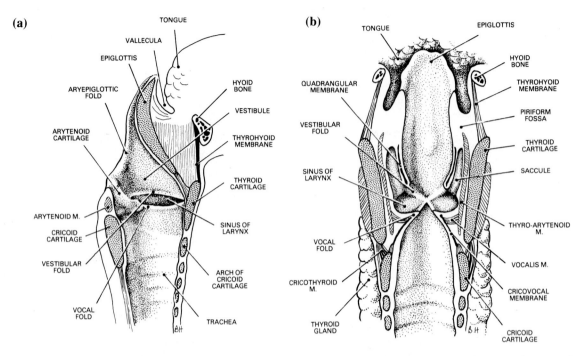

Figure 199   (a) The interior of the left side of the larynx in sagittal section. (b) The interior of the anterior part of the larynx in coronal section.

The Interior of the Larynx. This is divided into three parts by two pairs of folds lying approximately anteroposteriorly and projecting into the cavity of the larynx. The upper are called the *vestibular folds (false vocal cords)* and the lower the *vocal folds (true vocal cords)* (figure 199).

The part of the larynx above the vestibular folds is called the *vestibule*. Its upper limit is the opening of the larynx which communicates with the laryngopharynx. It is bounded anteriorly by the upper edge of the epiglottis, laterally by the aryepiglottic folds containing the aryepiglottic muscle and the *cuneiform cartilages*, and posteriorly by the arytenoid cartilages with the corniculate cartilages and the mucous membrane between them. The anterior wall of the vestibule is much longer than the posterior wall because of the upward projection of the epiglottis. The tubercle or lower part of this cartilage projects into the cavity of the vestibule.

The lower limit of the vestibule is defined by the vestibular folds and leads into the second part of the larynx through the space between the folds

(rima vestibuli). Each fold consists of fibrous tissue, the *vestibular ligament*, covered by mucous membrane and is attached anteriorly to the inner aspect of the lamina of the thyroid cartilage near the midline just above the attachment of the vocal fold, and posteriorly to the anterolateral surface of the arytenoid cartilage.

There is a considerable amount of loose connective tissue in the aryepiglottic folds and walls of the vestibule. Swelling due to effusion of fluid into the tissue can cause obstruction to breathing.

The middle part of the larynx is limited above by the vestibular folds and below by the vocal folds and is called the *ventricle (sinus)* of the larynx. Anteriorly the ventricle leads upwards into a space called the *saccule* which is lateral to the vestibular folds. The thyro-arytenoid muscle is lateral to the ventricle and saccule. There are also some muscle fibres medial to the saccule between it and the vestibular fold. These fibres may be responsible for the closing of the vestibular folds in swallowing and may enable the folds to be used in speech in certain circumstances. The saccule contains a large number of mucous glands and the muscle fibres related to it can press on the saccule and force the secretion on to the vocal folds which have no glands or goblet cells. The size of the saccule varies in different animals and in many apes it extends into the neck and even into the axilla.

The vocal folds are attached anteriorly near the midline to the inner surface of the lamina of the thyroid cartilage and posteriorly to the vocal process of the arytenoid cartilage. The vocal folds and arytenoid cartilages form the *glottis*. The space between them is called the *rima glottidis* which is described as extending backwards between the arytenoid cartilages thus forming an anterior *intermembranous part* and a posterior *intercartilaginous part*. The vocal fold is strikingly pearly white in the living because the stratified squamous epithelium which covers the fold is tightly bound to the underlying tissue and is avascular. Within the vocal fold there are the vocal ligament, which is the upper edge of the conus elasticus, and the vocalis muscle which is lateral to the ligament. The rima glottidis is longer in the male than in the female, about 2.4 cm as compared with about 1.8 cm.

The part of the larynx below the vocal folds has no special features. The inner surface of the conus elasticus and cricoid cartilage, covered by mucous membrane, forms its walls. Its cavity is continuous inferiorly with that of the trachea.

Most of the larynx is covered by ciliated mucous columnar epithelium. Stratified squamous epithelium is found over the vocal folds, along the upper edge of the aryepiglottic folds and the anterior surface of the epiglottis. Reference has already been made to the mucous glands in the pits of the epiglottis and in the saccule. They are also found in the aryepiglottic folds near the arytenoid cartilages. The taste buds on the posterior surface of the epiglottis are supplied by the vagus nerve.

The Functions of the Vocal Folds. The vocal folds can be abducted (moved away from the midline) by the posterior crico-arytenoid muscles and adducted (moved towards the midline) by the lateral crico-arytenoid, thyro-arytenoid and arytenoideus muscles (figure 200). In quiet respiration the vocal folds are in a midposition between abduction and adduction. In deep and forced respira-

tion they are widely abducted. They are adducted during swallowing.

Voiced speech as compared with voiceless speech (whispering) requires the adduction of the vocal folds and sufficiently forceful expiration to separate them at a fundamental frequency which although it can be varied from 60 to 500 Hz is about 120 Hz in men, 225 Hz in women and 265 Hz in children. In normal speech an individual varies the pitch within an octave. The actual sound produced is the resultant of the fundamental and the harmonics.

The adduction and abduction of the vocal folds in speech are not due to the laryngeal muscles but to the expiratory air exerting sufficient pressure to separate the vocal folds. They come together again because of their elasticity and the fall in pressure below the folds due to their opening. This fall in pressure also produces a suction effect which results in their being adducted again (*Bernoulli effect*).

The vocal folds can also be made more or less tense and to a limited extent lengthened or shortened. Their operating length, however, can be considerably changed as can their thickness. All three factors — tension, length and thickness — affect the pitch of the voice and are varied by the laryngeal muscles. The main muscle altering the tension is the cricothyroid. The vocalis muscle is chiefly responsible for altering the operating length and thickness. The obvious example of a change in length affecting the pitch of the voice is the change at puberty in the male voice due to a comparatively sudden lengthening of the vocal folds caused by the male sex hormones. In falsetto singing only the front half of the vocal folds are operating and they are very thin. The hoarseness which follows the accidental cutting of the external laryngeal nerve is due to the paralysis of the cricothyroid muscle.

If the recurrent laryngeal nerve is cut on one side the affected vocal fold lies in the midposition between abduction and adduction but voiced sounds are possible because the normal vocal fold can be pulled across the midline so that the rima glottidis is closed. If both recurrent laryngeal nerves are cut or otherwise interrupted, the vocal folds cannot be brought together and only whispering is possible. Strong muscular effort is impossible because the larynx (glottis) cannot be closed.

A markedly higher pitch is achieved by lifting the larynx so that the column of air above the vocal folds is shortened. This upward movement can be easily demonstrated on oneself by placing a finger on the laryngeal prominence and singing a low and then a high note.

Increased loudness of the voice is achieved by increasing the pressure of the expiratory airstream so that the vocal folds are more widely separated in each cycle of the frequency.

Phonemes in the English Language. A *phoneme* (*phonema* = *voice* or *word*, Greek) is defined as the smallest unit of significant contrastive sound in a given language or dialect. In English there are about 20 different vowel sounds and the differences between them depend on the shape of the mouth and lips and the position of the tongue as well as the length of time given to producing the sound.

There are about 25 consonants and these sounds depend on which part or parts of the mouth are used and how they are used. (The phonetic symbols are in brackets.) P (p) and B (b) are labial sounds, D (d) and T (t) involve the tip of the tongue and the anterior edge of the hard palate,

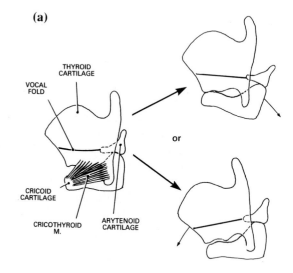

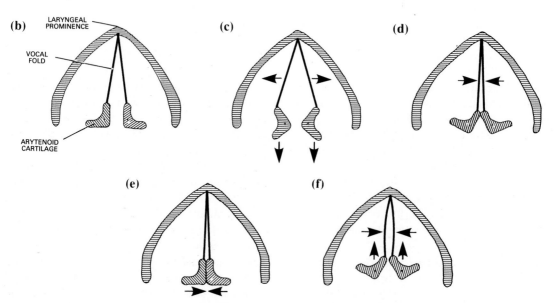

Figure 200   The action of the intrinsic laryngeal muscles on the vocal folds: (a) the cricothyroid (increased tension); (b) the vocal folds in quiet respiration; (c) the posterior crico-arytenoid (abduction and increased tension); (d) the lateral crico-arytenoid (adduction); (e) the arytenoideus (adduction); (f) the thyro-arytenoid (adduction and decreased tension).

TH (ɵ) as in *thigh* involves the tongue and front teeth, G (g) and K (k) involve the back of the tongue and palate and M (m), N (n) NG (ŋ) are nasal sounds produced with the palate lowered. L (l), R (r) involve the tongue and anterior part of the palate in a different way from D (d) and T (t). One should compare the TH (ɵ) in *thin* with the TH (ʒ) in *this* and the difference between S (s) and Z (z).

Good examples of differences in the phonemes of English speaking groups are (1) the Scottish phoneme CH (x) in *loch* which is not included among southern English phonemes; (2) the English phonemes AU (ɔː) in *caught* and O (ɔ) in *cot* which are not distinguished as separate phonemes in Scottish pronunciation.

A detailed analysis of vowels and consonents cannot be given here but it is obvious that recognisable speech involves complicated, intricate activity of the muscles of the tongue, palate, jaws and lips working in a coordinated manner. The activity of these muscles in speech is only one aspect of language which also embraces understanding what is being said, writing and reading as well as speaking. Paramount in language is the role of the human cerebral cortex.

Laryngoscopy. By introducing a mirror through the mouth and placing it behind the back of the tongue the larynx can be inspected. The appearance is shown in figure 201. The epiglottis and the aryepiglottic folds with the elevations produced by the cuneiform and corniculate cartilages can be seen. The piriform fossae are visible. In the cavity of the larynx the pearly white vocal folds are easily identifiable and they come together when the subject makes a voiced sound such as '*Ah*'. The pink vestibular folds are less obvious above the vocal folds. The rings of the trachea may be seen beyond the vocal folds.

The Arteries and Nerves of the Larynx. The arteries come from the thyroid arteries, the *superior laryngeal* from the superior thyroid and the *inferior laryngeal* from the inferior thyroid. The muscles are innervated by the recurrent laryngeal nerve, except the cricothyroid which is supplied by the external laryngeal nerve. Because the external laryngeal nerve runs with the superior thyroid artery and the recurrent laryngeal nerve with the

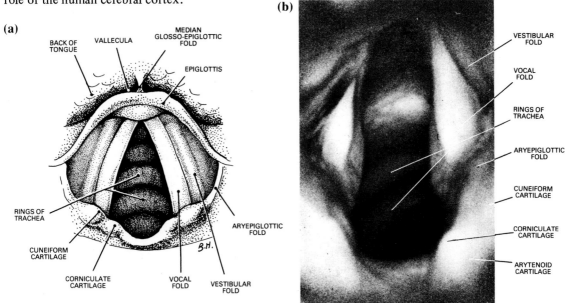

Figure 201 The larynx as seen with a laryngoscope: (a) diagram; (b) actual photograph.

inferior thyroid artery they are at risk in thyroid-ectomy. The sensory nerve supply of the lining of the larynx above the vocal folds comes from the internal laryngeal nerve which enters the larynx with the superior laryngeal artery through the thyrohyoid membrane. Below the vocal fold the sensory innervation comes from the recurrent laryngeal nerve which reaches the larynx by passing deep to the inferior constrictor together with the inferior laryngeal artery.

The Cervical Part of the Trachea (figures 150, 152)

The trachea extends from the cricoid cartilage, at the level of the sixth cervical vertebra, into the thorax, where it divides slightly to the right of the midline into the right and left main bronchi at the level of the fourth or fifth thoracic vertebra indicated anteriorly by the sternal angle. The thoracic part of the trachea is described on p. 51. Its total length is about 10 cm and it is about 2 cm wide. It is flattened posteriorly so that its lumen is D-shaped.

The trachea is superficial in the neck as compared with its position in the thorax. This is largely due to the thorax projecting anteriorly relative to the vertebral column and the backward curve of the thoracic vertebrae. In the neck the trachea is covered by skin and fascia. The anterior jugular veins which run downwards in the fascia have one or more cross-anastomoses in front of the trachea. The isthmus of the thyroid gland lies in front of the second, third and fourth tracheal rings, and the lobes of the gland lie laterally extending downwards to about the level of the sixth tracheal ring. On each side the common carotid artery is lateral to the trachea deep to the thyroid lobe. The oeso-phagus is posterior to the trachea and on each side the recurrent laryngeal nerve lies in the groove between them. The inferior thyroid arteries are lateral to the trachea and constitute its main blood supply.

24

The Autonomic Nerves and Lymphatic Vessels of the Head and Neck

The Sympathetic Ganglia and their Branches

The three ganglia of the cervical part of the ganglionated trunk together with their preganglionic and postganglionic components are described on p. 239. In summary the preganglionic fibres have their cell bodies in the lateral horn of the grey matter of the upper four or five thoracic spinal cord segments (mainly the first three). The postganglionic fibres (1) join the ventral rami of the cervical spinal nerves (they are distributed through the branches of the cervical and brachial plexuses and also the dorsal rami of the spinal nerves); (2) join the glossopharyngeal, vagus and hypoglossal nerves and are distributed with their branches; (3) form plexuses round the main arteries and their branches; (4) continue into the cranial cavity as the internal carotid nerve and the plexuses round the internal carotid and vertebral arteries; (5) descend into the thorax as cardiac branches.

The Parasympathetic Ganglia and their Branches

The parasympathetic preganglionic fibres emerge in the oculomotor, facial, glossopharyngeal and vagus nerves. The motor parasympathetic part of the vagus nerves, although the largest in the body, has no branches which end in the head and neck (its cervical cardiac branches go to the thorax) and is distributed almost entirely in the thorax and abdomen. The parasympathetic ganglia are related to branches of the trigeminal nerve. The ciliary ganglion in the orbit is attached to the nasociliary nerve (p. 274), the otic ganglion in the infratemporal fossa to the mandibular nerve (p. 207), the pterygopalatine ganglion in the pterygopalatine fossa to the maxillary nerve (p. 209) and the submandibular ganglion on the hyoglossus muscle to the lingual nerve (p. 223). Each ganglion has three nerves entering it, a sympathetic, a somatic motor or sensory and a parasympathetic. The otic ganglion has a motor branch from the nerve to the medial pterygoid muscle, and the other three ganglia receive a sensory contribution from a branch of the trigeminal nerve. Only the parasympathetic branch synapses in the ganglia. The other branches pass through without interruption.

The parasympathetic fibres in the oculomotor nerve synapse in the ciliary ganglion. The postganglionic fibres supply the ciliary muscle and the sphincter pupillae. The parasympathetic fibres in the facial nerve (1) synapse in the submandibular ganglion and its postganglionic fibres are secretomotor to the submandibular and sublingual salivary glands; (2) synapse in the pterygopalatine ganglion and its postganglionic fibres are secretomotor to the lacrimal gland. The preganglionic fibres from the glossopharyngeal nerve, after a complicated course (p. 207), synapse in the otic ganglion from which postganglionic fibres go to the parotid gland in the auriculotemporal nerve.

The Lymph Nodes, Lymphoid Tissue and Lymphatic Drainage of the Head and Neck

The Nodes. The arrangement of the lymph nodes is described on pp. 241–242. They are divided into superficial and deep. Most of the superficial nodes form a ring round the junction of the head and neck and the deep nodes lie along the internal jugular vein. Their afferent and efferent vessels have been described.

The Lymphoid Tissue. This refers to the palatine tonsils (p. 309), the pharyngeal tonsil (p. 309) and the lingual tonsil (p. 287). This ring of lymphoid tissue (*Waldeyer's ring*; Heinrich W.G. Waldeyer, 1836–1921, German anatomist) protects the beginning of the respiratory and alimentary tracts. The pharyngeal and palatine tonsils are frequently infected and enlarged. The significance of this has been discussed (p. 309).

The pharyngeal tonsil drains into the retropharyngeal lymph nodes. Lymph vessels from the palatine tonsil go mainly to the jugulodigastric (tonsillar) lymph node.

The Lymphatic Drainage of the Individual Parts of the Head and Neck. This is given in table 5.

The *lymphatic drainage of the tongue* is more complex. There is an intramuscular plexus of vessels draining into a submucosal plexus which drains in the following way. The vessels from the *tip* of the tongue pierce the mylohyoid muscle and go to the submental lymph nodes whose efferent vessels go mainly to the submandibular nodes. Some vessels go directly to the deep cervical nodes. The *side* of the tongue drains to the submandibular nodes and the *back* of the tongue directly to the deep cervical nodes. Vessels from the *central part* of the surface go to the right or left deep cervical nodes but some vessels go to the submandibular nodes. It is generally accepted that lymph from the right half of the tongue drains to nodes on the right side and those from the left half to nodes on the left. Lymph vessels near the midline may, however, cross to the opposite side.

All the vessels eventually end in the deep cervical lymph nodes. The jugulo-omohyoid (lingual) node was especially associated with the lymphatic drainage of the tongue but it is now known that vessels from the tongue also go to the jugulodigastric nodes.

Table 5

Structure	Nodes
Face scalp	
Anterior	→ facial → submandibular → deep cervical
Lateral	→ parotid → deep cervical
Scalp	
Posterior	→ occipital → deep cervical
Eyelids	
Medial	→ submandibular → deep cervical
Lateral	→ parotid → deep cervical
Chin	→ submental → submandibular → deep cervical
External ear	
Anterior	→ parotid → deep cervical
Posterior	→ retro-auricular → deep cervical
Middle ear	→ parotid → deep cervical
Neck	
Superficial	→ superficial cervical (anterior, lateral or posterior) → deep cervical
Deep	→ deep cervical
Floor of mouth (anterior), lower incisors	→ submental → submandibular → deep cervical or submental → deep cervical
Floor of mouth (lateral), teeth and peri-odontium (except lower incisors)	→ submandibular → deep cervical
Palatine tonsil	→ jugulodigastric (deep cervical)
Pharyngeal tonsil, nasopharynx paranasal sinuses, soft palate	→ retropharyngeal → deep cervical
Nasal cavity	
Anterior	→ submandibular → deep cervical
Posterior	→ retropharyngeal → deep cervical
Larynx (above vocal folds)	→ superior deep cervical
Larynx (below vocal folds), cervical trachea	→ laryngeal and tracheal → inferior deep cervical
Oropharynx, laryngeal pharynx, cervical oesophagus	→ deep cervical
Thyroid gland	
Upper part	→ laryngeal nodes
Lower part	→ tracheal nodes or superior mediastinal nodes

Part 5

The Vertebral Column

25

The Vertebral Column and Spinal Cord

The Vertebral Column as a Whole

The different parts of the vertebral column have been described, *cervical* (p. 186), *thoracic* (p. 3), *lumbar* (p. 59), *sacral* and *coccygeal* (p. 62). An articulated column consists of the bony vertebrae and the fibrocartilaginous *intervertebral discs* which form about one-quarter of the total height of the column. The column itself forms about two-fifths of the height of the whole body. Variations in total height reflect differences in the length of the lower limb much more than differences in the length of the vertebral column. The bodies of the vertebrae increase progressively in size from above downwards as far as the fifth lumbar vertebrae, below which they rapidly become smaller. This reflects the weight-bearing functions of the column and the transference of weight to the hip bones across the sacro-iliac joints.

The whole vertebral column has a number of curves. The cervical and lumbar vertebrae show a curve with the convexity anterior, and the thoracic vertebrae and sacrum curve in the opposite direction — their convexity is posterior. Until late in fetal life the whole vertebral column is curved with its concavity anterior (figure 202). The cervical curve appears late in fetal life and is more accentuated when the baby holds its head up between 6 and 12 weeks after birth. The lumbar curve, convex anteriorly, appears when the baby sits up at about 6 months and becomes more marked when the baby stands and begins to walk at about 12 months. The thoracic and sacral curves are called *primary*

curves because they are a persistence of the original curve in the fetus. They are due to differences between the anterior and posterior heights of the vertebral bodies. The cervical and lumbar are *secondary curves* and are due to differences between the anterior and posterior heights of the discs.

An increase in the curvature of the thoracic vertebrae is called a *kyphosis* (*kyphos = hump-backed*, Greek) and an increase in the lumbar curve a *lordosis* (*lordos = bent so as to be convex in front*, Greek) although the normal lumbar curve is often referred to as the lumbar lordosis. An increase in the lumbar curvature may be the result of an attempt to move the centre of gravity of the body backwards, for example in pregnancy. A slight lateral curvature is common and is called *scoliosis* (*skolios = crooked*, Greek). A marked degree of scoliosis is pathological but the cause is frequently unknown. It can occur as a result of failure of development of one-half of one or two vertebral bodies or a paralysis of the posterior muscles of the vertebral column due, for example, to poliomyelitis. A shortening of one lower limb can result in a compensatory scoliosis.

The normal curves of the vertebral column give it a resilience to vertical forces which are absorbed by the giving way and recovery of the arches of the column.

The *lumbosacral angle* (figure 56(d)) between the fifth lumbar and first sacral vertebrae is not a part of the curvatures of the column and measures about $150°$ (the angle between vertical lines through

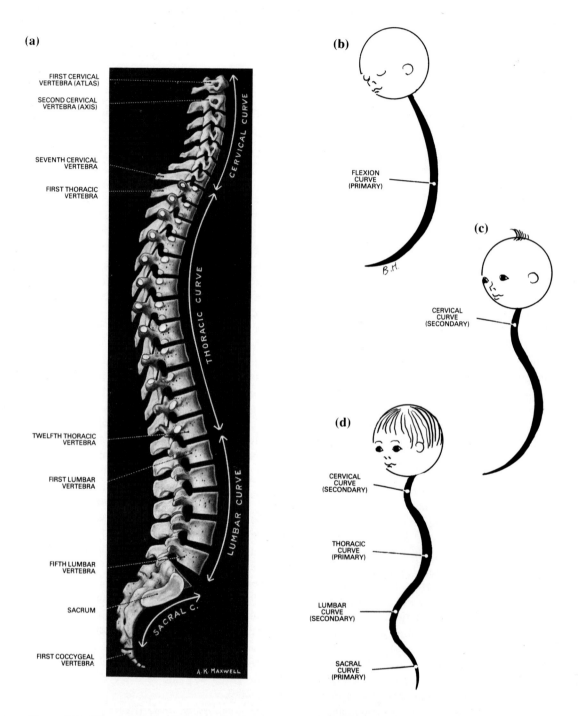

Figure 202   The curvatures of the vertebral column: (a) the adult (reproduced from *Hamilton's Textbook of Human Anatomy* by courtesy of the Editors and The Macmillan Press); (b) the single curve of the column which is present until late in fetal life; (c) the development of the cervical secondary curve at about 3 months; (d) the development of the lumbar secondary curve at about 6 months to 1 year.

the body of the fifth lumbar vertebra and the body of the first sacral vertebra).

The Vertebral Joints

The Joints between the Bodies. From the second cervical vertebra to the fifth lumbar each body of a vertebra articulates with the body immediately inferior to it by means of a secondary cartilaginous joint (figure 203). The adjacent surfaces of the bodies are covered by hyaline cartilage and are held together by an intervertebral fibrocartilaginous disc. The discs are narrowest in the upper thoracic region.

Each disc has an outer fibrous part, the *anulus fibrosus*, and an inner more jelly-like fibrous tissue,

the *nucleus pulposus*. The anulus consists of layers of collagen whose fibres run obliquely between the vertebrae. The fibres of one layer run in a different direction to that of the fibres of an adjacent layer. With advancing age the nucleus pulposus becomes less fluid and more fibrous until the whole disc resembles the anulus. Because fluid is lost from the discs during the day an individual may be 1–2 cm shorter at night than in the morning. The discs also become thinner with age so that the joint spaces become narrower and an individual's height decreases. Except for its outermost part, the discs are avascular and obtain their nutrition from the spongy bone of the vertebral bodies.

The discs are firmly bound to the edges of the hyaline cartilage and the bodies of the vertebrae and give stability to the vertebral column. Limited

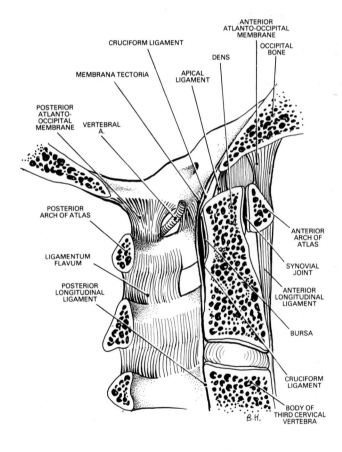

Figure 203   A sagittal section through the upper three cervical vertebrae to show the joints between the bodies of the vertebrae and the various ligaments between the vertebrae. Some of the ligaments of the atlas and axis are also shown.

movement between the adjacent vertebrae is possible because of the obliquity of the fibres forming the disc. One side of the disc can be compressed and the other stretched without lengthening the fibres. The discs, which can be compressed and regain their shape, also act as shock absorbers, for example when heavy weights are carried, and when jumping or running.

The *anterior longitudinal ligament* extends anterior to the bodies from the anterior arch of the atlas to the sacrum (figure 203). It is a thick, wide band and is attached to the vertebral bodies and intervertebral discs. This ligament is strong enough to support the vertebral column if, in the prone position, only the shoulders and pelvis are supported and the trunk is allowed to sag between them. Advantage is taken of this in the treatment of a crush fracture of the vertebrae. The *posterior longitudinal ligament* (figure 203), much weaker than the anterior, extends from the occipital bone posterior to the vertebral bodies to the sacrum (the part from the second cervical vertebra to the occipital bone is called the *membrana tectoria*) (figures 203, 204). This ligament is attached to the discs where it is fairly wide but is only loosely attached to the vertebral bodies where it is narrow. Veins from the bodies join the plexus of veins in the vertebral canal and separate the ligament from the adjacent bone.

Prolapsed or herniated disc is common and most frequently affects the discs between the fourth and fifth lumbar, and fifth lumbar and first sacral vertebrae. The discs between the fifth and sixth, and sixth and seventh cervical vertebrae also prolapse but much less frequently. The remaining discs are rarely affected. Usually the anulus tears posterolaterally and the nucleus is squeezed out where the disc is related to the intervertebral foramen so that a spinal nerve is pressed on. The muscles supplied by the nerve are weak and pain radiates along the distribution of the nerve. The nerves frequently affected are the fourth or fifth lumbar and the sixth or seventh cervical nerves.

The Zygapophyseal Joints. These are the joints between the articular processes. They are described as plane, synovial joints although in the lumbar region they have curved surfaces. The plane of the cervical joints is oblique and the superior articular process faces backwards, upwards and slightly outwards. The plane of the thoracic joints is more or less coronal and that of the lumbar joints begins posteriorly in the sagittal plane and then curves medially.

In the cervical region the zygapophyseal joints are behind the transverse processes and form a pillar of bone which is weight-bearing. In the

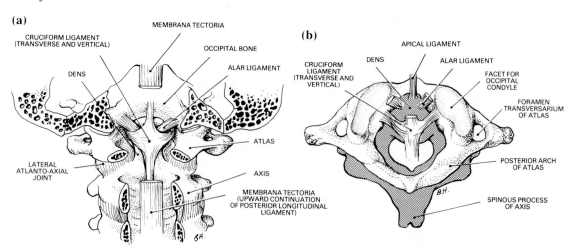

Figure 204   (a) A posterior view of the ligaments between the axis, atlas and occipital bone.
(b) A superior view of the atlas and axis.

thoracic region these joints lie in front of the transverse processes and in the lumbar region they again lie posterior to these processes. The intervertebral foramina lie anterior to the zygapophyseal joints and arthritic changes in these joints may produce bony projections (*osteophytes*) which may press on the spinal nerve in the foramen. The joints between the occipital bone and atlas, and atlas and axis lie anterior to the first and second cervical spinal nerves.

In the cervical vertebrae a joint-like structure may be found between the lateral parts of adjacent bodies where the lower body turns upwards and fits into the edge of the upper. Some authorities regard these joints as a degenerative split in the adjacent part of the intervertebral disc. Whatever they may be, they lie in front of the intervertebral foramen, can undergo arthritic changes and affect the relevant spinal nerve.

Several ligaments pass between the vertebrae. *Supraspinous ligaments* join the tips of the spinous processes and extend from the external occipital protuberance to the sacrum. In the neck region, from the occipital bone to the seventh cervical spinous process, the supraspinous ligament is called the *ligamentum nuchae* and takes the form of a fibro-elastic sagittal septum to which muscles are attached (*nucha = spinal marrow*, hence the *spinal cord*, Arabic; because the nape of the neck was used as a means of treating the spinal cord, *nucha* came to mean the *nape of the neck*). There are *interspinous* and *intertransverse ligaments* between the spinous processes and transverse processes respectively. The *ligamenta flava* (*flavus = yellow*, Latin) are yellow elastic ligaments extending from the internal surface of one lamina downwards to the upper edge of the lamina below (figure 203). They are attached along the whole length of the laminae. These ligaments are stretched in forward bending of the vertebral column and control the movement to some extent. They help the column to return to the vertical position.

The Atlanto-occipital Joints. Each of these is a synovial joint between the condyle of the occipital bone and the facet on the upper surface of the lateral mass of the atlas. The occipital facets are convex and the atlantal facets are concave. The two joints may be regarded as a single ellipsoid joint because the long axis of each joint is oblique pointing laterally from in front backwards. Movements therefore are about transverse and anteroposterior axes, and rotation about a longitudinal axis does not occur.

The *anterior atlanto-occipital membrane* (figure 203) is attached superiorly to the anterior edge of the foramen magnum and inferiorly to the anterior arch of the atlas. The *posterior atlanto-occipital membrane* (figure 203) is attached superiorly to the posterior edge of the foramen magnum and inferiorly to the upper border of the posterior arch of the atlas. Behind the lateral mass the posterior membrane arches over the vertebral artery and the first cervical nerve which is between the artery and the bone.

The Median Atlanto-axial Joint (figure 203). This is a synovial joint of the pivot type between the dens of the axis, and the ring formed by the posterior surface of the anterior arch of the atlas and the transverse part of the *cruciform ligament*. The joint is in two parts, an anterior with a loose capsule between the anterior part of the dens and the anterior arch of the atlas, and a posterior between the posterior groove of the dens and the ligament.

The Lateral Atlanto-axial Joints (figure 204(a)). These joints, one on each side, are between the almost flat, circular facets on the inferior surface of the lateral mass of the atlas and corresponding facets on the bone at the side of the dens of the axis. The upper end of the anterior longitudinal ligament is attached to the anterior surfaces of the atlas and axis. The laminae of the axis are attached to the posterior arch of the atlas by ligamenta flava.

Several ligaments pass between the axis and occipital bone inside the vertebral canal (figures 203, 204). An *alar ligament* on each side passes obliquely from the side of the upper part of the dens to the medial side of the occipital condyle. The *apical ligament* passes upwards in the midline from the apex of the dens to the anterior edge of the foramen magnum. The *cruciform ligament* has a *transverse part* which is the ligament already described as passing between the medial sides of the lateral masses of the atlas and behind the dens. The *vertical part* is attached inferiorly to the back of the body of the axis, and superiorly to the basilar part of the occipital bone inside the edge of the foramen magnum. The membrane tectoria covers the vertical part of the cruciform ligament and is the upward continuation of the posterior longitudinal ligament.

The Muscles of the Vertebral Column (figure 205)

There are posterior muscles lying on the sides of the column from the occipital bone to the sacrum, and anterior muscles which are found only in the cervical and lumbar regions. The posterior muscles are deep to the muscles passing between the vertebral column and the pectoral girdle (the trapezius, levator scapulae, rhomboids and latissimus dorsi). The *serratus posterior superior* is deep to the rhomboids and runs downwards and laterally from the ligamentum nuchae and spinous processes of the upper three thoracic vertebrae to the upper four ribs. The *serratus posterior inferior* (figure 14(c)) is deep to the latissimus dorsi and passes upwards and laterally from the spinous processes of the last two thoracic and first two lumbar vertebrae to the lower ribs. They are regarded as respiratory muscles and are supplied by the intercostal nerves.

The Posterior Vertebral Muscles. These muscles are covered by a layer of dense fascia (the thoracolumbar fascia) which in the thoracic region is attached medially to the thoracic spinous processes and laterally to the angles of the ribs.

In the lumbar region the fascia is in three layers (figure 63). The posterior layer is attached medially to the lumbar and sacral spinous processes, the middle layer to the tips of the lumbar transverse processes and the anterior layer to the middle of the anterior surface of the lumbar transverse processes. The middle and anterior layers surround the quadratus lumborum muscle. The upper edge of the anterior layer forms the lateral arcuate ligament to which part of the diaphragm is attached. The latissimus dorsi is attached to the posterior

layer, and the internal oblique and transversus abdominis muscles of the abdominal wall to the conjoined three layers. Inferiorly the fascia is attached to the iliac crest and the iliolumbar ligament.

The posterior muscles are divided into two main groups called the *erector spinae (sacrospinalis)* and *transversospinalis*. The erector spinae is subdivided into lateral, intermediate and medial parts, each of which is divided into three groups according to their level — lumbar, thoracic and cervical. Needless to state each of these nine muscles has a name. (This subdivision has existed at least since Andreas Vesalius, 1514–64, published his *De Humani Corporis Fabrica* in 1543.) The inferior part of the erector spinae has a tendinous attachment to the back of the sacrum, the adjacent iliac crest and the lumbar spinous processes. The lateral part of the muscle (*iliocostalis*) (figure 205(a)) is attached to the angles of the ribs and the transverse processes of the lower four cervical vertebrae. The intermediate part (*longissimus*) (figure 205(a)) is attached to the lumbar, thoracic and cervical transverse processes and the posterior surfaces of the ribs between the tubercle and angle. Its most superior part, the *longissimus capitis*, is attached to the back of the mastoid process of the temporal bone deep to the splenius capitis.

The medial part of the erector spinae (the *spinalis*) is attached to the spinous processes of the lumbar, thoracic and cervical vertebrae (figure 205(b)).

The fibres of the erector spinae are on the whole vertical and their superficial fibres span several vertebrae. The fibres of the transversospinalis, as the name implies, run from the transverse processes to the spinous processes and are usually oblique and short (figure 205(b)). There are three layers of muscles — *semispinalis*, *multifidus* and *rotatores*. The most superior part of the superficial layer is called the *semispinalis capitis*, which is attached to the occipital bone between the superior and inferior nuchal lines. There are also small slips of muscles between adjacent spinous processes and adjacent transverse processes.

There are two muscles in the neck which are superficial to the erector spinae and transversospinalis. The *splenius capitis* (figure 205(a)) runs

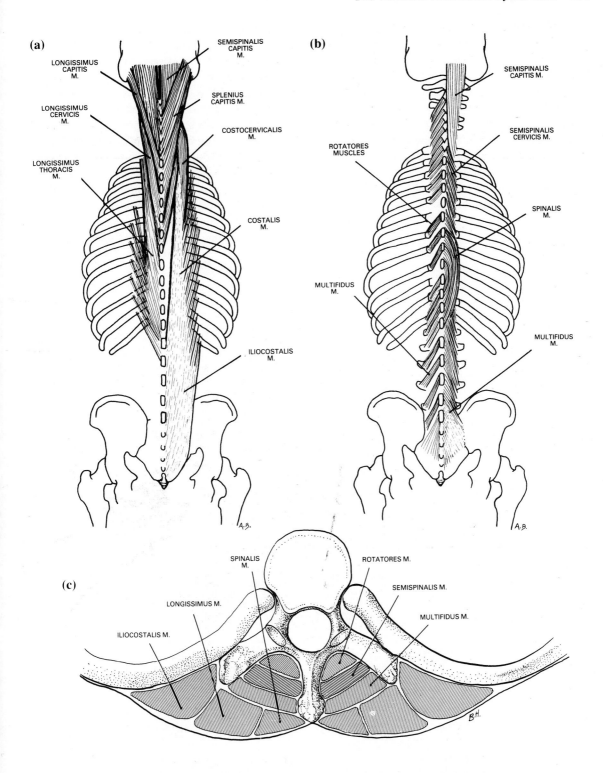

Figure 205 **The vertebral muscles: (a) longitudinal superficial; (b) longitudinal deep; (c) transverse.**

obliquely from the lower half of the ligamentum nuchae and upper thoracic spinous processes to the mastoid process and adjacent part of the occipital bone deep to the sternocleidomastoid and superficial to the longissimus capitis (*splenius = bandage*, Latin). The *splenius cervicis* passes obliquely from the spinous processes of the upper thoracic vertebrae to the transverse processes of the upper cervical vertebrae.

All the posterior vertebral muscles are supplied by dorsal rami of the spinal nerves. The actions of the muscles are described in the section on the movements of the vertebral column.

The Suboccipital Muscles (figure 206). This group of small muscles is attached to the axis, atlas and occipital bone. They lie deep to the semispinalis capitis and form a region called the *suboccipital*

triangle. The triangle is formed by (1) the *inferior oblique muscle* passing from the spinous process of the axis to the transverse process of the atlas; (2) the *superior oblique muscle* passing from the transverse process of the atlas to the occipital bone; (3) the *rectus capitis posterior major*, which is attached to the spinous process of the axis and to the occipital bone. There is in addition a small muscle medial to the rectus capitis posterior major called the *rectus capitis posterior minor*, which is attached inferiorly to the posterior tubercle of the atlas and superiorly to the occipital bone.

Within the triangle there are the posterior arch of the atlas, the posterior atlanto-occipital membrane, and the vertebral artery. The dorsal ramus of the first cervical spinal nerve which supplies all the muscles of the suboccipital triangle appears between the artery and the arch (figure 206). The

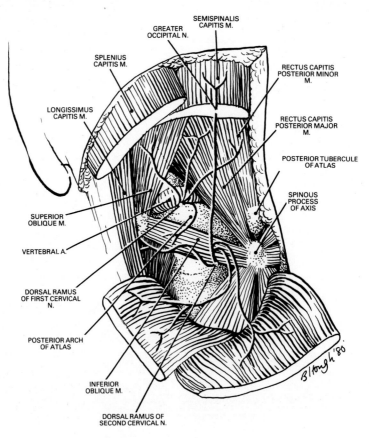

Figure 206   The suboccipital triangle.

dorsal ramus of the second cervical spinal nerve emerges below the inferior oblique muscle and divides into muscular branches which supply adjacent muscles. After piercing the semispinalis capitis it continues upwards into the posterior part of the scalp as the sensory *greater occipital nerve*.

The Anterior Vertebral Muscles. These have already been described. The lateral anterior prevertebral muscles in the neck include the *scalenus anterior*, *scalenus medius* and *scalenus posterior* which are attached to the anterior and posterior tubercles of the transverse processes of some of the cervical vertebrae and after passing downwards are attached to the first and second ribs (p. 230). The *longus colli* and *longus cervicis* are more medial (p. 229 and figure 157). There are two short muscles between the atlas and occiput, the *rectus capitis anterior* and the *rectus capitis lateralis* (p. 229). All these muscles are supplied by the ventral rami of one or more cervical spinal nerves.

The *psoas major* and *minor* and the *quadratus lumborum* (figure 88) may be regarded as anterior vertebral muscles on the posterior abdominal wall (p. 106). The psoas major is attached to the bodies and transverse processes of the lumbar vertebrae and passes downwards and somewhat laterally to sweep round the lateral side of the inlet of the pelvis. It enters the thigh deep to the inguinal ligament and becomes attached to the lesser trochanter of the femur. The psoas minor is attached to the twelfth thoracic and first lumbar vertebrae, passes downwards on the psoas major and is attached to the iliopectineal eminence. The quadratus lumborum is attached to the twelfth rib above, the iliac crest below and the transverse processes of the lumbar vertebrae medially. All three muscles are innervated by ventral rami of the upper lumbar nerves.

The Movements of the Vertebral Column

The basic movements are *flexion* (forward bending) and *extension* (backward bending) about a transverse axis, *lateral flexion* or *bending* to the right or left about an anteroposterior axis and *rotation* to the right or left. The amount of movement between adjacent vertebrae is small and the summation of each movement gives the vertebral column a considerable flexibility. Flexion of the vertebral column from the upright position if measured by the ability to touch one's toes includes flexion at the hip joints. Flexion in the cervical and lumbar regions is greater than in the thoracic region due to the thicker intervertebral discs and the plane of the zygapophyseal joints in the former and also limitation of thoracic movement due to the ribs and sternum. However, only $3°$ of flexion between adjacent thoracic vertebrae adds up to about $30-35°$ of flexion between the first and twelfth.

It has been estimated that total flexion in the cervical region amounts to about $45°$. In this movement each cervical vertebra slides upwards and then tilts forwards on the vertebra below. Extension in the cervical region is about $80°$. The least movement is between the seventh cervical and first thoracic vertebrae. In the upright position flexion is controlled by the posterior neck muscles of both sides which act against the weight of the head and neck (the trapezius, splenius capitis, longissimus capitis, semispinalis capitis and most of the short muscles in the suboccipital region). In the supine position (lying on one's back) the anterior muscles of both sides (the sternocleidomastoid, longus capitis, longus colli, the scalene muscles, the short muscles between the atlas and occiput) flex the head on the atlas and the cervical vertebrae on each other. In extension the reverse occurs — in the upright position the anterior muscles control extension and in the prone position (lying on one's face) the posterior muscles produce extension.

Combined flexion and extension in the thoracic part of the vertebral column amounts to about $40-50°$. The rib cage, the zygapophyseal joints and the long spinous processes all contribute to limiting these movements. Flexion in the upright position is controlled by the posterior vertebral muscles of both sides, and in the supine position is brought about by the anterior abdominal muscles of both sides especially the rectus abdominis. Extension in the upright position is controlled by the anterior abdominal muscles and in the prone position is produced by the posterior vertebral muscles.

Flexion in the lumbar region amounts to about 55° and extension to about 30°. The muscles controlling or producing these movements are the same as those involved in flexion and extension in the thoracic region with the addition of the psoas muscles, which are active flexors in the supine position and control extension in the upright position. There is less movement at the thoracolumbar junction than between the lumbar vertebrae and there is most movement at the lumbosacral joint. The range of movement is reduced with advancing age and at 65 years is about a half or one-third of the range at the age of 10 years.

Lateral flexion to the right and left is more marked in the cervical region (about 40° to one side) than in the thoracic and lumbar regions (about 25°). In the upright position one would expect lateral bending to the right to be controlled by the muscles on the left side of the vertebral column. It has been found, however, that contraction of the muscles on the right side is required to pull the vertebral column into lateral bending to the right. Lateral bending to the left similarly requires the contraction of the left muscles of the vertebral column. This implies that in some respects the vertebral column has an inherent stability due to the arrangement of its joints and ligaments. Lateral bending is associated with rotation of the vertebrae to the opposite side. This is most marked in the thoracic region where a rotation of 20° occurs in lateral bending. This is not seen in the lumbar region where practically no rotation occurs. Scoliosis (p. 325) is always associated with rotation.

Rotation is most marked in the cervical region and amounts to about 90° to the right or left. Of this about 45° takes place between the atlas and axis. It is estimated that there are about 35° of rotation to one side in the thoracic region and very little in the lumbar region (about 10–15°).

Rotation is brought about by the oblique muscles. Posterior muscles, which pass obliquely upwards and outwards behind the axis of movement, for example the splenius capitis, iliocostalis, longissimus, rotate the vertebrae to the same side. Anterior muscles which pass upwards and inwards in front of the axis of movement, for example the scalene muscles, also produce rotation to the same side. Posterior muscles which pass upwards and inwards behind the axis of rotation produce rotation to the opposite side, for example the trapezius and transversospinalis. Anterior muscles passing upwards and outwards in front of the axis of movement produce rotation to the opposite side, for example the sternocleidomastoid. Some of the anterior abdominal muscles are involved in rotation. For example, the right external oblique and the left internal oblique rotate the trunk to the left.

Movements between the atlas and skull and atlas and axis are more complicated than would appear from the foregoing description. The alar ligaments, passing laterally from the dens to the occipital condyle, would prevent rotation were there not a descent of the atlas due to the convex surfaces of the facets of the lateral atlanto-axial joints. This slackens the ligaments and the slackening is increased by a backward tilting of the atlas. The small muscles of this region contain a large number of muscle spindles. This makes possible the fine adjustment of the position of the head so that the eyes can be used more efficiently.

The Contents of the Vertebral Canal

These include the spinal cord, the spinal nerve roots and the beginnings of the spinal nerves, the meninges of the cord and the blood vessels.

The Spinal Cord and Spinal Nerves. The cord is about 45 cm long and extends from the foramen magnum to about the level of the disc between the first and second lumbar vertebrae. The lower end of the cord is cone-shaped (*conus medullaris*) and the apex of the cone continues downwards as the *filum terminale* (*terminal thread*), which together with the meninges extends into the sacral canal and eventually fuses with the back of the coccyx. Early in fetal life the spinal cord is the same length as the vertebral canal. The vertebral column grows in length much more than the cord and early in childhood the cord reaches its adult level. Due to this differential growth the roots of the spinal nerves which originally pass horizontally to their appropriate intervertebral foramen become more oblique towards the lower end of the spinal cord, with the result that the lumbar and sacral nerve roots pass downwards round the filum terminale towards their foramina and form the *cauda equina (horse's tail)* in the lower lumbar and sacral part of the vertebral canal.

The spinal cord is nearly circular in section and is about 1 cm in diameter with two enlargements: (1) in the lower cervical region for the nerve supply of the upper limb; (2) in the lumbar region for the nerve supply of the lower limb. Emerging from the spinal cord on each side there are the ventral and dorsal rootlets which form the 31 pairs of spinal nerves (eight cervical, 12 thoracic, five lumbar, five sacral and one coccygeal). The rootlets having emerged from the ventrolateral and dorsilateral aspects of the cord form the ventral and dorsal roots (figure 10). Each dorsal root has a ganglion on it (the dorsal root ganglion) and a ventral and dorsal root unite to form a spinal nerve at the interverte-bral foramen. The result is that the cauda equina is formed by the roots of the lumbar and sacral nerves.

A section of the spinal cord at any level has certain common features (figure 207). The fluted column of grey matter appears in the form of the letter H with narrow, somewhat elongated *dorsal horns*, bulbous shorter *ventral horns* and a small

central canal in the cross-limb of the H. The white matter surrounds the grey in the form of columns and between the two *dorsal columns*, the *posterior median septum* extends from the posterior surface to the grey matter. Anteriorly the *anterior median fissure* separates the anterior columns.

There are eight cervical nerves because the first emerges above the first cervical vertebra and the eighth below the seventh cervical vertebra. Inferior to this vertebra a spinal nerve emerges below its corresponding vertebra. The level of the origin of the upper cervical nerves from the spinal cord more or less corresponds to the level of their inter-vertebral foramina. The lower cervical nerves emerge from their intervertebral foramina at a level about one vertebra lower than their segmental origin. The differences in level of the middle thoracic spinal nerves is about two vertebrae and the lower thoracic about three. The lower lumbar and sacral nerve roots emerge from the spinal cord at about the level of the first lumbar vertebra.

The Spinal Meninges (figure 207). The *dura mater* is the outermost of the meninges and extends from the foramen magnum to the filum terminale with which it fuses at about the level of the second sacral vertebra. It is a tough fibrous membrane

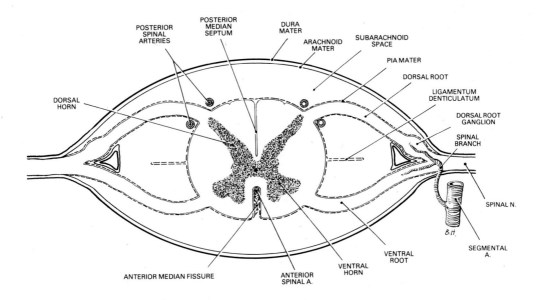

Figure 207   A transverse section of the spinal cord, its meninges and arteries.

which is continuous with the inner layer of cranial dura mater. The roots of the spinal nerves take a sheath of dura mater with them and the dura fuses with the epineurium of the spinal nerves and is attached to the periosteum at the edge of the intervertebral foramen. Between the dura and the vertebral canal there is the *epidural space* which contains thin-walled veins and fat. The quantity of semifluid fat in the space and blood in the veins varies with changes in the intrathoracic and intra-abdominal pressure.

Caudal analgesia involving only the sacral nerves can be achieved by injecting an anaesthetic into the epidural space through the sacral hiatus which is about 5 cm behind the tip of the coccyx. The roots of the appropriate nerves are anaesthetised as they form the cauda equina in the sacral canal. This is used in obstetrics in order to anaesthetise that part of the perineum innervated by the second, third and fourth sacral nerves.

The *arachnoid (mater)* of the spinal cord is a thin delicate membrane lining the dura mater. It is continuous with the arachnoid of the brain and extends for a short distance along the emerging spinal nerve rootlets. Between it and the underlying pia mater there is the *subarachnoid space* containing the *cerebrospinal fluid*. The subarachnoid space ends inferiorly at the level of the second sacral vertebra. Because of this the procedure called *lumbar puncture* can be used to obtain a specimen of cerebrospinal fluid without danger to the spinal cord. A hollow needle is inserted in the midline between the spinous processes of the third and fourth or fourth and fifth lumbar vertebrae. (With the back flexed the transverse plane through the highest points of the iliac crests is usually at the level of the space between the third and fourth lumbar spinous processes.) Lumbar puncture can also be used to inject substances into the subarachnoid space, for example penicillin.

The third of the meninges is the *pia mater*, which is closely applied to the surface of the spinal cord and enters the anterior median fissure. It also forms the posterior median septum in the midline of the posterior half of the spinal cord. The pia mater, arachnoid and an extension of the subarachnoid space are carried into the spinal cord with branches of the spinal arteries which lie on

its surface. The superficial part of the pia mater consists of loose connective tissue containing large numbers of blood vessels. Its deeper part is closely related to the non-neuronal elements (*glia*) of the spinal cord.

On each side the pia mater extends laterally as the *ligamentum denticulatum*, a longitudinal septum which has a lateral free edge except for the regular tooth-like processes which are attached to the arachnoid and dura between the upper 21 spinal nerves. The highest is attached at the level of the foramen magnum and the lowest at the level of the twelfth thoracic nerve. The first lumbar nerve as it passes to its intervertebral foramen can be identified because it crosses the last tooth of the ligament.

The Blood Supply of the Spinal Cord. The arteries to the spinal cord are from two main sources. The longitudinal arteries from the vertebral artery arise near the foramen magnum. The *anterior spinal artery* is formed by the union of a branch from each vertebral artery and runs downwards next to the anterior median fissure (figure 207). The *posterior spinal arteries*, one or two on each side, run downwards near the emerging dorsal rootlets. The second group of arteries are *segmental* and come from the spinal branches of the cervical, vertebral, posterior intercostal, lumbar and sacral arteries. They are most evident in the region of the spinal cord enlargements. An anterior branch of a segmental artery in the region of the twelfth thoracic vertebra is specially important because it is large and is the main blood supply to the anterior part of the cord below that level.

The Vertebral Venous Plexuses (figure 208). The plexuses lie in semifluid fat within the vertebral canal and outside the dura mater in the epidural space. There are two anterior longitudinal veins on the posterior surfaces of the vertebral bodies and two posterior longitudinal veins on each side of the midline anterior to the vertebral arches. These longitudinal channels (1) have large numbers of cross-connections and anteroposterior communications, with each other; (2) receive the veins from the spinal cord and the basivertebral veins from the vertebral bodies; (3) communicate with the

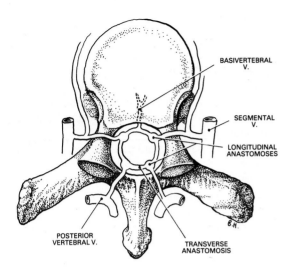

Figure 208   The vertebral venous plexuses.

vertebral, posterior intercostal, lumbar and sacral veins through intervertebral segmental veins; (4) anastomose with external venous plexuses on the anterior surfaces of the vertebral bodies and posterior surface of the laminae. The vertebral venous plexuses communicate superiorly with the intracranial venous sinuses and inferiorly with the pelvic veins. The vessels of the plexuses are thin-walled with no valves. Blood can flow in both directions and its volume can be changed with changes in intrathoracic and intra-abdominal pressure. The communications with the pelvis make it possible for cancer, infection and emboli to spread from the pelvis to the vertebral column and even the cranial cavity.

The veins of the spinal cord take the form of longitudinal vessels in the midline anteriorly and posteriorly and near the nerve roots. They have numerous anastomoses and drain into the internal vertebral plexus and segmental veins which go to the vertebral, intercostal and lumbar veins. Superiorly the veins communicate with the intracranial veins.

Some Further Considerations

The commonest congenital abnormalities have been described. They include some form of cervical rib related to the seventh cervical vertebra varying in its structure and length. Its motor and sensory effects on the branch of the first thoracic nerve which passes over it to the brachial plexus are referred to on p. 189. A unilateral lumbar rib related to the first lumbar vertebra is also a frequent anomaly (p. 64). Partial or complete fusion of the fifth lumbar vertebra with the sacrum and partial or complete separation of the first sacral vertebra to form an additional lumbar vertebra also occur.

One or more vertebral bodies may develop on only one side (*hemivertebra*) so that the vertebral column is concave on the undeveloped side. This is one cause of scoliosis. Failure of fusion posteriorly of the two halves of the vertebral arch, usually in the lower lumbar and sacral region, results in spina bifida. If only the bone is affected there may be no motor or sensory defects. Often the meninges, spinal cord and lumbar and sacral nerves are affected, resulting in sensory and motor defects of the lower limbs and disturbance of bladder and bowel functions.

Spondylolisthesis, in which the fifth lumbar vertebra together with the trunk slides forwards and downwards towards the pelvis, is often due to faulty development of the neural arch anterior to the inferior articular processes. The result is that the posterior half of the fifth lumbar vertebra is left behind, articulating with the superior sacral articular processes and attached to the ilia by the iliolumbar ligaments, and the body moves downwards and forwards. The marked angle between the fifth lumbar and first sacral vertebrae, in spite of the thick intervertebral disc, assists the downward and forward movement. The lumbar lordosis is accentuated, the height of the affected individual is decreased and because of the tension on the nerves forming the cauda equina there are motor and sensory defects along their distribution.

Injuries to the vertebral column can be very serious because of their effects on spinal nerves or their roots, and on the spinal cord. Fracture-dislocation of the upper cervical vertebrae usually causes death because of damage to the spinal cord. A less serious injury affecting adjacent cervical vertebrae is a dislocation of the articular processes on one side. An inferior articular process slides upwards and forwards too far and becomes wedged in the groove in front of the superior articular process of the vertebra below. This usually causes pressure on the spinal nerve between the two vertebrae. A bilateral dislocation of this type usually results in damage to the cord.

Compression-fractures of the bodies of the thoracic vertebrae occur due to excessive flexion arising from pressure on the shoulders, as in a roof fall in a mine, and affects the lower vertebrae (about the level of the tenth thoracic) where there is greatest mobility. In the absence of fracture of the articular processes the spinal cord and nerves escape injury. If the cord is injured, sensation and movement in the lower limbs are decreased or lost, and bladder, rectal and genital functions are affected.

Injury to the intervertebral discs has already been referred to (p. 328). This is thought to be due to lifting heavy weights by means of straightening the flexed trunk. In this situation the disc is compressed anteriorly and tensed posteriorly to an excessive degree. The result is that the anulus fibrosus is torn. This most commonly affects the disc between the fourth and fifth lumbar or fifth lumbar and first sacral vertebrae. The disc is damaged posterolaterally and the nucleus pulposus is squeezed out and presses on the fourth or fifth lumbar nerve. There is pain along the distribution of the nerve and the muscles supplied by the nerve are weakened. If the tear is central some of the roots forming the cauda equina may be affected. The other commonly affected discs are those between the fifth and sixth and sixth and seventh cervical vertebrae. A central prolapse of the nucleus pulposus through the anulus pulposus may press on the spinal cord. It is thought that these two regions are most commonly affected because they lie where there is considerable movement and where the curves of the vertebral column are changing direction. It is important that workers learn how to lift and carry heavy weights with the minimum flexion strain on the vertebral column.

Low back pain is common but only a small percentage of cases is due to prolapsed discs. It may be brought on by a sudden movement of the vertebral column, especially flexion. Any of the ligaments may be torn, the synovial membrane may be nipped between the articular processes or only the outer fibres of the anulus are damaged without a prolapse of the nucleus. All these structures except the inner part of the synovial membrane have a sensory innervation associated with pain. The cause of most cases of low back pain is not known and is not related to work involving lifting heavy weights.

A spinal nerve in the intervertebral foramen lies behind the body and intervertebral disc and in front of the zygapophyseal joint. Degeneration of the disc results in a narrowing of the foramen and arthritic changes in the joints may result in osteophytic outgrowths from the edges of the bones forming the joints. Pressure on the spinal nerve leads to sensory and motor disturbances along its distribution. This most commonly occurs in the lower cervical and lower lumbar regions of the vertebral column.

Part 6

The Upper Limb

26

The Shoulder Region

Man is the only primate in whom the upper limb normally has almost no locomotor function. The upper limb is completely free for use in grasping and moving objects and also for carrying out skilled, accurate, delicate movements such as are involved in writing and many occupations. For this purpose the hand has an especially rich nerve supply both motor and sensory. These skills depend, however, on the large motor and sensory representation of the hand in the human cerebral cortex. It has been suggested that the characteristic upright posture adopted by man probably more than two million years ago freed the upper limb for additional functions and, as a result of this, the human brain developed and enlarged into its present form.

The upper limbs develop as outgrowths from the body wall when the embryo is about 4 weeks old. The limb develops at the level of the lower cervical and first thoracic segments and very early on the segmental nerves grow into the limb bud which eventually differentiates into an upper arm, forearm and hand in that order.

The upper limb is attached to the trunk by the pectoral girdle, consisting of the clavicle and scapula which articulate with the axial skeleton only at the sternoclavicular joint. Elsewhere the girdle is attached to the head, neck and thorax almost entirely by muscles. As a result the pectoral girdle can move on the trunk and the mobility of the upper limb is greatly increased.

Distal to the pectoral girdle the upper limb is formed by the upper arm (*brachium*), forearm (*antebrachium*), wrist (*carpus*) and hand. (The *upper arm* is the best term for this part of the limb because the word *arm* is confused with the whole limb.) The upper arm articulates with the scapula at the shoulder joint, the forearm with the upper arm at the elbow joint and the hand with the forearm at the wrist joint.

The Pectoral Girdle and Humerus

The pectoral girdle consists of the *clavicle* and *scapula*.

The clavicle (figures 2, 3, 4, 209)

Commonly called the *collar bone*, the clavicle is elongated and tubular with a rounded medial end which articulates with the upper lateral angle of the manubrium sterni and the first costal cartilage (the *sternoclavicular joint*), and a flattened lateral end which articulates with the medial edge of the acromion of the scapula (the *acromioclavicular joint*). Laterally the anterior border of the clavicle is concave and medially it is convex. The inferior surface is roughened at either end for ligaments. The lateral area has a posterior *conoid tubercle*. Between the two ligamentous areas there is a groove for the subclavius muscle.

The clavicle acts like a strut, holding the upper limb away from the body. When it is fractured, most commonly at the junction of the outer and middle thirds, the weight of the upper limb carries the outer fragment downwards and inwards.

(a)   STERNAL
           END   ACROMIAL
                                                                                  END

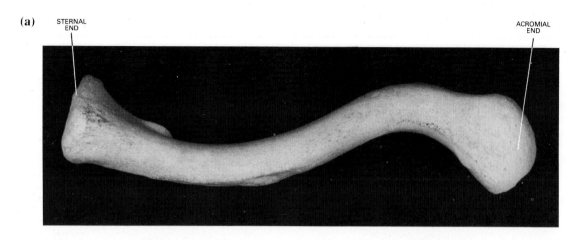

(b) STERNAL   FOR COSTO-   FOR CORACO-   ACROMIAL
         END   CLAVICULAR LIGAMENT   CLAVICULAR LIGAMENT   END

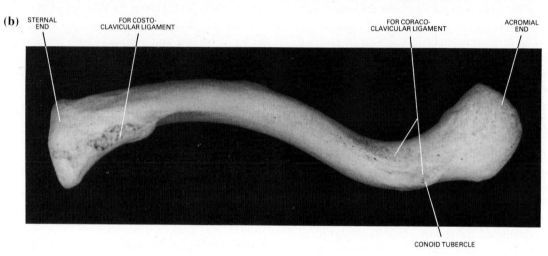

CONOID TUBERCLE

Figure 209   The left clavicle: (a) superior surface; (b) inferior surface.

The clavicle *ossifies* before any other bone in the body in the fifth week of intra-uterine life in mesenchyme. It is therefore usually described as ossifying in membrane because there is no cartilaginous precursor. Shortly after ossification has begun, cartilage appears at each end of the bone and growth occurs at the ends in the usual manner of longitudinal growth in long bones (p. 345). An epiphysis appears at the sternal end at about 16 or 17 years and fuses with the rest of the clavicle at about 25 years.

The scapula (figures 2, 3, 210)

Commonly called the *shoulder blade*, the scapula is a triangular bone which lies on the posterolateral surface of the thoracic cage extending from the second to the seventh ribs. It has a vertical *medial border* which is about 8 cm from the midline, a more or less horizontal *superior border* on which there is the *scapular notch*, and an oblique *lateral border* passing downwards and inwards to meet the medial border. The *angles* of the triangle are called *superior* (above and medial), *inferior* (below and medial) and *lateral* (above and lateral). At the lateral angle there is a pear-shaped concave area, the *glenoid cavity*, which is narrower above and has a raised edge. The *supraglenoid* and *infraglenoid tubercles* are on the upper and lower borders of the glenoid cavity respectively. The

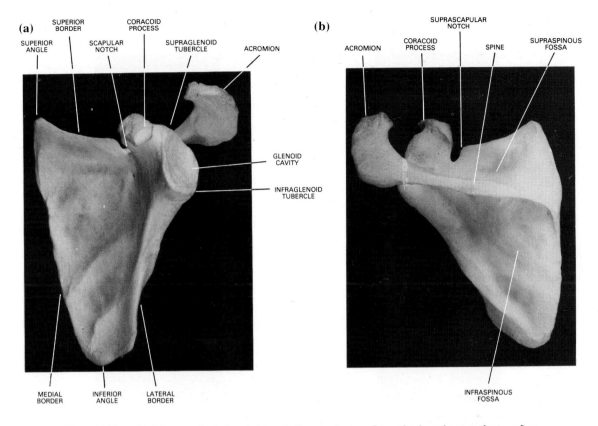

(a)

SUPERIOR
ANGLE

SUPERIOR
BORDER

SCAPULAR
NOTCH

CORACOID
PROCESS

SUPRAGLENOID
TUBERCLE

ACROMION

GLENOID
CAVITY

INFRAGLENOID
TUBERCLE

MEDIAL
BORDER

INFERIOR
ANGLE

LATERAL
BORDER

(b)

SUPRASCAPULAR
NOTCH

ACROMION

CORACOID
PROCESS

SPINE

SUPRASPINOUS
FOSSA

INFRASPINOUS
FOSSA

Figure 210   The left scapula: (a) costal (ventral, anterior) surface; (b) dorsal (posterior) surface.

head of the humerus articulates with the glenoid cavity which with the scapula in its normal position faces as much forwards as laterally.

The main part of the scapula has two surfaces. The *costal surface* is anterior, lies on the ribs and is slightly concave (the *subscapular fossa*). It has several ridges on it. The *dorsal surface* has a more or less horizontal shelf projecting backwards. This is the *spine of the scapula* which divides the dorsal surface into an upper quarter called the *supraspinous fossa* and a lower three-quarters called the *infraspinous fossa*. The fossae communicate round the lateral border of the spine medial to the glenoid cavity. The spine itself has a posterior edge with upper and lower borders. If followed laterally these borders separate widely as the spine turns forwards to form the acromion (*acros = topmost, omos = shoulder*, Greek) which has medial and lateral borders. The facet for the lateral end of the

clavicle is on the medial border.

The coracoid process (*corax = raven*, Greek; refers to the beak) projects forwards from the lateral end of the upper border of the scapula lateral to the scapular notch.

The scapula *ossifies* in cartilage at about the eighth week of intra-uterine life from a primary centre for the main part of the bone and the spine. There are several secondary centres most of which appear at puberty and fuse at about 25 years (the inferior angle, medial border, acromion, and lower part of the glenoid cavity). The major part of the coracoid process has a secondary centre which appears at 1 year after birth and fuses with the rest of the scapula at 14 years. Before this fusion another secondary centre for the coracoid process and adjacent part of the glenoid cavity appears. Fusion in this region is complete by 14 years.

(a)

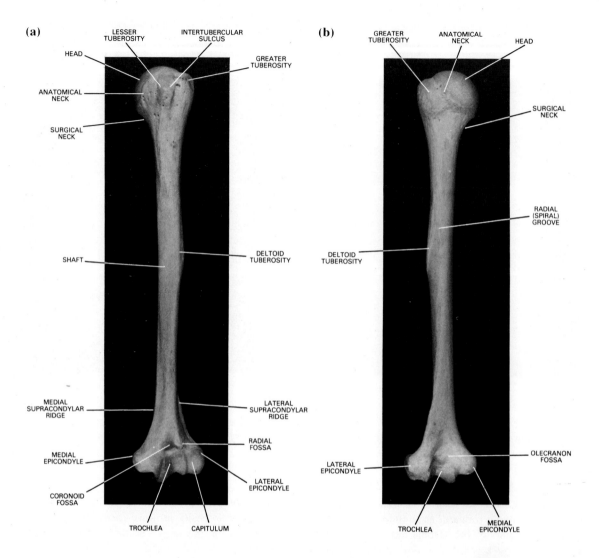

(b)

Figure 211   **The left humerus: (a) anterior view; (b) posterior view; (c) ossification.**

The humerus (figure 211)

This is the bone of the upper arm. In the anatomical position the bone appears twisted so that the upper end, the *head*, faces backwards. The main part of the bone, the *shaft*, is more or less cylindrical in its upper part but becomes flattened lower down and triangular in section with a broad *posterior surface* and *anterolateral* and *anteromedial surfaces*.

The upper end has a round head which faces medially and backwards and articulates with the glenoid cavity. The head is separated from the rest of the bone by a shallow groove, the *anatomical neck*. The *greater tuberosity* is a prominence on the lateral side of the head and anatomical neck. The *lesser tuberosity* is a smaller prominence in front of the head and neck. Between the prominences is the vertical *intertubercular sulcus* which continues on to the shaft beyond the tuberosities. The slightly constricted part of the shaft just distal to the tuberosities is called the *surgical neck* because it is one of the commoner sites of fractures of the humerus.

The shaft of the humerus has on the middle of

(c)

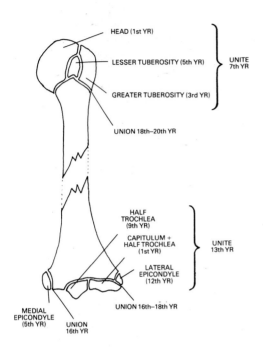

HEAD (1st YR)

LESSER TUBEROSITY (5th YR)

GREATER TUBEROSITY (3rd YR)

} UNITE 7th YR

UNION 18th–20th YR

HALF TROCHLEA (9th YR)

CAPITULUM + HALF TROCHLEA (1st YR)

LATERAL EPICONDYLE (12th YR)

} UNITE 13th YR

MEDIAL EPICONDYLE (5th YR)

UNION 16th YR

UNION 16th–18th YR

its lateral surface a V-shaped raised area called the *deltoid tuberosity*. On its posterior surface, passing downwards and laterally, there is the *groove for the radial nerve*. The lateral and medial borders of the shaft form the *lateral* and *medial supracondylar crests* as they pass downwards towards the lower end of the humerus.

The distal end is called the *condyle* (*condylos* = knob, *knuckle*, Greek). Above the articular area anteriorly there are two hollows, a small lateral *radial fossa* and a larger medial *coronoid fossa*. Posteriorly there is the single deep *olecranon fossa*. The articular area on the distal surface of the condyle is divided into a lateral rounded *capitulum* which faces forwards and does not extend on to the back of the condyle and a medial *trochlea* (*trochlea* = *pulley*, Latin). The trochlea extends on to the posterior surface and is separated laterally from the capitulum by a ridge. On the medial side the ridge separating the trochlea from the projection called the medial epicondyle is much more marked. The groove running anteroposteriorly in the trochlea divides it into a larger medial and smaller lateral area.

The lateral supracondylar crest ends in a prominence, the *lateral epicondyle*, which is the non-articular area lateral to the capitulum. On the medial side of the condyle there is a much larger projection called the *medial epicondyle* which has the vertical groove for the ulnar nerve on its posterior surface.

The main features of the *ossification of a long bone* are as follows. A cartilaginous model of the bone is formed at about 6 weeks of intra-uterine life. The cartilage is replaced by bone, hence the term *endochondral ossification*. This process begins in the outer part of the middle of the shaft at about 7 or 8 weeks of intra-uterine life (the *primary centre of ossification*) and spreads proximally and distally. At birth the *shaft* or *diaphysis* consists of bone and the ends (the *epiphyses*) are usually cartilaginous. At various times after birth one or more *secondary centres of ossification* appear in the middle of the epiphysis or epiphyses and extend outwards. The epiphysis remains separated from the diaphysis by a plate of cartilage (the *epiphyseal* or *growth plate*) and growth in length continues until about 18 years in the male and 16 years in the female when the epiphysis fuses with the diaphysis and the growth plate is ossified.

One end of the bone grows more rapidly and fuses later than the other end and is called the *growing end*. It is important to note that growth takes place at both ends. The growing end usually begins to ossify before the opposite end and the main nutrient artery of the bone is directed away from the growing end. In the upper limb the growing ends are at the shoulder and wrist and in the lower limb they are at the knee (figure 259). The appearance of primary and secondary centres of ossification as well as the fusion of epiphysis with the shaft occur earlier in females than in males.

Short long bones, such as the metacarpals of the hand, the metatarsals of the foot and the phalanges, develop and ossify in a similar way but have an epiphysis at only one end. *Short bones* such as the carpal (wrist) and tarsal (foot) bones develop by endochondral ossification and in a manner similar to the way in which the epiphysis of a long bone ossifies.

A knowledge of the ossification of bones enables one to understand certain aspects of growth and to interpret X-rays. In some circumstances ossification is the main means used to establish the age of an individual and the stage of ossification may reflect his or her nutritional status. Certain diseases affect only epiphyses and injuries can involve the epiphyseal cartilage with marked effects on the growth of the bone.

The humerus *ossifies* in cartilage from a primary centre in the shaft which appears at about 8 weeks of intra-uterine life. At birth both ends are cartilaginous. The proximal end is the growing end.

There are three secondary centres in the proximal end and four in the distal, as indicated in figure 211(c). The times given for the beginning of ossification are approximate. The epiphyseal centres at the proximal end form one epiphysis by 7 years which joins the shaft at about 18 years in males. The lateral three at the distal end fuse together but the epiphysis for the medial epicondyle remains separate (there is often a tongue of bone extending downwards from the shaft between the medial epicondyle and the trochlea). These epiphyses fuse with the shaft at about 16 years in males. In injuries involving the elbow region the separate epiphysis of the medial condyle has to be kept in mind. The age of the patient, the appearance of the edges of the apparent fracture and X-raying the uninjured side help to make a diagnosis.

The Skin and Surface Features of the Shoulder Region

The Skin

Over most of the shoulder region the skin shows no special features except in the axilla (the armpit) where it is invariably hairy after puberty and contains apocrine sweat glands. In the axilla the deep surface of the skin is attached to the underlying tissue.

The skin above the clavicle is supplied by the fourth cervical spinal cord segment through the supraclavicular nerves (C3, 4). Over the shoulder and extending down the lateral side of the upper arm the segment is the fifth cervical and the nerve supplying this area is the upper lateral cutaneous nerve of the upper arm (C5), a branch of the

axillary nerve. Below the clavicle the skin on the chest is supplied by the first and second thoracic segments through the first and second intercostal nerves (T1 and 2). Both segments pass into the axilla and down the medial side of the upper arm with the first thoracic segment lateral to and extending further than the second. A branch from the second intercostal nerve and the medial cutaneous nerve of the upper arm carry the fibres of the second and first thoracic segments respectively.

There is a considerable overlap of the innervation of the skin by neighbouring segments. For example, the main area innervated by the first thoracic segment is on the medial side of the upper arm but it extends upwards into the axilla and across to the thorax, and downwards into the upper part of the medial side of the forearm. The upper part of this area is overlapped by the second thoracic segment and the lower part by the eighth cervical.

The Surface Markings

Anteriorly, lateral to the midline jugular notch, *the* medial end of the clavicle *projects above the level of the articular area for the clavicle on the manubrium. The groove due to the* sternoclavicular joint *can be felt. The whole of the* clavicle *is subcutaneous and its medial forward convexity and lateral forward concavity can be followed to the flat, lateral end which is slightly higher than the* acromion *and indicates the position of the* acromioclavicular joint. *The curve from the neck to the shoulder is formed by the* trapezius muscle. *The acromion is subcutaneous and if followed backwards and then medially leads to the* spine of the scapula *which is also subcutaneous. The medial end of the scapular spine is normally at the level of the spinous process of the third thoracic vertebra. The* inferior angle of the scapula *is at the level of the seventh thoracic spinous process and is easily felt. In various movements involving the shoulder girdle the inferior angle can usually be seen to move. The extent to which the scapula projects backwards from the chest wall is very variable. If the head and neck are bent forwards the* spinous processes *of the* seventh cervical *and* first *and* second thoracic vertebrae *are visible.*

The roundness of the shoulder is due to the underlying muscle, the deltoid, *and the* upper end of the humerus. *If the muscle wastes and/or the head is dislocated the roundness is lost. In the anatomical position the* greater tuberosity *is felt laterally and the* lesser tuberosity *anteriorly. The* coracoid process *is palpable below the lateral third of the clavicle in a hollow between the deltoid laterally and the* pectoralis major *medially. This hollow is called the* infraclavicular fossa. *Above the clavicle between the trapezius laterally and the* sternocleidomastoid *medially there is the* greater supraclavicular fossa *(the* lesser *is between the sternal and clavicular heads of the sternocleidomastoid muscle) in which the chief structures are the* subclavian vessels *and* trunks of the brachial plexus *and some of their branches (p. 277).*

The *breast* is described on p. 12 in the section on the thorax.

The Anterior and Lateral Muscles of the Shoulder Region (figure 212)

The Pectoralis Major. This is a large muscle on the anterior thoracic wall and has two heads (figure 212(a)). The *clavicular head* is attached to the medial half of the anterior surface of the clavicle. The *sternocostal head*, attached to the anterior surface of the sternum and upper costal cartilages, extends downwards on to the rectus sheath. The fibres pass laterally to the humerus. The sternocostal head twists as it approaches the bone and passes deep to the clavicular head. Both heads are attached to the lateral lip of the intertubercular groove. The muscle is supplied by the lateral (C5, 6, 7) and medial (C8, T1) pectoral nerves from the lateral and medial cords respectively of the brachial plexus.

Acting together, the two heads adduct and medially rotate the upper arm at the shoulder joint.

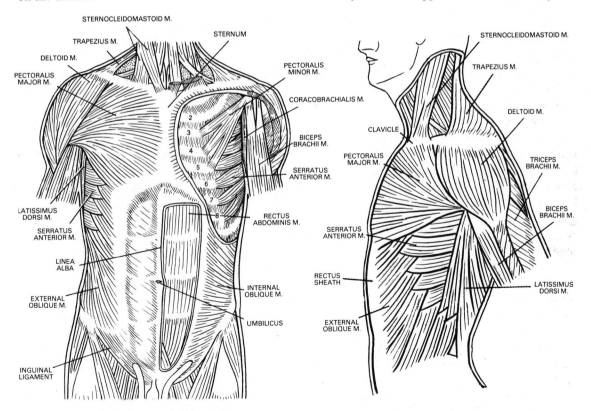

Figure 212 (a) The muscles of the front of the chest and upper part of the upper arm (the pectoralis major and deltoid have been removed on the left side). (b) A lateral view of the superficial muscles of the left upper arm.

The clavicular head is a flexor of the upper arm from the anatomical position and the sternocostal head extends the flexed upper arm. If the humerus is fixed the pectoralis major may assist the expansion of the thoracic cage in forced respiration.

The Pectoralis Minor. This muscle is deep to the pectoralis major (figure 212(a)). It is attached to the anterior surfaces of the third, fourth and fifth ribs, and passes upwards and laterally to be attached to the medial border of the coracoid process. Its nerve supply is mainly from the medial pectoral nerve. The pectoralis minor pulls the scapula forwards round the chest wall and rotates the scapula so that the glenoid cavity looks downwards. (Its line of pull is below the axis of rotation.)

The Subclavius. As its name implies, this muscle is inferior to the clavicle. It is attached to the inferior surface of that bone and passes downwards and medially to the first rib and costal cartilage. Its nerve supply is from the upper trunk (C5, 6) of the brachial plexus and its action is probably to pull the tip of the shoulder downwards.

The *clavipectoral fascia* extends from the clavicle to the pectoralis minor. It splits to enclose the subclavius and also surrounds the pectoralis minor. More laterally the clavipectoral fascia is attached to the fascia round the axillary blood vessels. The fascia is pierced by the cephalic vein as it passes to the axillary vein, the acromiothoracic artery as it becomes superficial, the lateral pectoral nerve as it goes to supply the pectoralis major and lymphatic vessels passing from the infraclavicular lymph nodes to the axillary nodes.

The clavicle, subclavius muscle, clavipectoral fascia and pectoralis minor form a continuous layer deep to the pectoralis major in front of the contents of the axilla.

The Deltoid (figures 212, 213). As the name suggests it is a triangular muscle with the base superior and the apex inferior, like an inverted capital delta in Greek. The upper attachment of the muscle is to the lateral half of the anterior surface of the clavicle, the outer border of the acromion and almost the whole of the lower edge of the scapular

spine. The fibres pass downwards and converge on to the deltoid tuberosity on the middle of the outer surface of the shaft of the humerus. The muscle is supplied by the axillary nerve (C5, 6) from the posterior cord of the brachial plexus.

The anterior and posterior fibres are straight. The middle fibres from the acromion form a multipennate muscle; that is, there are more or less parallel tendinous intersections to which short oblique muscle fibres are attached. The whole muscle is the main abductor of the humerus at the shoulder joint. The anterior fibres flex and medially rotate the humerus and the posterior fibres extend and laterally rotate the humerus at the shoulder joint.

The Posterior Muscles of the Shoulder Region (figure 213)

There are two large, superficial muscles which cover a number of muscles either joining the scapula to the vertebral column or the scapula to the humerus.

The Trapezius (figure 213). A *trapezium* is an irregular four-sided figure. Perhaps both muscles form a trapezium since each is triangular. The muscle has a long midline attachment to the external occipital protuberance, the ligamentum nuchae and the spinous processes of the seventh cervical and all the thoracic vertebrae. The upper fibres pass laterally and downwards to the lateral half of the posterior surface of the clavicle, the middle fibres pass directly laterally to the medial border of the acromion and the inferior fibres laterally and upwards to the upper border of the spine of the scapula. The trapezius is supplied by the spinal accessory nerve. The cell bodies of the fibres supplying the muscle are in the lateral horn of the upper cervical segments of the spinal cord. The spinal accessory nerve also supplies the sternocleidomastoid and reaches the trapezius by passing downwards and backwards across the posterior triangle (p. 238).

Both trapezius muscles brace back and shrug the shoulders and extend the head. A paralysed trapezius results in a dropped shoulder. One trapezius turns the head to the opposite side and tilts the

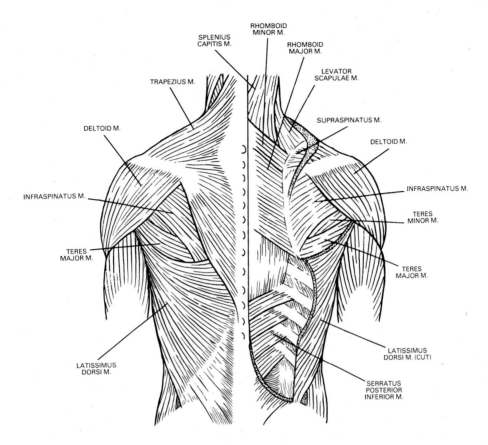

Figure 213 A posterior view of the muscles of the upper arm (the trapezius and lower medial part of the latissimus dorsi have been removed on the right side).

head towards the shoulder of the same side. The lower fibres attached to the *upper* border of the scapular spine rotate the scapula so that the glenoid cavity faces upwards. This action can only be performed in conjunction with the serratus anterior.

The Latissimus Dorsi (figure 213). This also has a long midline origin from the spinous processes of the lower thoracic vertebrae and the lumbar and sacral vertebrae through its attachment to the posterior layer of the thoracolumbar fascia. Its upper part is deep to the lower part of the trapezius. The latissimus dorsi is also attached to the iliac crest. As the muscle passes upwards and laterally towards the humerus it is joined by muscular slips from the lower four ribs and some fibres from the inferior angle of the scapula. The muscle ends in a

tendon which winds round the lower border of the teres major muscle and also twists so that the lowest fibres of the latissimus dorsi become uppermost. The tendon is attached to the floor of the intertubercular sulcus behind the tendon of the long head of the biceps brachii which lies in the groove. The latissimus dorsi forms part of the posterior wall of the axilla and is innervated by a branch of the posterior cord of the brachial plexus, the thoracodorsal nerve (C6, 7, 8).

The muscle is an extensor and medial rotator of the humerus at the shoulder joint. It also contracts in coughing, that is it assists expiration against an obstruction.

Deep to the latissimus dorsi the *serratus posterior inferior* runs upwards and laterally from the thoracolumbar fascia to the lower ribs (p. 330).

The Levator Scapulae, Rhomboid Minor and Rhomboid Major (figure 213). These three muscles, deep to the trapezius, are attached to the vertebrae and the medial border of the scapula. The *levator scapulae* is attached to the transverse processes of the upper four cervical vertebrae and passes downwards and backwards to the upper part of the medial border of the scapula. It is almost vertical and its action is to lift the scapula as in shrugging the shoulders. Its nerve supply is from the ventral rami of the upper cervical nerves.

The *rhomboid muscles* (the *minor* is above the *major*) are attached medially to the spinous processes of the lower cervical and upper thoracic vertebrae, pass downwards and laterally and are attached to the medial border of the scapula, the minor to the area opposite the scapular spine. They are active in bracing back the shoulders and can rotate the scapula so that the glenoid cavity faces downwards. Normally they would be active only in a resisted movement of restoring to the neutral position a scapula already rotated so that the glenoid cavity faces upwards. The rhomboid muscles are innervated by a branch of the fifth cervical nerve (dorsal scapular nerve).

The Supraspinatus, Infraspinatus, Teres Minor and Teres Major (figure 213). These four muscles join the scapula to the upper end of the humerus. The *supraspinatus* is attached to the supraspinous fossa of the scapula and passes laterally below the acromion and above the head of the humerus to end in a tendon which is attached to the facet on the upper part of the greater tuberosity and also to the capsule of the shoulder joint. The *infraspinatus* is attached to the infraspinous fossa and passes laterally and upwards. Its tendon is attached to the upper of the two facets on the back of the greater tuberosity and to the capsule of the shoulder joint. The *teres minor* is attached to most of the lateral border of the scapula inferior to the glenoid cavity and passes laterally to the lower of the two facets on the back of the greater tuberosity and about 2 cm of the bone below the facet. This muscle is also attached to the capsule of the shoulder joint. The supra- and infraspinatus are supplied by the suprascapular nerve (C5, 6) from the upper trunk of the brachial plexus and the teres minor by the

axillary nerve (C5, 6). Both this nerve and the nerve to the rhomboids have their origin in the neck above the clavicle and reach the muscles by passing laterally across the posterior triangle and then deep to the trapezius.

The supraspinatus is an abductor at the shoulder joint. Its role in this movement is discussed with movements at that joint. The infraspinatus and teres minor are lateral rotators of the humerus at the shoulder joint.

The *teres major* is attached to the lower part of the lateral border of the scapula and the posterior surface of the inferior angle (*teres = round*, Latin). The muscle runs laterally and upwards and reaches the anterior aspect of the upper end of the humerus to become attached to the medial lip of the intertubercular sulcus. As it passes forwards the tendon of the teres major lies in front of the long head of the triceps brachii which passed downwards from the infraglenoid tubercle of the scapula. The teres minor lies behind the long head. The way in which the latissimus dorsi winds round the lower border of the teres major to reach the floor of the intertubercular sulcus has already been described.

The teres major is an extensor and medial rotator of the humerus. With the upper arm abducted at the shoulder joint the teres major and the latissimus dorsi adduct the humerus against resistance. The teres major receives its nerve supply from the posterior cord of the brachial plexus through the lower subscapular nerve (C6, 7).

The Subscapularis and Serratus Anterior. These muscles are related to the costal (anterior) surface of the scapula. The *subscapularis* is a multipennate muscle attached to the ridges on the costal surface of the scapula. The muscle fibres pass upwards and laterally and are attached by a tendon to the lesser tuberosity of the humerus and to the capsule of the shoulder joint.

Together with the supraspinatus, infraspinatus and teres minor, the subscapularis forms the *rotator cuff*, a slightly misleading name because the supraspinatus is an abductor. This cuff of muscles helps to keep the disproportionately large head of the humerus in the shallow glenoid cavity during movements at the shoulder joint.

The subscapularis is supplied by the upper and

lower subscapular nerves (C5,6) from the posterior cord of the brachial plexus and is a medial rotator of the humerus at the shoulder joint.

The *quadrilateral (quadrangular) space* (figure 216) lies between the subscapularis superiorly, the teres major inferiorly, the shaft of the humerus laterally and the long head of the triceps medially. Behind the subscapularis, the capsule of the shoulder joint and the teres minor lie above the space through which the axillary nerve and the posterior circumflex artery pass. The most important of the superior relations is the shoulder joint because dislocation of the joint is downwards and not infrequently injures the nerve. Fractures in the region of the surgical neck of the humerus may also involve the nerve with resultant paralysis of the muscles supplied by the nerve, namely the deltoid and teres minor.

The *serratus anterior* (figure 212(a), (b)) arises by digitations from the sides of the upper eight ribs and passes backwards round the chest wall to be attached to the medial border of the scapula. The lower four digitations are attached near the inferior angle. The long thoracic nerve from the deep aspect of the fifth, sixth and seventh cervical spinal nerves runs downwards from the lower part of the posterior triangle on to the outer surface of the muscle and supplies it from its superficial surface. The nerve lies on the medial wall of the axilla where the lymph nodes draining the breast and upper limb are situated and may be damaged in surgical removal of the nodes.

The serratus anterior holds the scapula close to the chest wall, pulls the scapula forwards round the chest wall and by its action on the inferior angle rotates the scapula so that the glenoid cavity faces upwards. This last movement takes place when the upper limb is raised vertically alongside the head. If the nerve to the serratus anterior is damaged the inferior angle and medial border of the scapula project from the thoracic wall (*winging of the scapula*). This is greatly exaggerated in any movement which involves the muscle. The serratus

anterior because of its attachment to the ribs is regarded as an accessory muscle of respiration.

If the scapula is pulled forwards round the chest wall by the serratus anterior, an area called the *ausculatory triangle*, which is directly related to the chest wall without the intervention of muscles, lies between the trapezius above, the latissimus dorsi below, and the medial border of the scapula laterally.

The Biceps Brachii, Triceps Brachii (Long Head) and Coracobrachialis. These muscles begin in the region of the shoulder joint but belong to the upper arm. The *biceps brachii* has a *long head* whose tendon is attached to the supraglenoid tubercle and a *short head* which has a common attachment with the coracobrachialis to the tip of the coracoid process (figure 212(a)). The long tendon passes laterally and forwards over the head of the humerus inside the capsule of the shoulder joint and outside its synovial membrane. As it emerges from the capsule the tendon takes a sleeve of synovial membrane with it and is joined lower down by the short head of the muscle.

The *long head* of the *triceps brachii* (figure 216) is attached to the infraglenoid tubercle of the scapula and passes downwards in front of the teres minor and behind the teres major to join the lateral head on the back of the upper arm. The biceps and triceps brachii are described in more detail with the upper arm.

The *coracobrachialis* has an upper attachment to the tip of the coracoid process in common with the short head of the biceps brachii, and is attached inferiorly to the middle of the medial surface of the humerus. The musculocutaneous nerve (C5, 6, 7) enters the medial side of the muscle, passes through it and supplies it. The nerve is a branch of the lateral cord of the brachial plexus. The coracobrachialis is a weak flexor of the upper arm at the shoulder joint. In this movement the clavicular head of the pectoralis major and anterior fibres of the deltoid are much more important.

27

The Axilla

The *axilla* or *armpit* is a space bounded by anterior, posterior, lateral and medial walls. It extends upwards towards the neck with which the axilla communicates by means of a triangular space (the *apex* of the axilla) formed anteriorly by the clavicle, posteriorly by the upper border of the scapula and medially by the first rib (figure 4). Through this space the main blood and lymphatic vessels and nerves of the upper limb pass from and to the neck. The many lymph nodes in the axilla, together with the vessels and nerves, are embedded in fat.

The Walls of the Axilla

The anterior and posterior walls are mainly muscular. The *anterior wall* is formed superficially by the pectoralis major. *Its lower border forms the* anterior axillary fold *which can be palpated.* Deep to the pectoralis major there is another layer of structures forming part of the anterior wall, the clavicle, the subclavius, the clavipectoral fascia and the pectoralis minor.

The *posterior wall* is formed from above downwards by the subscapularis, latissimus dorsi and teres major muscles. More medially the lower border of the posterior wall is formed by the latissimus dorsi as it winds round the teres major. *The posterior wall descends to a lower level than the anterior and can be palpated as the* posterior axillary fold. *The* midaxillary line *is indicated by a vertical line on the thoracic wall midway between the axillary folds.*

The *lateral* and *medial walls* are bony with a muscle related to the bone. The lateral is formed by the shaft of the humerus and coracobrachialis, and the medial by the upper ribs and serratus anterior. *The lower part of the head and the medial side of the shaft of the humerus, and the upper ribs, can be palpated with the fingers in the axilla.*

The Axillary Artery and Vein (figure 214)

At the lateral border of the first rib the subclavian artery continues as the *axillary artery* and the *axillary vein* becomes the subclavian vein. The axillary artery extends to the lower border of the teres major where it becomes the *brachial artery*. The axillary vein which begins at the lower border of the teres major is a continuation of the *basilic vein*, a superficial vein of the forearm which perforates the deep fascia at the middle of the upper arm and continues upwards medial to the brachial artery. The axillary vein is medial to the axillary artery and both are crossed anteriorly by the pectoralis minor which traditionally divides the axillary artery into three parts.

The *main relations* of the axillary artery are as follows. The axillary vein lies medially and slightly anteriorly along its whole length. The two layers of the anterior wall of the axilla are anterior and the three muscles of the posterior wall are posterior. Since the artery crosses from the medial to the lateral wall, the first intercostal space, the serratus anterior and the long thoracic nerve are

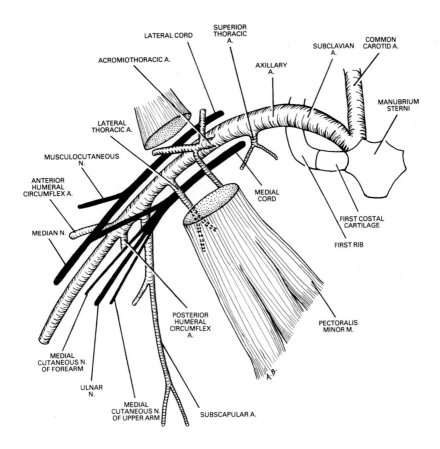

Figure 214   The axillary artery and part of the brachial plexus.

posterior to the first part of the axillary artery. The last part of the axillary artery is covered only by skin and fascia, that is inferior to the lower border of the pectoralis major, because the posterior wall reaches a lower level than the anterior wall. The coracobrachialis is lateral to the artery.

The *cords of the brachial plexus* are named in terms of their relation to the axillary artery, *lateral*, *posterior* and *medial*. The cords divide into their main branches deep to the pectoralis minor. The branches of the lateral cord, the *musculocutaneous nerve* and the *lateral head of the median nerve*, are lateral to the artery. The posterior cord continues as the *radial nerve* and gives off the *axillary nerve* both of which are posterior to the artery. The axillary nerve passes backwards between the subscapularis and teres major muscles. The medial cord continues medial to the artery as the *ulnar*

nerve. The *medial head of the median nerve* arises from the medial cord and crosses anterior to the artery to join the lateral head and form the *median nerve*. The other two branches of the medial cord, the *medial cutaneous nerves of the forearm* and *upper arm* lie medial to the artery, the former between the artery and vein and the latter medial to the vein.

The axillary vessels (and the brachial plexus) carry a continuation of the prevertebral part of the deep cervical fascia into the axilla. Medially this *axillary sheath* fuses with the clavipectoral fascia below the pectoralis minor. Infection in the axilla if deep to the axillary fascia may spread upwards into the neck. If superficial to the fascia an abscess spreads between the pectoral muscles and points either inferiorly at the lower border of the pectoralis major (the anterior axillary fold) or superiorly between the deltoid and pectoralis major.

Most of the *branches of the axillary artery* go to the walls of the axilla. The *subscapular artery* runs downwards on the posterior wall, the *superior* and *lateral thoracic arteries* go to the medial wall (the thorax) and the *acromiothoracic artery* to the anterior wall passing above the pectoralis minor. The subscapular artery is the largest branch and reaches the inferior angle of the scapula where it anastomoses with arteries on the chest wall and scapula. The *circumflex scapular artery*, a large branch of the subscapular artery, passes backwards next to the lateral border of the scapula through the *triangular space* which lies between the sub-scapularis above, the teres major below and the long head of the triceps brachii laterally.

The acromiothoracic artery gives branches to the pectoral muscles, the deltoid and the region of the acromion, including the acromioclavicular joint. The shoulder joint and neighbouring structures are supplied by the *anterior* and *posterior circumflex humeral arteries*. These arteries wind round the surgical neck of the humerus, the anterior passing laterally in front of the humerus and then backwards deep to all the muscles and the posterior passing backwards through the quadrilateral space with the axillary nerve.

The circumflex arteries in the region of the acromion anastomose with each other and with branches from the suprascapular and acromio-thoracic arteries. A number of arteries form the *scapular anastomosis* which links the subclavian artery with the third part of the axillary artery (figure 216). These are the suprascapular and trans-verse cervical branches of the subclavian artery, and from the axillary artery the subscapular artery and its circumflex scapular branch.

The *axillary vein*, which is regarded as a con-tinuation of the basilic vein beyond the lower border of the teres major, receives tributaries cor-responding with the branches of the artery. In addition the two *brachial veins* accompanying the brachial artery join the basilic vein after it pierces the deep fascia. The *cephalic vein*, the other large superficial vein, pierces the clavipectoral fascia and enters the terminal part of the axillary vein. The lateral axillary lymph nodes are closely related to the vein. The axillary vein becomes the subclavian vein at the outer border of the first rib.

The Brachial Plexus (figures 214, 215)

The formation of the brachial plexus in the lower part of the neck in the posterior triangle is des-cribed on p. 227. Briefly, the plexus is usually formed by the ventral rami of the fifth to the eighth cervical and first thoracic spinal nerves which emerge between the scalenus anterior and scalenus medius. These ventral rami constitute the *roots* of the plexus, a confusing name. The ventral rami join and form the *upper* (C5, 6), *middle* (C7) and *lower* (C8 and T1) *trunks*, which lie above the subclavian artery. The lower trunk lies just above the artery. *(The trunks can be palpated above the artery whose pulsations can be felt above the middle third of the clavicle, especially if the head is bent laterally to the same side to relax the muscles.)* The roots and trunks give off four branches, the more important *suprascapular* (C5, 6) and *long thoracic nerves* (C5, 6, 7) and less important *nerve to the rhomboids (dorsal scapular)* (C5) and *nerve to the subclavius* (C5, 6) (figure 155).

Deep to the clavicle the trunks divide into *anterior* and *posterior divisions* and inferior to the clavicle the divisions join to form *cords*. All the posterior divisions join to form the *posterior cord*, the anterior divisions of the upper and middle trunks join to form the *lateral cord* and the anterior division of the lower trunk continues as the *medial cord*. The cords are named according to their rela-tion to the axillary artery, although at the begin-ning of the artery the lateral and posterior cords are lateral and the medial cord is posterior to the artery, as can be expected from the relation of the trunks to the subclavian artery.

The lateral and medial cords give off one branch each before they divide into their terminal branches and the posterior cord gives off three branches. The *lateral* (C5, 6, 7) and *medial* (C8, T1) *pectoral nerves* come from the lateral and medial cords respectively and supply the pectoral muscles. The lateral pectoral nerve goes mainly to the pectoralis major and the medial supplies both the major and minor. The three branches from the posterior cord are the *upper* and *lower subscapular* and *thoraco-dorsal nerves* which supply the posterior wall of the axilla, the subscapularis, latissimus dorsi and the teres major. The upper subscapular nerve (C6, 7) supplies the subscapularis, the lower subscapular

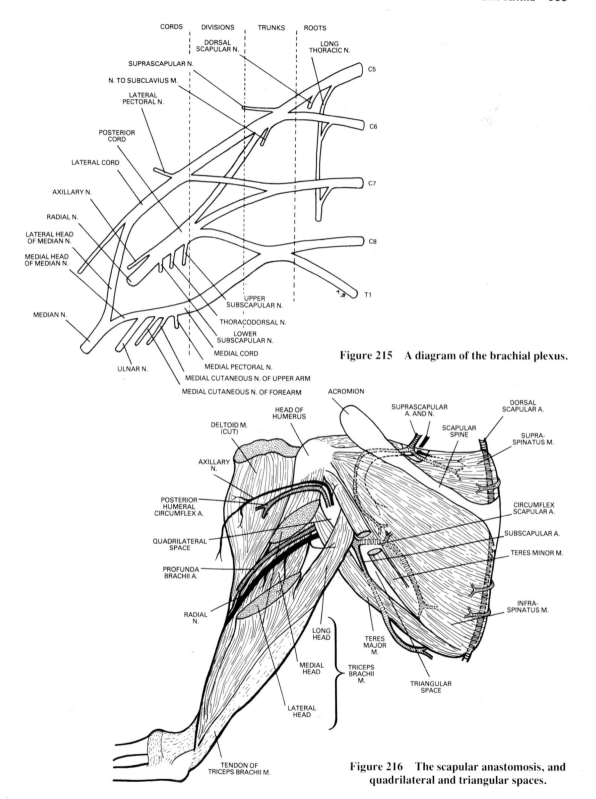

CORDS   DIVISIONS   TRUNKS   ROOTS

DORSAL SCAPULAR N.

SUPRASCAPULAR N.

N. TO SUBCLAVIUS M.

LATERAL PECTORAL N.

POSTERIOR CORD

LATERAL CORD

AXILLARY N.

RADIAL N.

LATERAL HEAD OF MEDIAN N.

MEDIAL HEAD OF MEDIAN N.

MEDIAN N.

ULNAR N.

LONG THORACIC N.

C5

C6

C7

C8

T1

UPPER SUBSCAPULAR N.

THORACODORSAL N.

LOWER SUBSCAPULAR N.

MEDIAL CORD

MEDIAL PECTORAL N.

MEDIAL CUTANEOUS N. OF UPPER ARM

MEDIAL CUTANEOUS N. OF FOREARM

Figure 215   A diagram of the brachial plexus.

DELTOID M. (CUT)

HEAD OF HUMERUS

AXILLARY N.

POSTERIOR HUMERAL CIRCUMFLEX A.

QUADRILATERAL SPACE

PROFUNDA BRACHII A.

RADIAL N.

ACROMION

SUPRASCAPULAR A. AND N.

SCAPULAR SPINE

DORSAL SCAPULAR A.

SUPRA-SPINATUS M.

CIRCUMFLEX SCAPULAR A.

SUBSCAPULAR A.

TERES MINOR M.

INFRA-SPINATUS M.

LONG HEAD

MEDIAL HEAD

LATERAL HEAD

TERES MAJOR M.

TRICEPS BRACHII M.

TRIANGULAR SPACE

TENDON OF TRICEPS BRACHII M.

Figure 216   The scapular anastomosis, and quadrilateral and triangular spaces.

(C5, 6) the subscapularis and teres major, and the thoracodorsal nerve (C6, 7, 8) the latissimus dorsi.

The lateral cord divides into the *musculo-cutaneous nerve* (C5, 6, 7) which enters the coraco-brachialis and the *lateral head of the median nerve* (C6, 7) which is joined by the *medial head of the median nerve* (C8, T1) from the medial cord. The *median nerve* continues downwards on the lateral side of the axillary and the upper part of the brachial arteries. These nerves are recognised by confirming that the musculocutaneous enters the coracobrachialis and that the median arises by two heads. The musculocutaneous nerve supplies the muscles of the front of the upper arm (the biceps brachii and the brachialis) as well as the coraco-brachialis and continues downwards as the *lateral cutaneous nerve of the forearm*.

The posterior cord divides on the subscapularis into the *axillary (circumflex) nerve* and the *radial nerve*. The axillary nerve (C5, 6) continues down-wards on the subscapularis to its lower border where it turns backwards and passes with the posterior humeral circumflex artery through the quadrilateral space below the subscapularis, the shoulder joint and the teres minor, medial to the surgical neck of the humerus. The nerve may be injured by dislocation of the shoulder joint or fracture of the neck of the humerus. The axillary nerve supplies the deltoid and the teres minor and gives off a cutaneous branch, the *upper lateral cutaneous nerve of the upper arm*, which is dis-tributed to the skin over the lower part of the deltoid. Damage to the axillary nerve, besides paralysis of the muscles, results in a sensory loss over the lower part of the deltoid.

The radial nerve (C5, 6, 7, 8, T1) continues downwards posterior to the axillary artery. At the lower border of the teres major the nerve passes backwards with the profunda brachii branch of the brachial artery between the long and medial heads of the triceps brachii and enters the radial groove on the posterior surface of the humerus between the lateral and medial heads of the triceps brachii. In the axilla the radial nerve gives off the *posterior cutaneous nerve of the upper arm*, which is dis-tributed to the posterior surface of the upper arm, and the *lower lateral cutaneous nerve of the upper arm* to the skin appropriate to its name. The radial

nerve is identified in the axilla by its position posterior to the artery, its large size and its con-tinuity with the posterior cord. The axillary nerve comes off the posterior cord much higher up than is usually appreciated and lies on the subscapularis for some distance before passing backwards in-ferior to that muscle.

The radial nerve can be damaged by the upper end of an old-fashioned crutch placed in the axilla (*crutch palsy*) or by pressure after falling asleep with the upper limb hanging over the back of a chair (*drunkard's palsy*). Extension at the elbow and wrist is lost and there is a loss of sensation over the skin of the middle of the back of the lower half of the upper arm and the back of the whole of the forearm.

The medial cord (C8, T1) gives off the *medial head of the median nerve*, the *ulnar nerve* and the *medial cutaneous nerves of the upper arm and forearm*. All of these nerves contain fibres from the eighth cervical and first thoracic spinal nerves. The medial head of the median nerves crosses the axillary artery anteriorly and joins the lateral head of the median nerve and the ulnar nerve lies medial to the axillary artery, between it and the vein, and continues downwards medial to the artery. The medial cutaneous nerve of the upper arm becomes medial to the axillary vein and is distributed to the skin on the medial side of the lower half of the upper arm and medial side of the elbow. The medial cutaneous nerve of the forearm continues downwards medial to the axillary and brachial arteries, becomes superficial about the middle of the upper arm and through anterior and posterior branches is distributed to the skin of the medial side of the forearm as far as the wrist.

The Axillary Lymph Nodes

These are described on p. 13. In summary (figure 217) there are *lateral nodes* along the axillary vein, *posterior nodes* along the subscapular vessels on the posterior axillary wall and *medial* or *pectoral nodes* deep to the lower border of the pectoralis major. The lymphatic vessels of the whole of the upper limb go to the lateral group, the lymphatic vessels from the breast and anterior wall of the

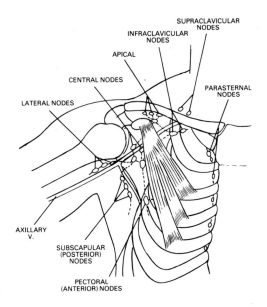

Figure 217   The axillary lymph nodes.

trunk above the umbilicus drain to the pectoral group, and the posterior walls of the axilla and trunk above the level of the umbilicus are drained by lymphatic vessels which go to the subscapular group. All these nodes drain to a *central group* embedded in the fat of the axilla and the central group drain to the *apical nodes* at its apex. From these the *subclavian lymph trunk* arises and on the right joins the *jugular lymph trunk* to form the *right lymph duct* which joins the beginning of the right brachiocephalic vein. On the left the subclavian lymph trunk usually joins the *thoracic duct*.

28

The Joints of the Shoulder Region

The *sternoclavicular joint* is between the medial end of the clavicle and the manubrium sterni and the *acromioclavicular joint* is between the lateral end of the clavicle and the acromion of the scapula. The scapula can move upwards, downwards, backwards and forwards on the chest wall without the involvement of the *glenohumeral joint*, which is between the head of the humerus and the glenoid cavity of the scapula. The movement of *lateral rotation of the scapula* in which the glenoid cavity faces upwards (the opposite movement is *medial rotation* and refers mainly to restoration of the scapula to the neutral position) normally takes place only in association with certain glenohumeral movements. The term lateral rotation refers to the inferior angle moving outwards.

The Sternoclavicular Joint (figure 218(a))

This is a synovial joint between the medial end of the clavicle and the upper lateral angle of the manubrium sterni and upper surface of the first costal cartilage. Because the articular surfaces are to some extent reciprocally concavoconvex the joint could be classified as a saddle joint. The clavicle projecting above the level of the manubrium and the joint space can be felt lateral to the jugular notch. The fibrous capsule lined by the synovial membrane is attached to the edges of the joint surfaces and is thickened anteriorly and posteriorly. The *costoclavicular ligament* lies immediately lateral to the joint and is attached to the inferior surface of the clavicle and the upper surface of the first costal cartilage and first rib. Its anterior fibres pass upwards and laterally and the posterior upwards and medially.

Within the joint there is a fibrocartilaginous disc which completely divides the joint into two cavities. The disc is attached to the fibrous capsule and also superiorly to the clavicle and inferiorly to the first costal cartilage.

The Acromioclavicular Joint (figure 218(b))

This is a synovial joint of the plane or gliding type between the lateral end of the clavicle and the medial surface of the acromion. The plane of the joint is oblique and faces laterally and downwards. The flat lateral end of the clavicle projects above the acromion. *This projection and the joint space can be felt.* The bones are held together by a fibrous capsule, and attached to the capsule superiorly there may be an incomplete disc between the joint surfaces.

Medial to the joint the *coracoclavicular ligament* passes between the lateral end of the inferior surface of the clavicle and the upper surface of the coracoid process. This ligament is in two parts — an anterior *trapezoid ligament* which runs backwards and laterally from the coracoid process and a posterior *conoid ligament* which runs upwards and medially from the posterior, medial edge of the coracoid process to the conoid tubercle of the clavicle.

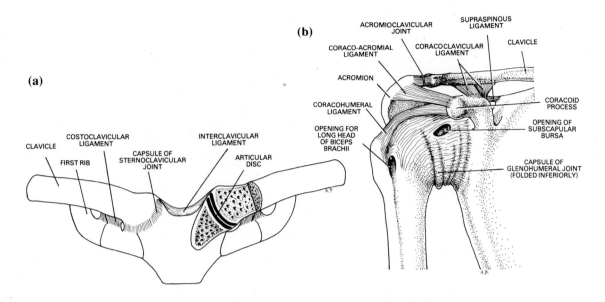

Figure 218 (a) **The sternoclavicular joints (the interior of the left sternoclavicular joint has been exposed to show the articular disc). (b) The right acromioclavicular and glenohumeral joints.**

The Movements of the Scapula on the Chest Wall

The scapula and clavicle can move upwards for a considerable distance, as in shrugging the shoulders, and downwards for a more limited distance. The scapula can be pulled forwards round the chest wall and backwards towards the midline as in bracing back the shoulders. In all these movements the lateral end of the clavicle moves with the scapula, and the medial end moves in the opposite direction on the fulcrum provided by the costoclavicular ligament.

Upward movement of the scapula in which the clavicle moves on the disc is produced by the upper fibres of the trapezius (the spinal accessory nerve), levator scapulae (C1–4) and rhomboids (C5). The inferior fibres of the trapezius pull the scapula downwards and may be assisted by the serratus anterior (the long thoracic nerve, C5, 6, 7).

Forward movement of the scapula round the chest wall in which the disc moves backwards with the medial end of the clavicle is largely due to the serratus anterior, which may be assisted by the pectoralis minor (medial pectoral nerve, C8, T1). This movement is used in attempts to push an object forwards with the outstretched upper limbs, and in lengthening the reach horizontally. Bracing the shoulders backwards is due to the trapezius and the rhomboids.

In dislocation of the acromioclavicular joint, usually accompanied by a torn coracoclavicular ligament, the clavicle dislocates upwards and outwards. This can be very unstable but wiring the clavicle to the acromion can result in reduced movements of the shoulder girdle (p. 362).

The Glenohumeral (Shoulder) Joint (figures 218(b), 219)

The Structure of the Glenohumeral Joint

This joint between the head of the humerus and the glenoid cavity is a synovial joint of the ball and socket type. The round head of the humerus is almost half a sphere and the glenoid cavity is shallow and somewhat narrowed superiorly. The cavity is deepened by the *glenoidal labrum*, a ring of fibrocartilage which is attached to the edge of the cavity, triangular in cross-section and about 4 mm deep (*labrum = brim, lip*, Latin).

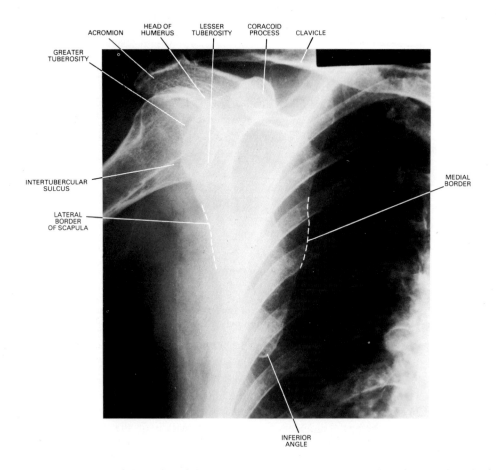

GREATER
TUBEROSITY

ACROMION
HEAD OF
HUMERUS
LESSER
TUBEROSITY
CORACOID
PROCESS
CLAVICLE

MEDIAL
BORDER

INTERTUBERCULAR
SULCUS

LATERAL
BORDER
OF SCAPULA

INFERIOR
ANGLE

Figure 219   An X-ray of the region of the shoulder joint (the humerus is abducted at the shoulder joint).

The fibrous capsule of the joint is attached medially to the edges of the glenoid cavity outside the labrum and laterally to the anatomical neck of the humerus, except inferomedially, where the capsule is attached to the shaft of the humerus about 2 cm below the neck. The tendons forming the rotator cuff (the teres minor and infraspinatus posteriorly, the supraspinatus superiorly and the subscapularis anteriorly) fuse with and strengthen the joint capsule.

The capsule is thickened superiorly and anteriorly to form the *glenohumeral ligaments* and also where it bridges the intertubercular sulcus and forms the *transverse ligament*. The *coraco-acromial ligament* lies above the joint and joins the lateral edge of the coracoid process to the acromion anterior to the acromioclavicular joint. The *coraco-humeral ligament* extends from the base of the coracoid process to the capsule in the region of the supraspinatus tendon.

The *synovial membrane* lines the capsule. Inferomedially the membrane extends from the capsule on to the bone and then upwards as far as the edge of articular cartilage. The long head of the biceps brachii is intracapsular and outside the synovial membrane and passes laterally over the head of the humerus and then downwards in the intertubercular sulcus. It takes with it a double fold of synovial membrane which extends beyond the transverse ligament for about 2 cm. The *bursa deep to the tendon of the subscapularis* near the glenoid cavity communicates with the joint cavity through an opening in the fibrous capsule and synovial membrane. Another important bursa (the *subacromial*) separates the acromion from the capsule of the joint and extends laterally below the deltoid muscle where it is called the *subdeltoid bursa*. This bursa may become diseased (*bursitis*) and affect the underlying tendon of the supraspinatus which may rupture.

The *arterial blood supply* of the joint is derived from branches of the acromiothoracic, anterior and posterior humeral circumflex and suprascapular arteries. The joint is *innervated* by branches from the axillary, suprascapular and lateral pectoral nerves.

The Movements at the Glenohumeral Joint

Because it is a ball and socket joint, movements about the three basic axes are possible, *abduction* and *adduction* about an anteroposterior axis, *flexion* and *extension* about a transverse axis, and *lateral* and *medial rotation* about a longitudinal axis. (Lateral and medial refer to the anterior surface of the humerus which turns to face laterally or medially in these movements.) In a joint in which flexion, extension, abduction and adduction can take place a movement called *circumduction* may be carried out. In this movement the limb is moved in such a way that the hand describes the base of a cone whose apex is the head of the humerus, in other words the upper limb is flexed, then abducted, then extended and finally adducted.

Since the glenohumeral joint is of the ball and socket type and the head of the humerus does not fit closely into the glenoid cavity, there is a wide range of movement. The movement of the upper limb in relation to the trunk is increased by scapular movements on the chest wall.

Because the glenoid cavity faces forwards as well as laterally it has been suggested that movements at the glenohumeral joint should be described in relation to the plane of the scapula; that is, flexion would be a forward and inward movement in a plane about midway between the coronal and sagittal planes and abduction an outward and forward movement at right angles to flexion.

It is proposed to ignore this problem because it is simpler to describe the movements in accordance with the accepted definitions of abduction, etc.

Abduction and Adduction. Abduction of the upper limb is a movement of the limb away from the body in the coronal plane. The limb can be moved through 180° so that it lies alongside the head. This involves movement at the glenohumeral joint and rotation of the scapula on the chest wall. Initially the humerus moves outwards due to the action of the deltoid (axillary nerve, C5, 6) and supraspinatus (suprascapular nerve, C5, 6). The deltoid exerts an upward force which without the assistance of the supraspinatus would not pull the upper limb outwards. Supraspinatus is needed for about 20°, after which the deltoid can continue to move the humerus. If the deltoid is paralysed due, for example, to injury to the axillary nerve, the supraspinatus is not strong enough as a rule to abduct the upper limb. If the supraspinatus is not functioning, for example due to rupture of its tendon, the deltoid on its own cannot initiate abduction. If the upper limb is abducted to 20° either passively or by leaning over to the side so that the limb hangs away from the body, the deltoid can continue abduction.

The stage of abduction at which the scapula begins to rotate so that the glenoid cavity faces upwards (lateral rotation) varies in different people. Usually the rotation is absent or slight during the first 50° and subsequently the humerus moves on the scapula and the scapula rotates at the same time. Of the total 180° of abduction, glenohumeral movement is involved in about two-thirds (120°) and rotation of the scapula in about one-third (60°). Rotation of the scapula is due to the contraction of the serratus anterior pulling mainly on the inferior angle of the scapula and the lower fibres of the trapezius acting on the upper border of the spine of the scapula. The interdependence of glenohumeral and scapular movement is interesting. For example, it is impossible for normal people to rotate the scapula laterally without glenohumeral movement. If the serratus anterior is paralysed due to injury of its nerve supply, the glenohumeral movement is limited to about 90°. In an operation called *arthrodesis* in which the humerus is fused to the glenoid cavity at an angle of 30° of flexion and abduction, the patient can lower the affected limb to the side of the trunk by medially rotating the scapula. It is now possible to abduct the limb through 90°, 30° to restore the scapula to its normal position and 60° by means of lateral rotation of the scapula. These two pathological situations have given rise to the misapprehension that 90° of abduction are due to glenohumeral movement and 90° to scapular rotation.

As the scapula is rotated laterally it also moves forwards and upwards to some extent. The lateral end of the clavicle also moves in the same direction and the whole clavicle twists about its long axis. This twisting is limited by the coracoclavicular ligament and the scapula then rotates at the acromioclavicular joint. This sequence of events can be seen by means of cineradiography. Although it is usually said that there is little movement at the acromioclavicular joint, orthopaedic surgeons found that in many cases of recurrent dislocation of the acromioclavicular joint treated by wiring the acromion and clavicle together, there was considerable limitation of abduction of the upper limb because the operation had effectively eliminated rotation of the scapula at that joint.

If the upper limb is abducted to 90° and then fully medially rotated, further abduction is impossible. This is due to tension on the tendons of the lateral rotators and the capsule. Some lateral rotation is required (the infraspinatus and teres minor) for full abduction to take place. It is often erroneously stated that lateral rotation is needed so that the greater tuberosity does not impinge on the acomion. X-rays show that even in full medial rotation at 90° these two bony processes are quite widely separated. Except for the trapezius all the muscles involved in abduction and lateral rotation are innervated by the fifth and sixth cervical segments — the deltoid and teres minor by the axillary nerve (C5, 6), the supraspinatus and infraspinatus by the suprascapular nerve (C5, 6) and the serratus anterior by the long thoracic nerve (C5, 6, 7). Injury to the upper trunk of the brachial plexus (C5, 6) (Erb's palsy) results in an inability to abduct and laterally rotate the upper limb at the shoulder (Wilhelm Erb, 1840–1921, Heidelberg neurologist) together with loss of some movements at the elbow, in the forearm and at the wrist. This injury

may occur in a baby as a result of the head being pulled backwards during labour in order to free the shoulder from the symphysis pubis.

In the anatomical position adduction of the upper limb at the shoulder joint is prevented by the trunk. If the limb is flexed or extended it can be moved towards the midline for about 20–30°. This movement if in front of the trunk is brought about by the pectoralis major (the lateral and medial pectoral nerves, C5, 6, 7, 8), and if behind the trunk mainly by the teres major (C5, 6).

Adduction, however, can refer to the restoration of the abducted limb to the anatomical position. This movement is controlled by the progressive relaxation of the muscles which are active in moving the upper limb to the fully abducted position — the serratus anterior, trapezius, deltoid and supraspinatus. Gravity is the force which lowers the limb. Reference has already been made to similar mechanisms elsewhere. For example, bending the trunk forwards from the upright position (flexion) is due to gravity controlled by the extensor muscles of the vertebral column. Muscles which act in order to produce a movement are called *prime movers* and the muscles which lengthen or relax at the same time are called *antagonists*. In many movements gravity replaces the prime movers and the movement is controlled by the antagonists.

If adduction from the abducted position is resisted the pectoralis major is strongly contracted, as in placing the hand on the waist with the elbow bent and pushing forcibly against the waist. The teres major and latissimus dorsi are also contracted in this movement.

Flexion and Extension. These movements take place in the sagittal plane about a transverse axis. In flexion the upper limb can be moved from the anatomical position through 180° so that it is alongside the head. The hand, however, faces backwards as compared with the final position of 180° of abduction in which the hand faces forwards. Flexion through 180° involves movement at the glenohumeral joint brought about by the anterior fibres of the deltoid, the clavicular head of the pectoralis major and the coracobrachialis (the last muscle is supplied by the musculocutaneous nerve, C6) and lateral rotation of the scapula due to the contraction of the serratus anterior and the lower fibres of the trapezius. With the upper limb flexed to 90° at the shoulder, unlike the limb abducted to 90°, medial rotation at the shoulder joint makes further flexion easier.

Extension from the anatomical position, movement backwards in the sagittal plane is limited to about 30° and is brought about by the teres major (subscapular nerve C6, 7), latissimus dorsi (the thoracodorsal nerve, C6, 7, 8) and the posterior fibres of the deltoid. Restoration of the flexed limb to the neutral position involves gravity under the control of the relaxing flexor muscles. Against resistance not only these three muscles but also the sternocostal part of the pectoralis major are involved. This very powerful movement is seen in swinging a hammer downwards from above the head or attempting to pull oneself upwards on a rope, although the correct way of climbing a rope involves the muscles of the lower rather than those of the upper limbs.

Lateral and Medial Rotation. These movements take place around a longitudinal axis. In lateral rotation the anterior surface of the humerus is turned laterally and the movement is due to the action of the infraspinatus, teres minor and posterior fibres of the deltoid. The range of movement is best tested with the forearm bent to a right angle at the elbow in order to eliminate the confusing effect of rotation of the forearm. From the anatomical position the humerus can be rotated laterally about 40–50°.

In medial rotation the anterior surface of the upper arm is turned medially and the movement is produced by a number of muscles — the subscapularis (the subscapular nerves, C5, 6), pectoralis major, teres major, latissimus dorsi and anterior fibres of the deltoid. The movement from the anatomical position is limited to some extent by the trunk and is about 50°. This is increased if the upper arm is flexed or abducted.

Rotation is the movement which is most commonly affected by pathological conditions of or injury to the shoulder joint. It has been said that if the middle of the back can be scratched from above (lateral rotation) and below (medial rotation) a satisfactory range of rotation is present.

Because the large head of the humerus does not fit closely into the shallow glenoid cavity, the glenohumeral joint is the most frequently dislocated in the body. The head of the humerus, especially if the humerus is abducted, is dislocated downwards where the capsule is unsupported and then moves forwards. The axillary nerve may be damaged with the result that the deltoid is partially or completely paralysed and there is a loss of sensation in the skin over the lower part of the deltoid. Both dislocation of the shoulder joint and wasting of the deltoid produce a typical flattening of the shoulder laterally as compared with the normal side.

In abduction at the shoulder joint, the subscapularis, infraspinatus and teres minor are active in order to prevent the head of the humerus moving upwards due to the action of the deltoid. Muscles which contract in order to prevent an unwanted movement due to the prime movers are called *synergists*. The term *fixators*, often used synonymously with synergists, should be used to describe muscles which contract in order to prevent movement at a joint not acted on by the prime movers. For example, when writing on a blackboard it is necessary to fix the joints in the shoulder region while moving the hand and fingers.

The terms flexion, extension, etc., describe the direction of the movement of one segment of the body relative to another but do not describe what is happening between the joint surfaces. The movements between the joint surfaces can be summarised as *sliding* or *translation*, and *spinning*. The shape of the joint surfaces determines to a large extent whether a sliding movement will result in rotation as well. No rotation occurs between flat surfaces. Flexion and extension at the glenohumeral joint are examples of a spin. Abduction and adduction and lateral and medial rotation at the shoulder joint are examples of a movement in which the head of the humerus slides on the glenoid cavity. That the head also rotates in a particular direction is due to the shape of the joint surfaces, the actions of the contracting muscles and the arrangement of the ligaments.

29

The Upper Arm and Forearm

The bone of the upper arm, the humerus, has already been described (pp. 344–346); the bones of the forearm are the radius and ulna, which in the anatomical position lie more or less parallel to each other with the radius on the lateral side. The muscles in the upper arm form an anterior flexor and posterior extensor group which move the forearm at the elbow. Similar groups in the forearm produce flexion and extension of the hand and digits. The nerves and arteries continue from the axilla into the more distal parts of the limb and the veins, deep and superficial, pass upwards from the forearm through the upper arm to the axilla. The cutaneous nerves of the forearm arise in the axilla and upper arm.

The Radius (figure 220)

The shaft of the radius, the lateral bone of the forearm, has a rounded *lateral surface* and *anterior* and *posterior surfaces* which meet medially in the sharp *interosseous border*, at the upper end of which there is a prominence, the *radial tuberosity*. The tuberosity is smooth anteriorly where it is related to a bursa and roughened posteriorly for the attachment of the tendon of the biceps brachii. The lower end of the interosseous border divides to form two ridges which extend to the *ulnar notch*, a concave articular area for the head of the ulna.

Extending downwards and laterally from the radial tuberosity on to the anterior surface there is an *oblique line* which ends about the middle of the lateral surface.

The upper end of the radius is called the *head*, which is separated from the shaft by the *neck*. The head has a proximal surface which is concave and articulates with the capitulum of the humerus. This articular area is continuous with an articular rim round the periphery of the head for articulation with the radial notch of the upper end of the ulna and an annular ligament attached to the edges of the notch. The radial tuberosity lies immediately distal to the medial side of the neck.

The distal end of the radius has four surfaces. The lateral surface continues distally as the *styloid process* above which there are two grooves for tendons going to the thumb. The *ulnar notch* for the head of the ulna is on the distal end of the medial surface. The lateral part of the anterior surface is subcutaneous and on it the radial artery can be palpated. This, as is well known, is the commonest site for counting the pulse rate. The posterior surface has a number of grooves for some of the extensor tendons. One of the ridges between the grooves is particularly prominent and is called the *dorsal tubercle* (*of Lister*; Joseph Lister, later Lord, 1827–1912, ought to be commemorated because of his contributions, made in Glasgow initially, to antiseptic and aseptic surgery.) The distal surface of the radius is concave for articulation with the scaphoid and lunate bones of the carpus.

The radius *ossifies* in cartilage. The primary centre of ossification for the shaft appears at about 8 weeks of intra-uterine life. At birth the ends of the radius are cartilaginous. The secondary centre

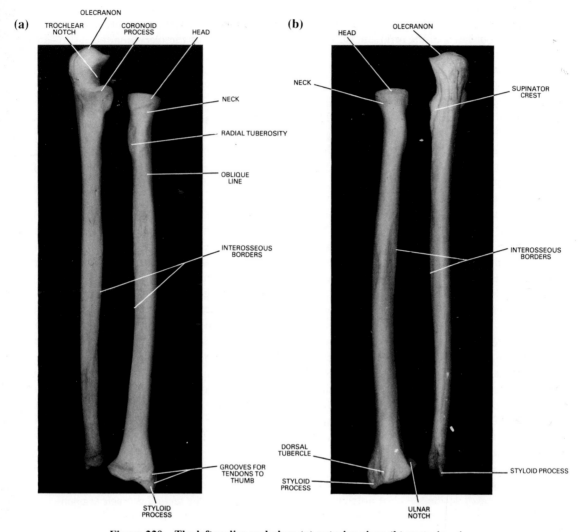

Figure 220   The left radius and ulna: (a) anterior view; (b) posterior view.

of ossification for the distal end appears at about the end of the first year and the centre for the proximal end at about 4 years. The distal end (the growing end) fuses with the shaft at about 20 years and the proximal end at about 18 years.

The upper epiphysis lies entirely within the capsule of the elbow joint and, because it is small relative to the annular ligament which encircles it, it is not uncommonly dislocated by traction.

The Ulna (figure 220)

The shaft of the ulna has three *surfaces*, an *anterior*

and *posterior*, which meet laterally at the *interosseous border*, and a rounded *medial surface*. The posterior border or surface is subcutaneous and can be palpated distally as far as the lower end of the bone which medially projects as the ulnar *styloid process*. The tip of the ulnar styloid process is about 2 cm proximal to the tip of the radial styloid process. This is an important difference because the radius is frequently fractured transversely about 3 cm proximal to its lower end, especially in middle-aged women who fall on to their outstretched hand. The distal fragment is displaced upwards and backwards and tilts forwards. This is called *Colles' fracture*, named after the same Dublin surgeon who described the superficial membranous fascia of the perineum (p. 163).

The lower end of the ulna is rounded and is called the *head*. It articulates laterally with the ulnar notch of the radius and distally with a *triangular fibrocartilage* which is attached to a pit on the lateral side of the junction of the styloid process with the head. The base of the cartilage is attached to the lower border of the ulnar notch of the radius. There is a groove on the posterior surface of the head.

The interosseous border at its upper end divides into two ridges which pass upwards to the anterior and posterior margins of the radial notch. The posterior ridge is called the supinator crest because the supinator muscle is attached to it.

The proximal end of the ulna has two processes projecting forwards, the upper *olecranon* and the lower *coronoid process* (*olene* = elbow, *cranion* = head, Greek). The *trochlear notch* lies between them (figure 220(a)). The upper surface of the olecranon has an anterior smooth area related to a bursa which lies between the capsule of the elbow joint and the triceps brachii, attached to the rough posterior area of this surface. The posterior surface of the olecranon is triangular, smooth and subcutaneous and is continuous with the subcutaneous posterior border of the ulna. There is a bursa between the subcutaneous area and the skin.

The coronoid process projects forwards and forms the lower part of the trochlear notch which articulates with the trochlea of the humerus. Immediately below the coronoid process there is a rough triangular area. Lateral to the process there is a horizontal concave articular area, the *radial notch*, which articulates with the rim of the head of the radius.

The trochlear notch has a median longitudinal ridge so that its articular area is convex from side to side and deeply concave from above downwards. The medial part of the trochlear notch projects forwards inferiorly and is directed anteriorly. The lateral part faces laterally.

The ulna *ossifies* in cartilage at about 8 weeks of intra-uterine life from a primary centre for the shaft. At birth the ends are cartilaginous. The distal epiphysis begins to ossify at about 5 years and fuses with the shaft at about 20 years. The proximal epiphysis, which is usually confined to the upper surface of the olecranon, begins to ossify at about 10 years and fuses with the shaft at about 18 years.

The Skin and Surface Markings

The skin of the upper arm and forearm shows no special features other than the arrangement of the hairs on the forearm. They are found mainly on the posterior surface and are directed from the lateral to the medial border. The arrangement of the dermatomes is as follows (figure 221). The lateral surface of the upper arm is innervated by the fifth cervical segment and the lateral surface of the forearm by the sixth cervical segment. This extends along the lateral side of the thumb. The seventh cervical segment innervates the skin of the index, middle and ring fingers and the area innervated by this segment extends proximally into the hand towards the middle of the wrist. The area innervated by the seventh cervical segment on the back of the hand extends further upwards on the forearm than on the anterior surface and almost reaches the elbow. The skin of the medial side of the hand (the little finger and forearm) is innervated by the eighth cervical segment and the medial side of the upper arm by the first thoracic segment except for an area of skin near the axilla which is innervated by the second thoracic segment.

This segmental innervation of the skin of the upper limb reflects its development as an outgrowth from the trunk opposite the fifth to the eighth cervical and first thoracic segments. The thumb or medial side is nearer the head and represents the *pre-axial border*, and the little finger or ulnar side the *postaxial border*. The *anterior* (*ventral*) and *posterior* (*dorsal*) *axial lines* run along the middle of the front and back of the upper arm and forearm respectively, and are defined as the lines where relatively widely separated dermatomes meet. There is little overlap of segmental innervation along these lines but there is considerable overlap where the skin is innervated by adjacent segments, for example in the hands. One can easily recall the dermatomes of the upper limb by remembering

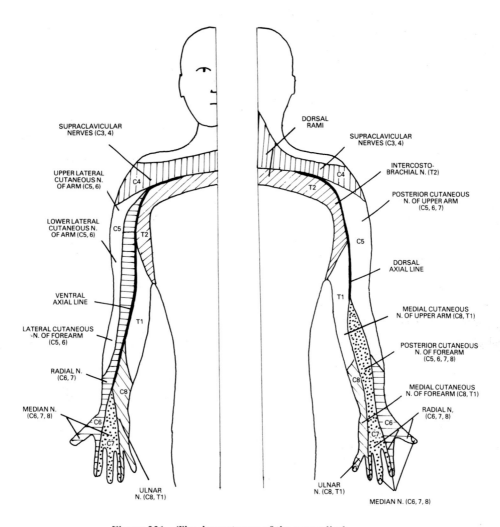

Figure 221   The dermatomes of the upper limb.

that the *middle* spinal cord segment of the brachial plexus (the seventh) innervates the skin of the *middle* finger.

It has been suggested that the dermatomes of the upper limb are differently arranged in that each dermatome is much more extensive longitudinally; for example the seventh cervical segment extends downwards along the whole length of the back of the upper limb from the midline of the back.

The names and segmental values of the nerves supplying the skin are shown in figure 221.

At the elbow the lateral *and* medial epicondyles *are subcutaneous and the* upper margin of the olecranon *can be felt in line with the epicondyles if*

*the forearm is fully extended. If the forearm is bent to a right angle, the olecranon is felt as the apex of a triangle with its base formed by a line between the epicondyles. These relationships are important and are altered in fractures of the olecranon and in fractures of the lower end of the humerus in which there is displacement of the lower part of the bone (*supracondylar fractures*). The* head of the radius *can be palpated about 2 cm distal and 1 cm medial to the lateral epicondyle and rotation of the forearm confirms this.*

The olecranon continues downwards into the subcutaneous posterior border of the ulna *and leads to the* ulnar styloid process. *The* radial styloid process, *larger than and 2 cm distal to the ulnar, is palpable on the lateral side of the wrist. The anterior surface and lateral border of the lower part of the radius are also subcutaneous. The* dorsal tubercle *of the radius 2 cm proximal and medial to the radial styloid process can be felt on the back of the wrist. The* head of the ulna *becomes very prominent on the posteromedial part of the wrist if the forearm is rotated inwards.*

The Superficial Veins

The *cephalic vein* runs along the whole length of the lateral side of the forearm and upper arm in the superficial fascia. The vein begins on the lateral side of the wrist by draining blood from the lateral part of the plexus of veins on the back of the hand. As the vein passes upwards it receives anterior and posterior tributaries in the forearm. At the elbow the cephalic vein lies anterolaterally, is superficial to the lateral cutaneous nerve of the forearm and gives off a large branch, the *medial cubital vein*, to the basilic vein (figure 222). The cephalic vein continues upwards in the upper arm on the lateral side of the biceps brachii, follows the anterior border of the deltoid into the deltopectoral groove between the two muscles and after perforating the clavipectoral fascia joins the axillary vein.

The *basilic vein* begins on the ulnar side of the wrist by draining the medial part of the superficial plexus on the dorsum of the hand. As the vein runs upwards on the medial side of the forearm it receives tributaries from both its surfaces and then passes on to the anteromedial part of the elbow where it receives the median cubital vein. At the elbow the branches of the medial cutaneous nerve of the forearm are superficial and deep to the vein. The basilic vein continues upwards on the medial side of the biceps brachii and about the middle of the upper arm it pierces the deep fascia to run upwards medial to the brachial artery and become the axillary vein at the lower border of the teres major. The basilic vein is joined by the brachial veins where it lies medial to the brachial artery.

There is often a large subcutaneous vein (the *median vein of the forearm*) running upwards on the front of the forearm towards the elbow, where

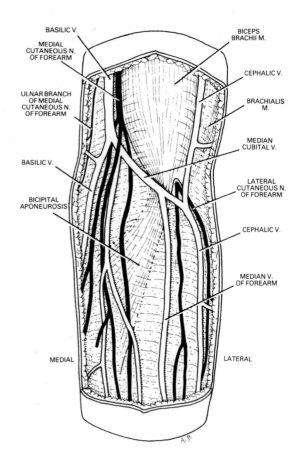

Figure 222   The superficial veins of the anterior aspect of the left elbow.

it joins the median cubital vein or basilic vein. Occasionally the median cubital vein is absent and the median vein of the forearm divides into lateral and medial branches which join the cephalic and basilic veins respectively.

The subcutaneous veins on the front of the elbow are important because they are used for obtaining specimens of blood and intravenous injection. They can be distended by circumferential pressure applied to the upper arm. Subcutaneous fat may obscure the distended veins but they can be almost invariably felt through the overlying tissues. It is unwise to attempt to insert a needle into a vein which is not visible or obviously palpable. The variation in the arrangement of the veins precludes depending entirely on one's anatomical knowledge of where a vein ought to be.

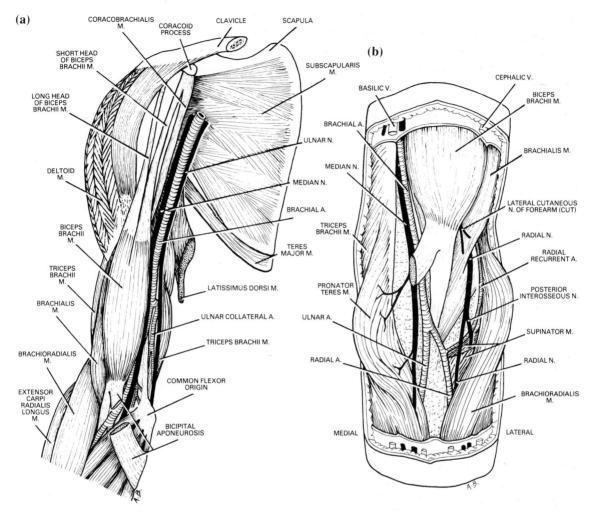

Figure 223 (a) The anterior aspect of the right upper arm. (b) The left cubital fossa.

The Upper Arm

Deep to the superficial fascia the structures of the upper arm are enclosed in a layer of deep fascia from which lateral and medial intermuscular septa pass inwards to the lateral and medial supracondylar ridges respectively. These septa to which the muscles are partly attached divide the upper arm into anterior (flexor) and posterior (extensor) compartments.

The anterior compartment (figure 223)

The Biceps Brachii. This muscle is attached by two heads to the scapula. The short head has a common attachment with the coracobrachialis to the tip of the coracoid process. The tendon of the long head is attached to the supraglenoid tubercle, passes anteriorly over the shoulder joint inside the capsule and outside the synovial membrane and runs downwards in the intertubercular sulcus where it lies between the pectoralis major and the latissimus dorsi. A sleeve of synovial membrane surrounds the tendon for about 2 cm distal to the capsule. In the upper third of the upper arm both heads become fleshy and unite to form the belly of the muscle. It ends in a tendon which twists laterally and is attached to the posterior part of the radial tuberosity. A bursa separates the tendon from the anterior half. In front of the elbow the tendon gives off a flat expansion, the *bicipital aponeurosis*, which passes downwards and medially over the brachial vessels and fuses with the deep fascia of the forearm.

The biceps brachii is supplied by the musculocutaneous nerve (C5, 6) and is a supinator and flexor of the forearm at the elbow. (*Pronation* is a movement in which the head of the radius rotates and its lower end crosses over to the medial side of the ulna so that the hand faces backwards. *Supination* is the restoration of the pronated forearm to the anatomical position in which the radius lies alongside the ulna and the hand faces forwards.) Inserting a corkscrew with the right hand and pulling the cork out involves the biceps brachii in the actions of supination and flexion. The actions of this muscle at the shoulder joint are not important. It is assumed that it assists flexion and prevents the head of the humerus moving upwards.

The Coracobrachialis (figure 223). This muscle has already been described (p. 351) and is attached distally to the middle of the medial side of the shaft of the humerus. The musculocutaneous nerve passes through it and supplies it. The muscle is a weak flexor of the humerus at the shoulder joint.

The Brachialis (figure 223). This muscle is attached to the anterior surface of the shaft of the humerus and extends upwards as far as the middle of the lateral surface where it embraces the attachment of the deltoid. The brachialis passes downwards in front of the elbow joint and is attached to the triangular area below the coronoid process of the ulna. It is supplied by the musculocutaneous nerve (C5, 6) and is a flexor of the forearm at the elbow joint. The muscle is also innervated by the radial nerve.

The Brachial Artery and Veins (figure 223). The *brachial artery* is a continuation of the axillary artery and extends from the lower border of the teres major to the level of the neck of the radius where it divides into the *radial* and *ulnar arteries*. The brachial artery is accompanied by two *brachial veins* (*venae comitantes, comitans = accompanying,* Latin) which are formed by the ulnar and radial

veins and join the basilic vein about the middle of the upper arm. The brachial artery lies medial to the biceps brachii muscle, on the lower end of the coracobrachialis and on the brachialis.

The median nerve is at first lateral to the artery and then crosses anterior to it. At the elbow the nerve is medial to the artery which is medial to the tendon of the biceps brachii, and the artery and nerve are deep to the bicipital aponeurosis. The ulnar nerve is medial to the upper part of the artery and then passes backwards into the posterior compartment. The radial nerve is posterior to the upper part of the artery and passes backwards between the long and medial heads of the triceps brachii.

The main branch of the brachial artery is the *profunda brachii* (figures 216, 224) which arises just distal to the teres major and accompanies the radial nerve as it passes backwards in the radial groove on the posterior surface of the humerus where the profunda gives off the *nutrient artery* to that bone. The profunda brachii gives off a branch which passes upwards and anastomoses with the arteries near the shoulder joint. The artery gives off two medial branches which descend towards the elbow joint on its medial side and take part in the anterior and posterior anastomoses in the region of the elbow. The upper branch accompanies the ulnar nerve and is called the *superior ulnar collateral artery*. The profunda brachii itself takes part in the anterior and posterior anastomoses on the lateral side of the elbow.

The brachial artery is superficial along its whole course unless it is overlapped by the biceps brachii and can be compressed against the middle of the medial surface of the humerus or the front of the humerus lower down. Its course can be determined by feeling it pulsating — the artery lies medial to the coracobrachialis and biceps brachii, and, in the front of the elbow, it lies medial to the tendon of the biceps brachii. The brachial artery at the elbow is used for measuring the blood pressure.

The brachial artery may divide high up in the upper arm in which case the median nerve passes between the two branches. One of the branches may be superficial to the bicipital aponeurosis and therefore immediately deep to the median cubital vein.

The Nerves in the Anterior Compartment (figure 223). Most of these have been described with the brachial artery. The *median nerve* is lateral to the artery, crosses anterior to it and then lies on its medial side. There are no branches of the median nerve in the upper arm. The *ulnar nerve* is medial to the artery and passes backwards through the medial intermuscular septum into the posterior compartment. The *radial nerve* is posterior to the artery and passes backwards medial to the humerus into the radial groove (figure 116).

The *musculocutaneous nerve* passes through the coracobrachialis, which it supplies, and lies between the biceps brachii and the brachialis, both of which it supplies. The nerve continues downwards into the forearm as the *lateral cutaneous nerve of the forearm*, becoming superficial below the level of the elbow where it lies deep to the cephalic vein. The nerve is distributed to both surfaces of the lateral side of the forearm as far as the base of the thumb.

The *medial cutaneous nerve of the upper arm* is medial to the brachial artery and after becoming cutaneous about the middle of the upper arm is distributed to the skin of its medial side below that level. The *medial cutaneous nerve of the forearm* becomes superficial at about the same level and divides into anterior and posterior branches which go to the skin of the forearm on the medial side. The anterior branch is usually anterior to the median cubital vein.

The Cubital Fossa (figure 223(b))

This is the hollow in the front of the elbow. It is triangular with a proximal base represented by an imaginary line between the two humeral epicondyles, a lateral boundary formed by the *brachioradialis* and an inferomedial boundary by the *pronator teres*. This is an important region because the superficial veins are used frequently for venepuncture and the brachial artery for measuring the blood pressure.

In the superficial fascia there are veins and cutaneous nerves. The cephalic vein is lateral, the basilic vein medial, and the median cubital vein passes from the cephalic to the basilic vein. The median vein of the forearm ends in the median cubital vein. The lateral cutaneous nerve of the forearm is deep to the cubital vein. The medial cutaneous nerve of the forearm, usually already branched, is both deep and superficial to the basilic vein.

The deep fascia covers the contents of the fossa and is reinforced on the medial side by the bicipital aponeurosis passing from the tendon of the biceps brachii downwards and medially to the deep fascia of the forearm.

Deep to the deep fascia the three main structures passing through the fossa from lateral to medial are the tendon of the biceps brachii going to the radial tuberosity, the brachial artery and the median nerve. The brachial artery divides at the level of the neck of the radius into the radial artery which passes downwards and laterally on the tendon of the biceps brachii and deep to the brachioradialis. The ulnar artery passes downwards and medially deep to the pronator teres. Within the fossa the radial and ulnar arteries give off recurrent branches to the elbow joint, and the ulnar artery gives off the common interosseous artery which divides into an anterior and posterior interosseous artery. The median nerve passes downwards between the two heads of the pronator teres. In the fossa the nerve gives off its branch to the pronator teres.

In the floor of the fossa there are from above downwards the brachialis, the capsule of the elbow joint and the supinator muscle. The brachialis tendon passes to the area below the ulnar coronoid process and the supinator is wrapped round the upper part of the radius. The radial nerve, lying laterally deep to the brachioradialis on the brachialis, divides into its two terminal branches. Its superficial branch, usually called the radial nerve, continues downwards deep to the brachioradialis. The deep branch passes backwards round the lateral side of the radius between the two layers of the supinator muscle and is called the posterior interosseous nerve.

There are frequently one or more lymph nodes in the cubital fossa above the trochlea of the humerus (*supratrochlear lymph node(s)*) to which efferent vessels from the medial side of the hand and forearm drain and from which vessels pass to the axillary nodes. The node or nodes may be more proximal and lie in the middle of the upper arm.

The posterior compartment (figures 116, 224)

The Triceps Brachii. This muscle as the name suggests has three heads, a *long head* from the infraglenoid tubercle, a *lateral head* from the back of the humerus above the radial groove and a *medial head* from the back of the humerus below the radial groove. The long and lateral heads join and run downwards superficial to the medial head. The three heads fuse and form above the elbow one tendon which is attached to the posterior part of

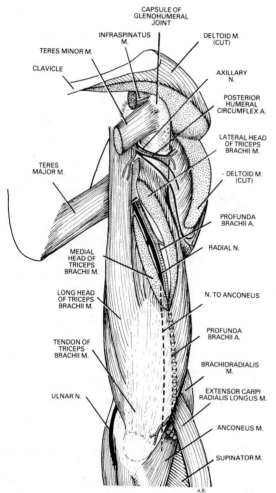

Figure 224   The posterior aspect of the right upper arm.

the upper surface of the olecranon. The tendon is separated from the capsule of the elbow joint by a bursa.

The triceps brachii is innervated by the radial nerve (C6, 7, 8). Each head has separate branches. The long and medial heads are supplied from the radial nerve as it enters the medial end of the radial groove. The nerve to the medial head (the *ulnar collateral nerve*) runs downwards next to the ulnar nerve. While in the radial groove the radial nerve gives off a branch which divides and supplies the lateral and medial heads and the anconeus muscle.

The triceps brachii is an extensor of the forearm at the elbow joint. The long head may support the shoulder joint inferiorly if the upper limb is held away from the body and against resistance may help to extend the humerus at the shoulder joint from the flexed position.

The Anconeus. This is a short muscle attached above to the back of the lateral epicondyle and inferiorly to the lateral side of the upper end of the ulna between the medial subcutaneous area and the supinator crest. Its direction is medial as well as downwards and in addition to extending the forearm at the elbow it can pull the ulna backwards and laterally, a movement which may occur in pronation of the forearm. The anconeus is supplied by a branch from the radial nerve (C7, 8) as it lies in the radial groove.

The Radial Nerve (figure 224). The radial nerve enters the posterior compartment by passing between the long and medial heads of the triceps brachii. The nerve then runs downwards and laterally between the lateral and medial heads in the radial groove and passes forwards through the lateral intramuscular septum into the anterior compartment where it lies on the lateral side deep to the brachioradialis on the brachialis.

While in the radial groove the radial nerve is accompanied by the profunda brachii artery and gives off a number of branches. The branches to the triceps brachii and anconeus have been described. The *posterior cutaneous nerve of the upper arm*, the *lower lateral cutaneous nerve of the upper arm* and the *posterior cutaneous nerve of the forearm* are given off in that order before the radial nerve reaches the lateral end of the radial groove and are distributed in the manner suggested by their names.

The radial nerve may be involved in fractures of the shaft of the humerus. If it is involved at the upper medial end of the groove, the triceps brachii and anconeus are affected as well as the muscles on the back of the forearm (the extensors of the hand and digits) which are supplied by a branch of the radial nerve. If the nerve is involved at the lower lateral end of the groove the triceps brachii is not affected but the posterior muscles of the forearm are. Paralysis of these muscles produces a condition described as a *wrist-drop* in which the hand cannot be extended at the wrist if the forearm is flexed and pronated.

The Ulnar Nerve. The ulnar nerve enters the posterior compartment by piercing the medial intermuscular septum medial to the biceps brachii about the middle of the upper arm. The nerve then runs downwards deep to the medial head of the triceps brachii and becomes subcutaneous where it lies in a groove on the back of the medial epicondyle. One of the branches of the profunda brachii artery and a branch of the radial nerve to the medial head of the triceps accompany the ulnar nerve as it passes downwards. There are no branches of the ulnar nerve in this part of its course other than a few small branches to the elbow joint.

The Forearm

The superficial veins (the cephalic laterally, basilic medially and median vein anteriorly) are described on p. 368 and reference has been made to the superficial nerves (the lateral, medial and posterior cutaneous nerves from the musculocutaneous, medial cord of the brachial plexus and radial nerve respectively). A layer of deep fascia surrounds the muscles of the forearm and is thicker posteriorly especially above where it receives an extension from the tendon of the triceps brachii. Anteriorly the bicipital aponeurosis extends from the tendon of the biceps brachii to the upper medial side of the forearm (figure 223). At the wrist there are special transverse bands, anteriorly the *flexor retinaculum* (*retinere* = *to retain*, Latin) and posteriorly the *extensor retinaculum*, which hold the tendons of the forearm muscles in position as they pass from the forearm into the hand.

There are anterior (flexor) and posterior (extensor) muscles in the forearm. The median, ulnar and radial nerves or their branches pass through the forearm into the hand, and the radial and ulnar arteries lie in the anterior (flexor) compartment.

The anterior muscles (figure 225)

These lie in three layers: (1) a superficial group all of which are attached to the common flexor origin on the anterior aspect of the medial epicondyle (the pronator teres, flexor carpi radialis, palmaris longus and flexor carpi ulnaris) and spread out as they pass distally; (2) an intermediate muscle, the flexor digitorum superficialis, attached to the radius and ulna as well as the common flexor origin; (3) a deep group, the flexor pollicis longus attached to the radius, the flexor digitorum profundus attached to the ulna and the pronator quadratus attached to both bones.

The Pronator Teres. One head is attached to the lower part of the medial humeral supracondylar ridge and the other to the medial side of the coronoid process. The two heads join and pass downwards and laterally to be attached to the middle of the lateral surface of the radius. The median nerve goes between the two heads and the ulnar artery deep to both heads as they pass downwards in the forearm. The radial artery and nerve lie on the muscle where it is attached to the radius.

The pronator teres is supplied by the median nerve (C6, 7) and its action is to pronate the forearm. It can also act as a flexor of the forearm at the elbow joint.

The Flexor Carpi Radialis. From the common flexor origin this muscle runs downwards and ends in a tendon which passes deep to the flexor retinaculum and is attached to the anterior surface of the bases of the second and third metacarpal bones. The median nerve (C6, 7) supplies the flexor carpi radialis which is a flexor and abductor of the hand at the wrist.

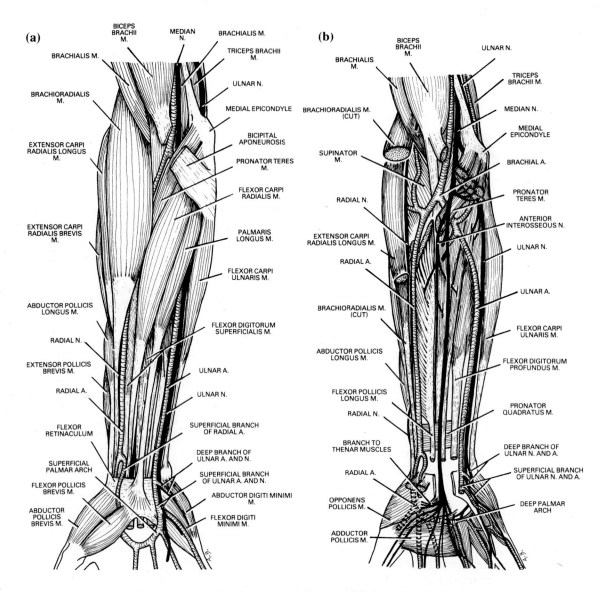

(a)

BICEPS BRACHII M.

BRACHIALIS M.

MEDIAN N.

BRACHIALIS M.

BRACHIORADIALIS M.

EXTENSOR CARPI RADIALIS LONGUS M.

EXTENSOR CARPI RADIALIS BREVIS M.

ABDUCTOR POLLICIS LONGUS M.

RADIAL N.

EXTENSOR POLLICIS BREVIS M.

RADIAL A.

FLEXOR RETINACULUM

SUPERFICIAL PALMAR ARCH

FLEXOR POLLICIS BREVIS M.

ABDUCTOR POLLICIS BREVIS M.

BRACHIALIS M.

TRICEPS BRACHII M.

ULNAR N.

MEDIAL EPICONDYLE

BICIPITAL APONEUROSIS

PRONATOR TERES M.

FLEXOR CARPI RADIALIS M.

PALMARIS LONGUS M.

FLEXOR CARPI ULNARIS M.

FLEXOR DIGITORUM SUPERFICIALIS M.

ULNAR A.

ULNAR N.

SUPERFICIAL BRANCH OF RADIAL A.

DEEP BRANCH OF ULNAR A. AND N.

SUPERFICIAL BRANCH OF ULNAR A. AND N.

ABDUCTOR DIGITI MINIMI M.

FLEXOR DIGITI MINIMI M.

(b)

BICEPS BRACHII M.

ULNAR N.

BRACHIALIS M.

BRACHIORADIALIS M. (CUT)

SUPINATOR M.

RADIAL N.

EXTENSOR CARPI RADIALIS LONGUS M.

RADIAL A.

BRACHIORADIALIS M. (CUT)

ABDUCTOR POLLICIS LONGUS M.

FLEXOR POLLICIS LONGUS M.

RADIAL N.

BRANCH TO THENAR MUSCLES

RADIAL A.

OPPONENS POLLICIS M.

ADDUCTOR POLLICIS M.

TRICEPS BRACHII M.

MEDIAN N.

MEDIAL EPICONDYLE

BRACHIAL A.

PRONATOR TERES M.

ANTERIOR INTEROSSEOUS N.

ULNAR N.

ULNAR A.

FLEXOR CARPI ULNARIS M.

FLEXOR DIGITORUM PROFUNDUS M.

PRONATOR QUADRATUS M.

DEEP BRANCH OF ULNAR N. AND A.

SUPERFICIAL BRANCH OF ULNAR N. AND A.

DEEP PALMAR ARCH

Figure 225   The front of the right forearm: (a) the superficial muscles; (b) the deep structures.

The Palmaris Longus. This muscle is often absent and if present may be found in only one forearm. It has a short muscular belly and a long tendon which crosses superficial to the flexor retinaculum and is attached to the palmar aponeurosis (the deep fascia of the palm). It is evolutionally a degenerating muscle as is evidenced by its long tendon and frequent absence. The muscle is supplied by the median nerve (C7, 8) and is a flexor of the hand at the wrist.

The Flexor Carpi Ulnaris. One head arises from the common flexor origin and the other from the medial side of the olecranon. The ulnar nerve passes forwards between the two heads from behind the medial epicondyle into the upper medial part of the forearm. The flexor carpi ulnaris is also attached to the posterior border of the ulna through an aponeurosis common to it and the flexor digitorum profundus and extensor carpi ulnaris.

The muscle ends in a tendon which is attached

to the pisiform bone and indirectly to the hamate and base of the fifth metacarpal bone by the piso-hamate and pisometacarpal ligaments. The ulnar nerve (C7, 8) supplies this muscle which is a flexor and adductor of the hand at the wrist.

The Flexor Digitorum Superficialis (Sublimis). It is attached to the common flexor origin, to the medial side of the coronoid process above the pro-nator teres, and to an oblique line on the front of the radius extending from the radial tuberosity to the attachment of the pronator teres. In the lower third of the forearm the muscle divides into four tendons which when they pass deep to the flexor retinaculum are arranged in two pairs. The super-ficial pair are the tendons to the middle and ring fingers and the deep pair those of the index and little fingers. In the hand the tendons separate and go to the medial four digits. At the base of the proximal phalanx each tendon divides and a tendon of the flexor digitorum profundus passes through the gap. The divided tendon of the superficialis muscle unites again behind the profundus tendon which lies in a groove formed by the superficialis tendon. The superficialis tendon divides again to become attached to the sides of the middle phalanx.

In the forearm the flexor digitorum superficialis lies between the superficial and deep group of muscles. The radial artery and nerve are superficial to it on its lateral side. The median nerve and ulnar artery pass deep to the muscle between its ulnar and radial attachments. The median nerve con-tinues downwards on its deep surface to which it is attached by fibrous tissue and at the wrist becomes more superficial and lies lateral to the superficialis tendons. In the palm the tendons are deep to the palmar aponeurosis and superficial vessels and digital nerves.

The flexor digitorum superficialis is innervated by the median nerve (C7, 8) and flexes the middle phalanx on the proximal and then the proximal phalanx on the metacarpal bone. It then becomes a weak flexor of the hand at the wrist. If, however, the fingers are held straight the flexor action of the superficialis (and the profundus) muscle on the hand is much greater.

The Flexor Pollicis Longus (figure 225(b)). Its proximal attachment is to the middle third of the anterior surface of the radius and the adjacent part of the interosseous membrane. The muscle ends in a tendon which passes deep to the flexor retin-aculum and is attached to the anterior surface of the base of the distal phalanx of the thumb. Its nerve supply is from the median nerve through the anterior interosseous nerve (C8) and its action is to flex the distal phalanx on the proximal, the proxi-mal phalanx on the first metacarpal bone and the first metacarpal on the trapezium.

The Flexor Digitorum Profundus. Its fibres are attached to the upper three-quarters of the anterior surface of the ulna, the adjacent area of the inter-osseous membrane and the aponeurosis, which is attached to the posterior border of the ulna. In the lower part of the forearm the muscle ends in four tendons of which the lateral to the index finger is most distinct. The tendons pass into the hand deep to the flexor retinaculum and deep to the tendons of the superficialis muscle. Each tendon passes through the corresponding divided tendon of the superficialis, rests on the re-united superficialis tendon and is attached to the anterior surface of the base of the distal phalanx (figure 234). The lumbrical muscles which are attached to the ten-dons in the palm are described with the muscles of the hand (p. 398).

The lateral half of the muscle which goes to the index and middle fingers is innervated by the anterior interosseous nerve, a branch of the median nerve, and the medial half, to the ring and little fingers, by the ulnar nerve (C8). The flexor digit-orum profundus flexes the terminal phalanges on the middle phalanges, the middle on the proximal and the proximal on the metacarpal bones. If the movement is carried out slowly, without undue force, no other muscles are involved in making a fist. If, however, the movement is performed quickly and/or forcibly other muscles assist in flexing the digits, for example the flexor digitorum superficialis. This is a general principle in relation to a movement in which more than one muscle can act as a prime mover. There is usually one muscle which is used for slow movements not involving much force. Other muscles are recruited for a rapid movement or a movement involving greater force.

This has been observed in the triceps brachii in that the medial head is used to extend the forearm and the lateral and long heads are recruited for rapid or forceful movements.

The Pronator Quadratus. This quadrilateral muscle is attached to the lowest quarter of the anterior surface of the ulna and passes laterally and slightly downwards to be attached to a similar area on the radius. The muscle is innervated by the anterior interosseous nerve (C8), a branch of the median nerve. As its name implies it is a pronator of the forearm.

The main blood vessels of the forearm (figure 225(b))

The brachial artery usually divides in the cubital fossa at the level of the neck of the radius into the *radial* and *ulnar arteries*.

The Radial Artery. The radial artery passes downwards on the tendons and muscles attached to the radius (the tendon of the biceps brachii, supinator, pronator teres, flexor digitorum superficialis, flexor pollicis longus and pronator quadratus) and directly on the radius above the wrist. In the upper half of the forearm the artery is deep to the brachioradialis muscle. In the lower half it is subcutaneous and can be palpated, especially over the lower quarter of the radius. Distal to the styloid process the artery runs backwards deep to the tendons of the abductor pollicis longus and extensor pollicis brevis into the hollow called the anatomical snuffbox. The artery then passes forwards between the first and second metacarpal bones into the palm of the hand. The superficial branch of the radial nerve is lateral to the artery in the upper two-thirds of the forearm. The nerve passes backwards deep to the brachioradialis to the back of the forearm. Two venae comitantes accompany the radial artery along its whole course.

The radial artery gives off a recurrent branch to the region of the elbow, muscular branches and a *superficial palmar branch* which goes into the palm superficial to the flexor retinaculum. The artery also gives off *palmar* and *dorsal carpal branches*.

The dorsal carpal branch arises in the snuffbox, runs medially deep to the extensor tendons and gives off *metacarpal branches* which divide into *digital branches*. The branches in the palm are described on p. 399.

The Ulnar Artery. The ulnar artery passes downwards and medially from its origin from the brachial artery. It runs deep to the pronator teres, flexor carpi radialis, palmaris longus and flexor digitorum superficialis and about the middle of the forearm runs straight downwards on the flexor digitorum profundus deep to the flexor carpi ulnaris. In the lower part of the forearm the artery is more superficial and lies between the flexor carpi ulnaris and the flexor digitorum superficialis. At the wrist it is superficial to the flexor retinaculum and lateral to the pisiform bone.

The median nerve is medial to the ulnar artery just distal to the elbow. As the nerve passes between the two heads of the pronator teres it crosses the artery anteriorly and becomes lateral to it. The ulnar nerve after entering the forearm runs downwards medial to the artery and accompanies it into the palm superficial to the flexor retinaculum.

The ulnar artery gives off anterior and posterior recurrent branches which pass upwards towards the elbow, supply the muscles of the region and take part in the anastomosis round the elbow.

The *common interosseous artery* arises about 2 cm below the origin of the ulnar artery, is about 1 cm long and divides into the *anterior* and *posterior interosseous arteries*. The anterior interosseous artery runs downwards on the anterior surface of the interosseous membrane with the anterior interosseous nerve, a branch of the median nerve. The artery supplies the deep muscles on the anterior and posterior aspects of the forearm, the latter by means of perforating branches. Above the pronator quadratus the artery, after giving off an *anterior carpal branch*, pierces the interosseous membrane to end on the back of the carpus. The posterior interosseous artery passes backwards above the upper border of the interosseous membrane and runs downwards with the posterior interosseous nerve between the superficial and deep layers of the posterior muscles of the forearm to the carpal region where it anastomoses with the anterior

The Upper Arm and Forearm   377

interosseous artery and branches of the radial and ulnar arteries.

The ulnar artery gives off muscular branches as it runs down the forearm and at the wrist gives off palmar and dorsal carpal branches.

The ulnar artery is accompanied by two venae comitantes which at the elbow join the radial venae comitantes to form the brachial veins. The ulnar veins receive blood from the hand and near the elbow receive anterior and posterior interosseous veins.

The nerves of the front of the forearm (figure 225(b))

These include the continuation of the median and ulnar nerves and the superficial branch of the radial nerve (usually referred to as the radial nerve).

The Median Nerve. In the cubital fossa the median nerve is medial to the brachial artery and continues downwards between the two heads of the pronator teres anterior to the ulnar artery which is deep to both heads. The median nerve, now lateral to the ulnar artery, passes deep to the flexor digitorum superficialis and continues downwards deep to and adherent to that muscle. Near the wrist the median nerve becomes more superficial, lateral to the tendons of the superficialis and lies between the palmaris longus which when present is medial and the flexor carpi radialis which is lateral. The median nerve passes into the palm deep to the flexor retinaculum. In the forearm the median nerve is accompanied by a branch of the anterior interosseous artery.

The median nerve supplies all the muscles of the forearm, except the flexor carpi ulnaris and the medial half of the flexor digitorum profundus, either directly, or indirectly through the anterior interosseous nerve which supplies the flexor pollicis longus, the lateral half of the profundus and the pronator quadratus. The *anterior interosseous nerve* is given off just above the pronator teres and runs downwards on the interosseous membrane between the flexor pollicis longus and the flexor digitorum profundus. The nerve ends on the deep surface of the pronator quadratus and gives branches to the

joints at the wrist.

The *palmar cutaneous branch* arises just above the flexor retinaculum and after piercing the deep fascia supplies the skin of the lateral and central parts of the palm.

The Ulnar Nerve. The ulnar nerve enters the forearm from behind the medial epicondyle by passing between the two heads of the flexor carpi ulnaris. The nerve runs downwards deep to the flexor carpi ulnaris on the flexor digitorum profundus on the medial side of the ulnar artery. In the lower half of the forearm the nerve and artery become more superficial and enter the palm lateral to the pisiform bone by passing anterior to the flexor retinaculum.

About the middle of the forearm a *palmar cutaneous branch* is given off and passes downwards to supply the skin on the medial side of the palm. A *dorsal branch* leaves the ulnar nerve about 5 cm above the wrist, passes backwards deep to the tendon of the flexor carpi ulnaris and is distributed as *dorsal digital nerves* to the sides of the little finger and the medial side of the ring finger as far as the distal interphalangeal joint. The ulnar nerve supplies branches to the medial half of the flexor digitorum profundus and to the flexor carpi ulnaris.

The Radial Nerve. The radial nerve in the cubital fossa lies deep to the brachioradialis and extensor carpi radialis longus on the brachialis. At the level of the lateral epicondyle the nerve divides into its two terminal branches, *superficial* and *deep*, usually called the *radial* and *posterior interosseous nerves.* The posterior interosseous nerve winds round the lateral side of the radius between the two layers of the supinator muscle and runs downwards between the superficial and deep muscles of the back of the forearm. The radial nerve continues downwards in the forearm on the lateral side of the radial artery but about two-thirds down the forearm the nerve leaves the artery and runs downwards and backwards deep to the brachioradialis. The nerve divides into four or five *dorsal digital nerves* which supply the two sides of the thumb, index and middle fingers and the lateral side of the ring finger as far as the interphalangeal joint of the thumb and the distal interphalangeal joints of the other digits. Because of the way in which any area of the skin is supplied by more than one nerve, division of the superficial branch of the radial nerve results in a loss of sensation over a small area of the skin about 2 cm in diameter, on the back of the hand proximal to the thumb and index finger.

The posterior muscles of the forearm (figure 226)

They are arranged in three groups: (1) two muscles attached to the lateral supracondylar ridge, the brachioradialis and extensor carpi radialis longus; (2) four muscles attached to the common extensor

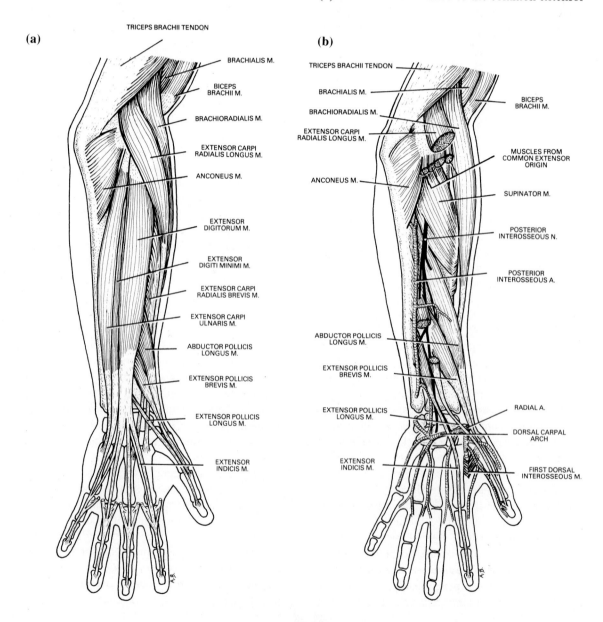

(a)

TRICEPS BRACHII TENDON

BRACHIALIS M.

BICEPS BRACHII M.

BRACHIORADIALIS M.

EXTENSOR CARPI RADIALIS LONGUS M.

ANCONEUS M.

EXTENSOR DIGITORUM M.

EXTENSOR DIGITI MINIMI M.

EXTENSOR CARPI RADIALIS BREVIS M.

EXTENSOR CARPI ULNARIS M.

ABDUCTOR POLLICIS LONGUS M.

EXTENSOR POLLICIS BREVIS M.

EXTENSOR POLLICIS LONGUS M.

EXTENSOR INDICIS M.

(b)

TRICEPS BRACHII TENDON

BRACHIALIS M.

BRACHIORADIALIS M.

EXTENSOR CARPI RADIALIS LONGUS M.

ANCONEUS M.

BICEPS BRACHII M.

MUSCLES FROM COMMON EXTENSOR ORIGIN

SUPINATOR M.

POSTERIOR INTEROSSEOUS N.

POSTERIOR INTEROSSEOUS A.

ABDUCTOR POLLICIS LONGUS M.

EXTENSOR POLLICIS BREVIS M.

EXTENSOR POLLICIS LONGUS M.

EXTENSOR INDICIS M.

RADIAL A.

DORSAL CARPAL ARCH

FIRST DORSAL INTEROSSEOUS M.

Figure 226   The back of the right forearm: (a) the superficial muscles; (b) the deep muscles.

origin on the lateral epicondyle, the extensor carpi radialis brevis, extensor digitorum, extensor digiti minimi and extensor carpi ulnaris (extensors of the wrist and digits other than the thumb); (3) five muscles in a deep plane and attached to the back of the radius and ulna, the supinator and the abductor pollicis longus to both bones, the extensor pollicis longus to the ulna, the extensor pollicis brevis to the radius and the extensor indicis to the ulna; except for the supinator these muscles are attached distally to the thumb or index finger. All these muscles also have attachments to connective tissue structures such as the ligaments of the elbow joint, the interosseous membrane and intermuscular septa and are supplied by the radial nerve or its deep terminal branch, the posterior interosseous nerve.

The Brachioradialis (figure 225). Its proximal attachment is to the upper two-thirds of the lateral supracondylar ridge. The muscle passes down the lateral side of the forearm and ends in a tendon which is attached to the lateral side of the lower end of the radius above the styloid process. At the elbow the muscle forms the lateral boundary of the cubital fossa and the radial nerve lies deep to it on the brachialis. The superficial branch of the radial nerve and the radial artery lie deep to the brachioradialis in the upper part of the forearm. The nerve passes backwards deep to the muscle and the artery becomes subcutaneous medial to its lower part.

The brachioradialis is supplied by the radial nerve (C6). Because of its line of pull it can pronate the forearm from the anatomical position to the midprone position and supinate the forearm from the fully prone position to the midprone position. In the midprone position it can flex the forearm at the elbow joint against resistance or in rapid movements.

The Extensors Carpi Radialis Longus and Brevis (figures 225, 226). The extensor longus is attached to the lower one-third of the lateral supracondylar ridge and the extensor brevis to the lateral epicondyle. They pass downwards on the lateral side of the forearm and lie in separate grooves on the back of the lower end of the radius deep to the ex-

tensor retinaculum. The longus tendon is attached to the posterior aspect of the base of the second metacarpal bone and the brevis tendon to a similar area on the third metacarpal bone. In the lower third of the forearm both muscles are crossed superficially by the abductor pollicis longus and extensor pollicis brevis as they pass laterally. Just distal to the radius, the tendon of the extensor carpi radialis longus is crossed superficially by the tendon of the extensor pollicis longus.

The longus muscle is supplied directly from the radial nerve and the brevis by the posterior interosseous nerve (mainly C7). These muscles extend and abduct the hand at the wrist. When the fist is tightly clenched they contract to prevent the hand being flexed by the flexors of the digits, that is they act as synergists preventing an unwanted action by the prime movers. The brevis tendon can be felt on the back of the wrist beyond the distal end of the radius when the fist is clenched. The longus tendon is covered in this position by the tendon of the extensor pollicis longus.

The Extensor Digitorum. This muscle is attached to the common extensor origin on the lateral epicondyle and, in the lower third of the forearm, divides into four tendons which go to the medial four digits. Deep to the extensor retinaculum the tendons lie in a groove on the back of the radius together with the tendon of the extensor indicis. On the back of the hand the tendons are joined by transverse bands. The most medial band between the tendons to the little and ring fingers may limit abduction of the little finger when the digits are fully extended and for this reason the band may be divided to increase the span of the fingers in pianists. The tendons of the extensor indicis and extensor digiti minimi are medial to and fuse with the respective common extensor tendons to the index and little finger.

The attachment of the extensor tendons of the medial four digits is complicated by their relation to an aponeurotic expansion, the *dorsal digital expansion* (figure 227), which extends in each digit from the metacarpophalangeal joint to the base of the distal phalanx, and by the attachment of the interosseous and lumbrical muscles to the expansion. The dorsal digital expansion has a tri-

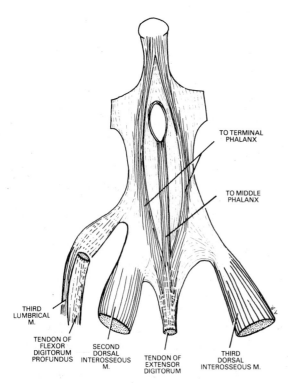

Figure labels:

TO TERMINAL PHALANX

TO MIDDLE PHALANX

THIRD LUMBRICAL M.

TENDON OF FLEXOR DIGITORUM PROFUNDUS

SECOND DORSAL INTEROSSEOUS M.

TENDON OF EXTENSOR DIGITORUM

THIRD DORSAL INTEROSSEOUS M.

Figure 227   A posterior view of the dorsal digital expansion of the right middle finger.

angular base at the level of the metacarpophalangeal joint. The extensor tendon blends with the middle of the base which forms part of the capsule of the joint. On the lateral side an interosseous and lumbrical muscle and on the medial side an interosseous muscle are attached to the base of the dorsal expansion. The base is also attached to the deep transverse metacarpal ligaments of the palm (p. 405). This band separates the tendon of a dorsal interosseous from the tendons of a palmar interosseous and lumbrical.

Further distally over the proximal interphalangeal joint the extensor tendon divides into three. The middle part, reinforced by the interosseous and lumbrical muscles is attached to the posterior aspect of the base of the middle phalanx. The lateral parts of the tendon are joined by the corresponding thickened edge of the dorsal digital expansion and after fusing are attached to the posterior surface of the base of the distal phalanx.

The extensor digitorum is supplied by the posterior interosseous nerve (mainly C7) and extends the digits at the metacarpophalangeal and proximal and distal interphalangeal joints. Flexion and extension at these joints can be carried out in various combinations of movements and are discussed on p. 410. Slow extension of the flexed digits as in straightening the digits after making a fist is brought about by the extensor digitorum (and extensor indicis and digiti minimi). A more rapid or more forceful extension involves the lumbrical and interosseous muscles which act at the interphalangeal joints.

The Extensor Digiti Minimi. Its upper attachment is to the common extensor origin and distally its tendon lies on the medial side of the little finger tendon of the extensor digitorum with which it fuses. Its nerve supply is from the posterior interosseous nerve (mainly C7) and its action is to extend the digit at the metacarpophalangeal and interphalangeal joints.

The Extensor Carpi Ulnaris. From the common extensor origin on the lateral epicondyle the muscle passes downwards to the medial side of the back of the forearm. Some of its fibres are attached to the posterior border of the ulna through the aponeurosis common to this muscle and the flexor digitorum profundus and the flexor carpi ulnaris. It forms a tendon which lies in the groove on the back of the lower end of the ulna and is attached to the posterior aspect of the base of the fifth metacarpal bone. The muscle is supplied by the posterior interosseous nerve (mainly C8) and is an extensor and adductor of the hand at the wrist.

The Supinator. The fibres of this muscle are in two layers between which the posterior interosseous nerve passes to the back of the forearm (figure 223(b)). The deep layer is horizontal, is attached to the supinator crest on the lateral side of the upper part of the ulna and winds round the upper part of the radius to which it is attached on its anterior, lateral and posterior surfaces. The superficial layer is more oblique and is attached to the common extensor origin and passes downwards round the upper end of the radius to become attached anteriorly at a lower level than the deep part.

The supinator is supplied by the posterior interosseous nerve (C6) and as the name suggests is a supinator of the forearm.

The Abductor Pollicis Longus (figure 226(b)). This muscle is attached to the posterior surfaces of the upper part of the radius and ulna. The muscle passes downwards and laterally, crosses superficial to the extensors carpi radialis brevis and longus and forms a tendon which lies in a groove on the lateral side of the lower end of the radius deep to the extensor retinaculum. The tendon is attached to the lateral side of the base of the first metacarpal bone.

The muscle is supplied by the posterior interosseous nerve (C8) which passes downwards superficial to the muscle with the posterior interosseous artery. It is the only digital muscle in the hand and foot which is attached to a metacarpal or metatarsal bone. Its action is to abduct the thumb at the carpometacarpal joint.

The Extensor Pollicis Brevis. Its upper attachment is to the posterior surface of the radius inferior to the attachment of the abductor pollicis longus. The muscle and tendon run downwards medial to the abductor and take a similar course, crossing superficial to the radial extensors of the wrist and the

radial artery. The tendon is attached to the posterior surface of the base of the proximal phalanx of the thumb.

The muscle is innervated by the posterior interosseous nerve (C8) and extends the thumb at the metacarpophalangeal and carpometacarpal joints.

The Extensor Pollicis Longus. This muscle is attached to the posterior surface of the ulna between the attachments of the abductor pollicis longus and extensor indicis. The muscle ends in a tendon which lies in a groove medial to the dorsal tubercle of the radius deep to the extensor retinaculum and passes along the back of the thumb to the posterior surface of the base of the distal phalanx of the thumb.

The muscle is innervated by the posterior interosseous nerve (C8) and extends the thumb at the interphalangeal, metacarpophalangeal and carpometacarpal joints of the thumb. The obliquity of the tendon results in the thumb being pulled backwards and rotated laterally as well as extended.

The Anatomical Snuffbox (figure 228). This refers to a hollow proximal to the base of the thumb, bounded laterally by the tendons of the abductor pollicis longus and extensor pollicis brevis and medially by the tendon of the extensor pollicis

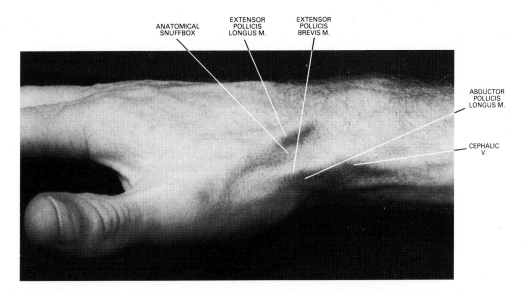

Figure 228 The right anatomical snuffbox.

longus. One presumes that it is called the *snuffbox* because snuff is deposited in this position before being sniffed. In the floor of the space it is possible to palpate proximally the radial styloid process, the lateral carpal bones (the scaphoid and the trapezium) and distally the base of the first metacarpal bone. The cephalic vein begins in the superficial fascia overlying the snuffbox and the terminal branches of the radial nerve can be felt as they pass across the tendon of the extensor pollicis longus. The radial artery lies in the hollow of the snuffbox. Of all the structures mentioned, clinically the most important is the scaphoid bone in so far as after an injury to the wrist, persistent pain on pressure in the snuffbox is characteristic of a fracture of this bone.

The Extensor Indicis. Its upper attachment is to the lower end of the posterior surface of the ulna. The muscle passes downwards medial to the extensor pollicis longus and ends in a tendon which passes deep to the extensor retinaculum together with the extensor digitorum. The indicis tendon is medial to the tendon of the extensor digitorum to the index finger and fuses with it proximal to the dorsal digital expansion. The muscle is supplied by the posterior interosseous nerve (C8) and is an extensor of the index finger.

The posterior interosseous artery and nerve (figure 226)

The artery is a branch of the common interosseous branch of the ulnar artery and passes to the back of the forearm between the radius and ulna above the upper border of the interosseous membrane. The nerve is one of the terminal branches of the radial nerve and reaches the back of the forearm by passing between the two layers of the supinator round the lateral side of the radius. The nerve with the artery lying medially passes down the back of the forearm between the superficial and deep muscles and supplies both groups. The nerve ends distally by supplying the joints of the carpus, and the artery ends by taking part in an anastomosis with the anterior interosseous artery and carpal branches of the ulnar and radial arteries.

30

The Elbow and Radio-ulnar Joints

The *elbow joint* is formed by the distal end of the humerus and the proximal ends of the radius and ulna. The *superior radio-ulnar joint*, between the head of the radius and the radial notch of the ulna and annular ligament, has a joint cavity continuous with that of the elbow joint. The *inferior radio-ulnar joint*, between the head of the ulna and the ulnar notch of the radius, has no communication with the wrist joint as a rule. The union by the interosseous membrane of the shafts of the radius and ulna is, by strict definition, a fibrous joint between the radius and ulna and is sometimes called the *middle radio-ulnar joint*.

The Elbow Joint (figure 229)

This is a synovial joint of the hinge type. The proximal surface of the joint is formed by the convex capitulum and pulley-like trochlea. The medial flange of the trochlea projects distally much more than the lateral. The trochlear notch has an upper olecranon part separated by a narrow ridge of bone which is not covered by articular cartilage. The concave upper surface of the radial head fits on to the convex surface of the capitulum.

The *capsular ligament* of the elbow joint is attached anteriorly to the humerus above the radial and coronoid fossae and posteriorly above the olecranon fossa. Inferiorly it is attached to the coronoid process and the annular ligament of the superior radio-ulnar joint. Laterally and medially the capsule is thickened by the *radial* and *ulnar*

collateral ligaments. The lateral and medial epicondyles, with their extensor and flexor areas respectively, are extracapsular.

The *radial collateral (lateral) ligament* is attached superiorly to the lateral epicondyle and inferiorly to the annular ligament. Its most posterior fibres are attached to the lateral side of the ulna. The *ulnar collateral (medial) ligament* has three bands, an anterior passing from the medial epicondyle to the medial side of the coronoid process, a posterior attached to the medial epicondyle and medial edge of the olecranon and an oblique passing between the olecranon and the coronoid process. The ulnar nerve as it lies in the groove behind the medial epicondyle is closely related to the ulnar collateral ligament. Almost all the muscles related to the elbow joint — the brachialis anteriorly, the triceps and anconeus posteriorly, the supinator and the muscles originating from the common tendon of the extensors laterally and those attached to the common tendon of the flexors medially — have an attachment to the capsule or collateral ligaments.

The *synovial membrane* lines the capsule and ends at the edges of the articular cartilage. Outside the synovial membrane and within the capsule there are *pads of fat* which move in and out of the radial, coronoid and olecranon fossae in movements at the joint. An extracapsular pad of fat on the medial side of the joint may be continuous with the intracapsular pad through a defect in the middle of the ulnar collateral ligament.

The *arteries* forming the anastomosis round the joint (p. 370) give branches to the joint. The *nerve*

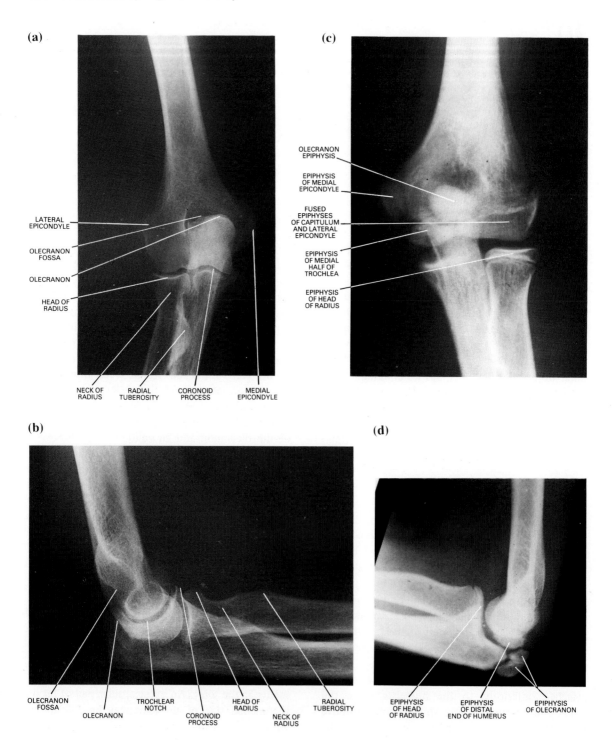

(a)

LATERAL EPICONDYLE

OLECRANON FOSSA

OLECRANON

HEAD OF RADIUS

NECK OF RADIUS   RADIAL TUBEROSITY   CORONOID PROCESS   MEDIAL EPICONDYLE

(c)

OLECRANON EPIPHYSIS

EPIPHYSIS OF MEDIAL EPICONDYLE

FUSED EPIPHYSES OF CAPITULUM AND LATERAL EPICONDYLE

EPIPHYSIS OF MEDIAL HALF OF TROCHLEA

EPIPHYSIS OF HEAD OF RADIUS

(b)

OLECRANON FOSSA

OLECRANON

TROCHLEAR NOTCH

CORONOID PROCESS

HEAD OF RADIUS

NECK OF RADIUS

RADIAL TUBEROSITY

(d)

EPIPHYSIS OF HEAD OF RADIUS

EPIPHYSIS OF DISTAL END OF HUMERUS

EPIPHYSIS OF OLECRANON

Figure 229   X-rays of the elbow joint: (a) anteroposterior with the elbow straight; (b) lateral with the elbow bent to a right angle; (c) and (d) anteroposterior and lateral of a boy aged 12 years.

supply is derived anteriorly mainly from the musculocutaneous nerve and posteriorly from the radial nerve. The ulnar and median nerves usually give twigs to the joint. As in all synovial joints the nerve fibres are vasomotor to a large extent but some subserve painful sensations and others, larger fibres, are mechanoreceptors, that is they give information about movements at the joint and the position in which it is held.

The *movements* at the elbow joint are flexion and extension. In flexion the forearm rotates about a transverse axis until the anterior surface of the forearm is in contact with the anterior surface of the upper arm. Thus contact of the soft parts limits further flexion. The main flexors are the brachialis, biceps brachii (both supplied by the musculo-cutaneous nerve, C5, 6) and the brachioradialis (supplied by the radial nerve, C5, 6). In slow movements not involving much force the brachialis is the main muscle used. Rapid or forceful movements recruit the biceps brachii and the brachioradialis. In very powerful flexion any of the muscles anterior to the joint, for example the pronator teres, may be involved. Extension is best defined as a restoration of the flexed forearm to the anatomical position and is brought about mainly by the triceps brachii and to some extent by the anconeus (both are supplied by the radial nerve, C7, 8). The medial head of the triceps brachii is the part used in slow movements and the lateral and long heads are involved in rapid and forceful movements. Extension is limited by the locking of the olecranon in the olecranon fossa. If the olecranon is fractured further extension is possible, although this is limited by the anterior part of the capsule and the muscles anterior to the joint.

In the anatomical position, with full extension at the elbow, the forearm deviates laterally and forms an angle, measured on the outer side, of about 160°. This is called the *carrying angle* and is due to the asymmetry of the trochlea of the humerus (the medial edge of the trochlea projects about 5 mm beyond the lateral) and the shape and direction of the articular areas of the trochlear notch (the lateral part of the articular area of the coronoid process faces laterally as well as upwards). When the forearm is fully flexed it is in line with the upper arm and the nearly symmetrical articular areas of the olecranon articulate with the anterior part of the trochlea. With the forearm fully extended at the elbow and rotated so that the thumb points forwards the carrying angle apparently disappears and the upper arm, forearm and hand are more or less in a straight line.

An interesting example of how the antagonists take over the functions of the prime movers without in any way interrupting a slow, smooth movement is well demonstrated at the elbow joint. If the upper limb is held at right angles from the body by abduction or flexion at the shoulder joint and the forearm is slowly flexed, the movement is at first brought about by the flexors of the elbow, mainly the brachialis. At some point when the forearm is approximately at a right angle to the upper arm, the brachialis relaxes and the triceps brachii contracts and controls further flexion. With the upper limb held in the same position at the shoulder extension of the forearm from full flexion is initially carried out by the triceps brachii, but beyond a right angle further extension is controlled by the brachialis, and the triceps brachii relaxes. One is completely unaware of the change of muscles controlling the movement and the movement is carried out smoothly and uninterruptedly.

Dislocation at the elbow joint is usually a backward movement of the ulna and is often associated with a fracture of the coronoid process. The forearm is in an extended position and the backward displacement leads to pressure on the brachial artery which may go into spasm and dangerously reduce the blood supply to the forearm and hand. This complication may arise in supracondylar fractures of the humerus in which the lower fragment is angulated forwards and the brachial artery is pressed on. The median nerve may be injured so that (1) pronation of the forearm; (2) flexion at the proximal interphalangeal joints of the medial four digits and distal interphalangeal joints of the index and middle fingers and interphalangeal joint of the thumb; (3) opposition of the thumb are lost. Flexion at the distal interphalangeal joints of the ring and little finger is retained. There is also a sensory loss on the lateral side of the palm and in the lateral three and a half digits anteriorly. In both supracondylar fractures and dislocations there is considerable swelling in the region of the elbow. In the former the normal alignment of the lateral and medial epicondyles and olecranon is not altered (p. 367), but in dislocations it is changed.

Fracture of the olecranon has to be considered when an apparently dislocated joint cannot be reduced. The joint is very unstable.

Dislocation may occur due to abduction of the forearm. This may be associated with tearing of the ulnar collateral ligament or more commonly an avulsion fracture of the medial epicondyle. The ulnar nerve may be damaged at the time of injury. Subsequently, if the fracture does not unite or the ligament not heal, the forearm may become more and more abducted. The ulnar nerve is stretched and sensory disturbances are found on the medial side of the hand and the little and ring fingers and weakness and paralysis of many of the small muscles of the hand. In addition the medial half of the flexor digitorum profundus is paralysed with a loss of flexion of the terminal phalanges of the ring and little fingers and the flexor carpi ulnaris is paralysed so that the hand is abducted when it is flexed at the wrist.

Reference has already been made to the possibility in a child of the dislocation of the head of the radius because the head is small, with the result that the annular ligament does not hold it in place very easily. In older people the annular ligament may be torn and the head dislocated forwards due to a fall on the hand with the forearm extended.

The Radio-ulnar Joints (figures 229, 230)

The *proximal (superior) radio-ulnar joint* is between the head of the radius and the fibro-osseous ring formed by the radial notch of the ulna and the annular ligament. The *distal (inferior)* is between the head of the ulna and the ulnar notch of the radius, and the *middle* between the shafts of the radius and ulna.

The Proximal (Superior) Radio-ulnar Joint

This is a synovial joint of the pivot type and its joint cavity is continuous with that of the elbow

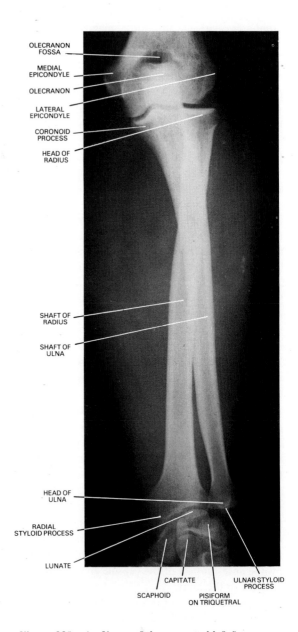

Figure 230   An X-ray of the pronated left forearm.

joint. The *annular ligament* is attached to the anterior and posterior edges of the radial notch and forms more than three-quarters of the ring in which the head of the radius lies. Posteriorly the ligament widens and is attached to adjacent areas of bone above and below the notch. Superiorly and laterally the annular ligament blends with the capsular ligament of the elbow joint and the radial collateral ligament. Inferiorly there are some loose fibres between the ligament and the neck of the radius which allow the head to rotate. The *quadrate ligament* is the name given to the fibrous tissue between the radius and ulna inferior to the joint.

Synovial membrane lines only the lower non-articular part of the annular ligament and turns upwards on the neck of the radius. Most of the annular ligament is lined by articular cartilage.

The Distal (Inferior) Radio-ulnar Joint

This is a pivot joint between the head of the ulna and the ulnar notch of the radius. The bones are held together by a *fibrous capsule* attached to the edges of the articular areas. Superiorly the capsule is continuous with the interosseous membrane and inferiorly with the capsule of the wrist joint. The *synovial membrane* lines the capsule and may extend upwards between the radius and ulna in front of the interosseous membrane (*recessus sacciformis*).

A triangular *articular disc* joins the distal ends of the radius and ulna. Its apex is attached to a pit on the lateral side of the proximal end of the styloid process of the ulna and its base is attached laterally to the lower edge of the ulnar notch of the radius. As a result the distal radio-ulnar joint is separated from the wrist (radiocarpal) joint but occasionally the disc is perforated. Anteriorly and posteriorly the disc is attached to the capsule of the wrist joint, superiorly it articulates with the head of the ulna and inferiorly it forms part of the proximal surface of the wrist joint.

The Middle Radio-ulnar Joint

The interosseous borders of the radius and ulna are joined by the interosseous membrane which passes obliquely downwards and medially from the radius to the ulna. Superiorly it has an upper free border which is about 3 cm distal to the radial tuberosity. Inferiorly it is attached to the posterior of the two lines into which the radial interosseous border divides and it blends with the capsule of the distal radio-ulnar joint. The deep muscles of the front and back of the forearm are attached to the membrane. The anterior interosseous nerve and vessels pass downwards on its anterior surface but posteriorly the vessels and nerve are related only to its lowest part. The anterior interosseous artery perforates the lower part of the membrane and lies on its posterior aspect and the posterior interosseous artery passes backwards above the upper border of the membrane.

There is a band of fibres attached to the radius distal to the radial tuberosity and running upwards and medially to the ulna in front of the attachment of the supinator. This is called the *oblique cord*.

The movements which occur at the radio-ulnar joints are *pronation* and *supination*. In pronation of the forearm the head of the radius rotates at the proximal radio-ulnar joint and the lower end of the radius swings over to the medial side of the ulna and, together with the hand, faces backwards. In supination the pronated forearm is restored to the anatomical position in which the radius and ulna are more or less parallel and the hand faces forwards. The main muscles producing pronation are the pronator teres and pronator quadratus (both are supplied by the median nerve, C7, 8). The muscles producing supination are the supinator and biceps brachii. The former is supplied by the radial nerve (C6), the latter by the musculo-cutaneous (C6). Slow and less powerful movements involve only the pronator quadratus and supinator.

The axis of the movements of pronation and supination can vary and is often erroneously stated to be through the centre of the head of the radius and the ulnar styloid process. It is obvious that if the index finger of the left hand is placed on the ulnar styloid process of the right wrist and the right forearm is pronated, the ulnar styloid moves laterally and backwards. The extent of the movement of the ulna can vary and it is said that the axis of movement of pronation and supination can pass through the head of the radius and any of the medial four digits. There is the problem of what causes the ulna to move and it has been suggested that the upper end of the ulna moves on the trochlea of the humerus (the two joint surfaces do not fit closely) and that the considerable movement of the distal end is the movement of the end of the long arm of a lever with the fulcrum at the elbow.

It has also been suggested that the anconeus can move the ulna in the way described.

The forearm can be pronated through about 160° from the anatomical position with the forearm extended, but medial rotation of the humerus at the shoulder joint can confuse the range of supination and pronation of the forearm. By flexing the forearm at the elbow this problem is eliminated. Likewise the range of lateral and medial rotation at the shoulder joint should be investigated with the forearm in the flexed position.

Supination as a rule is a more powerful movement than pronation. The threads of screws, corkscrews, etc., etc., are cut on the assumption that they will be inserted by supination of the right forearm.

Observation of many activities confirms how frequently the movements of pronation and supination are used. Loss of these movements is a marked disability and can occur as a result of cross-union between the radius and ulna following fracture of both bones. If the movements are lost it is best for the forearm to be fixed in the midprone position, that is with the palm of the hand facing medially.

31

The Wrist and Hand

Even the most cursory consideration of the extent to and the way in which the hand is used indicates its importance in every day life. The hand is a sensory and motor instrument capable of a very wide range of activities, ranging from the crude as in grasping an object in order to move it or wield it as a weapon, to the delicate as in movements involved in writing, painting, playing a musical instrument or spinning a cricket ball. There are few occupations in which a permanent defect of the hand does not amount to a considerable disability and the hand is particularly vulnerable because it is usually unprotected. It is liable to become infected or injured, and diseases of its joints are common. It can be indirectly affected by lesions of the peripheral and central nervous systems.

The Bones of the Wrist and Hand

The wrist or carpal bones collectively form the *carpus*. The distal carpal bones articulate with the *metacarpal bones*. The *phalanges* (two in the thumb and three in each of the other digits) form a *digit*. (The term *finger* should be avoided unless the finger is specified as the *thumb*, *index*, *middle*, *ring* and *little fingers*. If asked, most people say that there are four fingers and a thumb, but the *third finger* can mean a different finger to different people and the wrong finger has been amputated because of this.)

The carpal bones (the carpus) (figure 231)

These are arranged in two rows, a proximal consisting of, from lateral to medial, the *scaphoid*, *lunate*, *triquetral* and *pisiform* and a distal, the *trapezium*, *trapezoid*, *capitate* and *hamate* (*scaphe* = *boat*, Greek; *pisum* = *pea*, Latin; *caput* = *head*, Latin; *hamus* = *hook*, Latin). The scaphoid, hollowed medially to look like a boat, has a *tubercle* which is anterior and distal. Proximally the scaphoid articulates with the distal end of the radius and distally with the trapezium and trapezoid. Medially the scaphoid has a concave surface which together with the lunate articulates with the *head* of the capitate. The lunate articulates proximally with the distal end of the radius. The triquetral articulates proximally with the triangular articular disc of the wrist-joint. The proximal row of bones forms a convex articular surface which articulates with the concave area formed by the distal surfaces of the radius and triangular disc. The pisiform (like a split pea) articulates with the anterior surface of the triquetral.

The distal surfaces of the proximal row of bones form a sinuous articular area convex laterally and concave medially for the proximal surface of the distal row of bones; the trapezium and trapezoid articulate with the scaphoid, the head of the capitate with the scaphoid and lunate and the hamate with the triquetral. The distal surfaces of the distal row articulate with the bases of the metacarpal bones, the trapezium with the first, the trapezoid

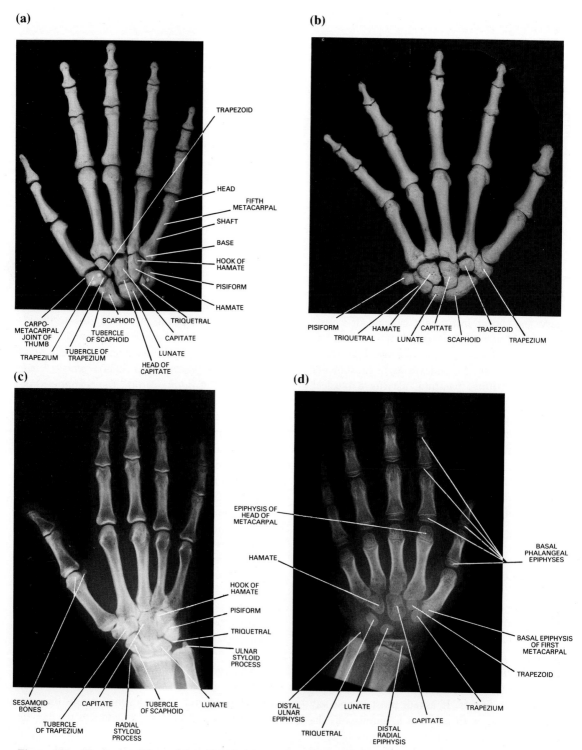

Figure 231   The bones of the wrist and hand: (a) anterior aspect; (b) posterior aspect; (c) X-ray of the adult wrist and hand; (d) X-ray of a child aged about 5 years.

with the second, the capitate with the third and the hamate with the fourth and fifth. The base of the second metacarpal is more proximal than that of the others and is slotted in between the trapezium and capitate with both of which it articulates.

The anterior aspect of the carpus has four projections. On the lateral side there are the tubercle of the scaphoid and the *tubercle (ridge) of the trapezium*, and on the medial side the pisiform and the *hook of the hamate. All four projections can be palpated. The tubercle of the scaphoid on the distal part of the bone is 2 cm medial and distal to the tip of the radial styloid process. The tubercle of the trapezium, more difficult to feel, is about 1 cm distal to the scaphoid tubercle. The pisiform is easily felt medially and is often seen in line with the tubercle of the scaphoid. The tendon of the flexor carpi ulnaris leads to the bone which may be regarded as a sesamoid bone in the tendon. The hook of the hamate, about 2 cm distal and slightly lateral to the pisiform, is more difficult to palpate.* The *flexor retinaculum* is attached to these four prominences and with the concave anterior surface of the carpus forms the *carpal tunnel* (figure 234). The long flexor tendons, the flexors digitorum superficialis and profundus, with the median nerve immediately deep to it on the lateral superficialis tendons, pass deep to the retinaculum. The flexor carpi radialis, lying in a groove on the trapezium, and the flexor pollicis longus are in the carpal tunnel.

The carpal bones *ossify* in cartilage. At birth all the carpal bones are cartilaginous. The capitate is the first to begin to ossify (early in the first year). The hamate begins to ossify late in the first year, the triquetral in the second and the lunate in the third. The scaphoid begins to ossify in the fourth year and the trapezium and trapezoid by the end of the fourth year. The ossification of the pisiform begins much later — in the 10th year. Excluding the pisiform it can be seen that the carpal bones usually ossify in an order indicated by a spiral, beginning with the capitate early in the first year, and passing successively to the hamate, triquetral, lunate, scaphoid, trapezium and trapezoid by the end of the fourth year. Ossification of the carpal bones is used as an indicator of physical development and state of nutrition. The time of commence-

ment of ossification and the degree of ossification of individual bones are delayed in slow physical development and malnutrition. X-rays of the carpal bones are compared with standard X-ray charts which were obtained by longitudinal studies of large numbers of children.

The carpal bones consist of an outer thin shell of compact bone and central spongy bone. The commonest injuries are fractures of the scaphoid and dislocation of the lunate. A fracture of the scaphoid may be complicated by the necrosis of the proximal part of the bone. This occurs because its blood vessels frequently enter the bone through the distal half (associated with the tubercle) and pass proximally so that a fracture across the middle of the scaphoid results in the proximal fragment losing its blood supply.

The metacarpal bones (figure 231)

Each bone has a *shaft*, a proximal *base* and a distal *head* which forms the prominence of the knuckle. The medial four metacarpal bones are similar in shape but the first metacarpal resembles in some ways a phalanx. The shaft of a metacarpal bone is curved with an anterior concavity and is triangular in section with lateral and medial ridges limiting the smooth posterior surface. The anterior border is rounded and marks off lateral and medial surfaces. The head has a distal, rounded, articular surface which extends further anteriorly than posteriorly and articulates with the base of a proximal phalanx. An anterior groove on the head lodges the flexor tendons. The base of each metacarpal bone has articular areas for the distal row of carpal bones and the bases of adjacent metacarpals.

The metacarpal bone of the thumb is shorter and broader than the others. The base has a proximal saddle-shaped articular facet, concave anteroposteriorly and convex from side to side for articulation with the trapezium. The lateral part of the articular surface is larger than the medial, as is the lateral part of the anterior surface as compared with the medial part. The carpometacarpal joint of the thumb is completely separate from the other carpometacarpal joints which are connected to each other by ligaments and by articulations between the sides of the adjacent bases of the metacarpals. The head of the first metacarpal, less rounded than that of the other metacarpals, has two small flattened areas anteriorly each of which articulates with a sesamoid bone embedded in the capsule of the metacarpophalangeal joint. The whole thumb is rotated through 90° so that its anterior surface faces medially. The second metacarpal bone is the longest mainly because its base is more proximal than that of the other metacarpals. It articulates with the trapezium and capitate as well as the trapezoid. These articulations help to make the second metacarpal bone immobile even to passive movement at its proximal end. The third metacarpal bone has a *styloid process* which is palpable and projects from the radial side of the posterior surface of the base. It is almost immobile at its carpometacarpal joint. The fourth and fifth metacarpal bones have no special features. They are shorter than the second and third and have a certain amount of mobility where they articulate with the hamate. (The fifth is more mobile than the fourth.)

The metacarpal bones *ossify* in cartilage and have a primary centre for the shaft which appears at about the seventh week of intra-uterine life. A secondary centre of ossification for the base of the first metacarpal and the heads of the other metacarpal bones appears at about 2 years and the epiphysis fuses with the shaft at about 17 years. There may be a pseudo-epiphysis at the head of the first metacarpal.

The phalanges (figure 231)

The thumb has a *proximal* and *distal phalanx* and the rest of the digits have a *proximal*, *middle* and *distal phalanx*. From their superficial appearance it would seem that it is the middle phalanx of the thumb which is missing but there is some evidence that the first metacarpal may be the bone which has disappeared; for example, the first metacarpal ossifies like a phalanx, with a basal epiphysis. The *proximal phalanges* have a shaft which is flat anteriorly and convex posteriorly. On the base of the phalanx there is a proximal, oval, concave articular area for the head of the metacarpal and on the head

there are two condyles making the surface concave from side to side and convex anteroposteriorly.

The shafts of the *middle phalanges* are similar to those of the proximal. They are smaller and can be recognised by the articular area on the proximal surface of the base having an anteroposterior ridge separating two concave areas for the condyles of the distal end of the proximal phalanx. The distal end of the middle phalanx has two condyles. A *distal phalanx* has a proximal facet on the base for the condyles of the head of the middle phalanx and is flatter than the other phalanges. Its distal end has on its anterior surface an elevation called the *tuberosity* which supports the pulp of the distal end of the finger.

The phalanges *ossify* in cartilage with a primary centre for the shaft which appears at about 7 weeks *in utero* and a secondary centre for the base which begins to ossify at about 2 years. The base joins the shaft at about 17 years.

The Palmar Aspect of the Hand

The general arrangement of the structures is as follows. The *skin* covers an especially thick layer of deep fascia called the *palmar aponeurosis*. Deep to the aponeurosis are the *superficial vessels and nerves* which continue distally as digital vessels and nerves. On each side of the palm there is an *eminence*, the *thenar* on the lateral side (thumb) and the *hypothenar* on the medial side (little finger), each formed by three small muscles (*thenar = palm of hand*, Greek). Deep to the vessels and nerves there are the *long flexor tendons*, four superficial and four deep. Associated with the deep tendons there are four *lumbrical muscles*. The flexor pollicis longus on the lateral side lies deep to the muscles of the thenar eminence.

Deep to the long flexor tendons there are *deep vessels and nerves* and the *adductor pollicis muscle*. In a deeper plane the four *palmar* and four *dorsal interossei muscles* are related to the metacarpal bones.

The skin

The skin of the palm of the hand and of the palmar

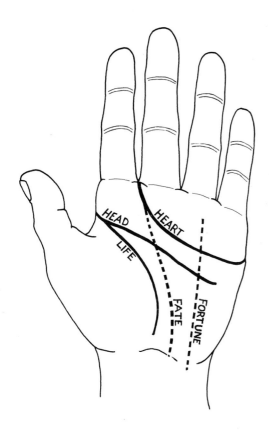

Figure 232   The flexure lines of the palm of the hand as used in palmistry.

surface of the digits shows some special features. It is firmly bound down to the underlying fascia. The typical creases in the palm, flexure lines *(figure 232), best seen on flexing the digits, are the* radial longitudinal crease *passing medial to the thenar eminence, the* proximal transverse crease, *which runs from the medial side of the palm (it does not reach the medial border) to the lateral border where it meets the radial longitudinal crease, and the* distal transverse crease, *which begins at the medial border and ends in the cleft between the index and middle fingers. These three creases are invariably present. Frequently there is an* intermediate longitudinal crease *which is medial to the radial longitudinal crease and joins the distal transverse crease, and a more* medial longitudinal crease *which runs in line with the ring finger.* The position and interpretation of these creases in palmistry are indicated in figure 232. The palmar creases (and the

finger-prints) of mentally deficient children suffering from *Down's syndrome (mongolian idiocy)* are different in their arrangement as compared with those of normal people (J.L.H. Down, 1828–96, English physician). The relationship between the syndrome and the palmar creases is obscure. Perhaps it should be added that the pattern found in Down's syndrome has also been found in people of very high intelligence. The sole of the foot and the toes also have creases and ridges and it has been reported that the Chinese examine the sole of the foot and not the palm of the hand — they are plantists not palmists.

There are also transverse creases at the wrist, the proximal *and* distal carpal creases. *The proximal is at the level of the ulnar styloid and the distal between the ulnar and radial styloid processes. The lunate lies between these creases, and the tubercle of the scaphoid and the pisiform on or just distal to the distal crease. There is often a third transverse crease proximal to the other two.*

There are digital creases, *a* proximal *which is about 2.5 cm distal to the metacarpophalangeal joint, a* middle *at the level of the proximal interphalangeal joint and a* distal *about 0.5 cm proximal to the distal interphalangeal joint. At the digital creases the skin is thinner than elsewhere and a penetrating wound through the crease is more likely to enter the underlying synovial sheath round the long flexor tendons (p. 400).*

There are also papillary ridges, *especially on the skin of the terminal phalanges. The arrangement of these ridges is specific for any individual so that finger-printing can be used for identification. There are numerous sweat glands in the skin of the palm and digits and their openings can be seen on the papillary ridges.*

The thickness of the epidermis of the different parts of the skin varies considerably and the stratum corneum is increased over areas subjected to pressure. There are no hair follicles in the skin of the palm and palmar surface of the digits.

Reference has already been made to the rich *sensory innervation of the fingers*, especially their tips, and most markedly those of the thumb and index finger. The nerves supplying the skin of the palm are the *palmar branch of the median nerve* over the thenar eminence and the lateral half of the palm (figure 233), and the *palmar branch of the ulnar nerve* over the hypothenar eminence and medial side of the palm. *Digital branches of the median nerve* supply the skin on the anterior surface of the lateral three and a half digits and also the skin over the posterior aspect of the distal phalanx including the nailbed. The *ulnar nerve* gives off *digital branches* to the skin of the anterior surface of the medial one and a half digits. These branches also supply the skin over the dorsal aspect of the terminal phalanx and the nailbed. The *radial nerve* supplies the skin over the back of the lateral part of the hand and the lateral three and a half digits as far as the distal interphalangeal joints and the *dorsal branch of the ulnar nerve* supplies the skin over the medial part of the dorsum of the hand and the medial one and a half digits as far as the distal interphalangeal joints. There is some variation in the sensory nerve supply of the skin on the lateral side of the ring finger. The ulnar nerve may supply this skin.

The *segmental innervation* of the skin of the hand and digits is as follows. The seventh cervical spinal cord segment supplies the skin of the index, middle and ring fingers and middle of the hand, both anteriorly and posteriorly. The sixth cervical segment supplies the skin over the thumb and lateral side of the palm and the eighth cervical that over the little finger and medial side of the palm (figure 221).

The palmar aponeurosis (figure 233)

The *palmar aponeurosis* covers the whole of the palm and is especially thick in the middle. It is much thinner over the thenar and hypothenar eminences. The *palmaris brevis* is a small muscle attached to the medial edge of the aponeurosis and the skin of the medial side of the palm of the hand. It is supplied by the ulnar nerve. Proximally the aponeurosis narrows towards the wrist and is continuous with the flexor retinaculum and the tendon of the palmaris longus. Distally the aponeurosis divides into four slips, the superficial fibres of which pass to the skin. Their deeper fibres divide into two and are continuous with the fibrous sheaths of the flexor tendons. Some of these fibres

pass dorsally to the region of the metacarpophalangeal joints. There are superficial transverse fibres forming the *superficial transverse metacarpal ligament* at the level of the clefts of the fingers. The digital vessels and nerves pass between the slips of the aponeurosis into the digits deep to this ligament.

From the lateral edge of the central part, a septum passes dorsally to the first metacarpal bone medial to the muscles of the thenar eminence and lateral to the flexor pollicis longus tendon. From the medial edge another septum to the fifth metacarpal bone passes lateral to the hypothenar muscles.

Contracture of the palmar aponeurosis which usually affects its medial half (*Dupuytren's contracture*) results in progressive flexion of the little and ring fingers at the metacarpophalangeal and proximal interphalangeal joints (Baron Guillame Dupuytren, 1777–1835, Paris surgeon; 15 structures and diseases are named after him). The distal phalanx is not flexed because the tips of the fingers press on the palm of the hand. Eventually there may be hyperextension of the distal phalanx due to this pressure. The condition occurs in elderly people and may be associated with work involving gripping implements which have hard handles, for example spades. The inability to extend the fingers even passively illustrates the strength of fibrous tissue. Treatment usually takes the form of removing the fibrous tissue but it tends to re-form and contract again.

The *flexor retinaculum* to which the proximal part of the palmar aponeurosis is attached is a strong, transverse band of fibrous tissue attached laterally to the tubercles of the scaphoid and trapezium and medially to the pisiform and hook of the hamate. Together with the anterior concave surface of the carpal bones the flexor retinaculum forms the *carpal tunnel* through which pass the long flexor tendons of the fingers and the median nerve. Compression of the nerve results in what is called the *carpal tunnel syndrome* in which the most characteristic symptoms are tingling and pins and needles in the digits supplied by the median nerve (the lateral three and a half digits). The patient may also complain of pain and weakness of the muscles in the hand supplied by the median

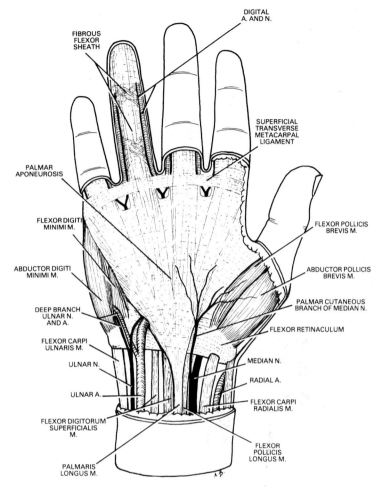

Figure 233 **The palmar aponeurosis, flexor retinaculum, fibro-osseous canals and thenar and hypothenar eminences of the right hand.**

nerve, especially the muscles of the thenar eminence. Usually the cause of this condition is not known but cutting the retinaculum, thus relieving the pressure on the nerve, results in a cure.

On the lateral side, the retinaculum splits to enclose the tendon of the flexor carpi radialis as it lies in the groove on the trapezium. On the medial side, the ulnar nerve and artery as they lie lateral to the pisiform are superficial to the retinaculum but are covered by a layer of fascia from the retinaculum. This explains why it is difficult to palpate the ulnar artery in this apparently superficial position. The palmar branches of the ulnar and median nerves and the palmaris longus tendon are also superficial to the retinaculum.

The superficial vessels and nerves (figure 234)

The *ulnar artery* and *nerve* enter the palm lateral to the pisiform bone and superficial to the main part of the flexor retinaculum and then run medial to the hook of the hamate. The artery gives off a *deep branch* and passes laterally deep to the palmar aponeurosis to form the *superficial palmar arch* which is completed on the lateral side by a branch of the radial artery. *The distal limit of the arch is indicated by a transverse line across the palm at the level of the web of the outstretched thumb. This is a better surface marking than the tip of the outstretched thumb which in many individuals is much more distal than the web.* The arch is super-

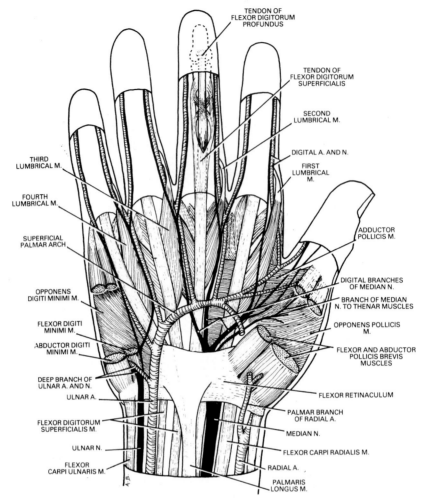

Figure 234: The superficial vessels and nerves of the palm, the long flexor tendons and the lumbrical muscles of the right hand.

ficial to the branches of the median nerve and lies on the long flexor tendons.

The arch gives off four branches which pass forwards to the digits. They each receive an anastomotic branch from the deeper metacarpal artery. The medial branch goes to the medial side of the little finger. Proximal to the webs each of the lateral three branches divides into two and forms *palmar digital arteries* to the adjacent sides of the little and ring, ring and middle, and middle and index fingers. Near the webs the palmar digital arteries become dorsal to the digital nerves. The palmar digital arteries anastomose with the much smaller dorsal digital arteries.

The ulnar nerve divides into a superficial and deep branch near the hook of the hamate. The

superficial branch divides into two nerves which supply the medial side of the little finger and the adjacent sides of the little and ring fingers. These *ulnar digital nerves* are posterior then anterior to the palmar digital arteries. The *deep branch* together with the deep branch of the ulnar artery passes between the muscles of the hypothenar eminence.

The *median nerve* just distal to the flexor retinaculum gives off a *muscular branch* to the three muscles of the thenar eminence and divides into three or four *digital branches*. The muscular branch may arise deep to the retinaculum and after appearing at its distal edge run upwards to the thenar eminence. It is sometimes referred to as the *recurrent branch*. The other branches run towards the digits and supply the two sides of the thumb, index

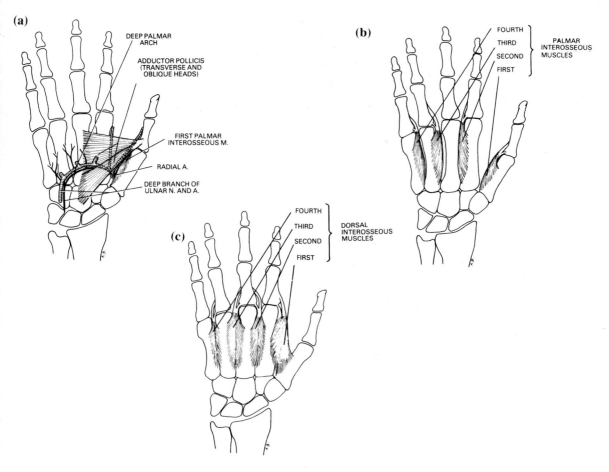

Figure 235   The deep vessels and nerves and the deep muscles of the right palm: (a) the deep palmar arch and the adductor pollicis muscle; (b) the palmar interossei; (c) the dorsal interossei.

and middle fingers and radial side of the ring finger. The way in which the median nerve gives off its branches varies. A lateral branch may supply both sides of the thumb and the radial side of the index finger and also the first lumbrical muscle, and a medial branch may supply the adjacent sides of the index and middle, and middle and ring fingers, and also the second lumbrical muscle. The nerves in the palm are deep to the superficial palmar arch and its digital branches, and in the fingers become anterior to the palmar digital arteries. These palmar digital nerves supply the skin over the back of the distal phalanx and also the nailbed as well as the sides and anterior aspects of the digits. They also supply the joints of the digits.

The thenar and hypothenar eminences (figures 233, 234)

Each eminence consists of three muscles with similar names, arrangements and attachments. Superficially and on the outer side there is an abductor, the *abductor pollicis brevis* and *abductor digiti minimi*. On the inner side of the abductor, there is a flexor, the *flexor pollicis brevis* and *flexor digiti minimi brevis*. Deep to these two muscles there is the *opponens pollicis* of the thenar eminence and the *opponens digiti minimi* of the hypothenar eminence. Proximally the three muscles on each side are attached to the lateral or medial part of the flexor retinaculum and its bony attachments, the tubercle of the scaphoid and tubercle of the trapezium laterally, and the pisiform and hook of hamate medially. Distally the abductors and flexors are attached to the outer side of the base of the proximal phalanx. The abductors send fibres into the dorsal digital expansion. There is always a sesamoid bone in the tendon of the thumb muscles at its attachment, and one in the little finger muscles in 70 per cent of the population. The opponens is attached to the side of the metacarpal bone, that of the thumb to the lateral side of the first and that of the little finger to the medial side of the fifth. Frequently the *flexor pollicis brevis* has a *deep head* which is attached proximally to the trapezoid and capitate, medial to the tendon of the flexor pollicis longus, and after passing deep to the tendon, joins the superficial part.

The thenar muscles are usually supplied by the median nerve (C8, T1) through its recurrent branch. The deep head of the flexor pollicis brevis is supplied by the deep branch of the ulnar nerve (C8, T1). There is frequently a connection between the median and ulnar nerves in the flexor pollicis brevis and the superficial and deep heads may be supplied by either nerve or both nerves. It has been estimated on the basis of a study of the effects of lesions of the median and ulnar nerves in the forearm, that the flexor pollicis brevis is innervated by the ulnar nerve as often as by the median nerve. The hypothenar muscles are supplied by the ulnar nerve (C8, T1).

The actions of the muscles of the thenar and hypothenar eminences are more or less what their names suggest. The effects they produce are more extensive on the thenar side because of the movements of the thumb at the carpometacarpal joint, as well as at the metacarpophalangeal joint. Since the thumb in the anatomical position is rotated through 90°, abduction is a movement anteriorly at right angles to the palm and flexion is a movement in the plane of the palm (figure 239(d)). The abductor pollicis brevis abducts the thumb and also medially rotates it to a variable extent. The flexor pollicis brevis flexes the thumb at the metacarpophalangeal and carpometacarpal joints. The opponens pollicis rotates the thumb medially at the carpometacarpal joint in the movement of opposition (figure 239(e)). The abductor digiti minimi pulls the little finger away from the ring finger in the plane of the palm (abduction and adduction of the fingers at the metacarpophalangeal joints are related to the middle finger and are discussed on p. 412). The flexor digiti minimi brevis flexes the little finger at the metacarpophalangeal joint and the opponens digiti minimi laterally rotates the fifth metacarpal bone to a slight extent as in cupping the hand.

The long flexor tendons and lumbrical muscles (figure 234)

These tendons lie in the middle of the palm. The tendons of the flexor digitorum profundus have the lumbrical muscles attached to them, the first to the lateral side of the tendon of the index finger, the second to the lateral side of the tendon of the middle finger and the third and fourth to the adjacent sides of the tendons of the middle and ring, and ring and little fingers. Each lumbrical muscle ends in a tendon which passes distally, winds round the lateral side of the proximal phalanx and is inserted into the dorsal digital expansion. The lateral two lumbrical muscles are usually innervated by the median nerve (C8, T1) and the medial two by the deep branch of the ulnar nerve (C8, T1). The median nerve may supply the third and the ulnar nerve the first and second lumbrical muscles.

The lumbrical muscles flex the digits at the metacarpophalangeal joints and extend them at the interphalangeal joints.

The way in which a superficialis tendon splits and allows the profundus tendon to pass through it and then re-form behind the profundus tendon is described on p. 375. A superficialis tendon splits again and is attached to the sides of a middle phalanx and a profundus tendon is attached to the anterior aspect of the base of a distal phalanx.

Beyond the metacarpal bones the long flexor tendons are enclosed in a fibro-osseous canal formed posteriorly by the anterior surface of the phalanges and laterally and anteriorly by fibrous tissue attached to the sides of the phalanges arching over the tendons (figure 233). The fibrous tissue is thinner opposite the joints. Each canal is lined by a synovial sheath which is reflected round the two tendons. As they lie in the fibro-osseous canals the tendons are joined to the phalanges by thin bands of connective tissue containing small blood vessels. These are called *vincula* (*vinculum = chain*, Latin). Short vincula pass between the tendons and the proximal and middle phalanges, and long vincula are attached to the tendons, where the superficialis splits, and to the proximal phalanges.

The tendon of the flexor pollicis longus lies medial to the opponens pollicis, enters a fibro-osseous canal similar to that of the other four digits and has a synovial sheath arranged somewhat differently from those of the long tendons of the other digits (p. 402 and figure 236).

The deep vessels and nerves (figure 235(a))

Deep to the long flexor tendons the deep branch of the ulnar nerve from the medial side and the deep palmar arch from the lateral side run across the palm. The *deep branch of the ulnar nerve* with the deep branch of the ulnar artery passes deeply between the abductor digiti minimi and flexor digiti minimi brevis, then laterally deep to the long flexor tendons where it lies next to the deep palmar arch. The nerve supplies the muscles of the hypothenar eminence, the third and fourth lumbrical muscles, all the interossei, the adductor pollicis, the deep head of the flexor pollicis brevis and frequently its superficial head.

The *deep palmar arch* is a continuation of the radial artery. The radial artery lies on the dorsum of the hand in the anatomical snuffbox and passes anteriorly between the two heads of the first dorsal interosseous muscle near the proximal end of the first metacarpal space. The artery then turns laterally and passes deep to the oblique head of the adductor pollicis then between its two heads as the deep palmar arch which is completed medially by the deep branch of the ulnar artery. This arch is about 1 cm proximal to the superficial palmar arch, just beyond the hook of the hamate. The deep palmar arch gives off three *palmar metacarpal arteries* which pass distally and anastomose with the more superficial digital arteries, three *perforating branches* which pass dorsally and anastomose with the dorsal metacarpal arteries and recurrent branches which run proximally to anastomose in front of the wrist.

The extensive anastomoses between the branches of the palmar arches make it difficult to control bleeding from an injury to either of them. Even tying both the radial and ulnar arteries in the forearm may be unsuccessful because of the carpal anastomoses and it may be necessary to tie the brachial artery at the elbow.

The deep muscles of the hand (figure 235)

These are the adductor pollicis and interossei. The *adductor pollicis* has two heads, a *transverse* and an *oblique*. The transverse head is attached to the anterior surface of the shaft of the third metacarpal bone and the oblique head to a proximal continuation of this, mainly the capitate (its attachment spreads to neighbouring structures, for example the bases of the second and third metacarpals and the anterior carpal ligaments). Both heads converge and join a common tendon which contains a sesamoid bone where it is attached to the medial side of the base of the proximal phalanx. Some of the lateral fibres of the oblique head pass deep to the tendon of the flexor pollicis longus and join the deep head of the flexor pollicis brevis.

The adductor pollicis is supplied by the deep branch of the ulnar nerve (C8, T1). Its action in the anatomical position would be to press the side of the thumb to the side of the index finger. Its main use is to press the tip of the abducted thumb to the tip of the index finger as in the movement called opposition (p. 409).

The Palmar Interossei. There are four of these muscles (figure 235(b)). The first and second are attached to the medial side of the shafts of the first and second metacarpal bones respectively. The muscles end in tendons which pass distally and are partly attached to the medial side of the proximal phalanx of the thumb or index finger. Each tendon proceeds dorsally and is attached to the extensor expansion of its own digit. The third and fourth palmar interossei are attached to the lateral side of the shafts of the fourth and fifth metacarpal bones respectively. Their tendons are attached partly to the lateral side of the base of the proximal phalanx of the ring or little fingers and partly to their own extensor expansion.

The four muscles are innervated by the deep branch of the ulnar nerve (C8, T1). When describing adduction and abduction of the medial four digits, an imaginary longitudinal axis through the middle finger is used. The second, third and fourth palmar interossei adduct the second, fourth and fifth digits towards the middle finger respectively. The attachment of the muscles to the dorsal digital expansions enables them to assist in extension at the interphalangeal joints. The first palmar interosseus adducts the thumb and assists flexion at its metacarpophalangeal joint.

The Dorsal Interossei. Each of these four muscles is attached to the adjacent sides of two metacarpal bones and distally ends in a tendon (figure 235(c)). The first tendon is attached to the radial side of the proximal phalanx of the index finger and its extensor expansion. The second and third pass to the lateral and medial sides respectively of the middle finger and into its dorsal digital expansion on each side. The fourth is attached to the medial side of the base of the proximal phalanx and the dorsal expansion of the ring finger.

The dorsal interossei are supplied by the deep branch of the ulnar nerve (C8, T1). The first and fourth abduct the index and ring fingers respectively from the middle finger and the second and third abduct the middle finger from its own axis, the second to the radial side and the third to the ulnar side. The dorsal interossei also assist in extending the phalanges at the interphalangeal joints.

If one includes the abductor pollicis brevis and abductor digiti minimi, all the dorsal digital expansions have on each side in the region of the metacarpophalangeal joint the tendon of a muscle attached to them. It has been suggested that one of the functions of these extensions of the interossei or short abductors is to prevent the dorsal part of the capsule of the joint slipping to one or other side in movements of the phalanges.

The first dorsal interosseus bulges backwards if the side of the thumb is pressed against the side of the index finger. Lesions of the ventral ramus of the first thoracic spinal nerve or the ulnar nerve

result in wasting of the small muscles of the hand, and is most easily visible in this muscle. It is not easy to detect this wasting in the other small muscles although eventually the posterior aspects of the intermetacarpal spaces become depressed due to the wasting of the dorsal interossei.

The fascial spaces of the hand (figure 236)

These refer to regions of the palm which are enclosed by fibrous septa and their significance is related to the way in which infection spreads within the hand. The *midpalmar* space is formed by the *intermediate palmar septum* which runs from the deep aspect of the palmar aponeurosis to the shaft of the middle metacarpal bone by passing medially over the adductor pollicis muscle. There appears to be considerable debate as to whether the septum passes medial or lateral to the long flexor tendons of the index finger. The medial limit of the midpalmar space is the septum which passes to the fifth metacarpal bone. The midpalmar space contains the long flexor tendons to the middle, ring and little fingers, the lumbrical muscles attached to the profundus tendons and the superficial vessels and nerves. If this space is infected it can be drained by an incision into the web between the middle and ring fingers along the line of the third lumbrical muscle.

The *thenar space* (not a particularly good name) is lateral to the midpalmar space and is bounded laterally by the septum to the first metacarpal bone and medially by the intermediate palmar septum. It contains the adductor pollicis muscle, the first palmar and dorsal interossei, the long flexor tendon of the thumb and digital vessels and nerves to the thumb and index finger. If infected it is usually approached by a posterior incision through the first dorsal interosseus muscle.

The synovial sheaths of the long flexor tendons (figure 237)

Reference has already been made to the synovial membrane which lines the fibro-osseous canals of the digits. The arrangement of the sheaths in the

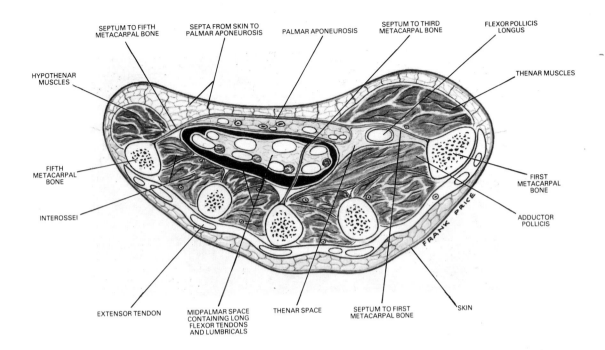

Figure 236   The fascial spaces of the hand.

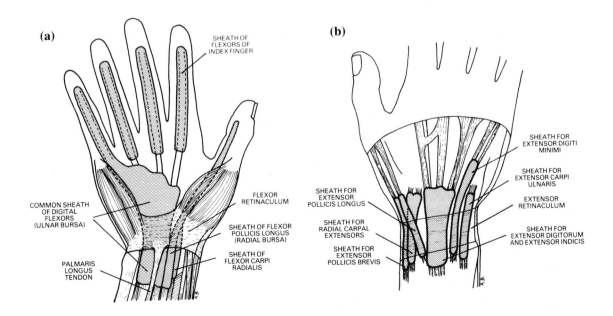

Figure 237   The synovial sheaths of the right wrist and hand: (a) flexor; (b) extensor.

region of the wrist and in the hand requires a more detailed description. The eight flexor tendons as they pass deep to the flexor retinaculum have a common synovial sheath. The sheath is invaginated by the tendons from the lateral side and there may be a thin septal process passing laterally from the medial part of the sheath between the superficial and deep tendons. The synovial sheath extends beyond the flexor retinaculum proximally about 2.5 cm and distally about 3 cm to the middle of the metacarpal bones. On the medial side the synovial sheath extends along the tendons of the little finger into the digit as far as the distal phalanx.

The tendon of the flexor pollicis longus has its own synovial sheath extending from about 2.5 cm proximal to the flexor retinaculum to the insertion of the tendon. The flexor carpi radialis also has a synovial sheath as it passes deep to the retinaculum.

The flexor tendons of the index, middle and ring fingers have synovial sheaths extending from the level of the metacarpophalangeal joint to the attachment of the tendons to the phalanges. Each synovial sheath lines a fibro-osseous canal and is reflected round the tendons. The vincula pass to the tendons between the lines of reflection.

Because of the synovial sheaths the tendons glide easily within the carpal tunnel and the fibro-osseous canals of the fingers. If the synovial sheath becomes infected, adhesions form between the tendons and the sheath and flexion movements are impossible or very limited. If the flexor tendons are cut retraction of the proximal ends makes union difficult and even after union adhesions may limit movement.

Infection of the tissues of the pad of the terminal phalanx of the digits may occur (*pulp-space infection*). This tissue consists of fat-filled spaces separated by fibrous septa passing between the skin and the periosteum of the bone. This condition is difficult to treat because of the loculation of the infected tissues. A possible complication of this infection is necrosis of the distal part of the phalanx because the swelling due to the inflammation presses on and closes the blood vessels supplying the bone. The proximal part of the bone survives because it receives its blood supply before the arteries enter the pulp space.

The Dorsum of the Hand

Most of the features of this part of the upper limb have already been described. The *skin* is comparatively mobile and with the digits extended shows over the back of the hand and joints transverse folds which allow flexion of the digits. If the skin and subcutaneous tissue become adherent to the deeper tissues due to an injury or a burn, flexion of the fingers is considerably reduced.

The skin on the dorsum of the hand is supplied on the lateral side by the *radial nerve (superficial branch)* and on the medial side by the *ulnar nerve (dorsal branch)*. These nerves also supply the skin on the posterior surface of the digits as far as the distal interphalangeal joint. Beyond these joints the skin of the lateral three and a half digits is supplied by the *median nerve* and that of the medial one and a half digits by the *superficial terminal branch of the ulnar nerve*.

Usually there are hairs on the skin on the back of the hand and proximal part of the digits. The hairs are directed from the lateral to the medial side and are fewer or absent in females. The hairs in the region of the base of the thumb are in the form of whorls. The direction and quantity of the hairs on the dorsal surface of the digits may be useful in identifying the side to which the digit belongs and the sex of the remains of a body. Pigmented areas in the skin are characteristically seen in older people.

There is a variable amount of *subcutaneous fat* in the dorsum of the hand and this influences the ease with which the veins forming the *subcutaneous venous plexus* can be used for an injection or the withdrawal of blood. The venous plexus drains laterally into the cephalic vein and medially into the basilic vein.

On the dorsum of the wrist the *deep fascia* is thickened and forms the *extensor retinaculum*, which is somewhat oblique because it is attached laterally to the anterior border of the radius and medially to the triquetral and pisiform bones. The retinaculum is also attached to the ridges on the back and lateral side of the distal end of the radius. Together with the bone these attachments form canals in which the extensor tendons run. As they do so they are enclosed in *synovial sheaths* in the following way (figure 237). On the lateral side of the styloid process one synovial sheath encloses the abductor pollicis longus and extensor pollicis brevis. The two radial extensors of the wrist have a common sheath lateral to the dorsal tubercle, and the extensor pollicis longus has its own synovial sheath medial to the tubercle. The extensor digitorum and extensor indicis have a common sheath. In the groove between the radius and ulna the extensor digiti minimi is enclosed in its own synovial sheath and the extensor carpi ulnaris is enclosed in a sheath where its tendon lies on the back of the distal end of the ulna. On the whole the synovial sheaths extend proximal to the retinaculum for a short distance (about 4 mm) and distally for about 1–2 cm beyond the retinaculum. The sheaths for the tendons to the thumb and carpal bones are shorter than those of the other tendons.

The *extensor tendons of the carpus and digits* are deep to the skin, superficial fascia and extensor retinaculum, the former passing to the bases of the second, third and fifth metacarpal bones and the latter into the dorsal digital expansion (pp. 379 and 380). Laterally the tendons of the abductor pollicis longus and extensor pollicis brevis on the radial side and the tendon of the extensor pollicis longus on the ulnar side form the boundaries of the *anatomical snuffbox* (p. 381). Branches of the superficial terminal branch of the *radial nerve* and dorsal branch of the *ulnar nerve* run forwards into the digits with the *dorsal metacarpal arteries* from the dorsal carpal branch of the radial artery. The arteries, however, do not extend as far distally as the nerves.

Between the metacarpal bones the four *dorsal interossei* are attached to the adjacent shafts. The first dorsal interosseus bulges posteriorly when the thumb is pressed against the index finger.

The Joints of the Wrist and Hand

The Radiocarpal (Wrist) and Intercarpal Joints (figure 238)

These joints are considered together because they function together. In all movements of the hand at the wrist there is movement at the radiocarpal (wrist) joint and between the carpal bones.

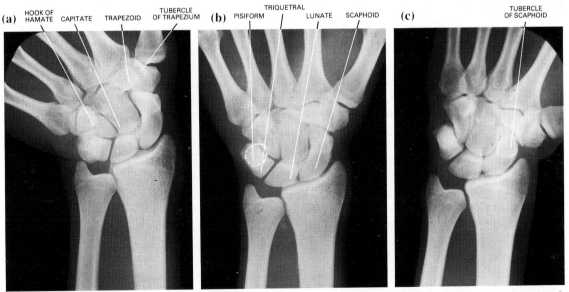

Figure 238 An X-ray of the wrist region: (a) the hand is adducted (ulnar deviation); (b) the hand is in the neutral position; (c) the hand is adducted (radial deviation). Note the changes in position of the various carpal bones.
(**Reproduced from** *Hamilton's Textbook of Human Anatomy* **by courtesy of the Editors and The Macmillan Press.**)

The *radiocarpal joint* is a synovial joint of the ellipsoid type, that is one articular surface is elliptical and concave (the distal surface of the radius and articular disc) and the other surface (formed by the proximal surfaces of the scaphoid, lunate and triquetral) is reciprocally convex. *The position of the joint is indicated by a line slightly convex proximally between the styloid processes of the radius and ulna.*

There are joints between the neighbouring bones of the proximal and distal rows of the carpus. There is also a sinuous joint between the two rows of carpal bones called the *midcarpal joint* (figure 238). The medial part of the midcarpal joint is formed by the convex proximal surfaces of the hamate and capitate, and the concave surfaces of the triquetral, lunate and scaphoid. More laterally the proximal surfaces of the trapezoid and trapezium articulate with the distal surface of the scaphoid at a joint whose surfaces are much more flat than those of the medial part.

The radiocarpal joint is enclosed in a *fibrous capsule* which is attached to the distal edges of the radius and ulna anteriorly and posteriorly. Laterally and medially it is attached to the radial and ulnar styloid processes respectively. More distally the capsule is attached to the proximal row of carpal bones anteriorly and posteriorly, and on the medial side to the triquetral and lateral side to the scaphoid. The fibrous capsule is thickened and thus strengthened anteriorly, posteriorly, laterally and medially to form appropriately named ligaments.

The joints between the sides of the individual bones of the proximal and distal rows of the carpal bones communicate with each other through the midcarpal joint, but *interosseous ligaments* separate this extensive joint cavity from the radiocarpal and carpometacarpal joints.

The *movements* which occur at the wrist and intercarpal joints take place at the same time. *Flexion* of the hand at the wrist (forward movement about a transverse axis for about 90°) involves movement at the wrist and midcarpal joints and movement at the latter joint is greater than at the former. The opposite is the case in *extension* in which the hand moves backwards for about 70° around a transverse axis and there is more movement at the radiocarpal joint than at the midcarpal joint. Flexion is limited by tension on the extensor tendons and is much reduced if the fingers are fully flexed. In other words the extensor tendons (and muscles) cannot lengthen sufficiently to allow full flexion of the hand and fingers at the same time. This is called *passive insufficiency*. The main muscles producing flexion are the flexor carpi radialis, supplied by the median nerve (C6, 7), and the flexor carpi ulnaris, supplied by the ulnar nerve (C7, 8). If present, the palmaris longus supplied by the median nerve (C7, 8) is also a flexor of the hand at the wrist. The main extensors are the extensor carpi radialis longus and brevis and the extensor carpi ulnaris supplied by the radial nerve or through its posterior interosseous branch (C7, 8).

In flexion the pisiform moves proximally almost 1 cm on the triquetral. The scaphoid not only moves about a transverse axis but also twists about its long axis so that the tubercle becomes less prominent in full flexion and more prominent in full extension.

Abduction and *adduction* of the hand in the region of the wrist take place about an anteroposterior axis and also involve both the radiocarpal and intercarpal joints. Abduction (*radial deviation*) is much more limited than adduction (*ulnar deviation*) because the radial styloid process extends further distally than the ulnar styloid. Abduction in which the hand moves away from the midline is brought about by the flexor carpi radialis and extensors carpi radialis longus and brevis. Adduction is due to the action of the flexor carpi ulnaris and extensor carpi ulnaris.

A study of X-rays of the carpal region with the hand abducted and adducted indicates the following movements of the carpal bones (figure 238). In abduction the proximal row moves medially on the distal surface of the radius and articular disc so that, for example, the lunate lies on the disc and the triquetral lies against the ulnar collateral ligament. There is much less movement at the midcarpal joint. In adduction there is more movement at the midcarpal than at the radiocarpal joint. The pisiform is pulled proximally towards the ulnar styloid process. Because the capitate rotates about an anteroposterior axis so that its distal part moves medially the hamate approaches the lunate and separates the capitate from the triquetral. In abduction the capitate comes close to the triquetral and separates the hamate from the lunate. In abduction and adduction the scaphoid not only moves from side to side, it rotates about a transverse axis so that the tubercle is more easily felt in abduction than in adduction.

A fall on the outstretched hand is more likely to result in the force on the hand being transmitted through the proximal part of the thenar eminence, then to the trapezium and trapezoid and then to the scaphoid. With the hand extended and abducted the scaphoid is rotated so that it lies anteroposteriorly rather than transversely and it is fractured across its waist. (There are other explanations as to why the scaphoid is the only carpal bone commonly fractured.) Reference has already been made to the characteristic pain on pressure in the anatomical snuffbox and the possible necrosis of the proximal fragment in this condition. The only other common injury to the carpal bones is an anterior dislocation of the lunate.

The Carpometacarpal and Intermetacarpal Joints (figures 231, 238)

The bases of the medial four metacarpal bones articulate on each side with each other and proximally with the distal surfaces of the trapezoid (the second metacarpal), the capitate (the third metacarpal) and the hamate (the fourth and fifth metacarpals). These joints on the whole are plane (gliding) synovial joints with the bones held together by a fibrous capsule lined by synovial membrane. Anterior and posterior thickenings of the capsule are described as palmar and dorsal ligaments. There is little movement at the carpometacarpal and intermetacarpal joints but there is some mobility of the fifth metacarpal on the hamate and a slight amount of movement at the fourth carpometacarpal joint. The third and second metacarpal bones are immobile at their carpometacarpal joints.

The *carpometacarpal joint of the thumb* is specially important because of the extensive movements which can occur at this joint. The joint is a saddle-shaped synovial joint between the base of the first metacarpal bone and the distal surface of the trapezium. The fibrous capsule of the joint is thickened laterally to form a lateral ligament and also anteriorly and posteriorly to form ligaments which run obliquely from the anterior and posterior surfaces of the trapezium to the medial side of the base of the metacarpal bone.

The movements which take place at this joint are described with the movements of the thumb.

The Metacarpophalangeal and Interphalangeal Joints

The *metacarpophalangeal joints* are between the head of a metacarpal bone and the base of a proximal phalanx. The articular surface of the metacarpal head is convex and fits into the concave surface of the phalangeal base. The joint may be described as either an ellipsoid or a ball and socket synovial joint. The articular area on the head of the metacarpal bone extends further on the palmar surface than on the dorsal.

The *fibrous capsules* of these joints have some special features. The anterior part is in the form of a thick fibrocartilaginous plate firmly joined to the base of the phalanx but loosely attached to the head of the metacarpal bone. The palmar surface of the plate is grooved for the flexor tendons. Laterally the plates are joined to the *deep transverse metacarpal ligaments* which lie between the second, third, fourth and fifth metacarpophalangeal joints. There is no deep transverse metacarpal ligament between the thumb and index finger. These ligaments separate the more superficial lumbrical muscles and digital vessels and nerves from the deeper interossei muscles. The dorsal digital expansion posteriorly and the palmar aponeurosis anteriorly also send slips which are attached to the deep transverse metacarpal ligaments.

The posterior part of the capsule is thin and is separated from the extensor tendon by a bursa. Laterally on each side a lateral ligament passes from the tubercles on the sides of the head of a metacarpal bone distally and forwards to the anterior aspect of the base of the phalanx.

The *interphalangeal joint of the thumb* and the *proximal and distal interphalangeal joints of the remaining digits* are condyloid joints structurally (the two convex condyles of the head of a phalanx fit into the two concave areas on the base of the adjacent phalanx) and hinge joints functionally (only movements about a transverse axis are possible). The capsules of the joints show similar features to those of the metacarpophalangeal joints in that (1) there is a palmar plate more firmly attached to the base of the more distal phalanx than to the head of the more proximal phalanx; (2) collateral ligaments laterally pass forwards as they pass distally. The extensor expansion forms the dorsal part of the capsule. There are differences, particularly the structures which are attached to the palmar plate of the metacarpophalangeal joints. These include the deep transverse metacarpal ligaments to which many other structures are attached. The result is that the metacarpophalangeal joints are linked in a way in which the interphalangeal joints are not. These differences may be significant in the treatment of stiffness of these joints following injury or in Dupuytren's contracture (p. 394).

The Movements of the Thumb (figure 239)

The terminology used to describe these movements

is confusing because the thumb is rotated medially through an angle of about 90°. This angle can be estimated by placing the thumb alongside the index finger and observing that the thumb nail faces almost laterally. In these circumstances *flexion* and *extension* refer to movements in the plane of the palm of the hand and *abduction* and *adduction* to movements at right angles to this plane. In addition to the thumb being already rotated, its length and the depth of the web between the thumb and the index finger influence the ease with which the tip of the thumb can be brought into contact with the tips of the other digits (*opposition*). Although the human thumb is not the most medially rotated or longest, nor has the deepest web of the primates, it has the greatest combination of these three features, so that opposition of the human thumb is more easily obtained as compared with the movement in other primates. The movement is not uniquely human.

At the *interphalangeal joint* of the thumb only *flexion* and *extension* take place. Flexion is brought about by the flexor pollicis longus (supplied by the median nerve, C8, T1) and extension by the extensor pollicis longus (supplied by the radial nerve,

(a)

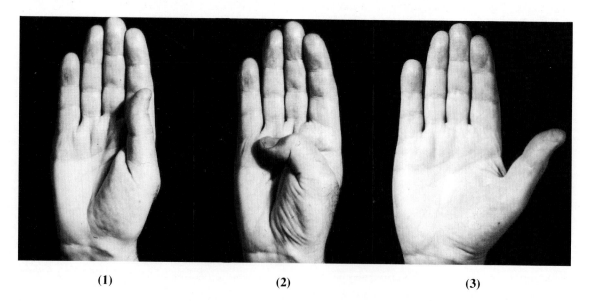

(1)   (2)   (3)

Figure 239   The movements of the thumb: (a) flexion and extension at all the joints.

(b)

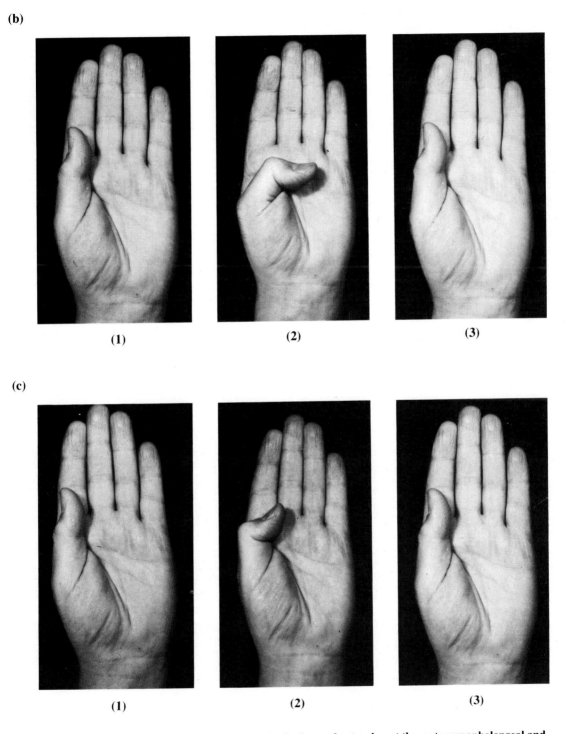

(1)   **(2)**   **(3)**

(c)

(1)   **(2)**   **(3)**

Figure 239 The movements of the thumb: (b) flexion and extension at the metacarpophalangeal and interphalangeal joints; (c) at the interphalangeal joint.

(d)

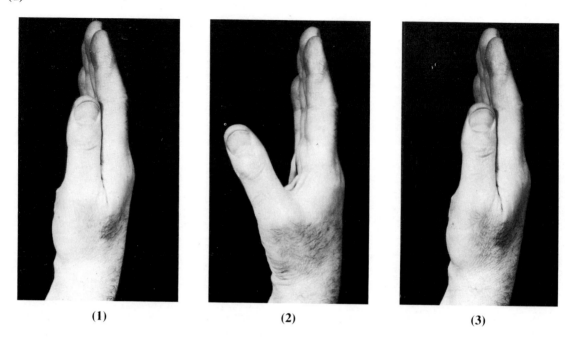

(1)   (2)   (3)

(e)

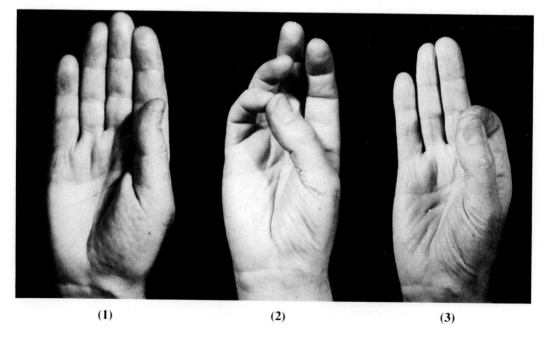

(1)   (2)   (3)

Figure 239   The movements of the thumb: (d) abduction and adduction; (e) opposition (reproduced from *Hamilton's Textbook of Human Anatomy* **by courtesy of the Editors and The Macmillan Press).**

C7, 8). The range of movement is very variable, particularly extension from the neutral position, and is in inverse ratio to the amount of extension at the metacarpophalangeal joint.

The main movements at the *metacarpophalangeal joint* of the thumb are *flexion* and *extension*. Flexion when associated with flexion at the interphalangeal joint is due to the continued action of the flexor pollicis longus unless the movements are rapid or forceful in which case the flexor pollicis brevis (supplied by the median nerve C8, T1) and the first palmar interosseus (supplied by the ulnar nerve C8, T1) contract. These two muscles can produce flexion at the metacarpophalangeal joint without flexion at the interphalangeal joint. This movement is difficult without some flexion at the carpometacarpal joint. Extension at the metacarpophalangeal joint is due to the extensor pollicis longus when extension at the interphalangeal joint is occurring at the same time. The extensor pollicis brevis (both extensors are supplied by the posterior interosseous nerve, C7, 8) is also involved, especially in movements occurring only at the metacarpophalangeal joint and in rapid, forceful movements. It must be emphasised that the movement of extension from the anatomical position takes place almost entirely at the carpometacarpal joint of the thumb.

There is considerable variation in the range of movement at the metacarpophalangeal joint of the thumb. The shape of the head of the first metacarpal bone is very variable and can be remarkably flat. A very flat head is associated with very much reduced flexion. Hyperextension at this joint is common and is more often found in the left hand than in the right, in women than in men, and in Indians than in Africans and Europeans. This movement is often referred to as *double-jointedness*, an odd term used to describe excessive movement, usually hyperextension, at any joint. Abduction is frequently accompanied by some medial rotation at this joint.

The saddle-shaped *carpometacarpal joint* of the thumb is the joint which gives this digit its range of mobility. Flexion, extension, abduction, adduction, rotation and opposition occur at this joint. *Flexion* from the anatomical position is not as marked as extension and is produced by the flexors pollicis longus and brevis if flexion takes place at the other two joints of the thumb at the same time. It is possible to produce flexion at this joint by the flexor pollicis brevis, although usually some flexion at the metacarpophalangeal joint occurs at the same time. *Extension* is due to the extensors pollicis longus and brevis.

Abduction, a movement away from the index finger at right angles to the plane of the palm, is due to the abductor pollicis brevis (supplied by the median nerve, C8, T1) and the abductor pollicis longus (supplied by the radial nerve, C7, 8). The latter muscle acts only at the carpometacarpal joint, the former also acts at the metacarpophalangeal joint so that the proximal phalanx is abducted relative to the metacarpal bone. *Adduction* of the thumb from the anatomical position results in pressing the thumb against the index finger and is due to the adductor pollicis (supplied by the ulnar nerve, C8, T1). The action of this muscle is more obvious in adducting the already abducted thumb against resistance, for example when pressing the tip of the thumb against the tip of the index finger.

The movement of *opposition*, so important in many activities involving the fingers, is defined as bringing the tip of the thumb against the tip or tips of any of the remaining digits. Initially in this movement the thumb is usually abducted and is then flexed, medially rotated and adducted. Flexion is produced by the flexors pollicis longus and brevis, medial rotation by the opponens pollicis (supplied by the median nerve, C8, T1) assisted by the flexor pollicis brevis, and adduction by the adductor pollicis. The medial rotation is also due to the shape of the joint surfaces producing a conjunct rotation, and the posterior oblique ligament which allows the lateral side of the metacarpal bone to rotate while fixing the medial side. In strong pressure between the tips of the thumb and the other digits, there is no flexion at the interphalangeal joint of the thumb, although the flexor pollicis longus is strongly contracted. *Restoration of the opposed thumb* to the anatomical position has no specific name and is largely due to the extensor muscles of the thumb. In this movement lateral rotation of the metacarpal bone is due partly to the shape of the joint surfaces and partly to the anterior oblique ligament.

The Movements of the Remaining Digits (figure 240)

As in the thumb, it is simpler to describe these movements by considering first the movements at the interphalangeal joints and then those that occur at the metacarpophalangeal joints. Only *flexion* and *extension* can occur at the *distal interphalangeal joints*. Flexion is produced by the flexor digitorum profundus (the lateral two tendons are

(a)

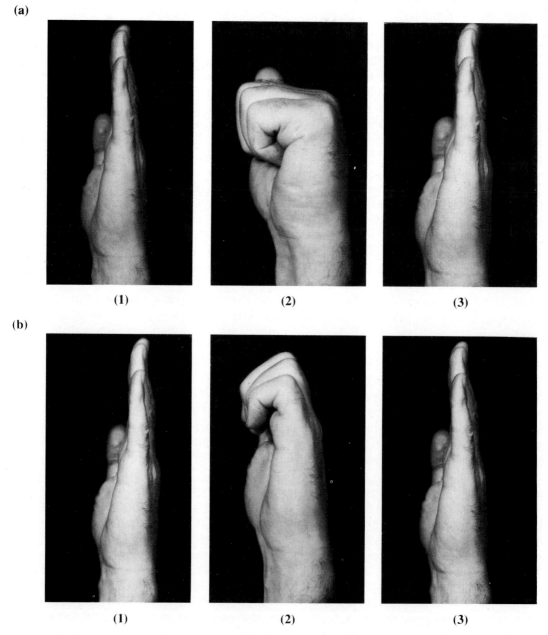

(1)   (2)   (3)

(b)

(1)   (2)   (3)

Figure 240   The movements of the digits excluding the thumb: (a) flexion and extension at all the joints at the same time; (b) flexion and extension at the interphalangeal joints.

supplied by the median nerve and the medial two by the ulnar nerve, C8, T1). Extension at these joints is produced by the extensor digitorum, including the extensor indicis and the extensor digiti minimi (all are supplied by the posterior inter-osseous nerve, a branch of the radial nerve, C7, 8). In rapid and/or forceful movements the interossei (supplied by the ulnar nerve, T1) and lumbrical muscles (supplied by the ulnar and median nerves, T1) are active.

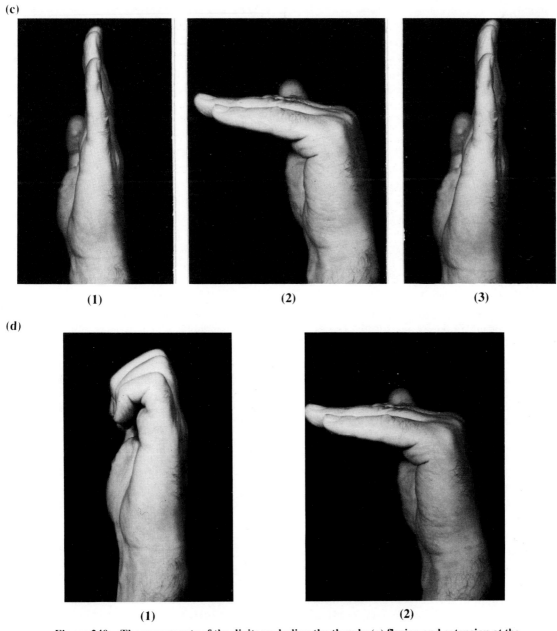

(c)

(1) **(2)** **(3)**

(d)

(1) **(2)**

Figure 240   The movements of the digits excluding the thumb: (c) flexion and extension at the metacarpophalangeal joints; (d) extension at the interphalangeal joints with simultaneous flexion at the metacarpophalangeal joints (reproduced from *Hamilton's Textbook of Human Anatomy* by courtesy of the Editors and The Macmillan Press).

Flexion at the *proximal interphalangeal joints* is due to the flexor digitorum profundus. The flexor digitorum superficialis (supplied by the median nerve, C7, 8) is involved only in rapid and/ or forceful movements. *Extension* at these joints is brought about by the same muscles as produce extension at the distal interphalangeal joints. At the *metacarpophalangeal joints abduction* and *adduction* are possible as well as *flexion* and *extension*. The latter movements are produced by the flexors digitorum profundus and superficialis and extensor muscles of the digits respectively. In the case of the little finger the flexor digiti minimi (supplied by the ulnar nerve, C8, T1) is also involved. The role of the lumbricals and interossei in flexion and extension movements at the metacarpophalangeal joints has evoked controversy. There is general agreement that the lumbrical muscles can produce flexion at these joints and it is suggested that the interossei can also assist in this movement.

Abduction and adduction of the digits at the metacarpophalangeal joints are movements related to a longitudinal axis through the middle finger (figure 235(b), (c)). The dorsal interossei are the abductors, the index finger being abducted by the first and the ring finger by the fourth. The little finger has its own abductor digiti minimi (supplied by the ulnar nerve, T1). The middle finger is abducted to the radial side by the second and to the ulnar side by the third dorsal interosseus. The palmar interossei are the adductors, the index finger is adducted by the second and the ring and little fingers by the third and fourth respectively.

When the fingers are flexed into the palm of the hand active abduction at the metacarpophalangeal joints is impossible, but passive abduction is possible if the long flexor tendons are relaxed. This inability to abduct actively may be due to the dorsal interossei being so relaxed that their contraction cannot take up the slack and produce any movement as well. This is called an *active insufficiency* of the muscles. Other explanations, however, have been put forward to account for this phenomenon.

During flexion there is an increasing radial deviation of the fingers so that the tips of the fingers meet the thenar eminence. This is due to the shape of the surfaces of the joints involved. The articular areas on the heads of the metacarpal bones are not parts of a perfect sphere and the two condyles on the heads of the phalanges are not equal in size or shape. Flexion movements therefore do not take place about a purely transverse axis.

The foregoing description of the movements applies to simultaneously flexing the fingers into the palm and extending them. There are different ways in which the fingers can be flexed and extended, as shown in figure 240. It is not proposed to analyse these in detail. However, the movement in which there is flexion at the metacarpophalangeal joints and simultaneous extension at the interphalangeal joints, although often called the *needle-threading movement*, is used very frequently in many skilled activities (figure 240(d)). This movement is used by males, who put the thread into the eye of a needle. Apparently females move the eye of the needle on to the thread.

The way in which objects are held by the hand varies with the purpose for which the object is used and its size, shape and weight. The *grip* has been classified in general terms into *precision* and *power* (figure 241). In the precision grip a small object is held between the thumb and index finger, or thumb and index and middle fingers, for example in holding a pen. If larger, for example in holding a round object like a cricket ball, the fingers are widely abducted at the metacarpophalangeal joints, the index finger is rotated in an ulnar direction and the ring and little fingers in a radial direction. There may be extension at the wrist. In the power grip, for example in holding a hammer, the object is held in the palm of the hand with the fingers flexed round it, deviated in an ulnar direction and rotated in a radial direction at the metacarpophalangeal joints. The thumb is pressed against the object either alongside or round it. There is slight extension at the wrist. A good example of the way in which the grip is changed according to the use to which a tool is put is the placing of a medium sized screwdriver into the head of a screw (precision grip) and the subsequent rotation of the screw (power grip). Other types of grip have been labelled *pincer* (holding an object between the thumb and index finger) and *hook* (carrying a case by the handle).

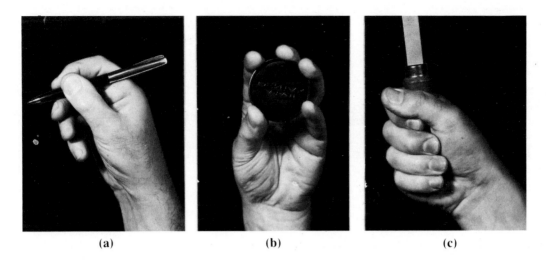

(a)   (b)   (c)

Figure 241   Precision and power grips: (a) precision grip as in holding a pen; (b) precision grip as in holding a round or spherical object; (c) power grip as in holding a hammer (reproduced from *Hamilton's Textbook of Human Anatomy* by courtesy of the Editors and The Macmillan Press).

32

The Venous and Lymphatic Drainage and Segmental Innervation of the Upper Limb

This is a summary of several topics which have already been dealt with in different regions and are therefore described briefly with reference to the appropriate chapters.

The Venous Drainage of the Upper Limb

The main veins of the limb are arranged as *superficial* and *deep* vessels. The main superficial veins of the forearm and arm are anterior, the *cephalic* on the lateral side and the *basilic* on the medial side (p. 368). There is usually a large *superficial median vein* running upwards on the front of the forearm. The arrangement of these three veins in front of the elbow is described on p. 368. The commonest is for the cephalic vein to send a branch upwards and medially (the *median cubital vein*) to join the basilic and for the median vein of the forearm to join the median cubital. The importance of the veins in front of the elbow has been emphasised.

The cephalic vein begins on the lateral side of the back of the wrist near the anatomical snuffbox by draining the *dorsal venous plexus* of the hand and ends by piercing the clavipectoral fascia inferior to the clavicle and joining the axillary vein. The basilic vein begins on the medial side of the back of the wrist by draining the dorsal venous plexus and becomes a deeper vein in the middle of the upper arm. At the lower border of the teres major it becomes the *axillary vein*. *Dorsal* and *palmar digital veins* drain into the *dorsal* and *palmar venous plex-*

uses respectively. The dorsal venous plexus goes to the cephalic and basilic veins and the palmar to the veins on the front of the forearm.

The *deep veins* correspond with the major arteries and their branches and are usually paired (*venae comitantes*). There are veins corresponding with the *superficial* and *deep palmar arches*. These veins receive *digital* and *metacarpal tributaries*. The deep palmar arch veins go to the *radial veins* accompanying the radial artery, and the superficial to the *ulnar veins*. The ulnar and radial veins join to form the *brachial veins*. *Interosseous veins* join the ulnar veins in the cubital fossa. The brachial vein ends in the *axillary vein* at the lower border of the teres major where the basilic vein changes its name to the axillary vein.

The axillary vein is usually a large single vein lying medial to the axillary artery and becomes the *subclavian vein* at the outer border of the first rib. Its relations and tributaries correspond with the relations and branches of the axillary artery (p. 352).

The Lymphatic Drainage of the Upper Limb

The *lymphatic vessels* are *superficial* and *deep*. The superficial vessels lie in the deeper part of the skin and follow the large superficial veins, the cephalic and basilic. The vessels from the hand tend to pass dorsally and the dorsal vessels of the forearm pass anteriorly to join the vessels in the front of the limb. The superficial vessels end in the *lateral nodes of the axilla* along the axillary vein, except for some vessels from the medial side of the forearm and hand which go to the *supratrochlear node(s)* (p. 371). Some vessels accompanying the cephalic vein end in the *infraclavicular nodes* lying between the deltoid and pectoralis major. Their efferents go to the *apical nodes* in the axilla or pass over the clavicle to the lowest *deep cervical nodes*.

The *deep lymphatic vessels* of the upper limb follow the main blood vessels and go to the lateral axillary nodes. Vessels from the scapular region go to the *posterior axillary nodes*.

The nodes of the axilla and the lymphatic drainage of the breast are described on p. 13.

The Segmental Innervation of the Upper Limb

The segmental innervation of the skin of the upper limb and the cutaneous nerves have been described on p. 366 and are summarised in figure 221. Division of a single spinal nerve does not lead to complete anaesthesia of the segment of skin supplied by the nerve because there is considerable overlap by neighbouring segments. Where adjacent segments are not supplied by consecutive spinal nerves, that is on either side of the *ventral* and *dorsal axial lines*, there is no overlap. Pressure on a cervical spinal nerve, for example the sixth or seventh, results in pain and disturbances of sensation along the distribution of the nerve. Prolonged pressure affects the muscles, which may become weak or paralysed.

The most common lesions in terms of segments affect (1) the upper trunk of the brachial plexus formed by the fifth and sixth cervical spinal nerves; (2) the first thoracic nerve. In the former the movements which are lost are abduction and lateral rotation at the shoulder joint, flexion at the elbow, supination of the forearm and extension of the hand at the wrist. If the first thoracic spinal nerve is affected (not infrequently the eighth cervical spinal nerve may also be involved) sensation on the medial side of the hand, forearm and upper arm may be altered or diminished and the small muscles of the hand waste, becoming weak and eventually paralysed. The segmental innervation of the muscles related to movements at the different joints are summarised in table 6.

Table 6

Joint(s)	Movements	Segmental innervation
Shoulder	Abduction and lateral rotation	C5, 6
	Adduction and medial rotation	C6, 7, 8
	Flexion	C5, 6
	Extension	Mainly C7, 8
Elbow	Flexion	C5, 6
	Extension	C7
Radio-ulnar	Pronation	C7, 8
	Supination	C6
Wrist	Flexion	C6, 7
	Extension	C6, 7
Digital	Flexion (long muscles)	C7, 8
	Extension (long muscles)	C7, 8
	Flexion and extension (hand muscles)	C8, T1

Part 7

The Lower Limb

33

The Hip Bone, Femur, Patella, and Anterior, Medial and Lateral Aspects of the Thigh

Although the basic structure of the lower limb is similar to that of the upper there are many differences which can be related to their different functions. Basically the lower limbs are used for maintaining the unique, human, bipedal, upright posture and for locomotion. For both these purposes much more strength and stability are required than is the case with the upper limb. The pelvic girdle, for example, is large and more or less immobile in relation to the trunk. The pectoral girdle bears much less weight and can move on the trunk. The pelvic girdle can only move with the vertebral column or on the lower limbs at the hip joints. The lower limbs transmit the weight of the body to the ground and have to transmit considerable forces in the opposite direction, for example when the heel meets the ground in every step in walking.

In view of their function one would expect the bones of the lower limb to be larger than the corresponding bones of the upper limb, for example the femur is much larger than the humerus. In order to prevent collapse or dislocation due to the forces to which they are subjected, joints in the lower limb are structurally more stable either due to the shape of the joint surfaces, for example the depth of the acetabulum of the hip bone as compared with that of the glenoid cavity of the scapula, or the number and strength of the ligaments, for example the knee and ankle joints, or the size of the muscles related to the joints.

Some additional and striking differences between the upper and lower limbs are the absence of pronation and supination between the two bones in the leg, the movements at the ankle are limited to flexion and extension, the sole of the foot can be turned inwards and outwards by movements between the bones within the foot (this to some extent replaces pronation and supination of the forearm) and the structure of the foot itself. The tarsus is a relatively much larger proportion of the foot than the carpus is of the hand, the phalanges are short, and the big toe, unlike the thumb, is not opposable.

The Hip Bone

This is described on p. 64. The main features of the hip bone relevant to the lower limb are shown in figure 242. The upper part is formed by the *ilium*, the posterior inferior part by the *ischium* and the anterior inferior part by the *pubis*. The main part of the ilium is called the *ala* and its upper border forms the *iliac crest* which ends anteriorly at the *anterior superior iliac spine* and posteriorly at the *posterior superior iliac spine*. The *iliac tubercle* is on the outer border of the iliac crest behind the anterior superior iliac spine below which there is a notch ending in the *anterior inferior iliac spine*. Posteriorly, inferior to the posterior superior iliac spine, the *posterior inferior iliac spine* bounds the deep *greater sciatic notch* which is converted into a foramen by the sacrospinous ligament.

The lower border of the greater sciatic notch is part of the ischium and the border of the notch

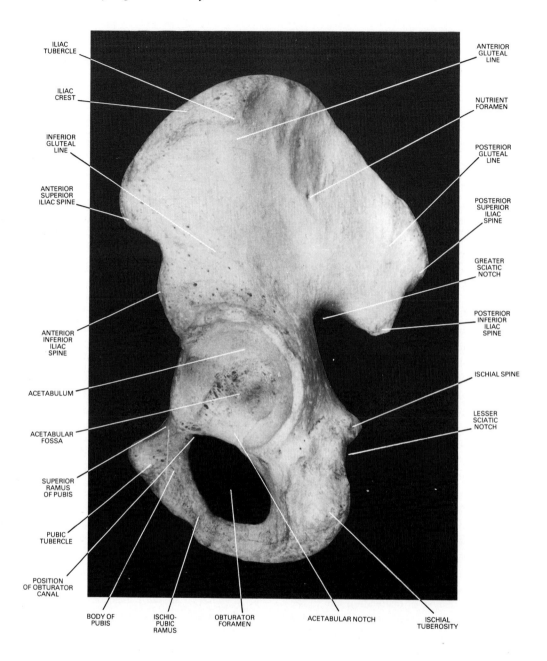

ILIAC
TUBERCLE

ILIAC
CREST

INFERIOR
GLUTEAL
LINE

ANTERIOR
SUPERIOR
ILIAC SPINE

ANTERIOR
INFERIOR
ILIAC
SPINE

ACETABULUM

ACETABULAR
FOSSA

SUPERIOR
RAMUS
OF PUBIS

PUBIC
TUBERCLE

POSITION
OF OBTURATOR
CANAL

ANTERIOR
GLUTEAL
LINE

NUTRIENT
FORAMEN

POSTERIOR
GLUTEAL
LINE

POSTERIOR
SUPERIOR
ILIAC
SPINE

GREATER
SCIATIC
NOTCH

POSTERIOR
INFERIOR
ILIAC
SPINE

ISCHIAL SPINE

LESSER
SCIATIC
NOTCH

BODY OF
PUBIS

ISCHIO-
PUBIC
RAMUS

OBTURATOR
FORAMEN

ACETABULAR NOTCH

ISCHIAL
TUBEROSITY

Figure 242   The outer aspect of the left hip bone.

ends below in the prominent *ischial spine*. Inferior to the ischial spine the shallow *lesser sciatic notch* is converted into the *lesser sciatic foramen* by the sacrospinous and sacrotuberous ligaments. The *ischial tuberosity* is the mass of bone inferior to the lesser sciatic notch. The upper part of the tuberosity is continuous superiorly with the *body of the ischium*, which forms part of the *acetabulum*. Anteriorly the tuberosity is continuous with the *ischial ramus*, which is continuous with the *inferior ramus of the pubis*, and together they form the *ischiopubic ramus*.

The ramus leads upwards and forwards to the *body of the pubis* which medially forms the *symphysis pubis* with the corresponding bone of the opposite side. The superior part of the pubic body has a *crest* which extends laterally to the *pubic tubercle* leading to the *superior ramus of the pubis*. The superior ramus extends laterally into the acetabulum. On the upper surface of the ramus there is the *pectineal line* ending laterally in the *iliopubic eminence* which marks the junction of the pubis with the ilium (figure 57(b)).

On the outer surface of the ala of the ilium there are three ridges. The *posterior gluteal line* is almost vertical and marks off a small rough area between it and the posterior iliac spines. The *anterior gluteal line* curves upwards and forwards from the edge of the greater sciatic notch to the iliac crest and has on it a large nutrient foramen. The *inferior gluteal line* lies about 3 cm above the acetabulum extending from the deepest part of the greater sciatic notch to between the two anterior iliac spines.

The *acetabulum* is a hemispherical hollow on the outer surface of the hip bone and is about 6 cm in diameter. It faces downwards and forwards as well as laterally. The prominent rim of the acetabulum is deficient inferiorly (the *acetabular notch*). The acetabulum has a horseshoe-shaped articular area between the limbs of which there is a rough area, the *acetabular fossa*. The fossa contains fat which lies between the synovial membrane and the capsule of the joint. The pubic bone forms the anterior one-fifth of the acetabulum, the ilium forms about two-fifths (the upper part) and the ischium about two-fifths (the lower posterior part).

The *obturator foramen* lies below and in front of the acetabulum and above the ischiopubic ramus. It is closed by the *obturator membrane* except superiorly where there is an opening completed above by the bony edge of the deep *obturator groove*.

The *ossification* of the hip bone is described on p. 67 and the *sex differences* on p. 129. The sex of a single hip bone is best determined by (1) estimating the subpubic angle ($<45°$ in the male; $> 45°$ in the female); (2) measuring the diameter of the acetabulum and the distance between the symphysis pubis and the edge of the acetabulum (in the male these are about equal; in the female the acetabulum is less than the second measurement); (3) looking at the greater sciatic notch (it is acute in the male; obtuse in the female).

The Femur (figure 243)

The *femur*, the bone of the thigh, has a shaft and upper and lower ends. The *upper end* consists of a rounded *head* forming more than half a sphere, a *neck* which is directed downwards, outwards and slightly forwards and two prominences, an upper lateral *greater trochanter* and lower medial *lesser trochanter*. The head articulates with the acetabulum at the hip joint and below and behind its centre has a depression for the attachment of the ligament of the head of the femur. The neck is at an angle of about 125° to the shaft (the angle is less in women than in men and greater in children) and is limited laterally by the *intertrochanteric line* in front and the *intertrochanteric crest* behind. There is a large number of foramina for blood vessels on the neck, especially superiorly and posteriorly.

The greater trochanter, subcutaneous and palpable, is quadrilateral in shape when looked at laterally. Medial to the posterior part of its upper border there is a deep depression, the *trochanteric fossa*. The posterior border of the greater trochanter continues downwards and medially as the prominent intertrochanteric crest on the middle of which there is the rounded *quadrate tubercle*. The lesser trochanter is a blunt pyramidal process projecting backwards and medially from the junction of the lower posterior part of the neck with the shaft.

The intertrochanteric line, which is anterior, separates the neck from the shaft and can be followed from the anterior upper angle of the greater trochanter to below the lesser trochanter, where it continues as the *spiral line* to the back of the shaft. This line joins the *linea aspera*, the vertical ridge on the back of the femoral shaft.

The *shaft* of the femur is cylindrical superiorly and flattened anteroposteriorly below. It is curved with an anterior convexity. In the erect position the shafts of the two femora are directed medially because the heads are separated by the width of

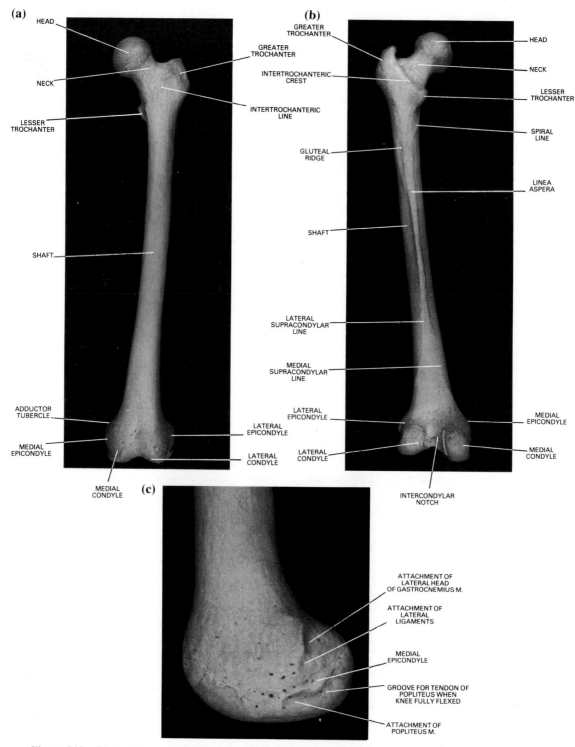

Figure 243 The left femur: (a) the anterior aspect; (b) the posterior aspect; (c) the lateral aspect of the lower end.

the pelvis and the lower ends usually meet at the knees. This obliquity is greater in women than in men because the female pelvis is relatively wider. On the middle of the posterior surface of the shaft there is the linea aspera, a vertical ridge of bone which inferiorly divides into the *lateral* and *medial supracondylar lines*. Between these lines there is a flat, triangular area, the *popliteal surface*. Superiorly the linea aspera divides into a lateral *gluteal ridge* which runs to the greater trochanter and a medial line which is continuous with the spiral line. The *adductor tubercle* is at the lower end of the medial supracondylar line and indicates the junction of the shaft with the lower epiphysis since the epiphyseal line passes through the tubercle. The linea aspera has a large number of muscles attached to it. It has considerable bulk and acts as a buttress for the concave aspect of the shaft. There is a large nutrient foramen on the linea aspera directed towards the upper end of the femur.

The *lower end* of the femur is irregular in shape with a *lateral* and *medial condyle* meeting anteriorly and separated posteriorly by the *intercondylar notch*. The distal and anterior surfaces of the condyles are smooth for articulation with the tibia inferiorly and the patella anteriorly. The two tibial articular areas are separated from the patellar area by a faint groove on each side. The lateral surface of each condyle is rough, subcutaneous and easily palpable and projects superiorly to form an *epicondyle*, *lateral* and *medial*. The medial condyle is at a lower level than the lateral. This is due to the obliquity of the shaft and the horizontal plane of the knee joint. The tibial articular area of the medial condyle is narrower and extends further forwards than that of the lateral condyle.

The adductor tubercle lies immediately above the medial epicondyle, both of which are palpable subcutaneously. The direction of the latter is a guide to the direction of the head, which is not palpable.

Above the lateral epicondyle there is usually a well marked circular depression to which the lateral head of the gastrocnemius is attached (figure 243(c)). The lateral ligament is attached to the lateral epicondyle itself, on which there may be a small pit. Inferior to the condyle there is a depression from which a groove passes upwards and backwards. The popliteus muscle is attached to the depression and its tendon lies in the groove when the leg is flexed on the thigh.

The intercondylar notch is separated from the articular areas of the condyles by the *intercondylar line* which bounds the patellar articular area posteriorly. The patellar articular area on the lateral condyle extends further forwards than that on the medial condyle. That the medial condyle is larger and lower than the lateral and has a tibial articular area which is greater than that of the lateral should not be confused with the fact that the lateral condyle projects further forwards than the medial.

The *ossification* and *structure* (figures 57(c), 244, 254, 259(c)) of the femur are of special importance, the former because it has been used to determine the age of a fetus in medicolegal work and the latter because it illustrates the relation between the structure and function of bone. The femur ossifies in cartilage from a primary centre which appears about the seventh week of fetal life. The secondary centre of ossification at the lower end appears about the 36th week of fetal life and was regarded as an indication of the viability of a fetus which was assumed to be incapable of an existence independent of its mother before that time. In more recent times this period for the viability of a fetus has been questioned, especially if viability refers to only the brief period during which a fetus of this age can survive. It is of interest that the possible length of a pregnancy which is normally accepted to be about 280 days (nine calendar or 10 lunar months) has been extended by a learned judge to as long as 360 days.

The upper end of the femur has secondary centres which appear (1) in the head during the first year; (2) in the greater trochanter about the third year; (3) in the lesser trochanter about the 13th year (figure 244(a)). They fuse separately with the neck and shaft at about 18 years of age. The lower end fuses with the shaft at about 20 years and is the growing end. The plane of the epiphyseal cartilage between the head and neck alters with age. Early on it is nearly horizontal but later it becomes more vertical so that the epiphysis is most likely to move between the age of 5 and 10 years (*slipped epiphysis*). A condition called *osteochondritis juvenalis*, which only affects epiphyses or ossifying bones, can affect the head of the femur. It cannot occur after the epiphysis has fused with the neck, that is after about 18 years.

The shaft of the femur consists of an outer layer of thick compact bone, thickened posteriorly, and a thin layer of spongy bone enclosing a medullary cavity. The ends of the bone have only a thin layer of compact bone enclosing a mass of spongy bone the trabeculae of which are arranged in a very definite manner especially in the upper end. Trabeculae pass from the upper part of the head to the inferomedial part of the neck and resist compression forces due to the weight of the body being transmitted through the head to the neck and thence to the shaft. Trabeculae arch from the lower part of the head deep to the greater trochanter to the lateral part of the shaft and resist bending forces. There is also a vertical ridge of compact bone, the *calcar femorale*, which passes from the medial side of the shaft from just above the lesser trochanter into the neck (*calcar* = *spur*, Latin).

(a)

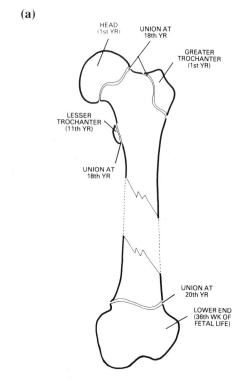

(b1)

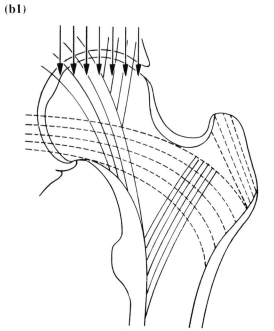

(b2)

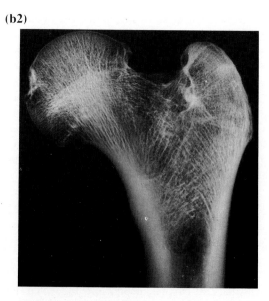

Figure 244   (a) The ossification of the femur: (b1) the theoretical forces of compression (continuous lines) and tension (dotted lines) in the head and neck of the femur (after M. G. Graveney, Physics Department, Guy's Hospital Medical School); (b2) the arrangement of the trabeculae in the head and neck of the femur as seen in a radiograph (reproduced from *Hamilton's Textbook of Human Anatomy* by courtesy of the Editors and The Macmillan Press).

This bone varies in size in different individuals and resists shearing stresses between the neck and shaft. Trabeculae between the neck and shaft near the greater trochanter resist the forces produced by the contraction of the muscles attached to the greater trochanter. A model designed to resist the stresses and strains to which the upper end of the femur is subjected, is very similar to the actual structure seen in an X-ray of this part of the bone (figures 244(b2), 254). At the lower end of the femur the trabeculae are arranged horizontally and vertically so that both compression and tension forces are resisted.

The neck of the femur is an upward extension of the shaft and the curves of both the neck and the shaft itself are examples of bony arches which give resilience to weight-bearing structures. The bone in the concavity of the neck and shaft is thickened in order to buttress the arches.

With advancing age bones show degenerative changes. One consequence is a thinning of the bone so that it becomes more fragile. In the case of the femur these changes can lead to a fracture of its neck as a result of a comparatively minor degree of indirect violence. Because the blood supply to the head of the femur is mainly through vessels which enter the neck, the head necroses and the fracture does not unite. These fractures are often treated by pinning together the neck and head. In a child, before the epiphysis of the head unites with the neck, the blood vessels entering the head through the ligament attached to its fossa are an important source of blood to the head.

The Patella (figure 245)

The patella, the largest sesamoid bone in the body, is embedded in the tendon of the quadriceps femoris. Its deep surface forms an articulation with the anterior intercondylar area of the lower end of the femur. Inferiorly this surface is non-articular and forms a triangular apex which distinguishes the lower from the upper border. The articular area has a vertical ridge which divides it into a larger lateral and smaller medial facet for articulation with the anterior areas of the lateral and medial femoral condyles. The difference in sizes of these articular areas distinguishes the lateral from the medial side.

The superficial surface of the patella, although covered by the tendon of the quadriceps femoris, is subcutaneous and easily palpated. The prepatellar bursa lies between the patella and the skin. There are foramina for blood vessels and also longitudinal

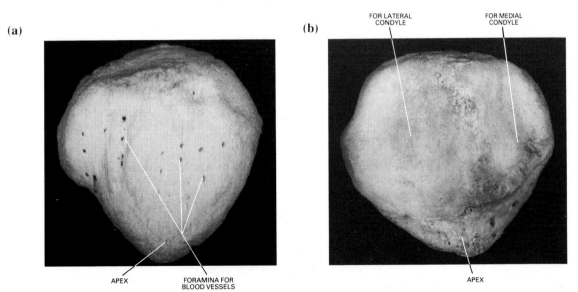

(a)

(b)

FOR LATERAL CONDYLE   FOR MEDIAL CONDYLE

APEX   FORAMINA FOR BLOOD VESSELS   APEX

Figure 245   The left patella: (a) the anterior aspect; (b) the posterior aspect.

ridges on the superficial surface. The patellar ligament, a continuation of the tendon of the quadriceps femoris, is attached to the apex of the patella.

The patella *ossifies* in cartilage from several
centres which appear between the third and sixth
years and rapidly fuse with each other. Ossification
is usually completed by puberty.

Although the patella is regarded as a structure
which improves the action of the quadriceps femoris because it acts like a pulley, it is claimed that
removal of the patella following its fracture does
not impair the function of the muscle either as an
extensor of the leg at the knee or as a stabiliser
when the weight of the body falls behind the transverse axis of the joint.

The Anterior, Medial and Lateral Aspects of the Thigh

The upper part of this region is related to the
abdominal wall and the hip, and the lower part
to the knee. The main vessels (the femoral artery
and vein) enter and leave the upper part of the
thigh. The femoral and obturator nerves are the
nerves of the anterior and medial parts of the thigh
but the main nerve of the lower limb (the sciatic)
enters the thigh at the back.

The surface markings and skin

The oblique inguinal fold *passing downwards and
medially, distal and parallel to the inguinal ligament, indicates the junction of the thigh with the
abdomen and the attachment of the membranous
layer of the superficial abdominal fascia to the
deep fascia of the thigh about 1 cm distal to the
inguinal ligament. The* anterior superior iliac spine
can be felt laterally and also the iliac crest *curving
backwards from the spine. The* pubic symphysis *is
palpable in the midline and the* pubic tubercle *can
be felt about 2 cm lateral to the midline on the
upper border of the pubic bone. The* greater trochanter *is felt laterally at the widest part of the hips,
about 12 cm below the iliac crest. On the medial
side of the thigh the subcutaneous* great saphenous
vein *can often be seen passing upwards from be-*

hind *the medial femoral condyle to the anterior
medial part of the thigh.*

The skin of the thigh is usually hairy except for
the upper medial part. A large number of cutaneous
nerves supply the skin (figure 275). The upper part
of the lateral side is supplied by the *iliac branch* of
the *iliohypogastric nerve* (L1). Lower down, the
skin on the middle of the outer side is supplied by
the *lateral femoral cutaneous nerve* (L2, 3). The
intermediate and *medial femoral cutaneous nerves*
go to the skin on the front and medial side of the
thigh (L2, 3). The skin of the upper medial aspect
of the thigh also receives branches from the *ilio-
inguinal nerve* (L1), the *genitofemoral nerve* (L2)
and the *obturator nerve* (L2, 3, 4). It is important
to know the *dermatomes*, the area of the skin
supplied mainly by one spinal nerve (figure 275).
A hand placed over the skin between the iliac crest
and the greater trochanter indicates the main area
supplied by the *first lumbar spinal cord segment.*
(This area extends further forwards than is indicated by the position of the hand.) The area supplied by the *second lumbar nerve* is indicated by a
hand placed on the middle of the lateral side of the
thigh. This area extends anteriorly and medially.
The area supplied by the *third lumbar nerve* is
indicated by placing the hand on the lower part of
the *medial* side of the thigh and extends to some
extent in all directions.

The superficial and deep fasciae

There may be a considerable amount of fat in the
subcutaneous tissue of the thigh. The nerves to the
skin can be seen passing downwards. The *lateral
femoral cutaneous nerve*, a direct branch of the
lumbar plexus, enters the thigh deep to the inguinal
ligament about 2 cm medial to the anterior superior
iliac spine, the *intermediate* and *medial femoral
cutaneous nerves* are branches of the femoral nerve
and arise distal to the inguinal ligament, and the
femoral branch of the *genitofemoral nerve* pierces
the deep fascia about 3 cm below and lateral to
the pubic tubercle.

On the medial side of the thigh the *great (long)
saphenous vein (saphena = a vein in the leg*, Latin;
from *sapin*, Arabic) runs upwards in the superficial

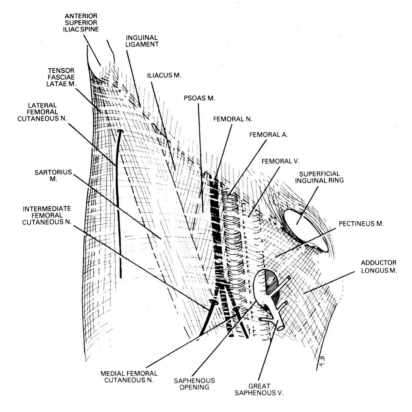

Figure 246   The fascia lata of the upper anterior part of the thigh.

fascia and pierces the deep fascia at the *saphenous opening* (figure 246) which is covered by thin perforated fascia, the *cribriform fascia* (*cribrum = sieve*, Latin). Superficial veins, the *superficial external pudendal* from the medial side and the *superficial external iliac* from the lateral side, enter the great saphenous vein before it passes through the saphenous opening. Small arteries from the femoral artery become superficial by passing through the cribriform fascia.

There are important *lymph nodes* in the superficial fascia inferior to the inguinal ligament. An *upper transverse group* receives lymphatic vessels from the skin of the lower half of the abdominal wall and the buttock, from the external genitalia and from the lower part of the anal canal and vagina. A *lower vertical group* along the terminal part of the great saphenous vein receives most of the superficial lymphatic vessels of the lower limb. The efferent vessels from these superficial nodes go either to the *deep inguinal nodes* along the

femoral vein or directly to the *external iliac nodes* (figure 100).

The *deep fascia* (the *fascia lata*) forms a very distinct fibrous sheath round the thigh (*latus = broad*, Latin) and is especially thickened on the lateral side where it forms the *iliotibial tract*. The iliotibial tract, as the name implies, is attached superiorly to the ilium along the outer border of its crest and inferiorly to the tibia just below its lateral condyle where it can be seen and palpated. At its attachment to the ilium, the iliotibial tract splits to enclose the tensor fasciae latae. This muscle passes downwards and backwards from the iliac crest into the tract to which it is attached. More posteriorly the major part of the gluteus maximus, the large muscle of the buttock, is inserted into the tract.

Superiorly, the fascia lata is attached at the back to the sacrum and coccyx, sacrotuberous ligament and ischial tuberosity and anteriorly to the inguinal ligament and ischiopubic ramus. Distally it is attached to the bony prominences round the knee joint — the condyles of the femur and tibia and head of the fibula — and several of the tendons round the joint, for example the tendon of the quadriceps femoris. Lateral and medial septa are described passing inwards towards the linea aspera separating, on the lateral side, the vastus lateralis from the short head of the biceps femoris, and on the medial side the vastus medialis from the adductor muscles.

The saphenous opening, through which the great saphenous vein passes to join the femoral vein, lies 3 cm below and lateral to the pubic tubercle. The lateral and medial edges of the opening are not in the same plane. The fascia lata forming the lateral boundary is sickle-shaped (the *falciform margin*; *falx = sickle*, Latin), is attached to the anterior surface of the femoral sheath and is more superficial than the fascia forming the medial boundary, which can be followed upwards deep to the femoral sheath over the underlying muscles towards the pubic bone. The saphenous opening is covered by the cribriform fascia and transmits the great saphenous vein, small arteries, branches of the femoral artery and lymphatic vessels. Operations on the great saphenous vein in the region of opening are common and a femoral hernia (p. 429) becomes superficial through this opening. Because of the arrangement of its margins the hernia is directed upwards and medially towards the pubic tubercle.

The femoral triangle

The front of the thigh is divided into an upper medial triangular area and a lower lateral area by the oblique *sartorius muscle* (figure 247). This muscle is attached superiorly to the anterior superior iliac spine and inferiorly to the upper part of the anteromedial surface of the tibia. It is supplied by the femoral nerve (L2, 3). Its action is to flex and laterally rotate the thigh at the hip and the leg at the knee. Its action is said to produce the position of the lower limb associated with the tailor who sat sewing on a table (*sartor = tailor*, Latin). Its actions, however, are unimportant in the movements of the lower limb, although its

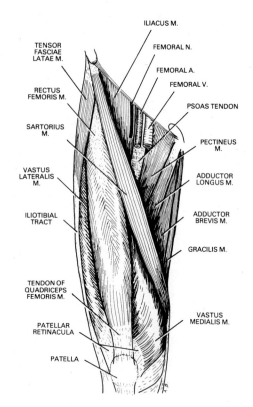

Figure 247   The anterior and medial aspect of the thigh.

long fibres, said to extend the whole length of the muscle, are frequently used for investigations into the properties of skeletal muscle. The region above and medial to the sartorius is called the *femoral triangle* and the region below and lateral contains the large quadriceps femoris muscle. Deep to the sartorius is the *adductor (subsartorial) canal of Hunter*. (John Hunter, 1728–93, a Scottish surgeon, deserves to be commemorated; his fame when he lived was such that his bust was placed in Leicester Square, London, together with busts of Newton, Reynolds and Hogarth and a statue to Shakespeare. The Hunterian Museum of the Royal College of Surgeons of England was founded by John Hunter.)

The *femoral triangle* is bounded inferiorly by the medial border of the sartorius, superiorly by the inguinal ligament and medially by the medial border of the adductor longus, which is attached above to the body of the pubis and below to the linea aspera. *The triangle can be seen as a hollow inferior to the inguinal ligament if the thigh is flexed, abducted and laterally rotated at the hip.* The saphenous opening is in the fascia lata, which forms a roof over the triangle. The main structures in the triangle are the femoral vessels in the femoral sheath, their branches and tributaries, and the femoral nerve lateral to the femoral sheath. The floor of the triangle is muscular and consists of, from the lateral to the medial side, the iliopsoas tendon and the pectineus and the adductor longus muscles.

The Femoral Sheath (figures 61, 65). The sheath, about 3–4 cm long, is formed by continuations from the abdomen of the fascia transversalis anteriorly and the fascia iliaca posteriorly. Distally it becomes continuous with the walls of the femoral vessels. The sheath is divided into three compartments. The lateral contains the femoral artery and the middle, the femoral vein; the medial compartment forms the *femoral canal*. The femoral branch of the genitofemoral nerve pierces the lateral wall of the sheath and the great saphenous vein pierces the medial wall. The upper end of the femoral canal is called the *femoral ring*, which is bounded anteriorly by the inguinal ligament, laterally by the femoral vein, posteriorly by the pectineal fascia on the pectineus muscle and medially by the lateral border of the lacunar ligament. There may be a lymph node in the femoral canal and lymphatic vessels pass through it. It has been suggested that its function is to allow expansion of the femoral vein due to variations in the venous return from the lower limb.

The femoral canal is the channel down which a *femoral hernia* passes. The protrusion of peritoneum, usually with a loop of small intestine, extends downwards and may become more superficial by passing through the saphenous opening. The swelling then extends upwards and medially towards the pubic tubercle. A femoral hernia is much less common than an inguinal in both sexes and is commoner in women than in men because of the wider space between the inguinal ligament and the pubic bone in the female pelvis. At operation the reduction of a femoral hernia, that is the replacement of the contents of the hernial sac of peritoneum, may be difficult. If the lacunar ligament has to be cut in order to enlarge the femoral ring the possibility of an abnormal obturator artery on the deep surface of the ligament must be kept in mind.

The Femoral Artery and Vein. The artery is a continuation of the external iliac artery beyond the inguinal ligament and *can be felt pulsating midway between the anterior superior iliac spine and the symphysis pubis*. The artery lies in the lateral compartment of the femoral sheath and passes downwards deep to the sartorius into the adductor canal. It enters the back of the thigh medial to the shaft of the femur through an opening in the adductor magnus and becomes the *popliteal artery*. In the femoral sheath the vein is medial to the artery but more inferiorly the vein is posterior. The femoral nerve is lateral to the artery outside the femoral sheath. The artery lies on the muscles of the floor of the femoral triangle – the iliopsoas, pectineus and adductor longus – before passing on to the adductor magnus.

A large branch, the *profunda femoris artery*, which arises in the upper part of the femoral triangle and lies behind the main artery with the femoral and profunda femoral veins intervening, passes deep to the adductor longus (figure 248). The profunda femoris artery gives off several *perforating branches* which pass through the adductor muscles to the back of the thigh. Its termination also perforates the adductor muscles and takes part in the anastomosis round the knee joint. The perforating arteries divide into ascending and descending branches and form a posterior anastomotic link between the arteries of the buttock and the branches of the popliteal artery at the back of the knee.

The femoral artery gives off superficial branches, the *superficial epigastric* running upwards and medially to the anterior abdominal wall, the *superficial external pudendal* running medially to the skin of the external genitalia and the *superficial circumflex iliac* passing laterally towards the anterior superior iliac spine. The *deep external pudendal branch* also passes medially to the region of the external genitalia.

The profunda femoris artery usually gives off the *medial* and *lateral circumflex arteries* but their

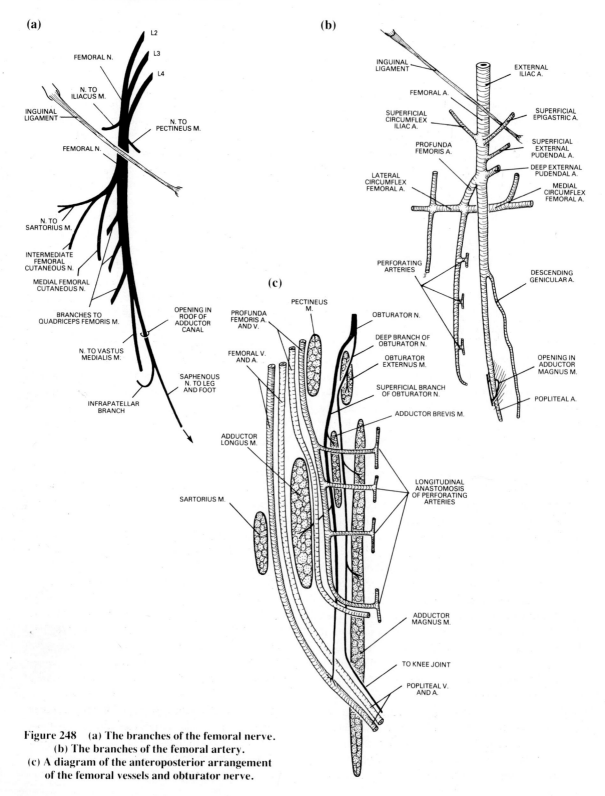

(a)

L2
L3
L4

FEMORAL N.

N. TO
ILIACUS M.

INGUINAL
LIGAMENT

N. TO
PECTINEUS M.

FEMORAL N.

N. TO
SARTORIUS M.

INTERMEDIATE
FEMORAL
CUTANEOUS N.

MEDIAL FEMORAL
CUTANEOUS N.

BRANCHES TO
QUADRICEPS FEMORIS M.

OPENING IN
ROOF OF
ADDUCTOR
CANAL

N. TO VASTUS
MEDIALIS M.

SAPHENOUS
N. TO LEG
AND FOOT

INFRAPATELLAR
BRANCH

(b)

INGUINAL
LIGAMENT

EXTERNAL
ILIAC A.

FEMORAL A.

SUPERFICIAL
CIRCUMFLEX
ILIAC A.

SUPERFICIAL
EPIGASTRIC A.

PROFUNDA
FEMORIS A.

SUPERFICIAL
EXTERNAL
PUDENDAL A.

LATERAL
CIRCUMFLEX
FEMORAL A.

DEEP EXTERNAL
PUDENDAL A.

MEDIAL
CIRCUMFLEX
FEMORAL A.

PERFORATING
ARTERIES

DESCENDING
GENICULAR A.

OPENING IN
ADDUCTOR
MAGNUS M.

POPLITEAL A.

(c)

PECTINEUS
M.

PROFUNDA
FEMORIS A.
AND V.

OBTURATOR N.

DEEP BRANCH OF
OBTURATOR N.

FEMORAL V.
AND A.

OBTURATOR
EXTERNUS M.

SUPERFICIAL BRANCH
OF OBTURATOR N.

ADDUCTOR
LONGUS M.

ADDUCTOR BREVIS M.

SARTORIUS M.

LONGITUDINAL
ANASTOMOSIS
OF PERFORATING
ARTERIES

ADDUCTOR
MAGNUS M.

TO KNEE JOINT

POPLITEAL V.
AND A.

**Figure 248   (a) The branches of the femoral nerve.
(b) The branches of the femoral artery.
(c) A diagram of the anteroposterior arrangement
of the femoral vessels and obturator nerve.**

origin is variable. They may arise by a common trunk or from the main femoral artery singly or by a common trunk. The medial circumflex femoral artery passes backwards on the medial side of the femur between the pectineus and the psoas tendon and through successive layers of muscles to reach the back of the thigh where it divides into transverse and ascending branches which anastomose with other arteries in this region. The lateral femoral circumflex artery passes laterally deep to the sartorius and rectus femoris muscles where it divides into ascending and transverse branches which take part in the anastomoses in the buttock and back of the thigh, and a descending branch which passes downwards as far as the knee. Both circumflex arteries give off branches which supply the neck and head of the femur.

The profunda femoris artery is the main source of blood to the muscles of the thigh. The artery and its branches take part in a chain of anastomoses on the back of the thigh from the buttock to the back of the knee. The gluteal arteries in the buttock come from the internal iliac artery and they anastomose with branches of the medial and lateral femoral circumflex arteries. The circumflex arteries anastomose down the back of the thigh with the series of perforating arteries, the lowest of which anastomoses with branches of the popliteal artery. Blockage of the external iliac or femoral artery need not result in the loss of the blood supply to the lower limb since blood can reach the limb from the internal iliac artery via the anastomoses on the back of the thigh. It should be added that if the cutting off of the blood supply is sudden, for example as a result of a penetrating wound severing the femoral artery (assuming that the haemorrhage is stopped almost immediately), it is unlikely that the anastomotic channels would open up quickly enough to save the limb. If, however, the obstruction is slow it is probable that the blood supply to the limb would be maintained through the anastomoses.

The *femoral vein* is the continuation of the popliteal vein at the opening in the adductor magnus. It continues upwards through the adductor canal and femoral triangle at first posterior and then medial to the femoral artery. It lies in the middle compartment of the femoral sheath. At the inguinal ligament the femoral vein becomes the external iliac vein. The profunda femoris vein, its largest tributary, joins the femoral vein about 6 cm inferior to the inguinal ligament. Other tributaries are the great saphenous vein and the medial and lateral femoral circumflex veins. The femoral vein has several valves, one of which is inferior to the entry of the profunda femoris vein. The deep inguinal nodes, receiving the lymph from almost the whole of the lower limb, are arranged vertically along the upper part of the femoral vein. These nodes drain to the external iliac nodes.

The Femoral Nerve (figure 248). The femoral nerve is a branch of the lumbar plexus and arises from the ventral rami of the second, third and fourth lumbar nerves. It emerges from the lateral side of the psoas muscle in the iliac fossa and, running downwards and laterally between the psoas tendon and iliacus, enters the thigh deep to the inguinal ligament and lateral to the femoral sheath. The nerve supplies the iliacus muscle in the iliac fossa and the pectineus above the inguinal ligament. About 3 cm distal to the ligament the femoral nerve gives off a number of branches (the *intermediate* and *medial femoral cutaneous nerves*, *nerves supplying* the sartorius and the quadriceps femoris and the hip and knee joints) and lateral to the femoral vessels continues into the adductor canal as the *saphenous nerve*. The branch supplying the vastus medialis enters the canal and ends in the muscle which forms the lateral wall of the canal. The saphenous nerve passes medially anterior to the femoral vessels, perforates the roof of the canal (the sartorius or adjacent fascia) and runs downwards on the medial side of the knee and leg alongside the great saphenous vein to the medial border of the foot as far as the ball of the big toe.

In general terms the femoral nerve supplies the flexors of the thigh at the hip (the psoas is supplied by the ventral rami of the second and third lumbar nerves as they pass through the muscle) and the extensors of the leg at the knee. The cutaneous branches of the nerve carry fibres supplying the dermatomes innervated by the second, third and fourth lumbar nerves (the dermatome of the fourth lumbar nerve is on the medial side of the leg and extends on to the medial side of the foot).

The Muscles (figure 247). The *iliacus*, which is attached to the iliac fossa, enters the thigh deep to the inguinal ligament and lateral to the *psoas* tendon. The two tendons join and are attached to the lesser trochanter and the bone immediately below. The psoas tendon is anterior to the hip joint and is separated from its capsule by a bursa which may communicate with the joint. These muscles are the most important flexors of the thigh at the hip and are also involved in flexing the trunk on the thighs, from the supine position. The psoas muscles also flex the lumbar part of the vertebral column. Both muscles are supplied by the second and third lumbar nerves, the iliacus by a branch of the femoral nerve. The psoas is also innervated by the first lumbar nerve.

The *pectineus* is attached to the upper surface of the superior ramus of the pubis (*pecten = comb*, Latin) and passes downwards and laterally in the floor of the femoral triangle to become attached to the femur lateral to and below the attachment of the iliacus. It is a flexor and adductor of the thigh at the hip and is supplied by the femoral nerve and sometimes additionally by the obturator nerve (L2, 3). The femoral sheath, particularly the femoral canal, lies on the pectineus. The fascia on the upper part of the muscle is continuous medially with the pectineal and lacunar ligaments.

The adductor region (figures 247, 248)

The *adductor longus* which forms part of the floor of the femoral triangle has a narrow attachment superiorly to the front of the body of the pubis (bone sometimes grows into the muscle to form a tubercle) and as it passes downwards and laterally widens to become attached to the middle third of the linea aspera. The *adductor brevis* lies deep to the adductor longus and pectineus and is attached to the body and inferior ramus of the pubis. It passes laterally and being more horizontal than the longus is attached to the linea aspera above the attachment of that muscle.

The *adductor magnus* has an extensive attachment to the ischiopubic ramus and ischial tuberosity. Its upper fibres from the pubic ramus are almost horizontal. The rest of the fibres from the

ischial ramus and tuberosity become more and more oblique as they pass to the linea aspera. The fibres from the ischial tuberosity are almost vertical and go to the adductor tubercle. There is a series of openings between the muscle and the femur for the passage of the perforating and terminal branches of the profunda femoris artery and for the femoral vessels. The opening for the femoral vessels is much larger than the others. The posterior surface of the adductor magnus may be regarded as the floor of the posterior aspect of the thigh on which the sciatic nerve and hamstring muscles descend towards the back of the knee.

The *gracilis* is a narrow strap-like muscle bounding the medial side of the thigh. It extends from the edge of the ischiopubic ramus to the upper lateral part of the medial surface of the tibia behind the sartorius.

The *obturator externus muscle* is attached to the external aspect of the obturator membrane and the bone on the medial side of the foramen. The muscle lies deep to the pectineus and adductor longus and is in the same plane as the adductor brevis. The muscle passes laterally and then winds upwards below the neck of the femur to become attached to the trochanteric fossa on the medial side of the greater trochanter.

All the muscles are supplied by the *obturator nerve* (L2, 3, 4) which, within the abdomen, emerges from the medial edge of the psoas muscle near the pelvic inlet. The nerve runs round the lateral wall of the bony pelvis above the obturator vessels about 1 cm inferior to the inlet, and leaves the pelvis through the obturator canal in the upper part of the obturator membrane. Before entering the adductor region of the thigh the nerve has already divided into an anterior branch which then lies in front of the obturator externus muscle and a posterior branch which perforates the muscle (figure 248). The anterior branch passes downwards deep to the adductor longus on the adductor brevis with the profunda femoris vessels and supplies the gracilis and adductors longus and brevis. It also gives a branch to the hip joint and the skin on the medial side of the lower part of the thigh and it may supply the pectineus.

The posterior branch of the obturator nerve supplies the obturator externus and runs downwards deep to the adductor brevis on the adductor magnus which it supplies. The posterior branch ends in the knee joint by passing with the femoral vessels through the adductor magnus into the popliteal fossa.

Both the femoral and obturator nerves supply the hip and knee joints and both come from the second, third and fourth lumbar spinal nerves. Pain due to disease in the lumbar region of the vertebral column or hip may be referred to the knee joint. Because of the way in which the obturator nerve is distributed it is possible to divide the anterior branch of the nerve to paralyse part of the adductor muscles. In children with marked spasticity of the adductor muscles resulting in an inability to abduct the lower limbs at the thigh, this operation reduces the effect of the spastic adductor muscles without paralysing them completely.

The *obturator artery*, after passing through the obturator canal, divides into two branches which encircle the foramen deep to the obturator externus on the membrane. These branches supply the muscles and anastomose with the medial circumflex and inferior gluteal arteries.

The obturator externus is a lateral rotator of the thigh at the hip. The remaining four muscles, as their name implies (the gracilis has been called the adductor gracilis), adduct the abducted thigh. In the upright position adduction at the hip is only possible after flexing or extending the thigh. When lying down, if one lower limb is abducted, the other limb can be adducted beyond the midline. The adductors are inactive in standing and show little activity in walking. It has proved difficult to give these powerful muscles an adequate function. Perhaps they are most useful for gripping when climbing a rope or the trunk of a tree. The sexual function which has been attributed to them cannot apply to both sexes.

The adductor (subsartorial) canal (of Hunter)

This refers to a canal formed by the vastus medialis on the lateral side and the adductors longus and magnus medially. It is roofed over by the sartorius muscle and the fascia passing between the adductors and the vastus medialis. Entering the canal

from above are the femoral vessels, femoral nerve or its continuation the saphenous nerve, and the nerve to the vastus medialis. The femoral artery passes through the opening in the adductor magnus where it becomes the popliteal artery and the popliteal vein becomes the femoral vein. The saphenous nerve pierces the roof of the canal and becoming superficial continues distally along the medial side of the knee, leg and foot. The nerve to the vastus medialis ends in that muscle. Within the canal the femoral artery gives off the *descending genicular artery (the arteria anastomotica magna)* which passes downwards and takes part in the anastomosis round the knee. Hunter claimed that if the femoral artery was tied for a popliteal aneurysm (*aneurysm = permanent dilatation of an artery due to a diseased wall*) it must be tied above the origin of this artery because it made such a large contribution to the anastomosis round the knee joint and to the popliteal artery.

The tensor fasciae latae and quadriceps femoris muscles (figure 247)

The *tensor fasciae latae* is attached to the anterior third of the outer border of the iliac crest. Its fibres extending for about one-third of the length of the thigh pass downwards and backwards into the iliotibial tract. It is a flexor and medial rotator of the thigh at the hip. After the limb has been abducted at the thigh the tensor fasciae latae may assist in further abduction, especially against resistance. Through the iliotibial tract, if the foot is off the ground, it flexes the leg at the knee. If the foot is on the ground it produces extension of the leg. The muscle is supplied by the superior gluteal nerve (L4, 5, S1) and is considered to be part of the gluteal musculature.

The *quadriceps femoris* consists of four parts. The *rectus femoris* has a straight head, attached to the anterior inferior iliac spine, and a reflected head attached to a groove above the acetabulum. The muscle is superficially bipennate and ends as an aponeurosis which is attached to the anterior part of the upper border of the patella and forms the central part of the quadriceps tendon.

The *vastus lateralis* and *vastus medialis* have

similar attachments to the lateral and medial sides of the femur respectively. The upper attachment of both muscles extends on to the front of the upper end of the femur along the intertrochanteric line. The vastus lateralis winds round the lateral side below the greater trochanter and along the lateral lip of the linea aspera down to the lateral supracondylar line. The vastus medialis winds round the medial side below the lesser trochanter and along the medial lip of the linea aspera and the medial supracondylar line. The vastus lateralis is attached to the lateral border of the patella, forms the lateral part of the quadriceps tendon and strengthens the lateral side of the capsule of the knee joint. The muscle fibres of the vastus medialis extend further distally than those of the vastus lateralis and its lowermost fibres reach the patella and are almost horizontal in their direction. The muscle is attached to the medial border of the patella and strengthens the medial part of the capsule of the knee joint. The *vastus intermedius* is attached to the anterior and lateral surfaces of the upper two-thirds of the shaft of the femur. Distally the intermedius, deep to the rectus femoris, is attached to the upper border of the patella.

The *quadriceps tendon*, the name given to that part of the quadriceps femoris attached to the patella, continues distal to the patella as the *patellar ligament*, which is attached proximally to the apex of the patella and distally to the tibial tuberosity.

The patella is a sesamoid bone in the quadriceps tendon. The *suprapatellar bursa*, which communicates with the cavity of the knee joint, lies between the quadriceps tendon and the femur and extends about 4–5 cm above the upper border of the patella. The *articularis genus muscle* is attached to the upper border of the bursa and the anterior surface of the femur. The ligamentum patellae is separated from the upper end of the tibia by the *deep infrapatellar bursa.*

The quadriceps femoris extends the leg on the thigh at the knee as in kicking a ball. However, its importance lies in its use as an extensor at the knee when the foot is fixed, as in standing up from the sitting position and walking up a slope or stairs. It also controls flexion at the knee in sitting down and in walking down stairs. In many activities the weight of the body falls behind the transverse axis of movement at the knee joint and a strong quadriceps femoris is required to prevent the knee giving way. This is what a patient complains of when the quadriceps is weak. In the upright position the weight falls in front of the knee joint and the quadriceps femoris is relaxed. Although the leg is extended on the thigh at the knee during the swing stage of every step, this movement is largely a passive swing and the quadriceps femoris contracts only at the end of the movement.

The quadriceps femoris is supplied by the femoral nerve (L2, 3, 4).

34

The Gluteal Region, Back of the Thigh and Popliteal Fossa

The main mass of the buttock consists of a variable amount of fat and the *gluteus maximus muscle*. Deep to the gluteus maximus there are several muscles and the vessels and nerves which emerge from the pelvis through the greater sciatic foramen. Appearing at the lower edge of the gluteus maximus, the *hamstring muscles* descend and diverge so that they form the upper boundaries of the hollow at the back of the knee, the *popliteal fossa*, which contains the continuation of the femoral vessels and the divisions of the main nerve of the lower limb, the sciatic nerve.

The Gluteal Region

The Skin and Surface Markings

The skin may be hairy, especially in males. A horizontal fold, due to the attachment of the skin to the underlying fascia, marks off the lower border of the buttock. This *gluteal fold* does not correspond with the lower border of the gluteus maximus which passes downwards and laterally and is oblique and deep to the fold.

The skin of the buttock has a multiple *nerve supply*. Its medial part near the midline is supplied by the dorsal rami of the *sacral spinal nerves*. More laterally it is supplied by the dorsal rami of the *lumbar nerves* which extend downwards (figure 275). The upper lateral part is supplied by the iliac branch of the *iliohypogastric nerve* (L1). The lower part of the skin receives fibres from the *posterior femoral cutaneous nerve* (S1, 2, 3). In terms of dermatomes the skin near the natal cleft is supplied by the fourth sacral nerve and more laterally by the third sacral nerve, which does not extend beyond the buttock (figure 275). The dermatome of the second sacral nerve extends from the lower edge of the buttock downwards along the middle of the back of the thigh and calf. The dermatome on the medial side of the thigh is supplied by the third lumbar nerve and on the lateral side by the second lumbar nerve. The dermatome of the medial side of the leg is supplied by the fourth lumbar nerve and of the lateral side by the fifth lumbar nerve. This arrangement of the dermatomes determines the *ventral* and *dorsal axial lines* which bound the dermatome of the second sacral nerve (the ventral is medial and the dorsal is lateral). There is little overlap of the innervation of the skin on either side of these lines.

The posterior part of the iliac crest ends at the posterior superior iliac spine *which is usually marked by a dimple. A line joining the two dimples almost invariably indicates the level of the spinous process of the* second sacral vertebra. *The greater trochanters are at the widest part of the hips. The* ischial tuberosity, *overlapped by the gluteus maximus in the upright position, can be easily felt if the thigh is flexed or the subject is in the sitting position, because the muscle slides away from the tuberosity in these situations. A line joining the anterior superior iliac spine to the ischial tuberosity normally touches the upper border of the greater trochanter.*

The Muscles (figure 249)

The Gluteus Maximus. This is a large quadrilateral muscle forming the main prominence of the buttock and consisting of strikingly coarse muscle bundles. It is attached to the back of the lower part of the sacrum and the coccyx and the sacro-tuberous ligament. Its upper fibres extend on to the adjacent area of the ilium between the posterior part of the iliac crest and the posterior gluteal line.

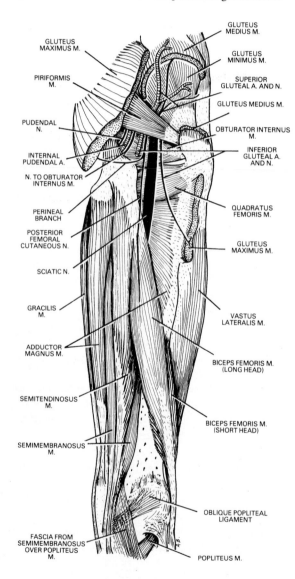

Figure 249　The gluteal region and hamstring muscles.

The fibres pass downwards and laterally and enter the iliotibial tract except for the deeper inferior part of the muscle which is attached to the gluteal tuberosity (ridge) between the greater trochanter and the linea aspera. There is usually a bursa between the muscle and the greater trochanter and one between it and the ischial tuberosity.

The gluteus maximus is superficial to the lower part of the gluteus medius and to the structures which emerge from the greater and lesser sciatic foramina. It also covers the origins of the hamstring muscles and the upper part of the adductor magnus. The proximal part of the posterior longitudinal anastomosis of the back of the thigh is deep to the muscle.

The size of the muscle is a reflection of the force required to straighten the flexed trunk on the thigh and straightening of the flexed thigh on the trunk in activities such as standing up, climbing and walking up stairs. In all these actions the muscle is assisted by the hamstrings attached to the ischial tuberosity. In fact the hamstrings are the primary extensors of the thigh at the hip. The gluteus maximus is an antigravity muscle and is active in the terminal part of flexing the trunk at the thigh and sitting down. In the standing easy upright position the gluteus maximus is relaxed. In walking on a flat surface it is active in the early part of the stance phase (p. 491). From the anatomical position the gluteus maximus can extend the lower limb at the hip. It is not active, however, unless the movement is rapid or performed with some force. The action of the muscle on the leg at the knee through the iliotibial tract depends on whether the foot is on the ground or free. If the former, the result is extension at the knee; if the latter, flexion of the leg at the knee occurs.

The gluteus maximus is supplied by the inferior gluteal nerve (L5, S1, 2). Intramuscular injections into the gluteus maximus must be given into its upper lateral part because of the danger of penetrating the muscle and injuring the sciatic nerve which is deep to the lower two-thirds of the muscle.

The Gluteus Medius and Minimus. The *gluteus medius*, partly deep to the maximus, is attached to the outer surface of the ala of the ilium between the posterior and anterior gluteal lines as far upwards as the outer border of the iliac crest. The muscle passes laterally over the greater trochanter and is attached by a tendon to its outer surface along an oblique line which passes downwards and forwards. The tendon is separated from the greater trochanter by a bursa.

The gluteus medius is an abductor of the thigh at the hip but its important function is to prevent the unsupported side of the body from falling when standing on one limb. The right gluteus medius contracts when standing on the right lower limb. This occurs in every step in walking and in going up and down stairs. If the gluteus medius is not functioning properly the unsupported side of the body descends when standing on one limb. This is seen in congenital dislocation of the hip and in many diseases affecting the head or neck of the femur. Malfunctioning or paralysis of the muscle affects the gait. Either the unsupported side falls in each step or the body is deliberately thrown upwards over the supporting limb in an exaggerated manner.

The *gluteus minimus* is deep and anterior to the medius. It is attached to the outer surface of the ala of the ilium between the anterior and inferior gluteal lines. In the upright position most of the muscle is anterior to the hip joint and its fibres are attached to the anterior surface of the greater trochanter. The minimus assists the medius in abduction and in keeping the body upright when the opposite limb is off the ground. It is probably the most important medial rotator of the thigh at the hip joint.

The superior gluteal nerve (L4, 5, S1) supplies both the medius and minimus and also the tensor fasciae latae.

The Piriformis, Obturator Internus and Quadratus Femoris.

These muscles are in the same plane as the gluteus minimus and are deep to the medius and maximus in that order from above downwards. The adductor magnus is immediately inferior to the quadratus femoris. The *piriformis* and *obturator internus* are described with the pelvis (p. 131). The *piriformis* is attached to the middle of the anterior surface of the sacrum, leaves the pelvis through the greater sciatic foramen and is attached to the upper border of the greater trochanter. The

piriformis is supplied by the second and third sacral nerves.

The *obturator internus* is attached to the inner surface of the obturator membrane and the surrounding bone. The muscle passes downwards and backwards and ends in a tendon which bends laterally at a right angle and leaves the pelvis through the lesser sciatic foramen. It is joined by two small muscles, the *superior* and *inferior gemelli*, which are attached to the spine and tuberosity of the ischium respectively, and the common tendon is attached to the upper border of the greater trochanter in front of the piriformis. The nerve to the obturator internus (L5, S1, 2) also supplies the superior gemellus.

The *quadratus femoris* is attached to the outer surface of the ischial tuberosity and passes laterally to be attached to the quadrate tubercle on the intertrochanteric crest. The nerve to the quadratus femoris (L4, 5, S1) also supplies the inferior gemellus.

All these muscles are lateral rotators of the thigh at the hip joint and are closely related to its capsule.

The Blood Vessels and Nerves (figure 249)

The nerves are branches of the sacral plexus and emerge through the greater sciatic foramen, and the blood vessels are branches or tributaries of the internal iliac vessels. They are all related to the piriformis. The *superior gluteal nerve* (L4, 5, S1) and *artery* are above the piriformis. The nerve supplies the gluteus medius, gluteus minimus and tensor fasciae latae. The artery supplies all the gluteal muscles. Its anastomosis with the inferior gluteal and lateral and medial femoral circumflex arteries forms the upper part of the anastomosis between the internal iliac and popliteal arteries. A branch also anastomoses with other arteries in the region of the anterior superior iliac spine. The superior gluteal vein has tributaries corresponding with the branches of the artery and ends in the internal iliac vein.

The vessels and nerves emerging at the lower border of the piriformis are conveniently grouped in the following way.

(1) The *inferior gluteal vessels* and *nerve* (L5, S1, 2) exit near the medial part of the lower border of the muscle and enter the gluteus maximus. The nerve occasionally also supplies the short head of the biceps femoris. The artery takes part in the anastomosis in the region of the hip joint and descends down the back of the thigh with the sciatic nerve which it supplies.

(2) The *sciatic* and *posterior femoral cutaneous nerves* emerge lateral to the inferior gluteal vessels and nerve. The sciatic nerve (L4, 5, S1, 2, 3), the largest nerve in the body, runs downwards in the middle of the thigh and divides about half way into the *tibial* (*medial popliteal*) and *common peroneal* (*lateral popliteal*) *nerves*. The sciatic nerve lies on the obturator internus, quadratus femoris and adductor magnus. It is deep to the gluteus maximus and is crossed superficially by the long head of the biceps femoris. *The course of the nerve in the thigh can be marked by a band 1.5 cm wide extending from midway between the ischial tuberosity and greater trochanter to the apex of the popliteal fossa.*

The sciatic nerve supplies branches to the hip joint and the hamstring muscles. The short head of the biceps femoris is supplied by the common peroneal nerve and the long head of the biceps, semimembranosus and semitendinosus by the tibial nerve. Although the sciatic nerve appears to be one nerve it consists of two divisions bound up in one connective tissue sheath. The two divisions may be separate along its whole course and emerge as two nerves from the pelvis.

The posterior femoral cutaneous nerve (S1, 2, 3) is posterior or medial to the sciatic nerve and runs downwards superficial to the biceps femoris and deep to the fascia lata, which it pierces at the back of the knee to continue subcutaneously as far as the middle of the back of the calf. The nerve gives sensory branches to the skin of the lower lateral part of the buttock and a perineal branch to the skin of the scrotum or labium majus and supplies the skin of the back of the thigh, knee and calf.

(3) The *pudendal nerve* (S2, 3, 4), *internal pudendal vessels* and *nerve to the obturator internus* (L5, S1, 2) emerge medial to the sciatic nerve, run downwards over the ischial spine and sacrospinous

ligament and enter the lesser sciatic foramen. The pudendal nerve and internal pudendal vessels run forwards in the pudendal canal on the lateral wall of the ischiorectal fossa. Their distribution is described with the perineum (chapter 12). The nerve to the obturator internus supplies that muscle on its perineal surface and also the gemellus superior.

(4) The *nerve to the quadratus femoris* (L4, 5, S1) passes downwards deep to the sciatic nerve and obturator internus and supplies its own muscle and also the gemellus inferior.

The Back of the Thigh (figures 249, 250)

Inferior to the gluteus maximus the main structures of the region are the diverging hamstring muscles. As they diverge they form the upper boundaries of the popliteal fossa. The sciatic and posterior femoral cutaneous nerves pass downwards in the

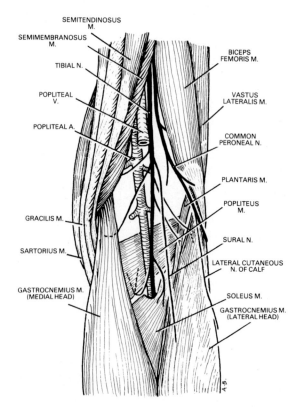

Figure 250   The popliteal fossa.

middle of the thigh and the femoral vessels enter its lower part through the opening between the adductor magnus and the femur.

The Hamstring Muscles. These comprise the *biceps femoris, semitendinosus* and *semimembranosus* and are attached to the ischial tuberosity which is divided into a superior and inferior area. The hamstrings are attached to the superior area, the *long head of the biceps femoris* and *semitendinosus* by a common attachment medially and the *semimembranosus* laterally. The long head of the biceps femoris passes downwards and laterally superficial to the semimembranosus and forms the upper lateral boundary of the popliteal fossa. It is joined by the *short head*, which is attached to the linea aspera in line with the attachment of the gluteus maximus. The tendon of the biceps femoris is attached to the head of the fibula on either side of the fibular collateral ligament of the knee joint. The common peroneal nerve is deep to the medial border of the tendon.

The semimembranosus passes downwards and medially and its tendon is attached mainly to a groove on the medial and posterior surfaces of the medial condyle of the tibia. By aponeurotic expansions the tendon is also attached to the upper part of the tibia, upwards and laterally to the posterior part of the capsule of the knee joint (the *oblique popliteal ligament*) and the posterior surface of the popliteus. Together with the tendon of the semitendinosus, the semimembranosus forms the upper medial boundary of the popliteal fossa. The tendon of the semitendinosus, much longer than that of the semimembranosus and about half the length of the muscle, lies in a groove on the posterior surface of the semimembranosus and is attached to the upper medial surface of the tibia behind the attachment of the sartorius.

The hamstrings are flexors of the leg at the knee joint. The muscles attached to the ischial tuberosity are extensors of the thigh at the hip joint or the trunk on the lower limb. The hamstrings are always active in extension of the lower limb at the thigh. If the movement is rapid or demands more power the gluteus maximus is recruited. The biceps femoris can laterally rotate the leg at the knee and the semimembranosus and semitendinosus can pro-

duce medial rotation if the knee is bent.

The hamstrings are supplied by the sciatic nerve (L5, S1, 2), the short head of the biceps femoris by the common peroneal nerve and the others by the tibial nerve.

The Popliteal Fossa (figure 250)

This is the hollow region on the back of the knee and is more easily seen on flexing the leg on the thigh. It is comparable with the cubital fossa on the front of the elbow but is diamond-shaped and not triangular. The diverging hamstrings form the upper lateral and medial borders. *The* tendon of the biceps femoris *passing to the* head of the fibula *can be felt on the lateral side and in front of it the lower end of the* iliotibial tract. *On the medial side the* tendon of the semitendinosus *is palpable and is posterior to the* tendon of the semimembranosus. *The* tendon of the vastus medialis *is medial to these two tendons and between the vastus medialis and the hamstrings the* adductor magnus tendon *going to the* adductor tubercle *can be felt in a deeper plane. In the midline the* popliteal artery *can be felt pulsating if the leg is bent at the knee. The lower converging boundaries of the popliteal fossa are formed by the* lateral *and* medial heads of the gastrocnemius muscle.

The *skin* over the fossa *is innervated* in the middle by the posterior femoral cutaneous nerve (S2), laterally by the lateral femoral cutaneous nerve (L2) and medially by the medial femoral cutaneous and obturator nerves (L3). In the superficial fascia, in addition to branches of these nerves, there is the *small (short) saphenous vein*. This vein begins on the lateral side of the dorsum of the foot, passes upwards behind the lateral malleolus and, moving medially, lies in the middle of the back of the popliteal fossa before piercing the deep fascia to end in the popliteal vein. The deep fascia roofing over the popliteal fossa is the lower posterior part of the fascia lata and has a large number of transverse fibres. The fascia is attached to the femoral and tibial condyles and laterally to the head of the fibula. It resists extension of the leg on the thigh in the upright position.

The *tibial (medial popliteal) nerve*, and the *popliteal vein* and *artery*, from superficial to deep, lie vertically in the middle of the fossa. The *tibial nerve* superiorly arises from the sciatic nerve deep to the hamstrings above the fossa, and inferiorly disappears deep to the converging heads of the gastrocnemius. In the fossa the nerve lies on the popliteus and crosses the vessels from the lateral to the medial side. In the lower part of the fossa the tibial nerve gives *muscular branches* to the gastrocnemius, soleus, plantaris and popliteus muscles. It also gives off *sensory branches*: (1) the *sural nerve*, which is joined by the sural communicating branch of the common peroneal nerve and descends on the lateral side of the leg, ankle and foot; (2) branches to the knee joint.

The *popliteal vein* is formed inferiorly at the lower border of the popliteus by the union of the *anterior* and *posterior tibial veins*. The vein receives the small saphenous vein and tributaries from the muscles and knee joint and continues upwards posterior to the artery to the opening in the adductor magnus through which it passes and becomes the *femoral vein*. The *popliteal artery* has a similar course to the vein and lies deep to it on the fat covering the lower surface of the femur and on the popliteus, at the lower border of which it divides into the *anterior* and *posterior tibial arteries*. In the fossa the artery gives off superior and inferior muscular branches and five branches to the knee joint − the medial superior and inferior, the lateral superior and inferior and the middle genicular. These articular branches also supply the adjacent muscles and take part in the anastomosis round the knee joint, superiorly and anteriorly with the descending branch of the lateral femoral circumflex and the descending genicular arteries, and superiorly and posteriorly with the lowest of the perforating branches of the profunda femoris artery. Inferiorly the genicular branches anastomose with branches of the anterior and posterior tibial arteries.

The *common peroneal (lateral popliteal) nerve*, the second main division of the sciatic nerve, enters the popliteal fossa at its apex and passes downwards and laterally deep to the biceps femoris and its tendon and superficial to the lateral head of the gastrocnemius. It continues round the neck of the fibula deep to the peroneus longus muscle and divides into the *superficial peroneal (musculocutaneous)* and *deep peroneal (anterior tibial) nerves. The nerve can be felt subcutaneously as it crosses the neck about 3 cm distal to the apex of the fibula.* At this site external pressure or involvement in a fracture of the adjacent fibula can affect the nerve.

The branches of the common peroneal nerve in the popliteal fossa are articular and cutaneous. The cutaneous branches are the *sural communicating*, which joins the sural branch of the tibial nerve, and the *lateral cutaneous nerve of the calf*.

The *floor of the popliteal fossa* is formed from above downwards by the popliteal surface of the lower posterior aspect of the femur, the posterior part of the capsule of the knee joint and the popliteus muscle covered by fascia.

Embedded in the fat in the fossa there are *lymph nodes* arranged along the popliteal vessels. The afferents to these nodes come from the lateral side of the foot (the little toe) and the leg, and their efferents go to the deep inguinal nodes in the femoral triangle. Inflammation of these nodes due to infection of the region drained by them may be a cause of pain in the back of the knee.

35

The Hip Joint

The hip joint is a ball and socket synovial joint between the head of the femur and the acetabulum of the hip bone. The head of the femur is somewhat larger than half a sphere. The acetabulum is deepened by a ring of fibrocartilage (the *acetabular labrum*) which is attached to its edge and bridges the notch on the lower part of the acetabulum. The labrum is triangular in section with the base attached to the bone. The diameter of the free edge of the labrum is less than that of the acetabulum and extends beyond the equator of the head so that it grips the head to some extent. The articular surface of the femoral head has a depression in it to which the *ligament of the head of the femur* is attached. The other end of this ligament is attached to the edge of the notch. The articular area of the acetabulum is shaped like a horseshoe with the opening of the shoe inferiorly. The concavity of the shoe is non-articular and roughened and contains a fibrofatty pad.

The Ligaments (figure 251). The *fibrous capsule* is attached medially to the hip bone outside and just beyond the edge of the acetabulum. Laterally the capsule is attached to the intertrochanteric line anteriorly and to the neck of the femur posteriorly, 1 cm medial to the intertrochanteric crest. The capsule therefore covers the whole of the femoral neck in front and only part of the neck behind. Longitudinal bands of fibres pass from the capsule to the neck anteriorly and superiorly. These bands are called *retinacula* and contain blood vessels which supply the neck and head of the femur. The fibrous capsule is thicker anteriorly and superiorly. The deeper fibres are arranged in a circular manner round the neck (*zona orbicularis*).

The capsule is strengthened by three ligaments (figure 251). The *iliofemoral ligament* is attached superiorly to the anterior inferior iliac spine and passes downwards and laterally in front of the joint to divide into two limbs so that it is referred to as the *Y-shaped ligament of Bigelow* (H.J. Bigelow, 1818–90, American surgeon). The limbs are attached to the upper and lower parts of the intertrochanteric line. The *pubofemoral ligament* is attached superiorly to the iliopubic eminence and superior ramus of the pubis and inferiorly to the anterior and inferior aspects of the neck of the femur. The *ischiofemoral ligament* is attached to the posterior part of the acetabulum, winds upwards and forwards over the neck of the femur to become attached to the greater trochanter at the upper end of the intertrochanteric line.

The *transverse ligament* bridges the gap formed by the acetabular notch and may be regarded as a non-cartilaginous part of the acetabular labrum. The *ligament of the head of the femur* is attached within the joint to the pit of the femoral head and inferiorly to the edges of the acetabular notch and the transverse ligament. The ligament of the head is outside the synovial membrane which forms a sheath round it. Before the epiphysis of the head fuses with the neck the vessels in this ligament form an important source of blood to the head.

The Synovial Membrane (figure 251(c)). This lines the fibrous capsule. Laterally it is reflected on to the neck of the femur and extends as far as the edge of the articular cartilage of the head. The synovial membrane covers both edges of the labrum, surrounds the ligament of the head of the femur and covers the fat over the non-articular area of the acetabulum, that is these structures are intracapsular but extrasynovial. The bursa deep to the tendon of the psoas may communicate with the joint through an opening between the iliofemoral and pubofemoral ligaments.

The Main Relations (figure 252). Anteriorly the straight head of the rectus femoris, the iliacus, the psoas tendon and the pectineus are in front of the capsule from above downwards. The femoral nerve lies between the iliacus and psoas tendons and the femoral artery and vein on the psoas tendon and pectineus.

Posteriorly from above downwards the piriformis, the obturator internus and the quadratus femoris lie close to the capsule. The nerve to the quadratus femoris is deep to the obturator internus and therefore lies directly on the capsule and the sciatic nerve is separated from the capsule by the obturator internus.

Superiorly the reflected head of the rectus femoris and the gluteus minimus lie on the capsule and *inferiorly* the obturator externus winds posteriorly below the capsule and lies between the capsule and the quadratus femoris.

(a)

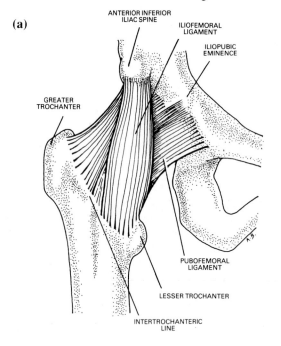

(b)

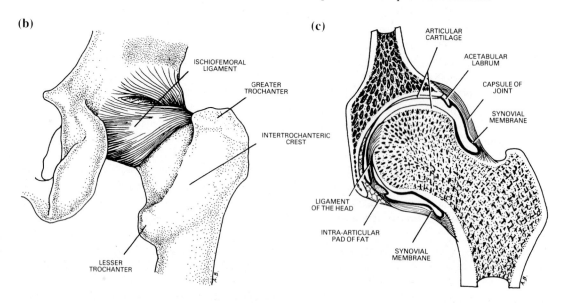

Figure 251   The ligaments of the hip joint: (a) iliofemoral and pubofemoral; (b) ischiofemoral; (c) a coronal section through the hip joint.

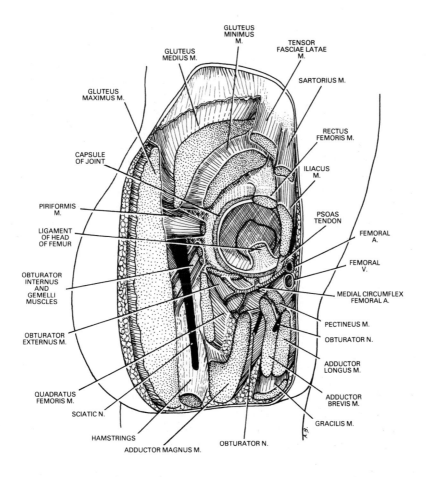

GLUTEUS
MINIMUS
M.

TENSOR
FASCIAE LATAE
M.

GLUTEUS
MEDIUS M.

SARTORIUS M.

GLUTEUS
MAXIMUS M.

RECTUS
FEMORIS M.

CAPSULE
OF JOINT

ILIACUS
M.

PIRIFORMIS
M.

PSOAS
TENDON

LIGAMENT
OF HEAD
OF FEMUR

FEMORAL
A.

FEMORAL
V.

OBTURATOR
INTERNUS
AND
GEMELLI
MUSCLES

MEDIAL CIRCUMFLEX
FEMORAL A.

OBTURATOR
EXTERNUS M.

PECTINEUS M.

OBTURATOR N.

ADDUCTOR
LONGUS M.

QUADRATUS
FEMORIS M.

ADDUCTOR
BREVIS M.

SCIATIC N.

GRACILIS M.

HAMSTRINGS

OBTURATOR N.

ADDUCTOR MAGNUS M.

Figure 252   The structures related to the hip joint as seen in a sagittal section.

The Blood and Nerve Supply. The *arteries* to the hip joint come from the gluteal, medial femoral circumflex and obturator arteries. The femoral and obturator *nerves* give branches to the joint but there are also twigs from the nerve to the quadratus femoris and superior gluteal nerve. Denervation of the joint is one means of treating a diseased hip joint causing pain on weightbearing and movement. It is necessary to divide all the nerves to the joint in order to produce a pain-free hip.

The Movements. Since the hip joint is of the ball and socket type, the basic movements are flexion and extension about a transverse axis, abduction and adduction about an anteroposterior axis, and lateral and medial rotation about a longitudinal axis. Movements, however, can take place about an infinite number of axes and flexion or extension is often combined with abduction, etc. The movements of flexion and extension may be regarded as a spin of the femoral head in the acetabulum and the other movements as a translation or sliding of the head so that the axis of movement changes as the head moves.

In the normal upright position *flexion* of the thigh at the hip joint, a forward movement in the sagittal plane, is possible through about 60°, if the knee is straight. With the knee bent so that the hamstrings are slack, further flexion of about 40° is possible. This is a very good example of passive insufficiency. Any additional flexion is only apparent and is due to flexion of the trunk, and by pulling on the bent leg, the front of the thigh can be brought against the front of the abdomen. The main flexors of the thigh at the hip are the iliacus and psoas. They can be assisted by the rectus femoris, pectineus and sartorius. The spinal nerves which are involved are mainly the second and third lumbar through the femoral nerve. Flexion of the trunk and pelvis involves flexion at the hip joints. In the upright position this is controlled by the extensor muscles of the trunk (erector spinae) and the extensors of the thigh at the hip, the hamstrings and the gluteus maximus. When lying supine the flexor muscles of the trunk and the psoas are the main muscles involved. Flexion controlled by the extensors also occurs in sitting down and going downstairs.

Extension of the thigh at the hip, a backward movement in the sagittal plane from the anatomical position, is limited to about 15°. Further apparent extension is due to extension at the vertebral column, especially in the lumbar region. The extensors are the hamstrings supplied by the sciatic nerve and the gluteus maximus supplied by the inferior gluteal nerve. The spinal cord segments involved are mainly the fifth lumbar and first and second sacral. Extension at the hips also includes restoration of the flexed pelvis and trunk to the upright position or straightening of the thigh as in standing up and going up stairs.

Abduction of the thigh at the hip, a movement away from the body in the coronal plane, is limited to about 40° due largely to tension of the adductors. The range of the movement is increased considerably if the thigh is also partially flexed at the hip. An apparent increase in abduction is produced by a lateral bending of the trunk to the opposite side. Abduction of the thigh, however, is not a movement commonly performed, except perhaps in a ballet, but it is curious that the 40° of slow abduction can be increased to about 70–80° if the lower limb is kicked outwards rapidly. The main abductors are the gluteus medius and minimus and tensor fasciae latae supplied by the superior gluteal nerve (L4, 5, S1).

Adduction in the anatomical position, a movement beyond the midline in the coronal plane, is impossible, but the flexed or extended limb can be adducted in front of or behind the opposite limb

for about 20–30°. The adductor muscles, longus, brevis and magnus, and gracilis, supplied by the obturator nerve (L2, 3, 4), produce the movement. Reference has already been made to the descent of the trunk at the hip which would occur when standing on one limb and is prevented by the gluteus medius of the supporting limb (p. 437).

Lateral rotation is a movement about a longitudinal axis through the head of the femur and intercondylar notch so that the anterior surface of the thigh faces laterally. The range of movement shows considerable variation, 40–80°, and the muscles producing the movement are piriformis, obturators internus and externus and quadratus femoris. The main spinal cord segments involved are L5 and S1. *Medial rotation* takes place about the same longitudinal axis so that the anterior surface of the thigh faces medially. There are about 40° of medial rotation and the movement is produced mainly by the gluteus minimus and tensor fasciae latae supplied by the superior gluteal nerve (L4, 5, S1).

When the range of movement at the hip joint is being estimated, it is important to determine that there is no movement of the pelvis or vertebral column. An apparent increase in flexion at the hip due to flexion in the lumbar region of the vertebral column has already been referred to. In a similar way a flexion deformity at the hip can be disguised by extension of the lumbar vertebrae. In each step in walking the extension at the hip is apparently increased by a rotation of the pelvis about a vertical axis equivalent to the medial rotation of the femur already described (figure 253).

Traumatic dislocation of the hip requires considerable violence in view of the depth of the acetabulum and the powerful ligaments which maintain its stability. Dislocation most commonly occurs in car accidents in which the lower end of the femur is struck with the thigh and leg flexed to about a right angle. The thigh is usually also medially rotated and slightly adducted. In this position the head of the femur is driven backwards through the capsule, on which it is partly resting, and frequently the posterior edge of the acetabulum is broken off.

Congenital dislocation of one or both hip joints is not uncommon and is associated with a shallow

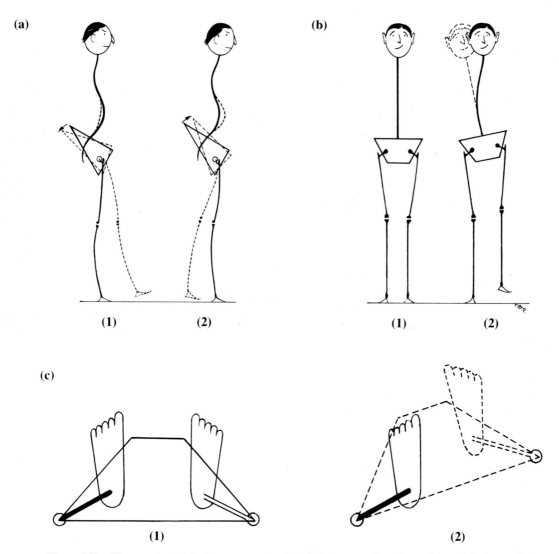

Figure 253 **The way in which the movements of the pelvis may affect the position of the lower limb:**
(a) (1) flexion at the lumbar vertebrae can produce apparent flexion at the hip joint, (2) extension at the
lumbar vertebrae can produce apparent extension at the hip joint; (b) (1 and 2) tilting of the pelvis through an
anteroposterior axis through one hip joint; (c) (1 and 2) rotation of the pelvis about a longitudinal axis through one
hip joint as seen from above (reproduced from *Hamilton's Textbook of Human Anatomy* **by courtesy of the Editors**
and The Macmillan Press).

acetabulum the edge of which is deficient superiorly. Usually the femoral head lies above the acetabulum with the result that a hollow can be felt distal to the middle of the inguinal ligament instead of the fullness produced by the normal position of the head. Early treatment by fixation of the head in the acetabulum with the femur abducted and laterally rotated (the opposite of

the position which is associated with traumatic dislocation) often produces a normal hip.

The head or neck of the femur is frequently involved in disease. *Slipped epiphysis* and *osteochondritis juvenalis* have already been referred to (p. 423). Tuberculosis of the head used to be common in children before the age of 5 years. *Osteoarthritis* in older and not so old people, a crippling

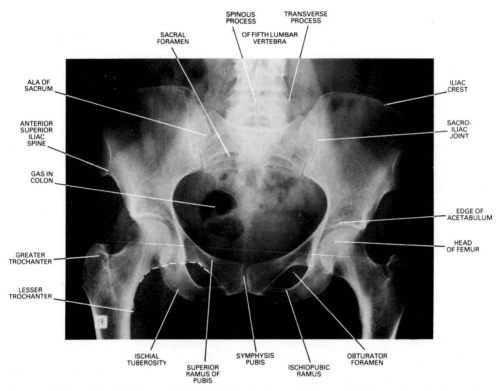

Figure 254   An X-ray of the hip joints. (The broken line is *Shenton's line* and is formed by the lower edges of the neck of the femur, the acetabulum and the superior ramus of the pubis. It is irregular in pathological conditions of the neck of the femur, for example a fracture.)

disease, is common. Replacement of the femoral head (and neck) with a prosthesis is frequently performed for this condition. Fracture of the femoral neck often results in necrosis of the head because it loses its blood supply and union does

not occur. In many of these conditions the gluteus medius of the affected side is unable to operate effectively. When the patient stands on one limb the unsupported side falls (*Trendelenberg's sign*; F. Trendelenberg, 1844–1924, German surgeon).

36

The Tibia, Fibula and Knee Joint

It is necessary to describe the tibia and fibula, especially their upper ends, in order to understand the structure and function of the knee joint. All the muscles which act at this joint have been described except three posterior muscles — the popliteus, gastrocnemius and plantaris.

The Popliteus (figures 250, 264). This muscle is attached by a tendon to a pit on the lateral side of the lateral condyle of the femur within the capsule of the knee joint and passes through the capsule obliquely downwards and medially to become attached to the upper part of the posterior surface of the tibia above the soleal line. As the tendon passes through the capsule it takes with it a prolongation of the synovial membrane. The deep surface of the upper lateral part of the muscle is attached to the posterior end of the lateral meniscus of the knee joint and the main part of the muscle is covered by an expansion of the tendon of the semimembranosus.

The popliteus is supplied by the tibial nerve (L4, 5, S1) by a branch which arises in the popliteal fossa, runs downwards superficial to the muscle and winds round its inferior border to enter its deep surface. The popliteus can flex the leg at the knee joint and rotate the tibia medially on the femur or rotate the femur laterally on the tibia. Because of its attachment to the lateral meniscus the popliteus may pull the posterior part of that structure backwards in flexion at the knee joint and prevent it from being crushed between the femoral and tibial condyles.

The Gastrocnemius (figures 250, 264). This is the superficial muscle of the back of the calf. Its upper attachment is by two heads, a lateral to a small pit on the lateral surface of the lateral condyle and a medial to a larger area on the posterior surface of the femur above the medial condyle. The two heads remain separate as far as the middle of the calf where they converge and form a common tendon with that of the soleus muscle, the tendo calcaneus (Achilles' tendon), which is attached to the middle of the posterior surface of the calcaneus. The soleus and the tendo calcaneus are considered in more detail on p. 467.

There is a bursa deep to the medial head of the gastrocnemius and often a sesamoid bone in the lateral head where it crosses the lateral femoral condyle. The gastrocnemius is supplied by branches of the tibial nerve (S1, 2). Together with the soleus, the gastrocnemius plantar flexes the foot at the ankle joint. A more important action of these muscles is seen in their moving the body on the foot as in standing on tiptoe or pulling the leg backwards on the foot when standing up or walking up stairs. Since the gastrocnemius arises from the femur it can flex the leg on the thigh at the knee joint. The two bellies of the gastrocnemius can be seen and felt in the upper part of the back of the calf in an individual standing on tiptoe.

The Plantaris. This muscle is the representative of a much larger muscle in animals. It has a short, narrow muscle belly of about 8 cm, and a long tendon about 30 cm in length. The muscular part is attached to the back of the femur above the lateral condyle and the tendon passes downwards obliquely between the gastrocnemius and soleus to fuse with the medial border of the tendo calcaneus. The plantaris is supplied by the tibial nerve (S1, 2) and makes a contribution to the action of the gastrocnemius at the knee joint and the tendo calcaneus at the ankle joint. The muscle may rupture at the junction of the muscle and tendon and this condition has to be considered as a possible cause of pain at the back of the knee.

The Tibia (figure 255)

The tibia is the medial bone of the leg. It articulates with the femur at the knee joint and transmits the weight of the body to the foot. The fibula does not articulate with the femur and is a much more slender bone than the tibia.

The *shaft* of the tibia is triangular in section and has a subcutaneous *anterior border* and *medial surface*. The *lateral surface* has muscles attached to it as has the *posterior surface*. The *interosseous border* separates the lateral from the posterior surface and extends upwards on to the lateral aspect of the upper end of the tibia. Inferiorly the border divides into two ridges.

The anterior border leads upwards to the *tibial tuberosity* on the front of the upper end of the bone and inferiorly, where the border is much less distinct, to the front of the *medial malleolus*. The *medial border* inferiorly passes behind the malleolus. At the upper limit of the lateral surface there is a facet for the head of the fibula. The *soleal line* passes downwards and medially on the posterior surface from the back of this facet. A vertical line extends downwards on the middle of the posterior surface and passes laterally to join the interosseous border. Medial to the vertical line and inferior to the soleal line there is a large opening for the *nutrient foramen* which is directed downwards. This opening is at the junction of the upper and middle thirds of the shaft. A fracture in the region of the junction of the middle and lower thirds often takes a long time to unite because of its poor blood supply.

The *upper end* of the tibia is expanded as compared with the shaft and curves backwards so that it overhangs the posterior surface of the shaft. It consists of two *condyles*, the upper surfaces of which are separated by an intercondylar area with an *intercondylar eminence* projecting upwards from its middle. The eminence consists of *lateral* and *medial tubercles*. Each *lateral* and *medial condyle* has a superior articular surface for the lateral and medial condyles of the femur respectively. The articular area on the lateral condyle is shorter, broader and more circular than that of the medial condyle. There is a shallow groove on the medial and posterior aspects of the medial condyle. The *tibial tuberosity* is a prominence in front of and below the two condyles. Its lower part is rough and its upper part is smooth, indicating that a ligament (patellar ligament) is attached to the lower part and a bursa separates the ligament from the upper part.

The lower end of the tibia is much smaller than the upper end, but since the shaft narrows as it passes downwards the lower end is relatively expanded compared with the adjacent part of the shaft. The medial side of the lower end continues downwards as the *medial malleolus*, the inner surface of which articulates with the medial side of the talus. This articular area is continuous with an articular area on the distal surface of the lower end of the tibia. This latter articular area is convex from side to side and concave from front to back, and fits the reciprocally curved superior articular surface of the talus. On the posterior surface of the distal end there is a groove passing downwards and medially for the tendon of the tibialis posterior. The *fibular notch* bounded by the divided lower end of the interosseous border is on the lateral surface.

The tibia *ossifies* in cartilage from a primary centre for the shaft which appears at about the seventh week of intra-uterine life, and from two secondary centres, one for the upper end, which usually appears just before birth, (figure 259(c), (d)) and one for the lower end, which appears during the first year of life. The upper epiphysis usually includes the tuberosity, which may, however, ossify from a separate centre. This is of some importance in that the tubercle is liable to be affected by the disease involving ossifying bones

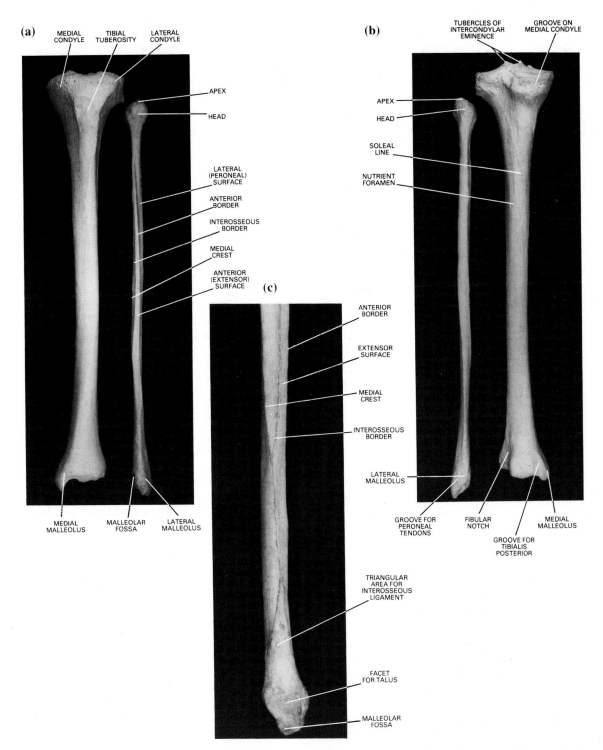

Figure 255   The left tibia and fibula: (a) anterior aspect; (b) posterior aspect; (c) the medial aspect of the lower half of the fibula.

(osteochondritis juvenalis), already referred to in relation to the head of the femur. The distal end fuses with the shaft at about 18 years and the proximal end at about 20 years. The tibia is weight-bearing and its upper and lower ends have vertical and horizontal trabeculae of bone arranged similarly to those in the lower end of the femur.

The Fibula (figure 255)

The fibula is the slender lateral bone of the leg and articulates superiorly with the tibia and inferiorly with the tibia and talus to form part of the ankle joint. The side to which a fibula belongs is most easily determined by distinguishing the lower end from the upper by the presence of a fossa on its medial surface. The fossa is inferior, medial and posterior. By placing the fibula in one's own leg with the fossa in the correct position one can determine whether the bone is from the right or left leg.

The *shaft* has three *surfaces, lateral, anterior* and *medial*, separated by three borders. The *anterior border* is found by following upwards the apex of the triangular area on the outer surface of the lower end. This border separates the lateral from the anterior surface. The *interosseous border* is determined by finding the rough triangular area above the articular area on the medial side of the lower end and following the apex upwards into a line which divides into two (figure 255(c)). The anterior of these lines is the interosseous border. The posterior line is the *medial crest* which separates two of the deep muscles in the back of the calf. The lower part of the shaft is apparently twisted so that the lateral surface is posterior in the lower third of the shaft and the posterior surface is medial.

The *proximal end* of the fibula, called the *head*, is irregularly cuboidal in shape and its upper surface, which is oblique, articulates with the inferior surface of the lateral tibial condyle. Posteriorly the head projects upwards to form the *apex (styloid process)* of the fibula. The narrow region between the head and shaft is often referred to as the *neck*.

The *distal end* of the fibula is called the *lateral malleolus* and has a subcutaneous lateral surface.

The tip of the lateral malleolus extends about 1 cm beyond the tip of the medial and this relationship is used to determine the possibility of displacement in fractures in this region. There is a vertical groove on the posterior surface of the lateral malleolus. The anterior part of the medial surface articulates with the lateral side of the talus. The smaller posterior part is hollowed out to form the *malleolar (digital) fossa*.

The fibula *ossifies* in cartilage from a primary centre for the shaft which appears about the seventh week of intra-uterine life. The proximal epiphysis begins to ossify at about 5 years (figure 259(c), (d)) and the distal at about 2 years. This is unusual in that the growing end of a long bone (the end which grows more and fuses later) begins to ossify before the other end. Even in animals in which the fibula is only a proximal sliver of bone, as in a horse, or completely absent, as in an ox, or weight-bearing, as in marsupials, this pattern of ossification is seen. The distal end fuses with the shaft at about 18 years and the proximal end at about 20 years.

The Knee Joint (figures 256–259)

The knee joint includes the joints between the patella and femur (*patellofemoral*) and between the condyles of the tibia and femur (*tibiofemoral*). The arrangement of the synovial membrane suggests that the human knee joint developed from three joints (patellofemoral and two tibiofemoral) but this has been questioned. The knee joint is a condylar synovial joint. The articular areas on the condyles of the femur are marked off from the patellar area by two faint grooves. The medial, condylar, articular area extends further forwards than that of the lateral so that it is more oval than the articular area on the lateral condyle. The articular areas of the femoral condyles are convex from front to back and also transversely, but the anteroposterior curve is much more marked posteriorly so that the outline of the curve is spiral.

The articular areas on the tibial condyles are comparatively flat, the medial being more oval anteroposteriorly than the lateral which is more round. The two menisci attached to the peripheral borders of the upper surface of the condyles of the tibia, because of their shape, deepen the socket presented by the tibia for the femur. The menisci are wedge-shaped, with the base of the wedge on the peripheral border.

The patellar articular surface of the femur is concave from side to side and convex antero-posteriorly. It extends further forwards on the lateral condyle than on the medial. It also extends backwards on to the front of the lateral edge of the articular area of the medial condyle. The articular surface of the patella is divided by a vertical ridge into a larger lateral and smaller medial area corresponding with the patellar areas on the condyles of the femur. A medial vertical strip may also be marked off corresponding with the articular area on the anterior part of the lateral edge of the medial condyle.

The Fibrous Capsule and Ligaments
(figures 256, 257)

Superiorly the fibrous capsule is attached posteriorly, laterally and medially to the femoral condyles and inferiorly to the tibial condyles just beyond their articular edges. On the lateral side the capsule covers the femoral attachment of the popliteus tendon which emerges from the capsule posteriorly and laterally. Anteriorly the capsule is replaced from above downwards by the quadriceps femoris tendon, patella and patellar ligament. Lateral and medial to these structures fibrous expansions of the vastus lateralis and vastus medialis fuse with the lateral and medial parts of the capsule respectively. These are called the *lateral* and *medial patellar retinacula*. In addition to the ligaments about to be described, the capsule is strengthened posteriorly by fibres from the tendons of the lateral and medial heads of the gastrocnemius, laterally from the iliotibial tract, and medially from the semimembranosus. The deep surface of the capsule is attached to the lateral surfaces of the menisci.

The Fibular and Tibial Collateral Ligaments.
The *fibular collateral ligament* is a rounded cord separate from the capsule and attached superiorly to

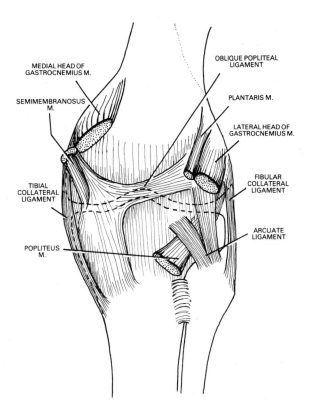

Figure 256   The posterior ligaments of the knee joint.

the lateral epicondyle of the femur above the attachment of the popliteus. Inferiorly it is attached to the head of the fibula where it is enclosed by a splitting of the tendon of the biceps femoris. The *tibial collateral ligament* is broad and flat and is attached superiorly to the medial epicondyle of the femur and inferiorly to the medial tibial condyle and the adjacent part of the medial surface of the shaft. Posteriorly the ligament blends with the underlying capsule.

The Oblique and Arcuate Popliteal Ligaments.
The *oblique ligament* is posterior and passes upwards and laterally from the back of the medial tibial condyle to the back of the lateral femoral condyle. It is regarded as an expansion of the semimembranosus tendon. The *arcuate popliteal ligament* is posterior and lateral and extends from the lateral epicondyle of the femur to the head of the fibula. Its medial part arches downwards on to the posterior part of the intercondylar area of the tibia.

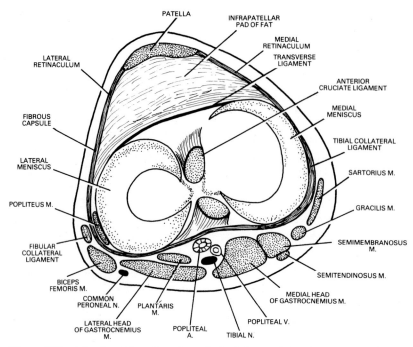

Figure 257   A horizontal section through the left knee joint above the menisci.

The Cruciate Ligaments (figures 257, 258). These ligaments lie within the capsule but outside the synovial membrane. Their names refer to their attachments to the tibia and the fact that they cross. The *anterior cruciate ligament* is attached to the intercondylar area of the upper surface of the tibia between the anterior ends of the two menisci. It passes backwards, laterally and slightly upwards and is attached to the medial surface of the lateral condyle of the femur. The *posterior cruciate ligament* is attached behind the posterior ends of the menisci to the posterior end of the intercondylar area. It passes forwards, medially and slightly upwards and is attached to the lateral surface of the medial condyle of the femur.

The Synovial Membrane and Bursae (figure 258)

The arrangement of the synovial membrane is complicated but is more easily understood if it is remembered that the joint was probably three joints (p. 450), that all so-called intra-articular structures are intracapsular and outside the synovial membrane and that, as in all synovial joints,

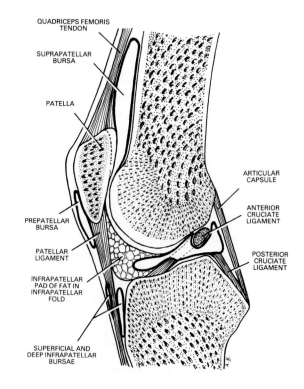

Figure 258   A sagittal section through the knee joint.

the synovial membrane ends at the edge of the articular cartilage. The synovial membrane lines the lateral and medial parts of the capsule. Posteriorly the membrane passes forwards from the capsule to pass round the cruciate ligaments which would appear to be invaginated into the capsule from behind. There may be a pocket of membrane passing between the ligaments from the lateral side. Laterally and medially the menisci project into the synovial membrane but the membrane does not cover the surfaces of the menisci and is continuous with the surface layer of the menisci.

Anteriorly above the patella the synovial membrane extends from the upper border of the patella deep to the quadriceps extensor tendon for about 5–7 cm, and turns backwards and then downwards on the anterior surface of the femur as far as the articular cartilage on the condyles. From the lateral and medial borders of the patella the synovial membrane passes backwards as two *alar folds* which come together as the *infrapatellar fold* which is attached to the anterior edge of the intercondylar notch. This may be regarded as the remains of the partition separating the patellofemoral joint from the tibiofemoral joints. The alar folds also extend downwards on to the anterior part of the upper surface of the tibia as the remains of the anterior part of the vertical partition between the two tibiofemoral joints. The space between the layers of these folds contains fat (the *infrapatellar pad of fat*).

There is a large number of bursae related to the knee joint. The following are important.

(1) The *suprapatellar bursa* lies above the patella, extends for about 5–7 cm above its upper border and communicates with the joint. If there is excess fluid in the knee joint the fluid in this bursa can be pushed down so that the patella floats away from the femur.

(2) The *prepatellar bursa* lies in front of the patella and is subcutaneous.

(3) The *superficial* and *deep infrapatellar bursae* are superficial and deep to the patellar ligament respectively.

Not uncommonly the prepatellar and superficial infrapatellar bursae become enlarged due to an excessive collection of fluid. The enlargements were called *housemaid's* and *parson's knee* respectively for doubtful connections with these occupations.

(4) The bursa deep to the medial head of the gastrocnemius usually communicates with the cavity of the joint. If this bursa is enlarged there is produced in full extension of the knee a sausage-shaped swelling extending laterally and upwards deep to the oblique popliteal ligament.

(5) The *popliteal bursa* is an extension of the synovial membrane round the popliteus tendon as it emerges from the capsule.

There may be a bursa between tendons, for example between the tendons of the semimembranosus and semitendinosus, or between a tendon and a ligament, for example between the fibular collateral ligament and the tendon of the biceps femoris, or between a tendon and the capsule, for example between the medial head of the gastrocnemius and the capsule.

The Intracapsular Structures

Some of these have been described – the cruciate ligaments and the tendon of the popliteus. In addition the *lateral* and *medial menisci (semilunar cartilages)* are crescentic pieces of fibrocartilage attached to the periphery of the articular surfaces of the lateral and medial tibial condyles by the adjacent deep parts of the capsule called the *coronary ligaments*. Both menisci have a deep peripheral border and a narrow inner edge and their upper femoral surface is concave and the inferior tibial surface is flat. The lateral meniscus is more rounded than the medial and its anterior and posterior ends lie within the ends of the medial which is more crescentic. The anterior cruciate ligament is attached between the anterior ends of the menisci and the posterior cruciate ligament behind their posterior ends. The medial meniscus is attached to the deep surface of the capsule and tibial collateral ligament. Posteriorly the lateral meniscus is separated from the fibular collateral ligament by the tendon of the popliteus which is attached to the meniscus. The posterior end of the lateral meniscus is attached to the lateral side of the medial epicondyle by ligaments which pass behind and in front of the posterior cruciate ligament.

The menisci are frequently injured and are the torn cartilages of famous sportsmen, especially footballers and cricketers. The medial meniscus is torn three times more often than the lateral. The injury to the meniscus is usually produced by a rotation of the slightly flexed femur on the fixed tibia so that the meniscus is crushed between the femoral and tibial condyles. The immediate effect is a swelling, due to haemorrhage and an effusion of fluid, and a locking of the knee due to the torn meniscus becoming wedged between the condyles. Although recovery takes place, in so far as the knee becomes mobile and the fluid is absorbed, repair of the cartilage is unlikely. Subsequently the torn piece of the meniscus may become wedged between the condyles with locking of the knee. Surgical removal of the meniscus is the common and successful treatment.

The Movements at the Knee Joint

Because of the medial rotation of the lower limb during embryonic development so that the big toe is medial, *flexion* is a backward movement of the leg on the thigh and *extension* is the restoration of the flexed leg to the neutral position. Flexion is associated with an initial rotation and extension with a terminal rotation about a longitudinal axis. If the leg is bent to a right angle it can be actively rotated medially and laterally on the femur. In all movements the menisci move with the tibia on the femur, although at the extremes of extension the anterior horns of the menisci are pushed forwards on the tibia.

From the neutral position with the foot off the ground the leg can be flexed, that is moved backwards on the femur until the back of the calf is in contact with the back of the thigh. At the beginning of flexion the tibia *rotates medially* on the femur and then slides backwards on the femoral condyles and becomes flexed because of the shape of the condyles. These are much more curved posteriorly than anteriorly so that flexion of the leg is more marked in the later part of the movement. The initial medial rotation of the tibia is due to the popliteus muscle (supplied by the tibial nerve, L4, 5, S1) and possibly the medial hamstrings, and is associated with the greater antero-posterior length of the medial femoral condyle as compared with that of the lateral. The popliteus also pulls the posterior end of the lateral meniscus backwards. The patella moves downwards on the patellar surface of the femur and tilts so that the upper part of the articular surface of the patella is in contact with the femur. In extreme flexion the medial edge of the patella is in contact with the medial condyle of the femur. The main flexors are the hamstring muscles (the semimembranosus, semitendinosus and biceps femoris) which are supplied by the sciatic nerve (L4, 5, S1, 2). The sartorius, gracilis and popliteus may assist in this movement and the gastrocnemius is involved in a resisted flexion movement at the knee joint. Due to the direction of their fibres, the fibular collateral and posterior part of the tibial collateral ligaments are slackened and the posterior cruciate ligament is taut in flexion.

From the position of full flexion, the leg can be extended on the thigh until the leg and thigh are in a straight line. The term *hyperextension* is often used for extension beyond this position, but 5–10° beyond a straight line can be regarded as normal. The tibia with the menisci slides forwards and becomes extended on the femur until the anterior edge of the articular area of the lateral femoral condyle is reached. The articular area of the medial condyle extends further forwards than that of the lateral and the terminal part of extension is accompanied by a lateral rotation of the tibia until the anterior edge of the medial condyle is reached. In full extension the anterior ends of the menisci are pushed forwards and a position is reached in which there is maximum contact between the femoral and tibial condyles. This is called the *close-packed position of maximum congruence*. This terminal screwing of the tibia on the femur in which the ligaments become taut, especially the anterior cruciate, fibular and tibial collateral and posterior ligaments, is referred to as *locking of the knee*. During this movement the patella is pulled upwards on the femur by the quadriceps femoris, which is the muscle extending the leg on the thigh and is supplied by the femoral nerve (L2, 3, 4).

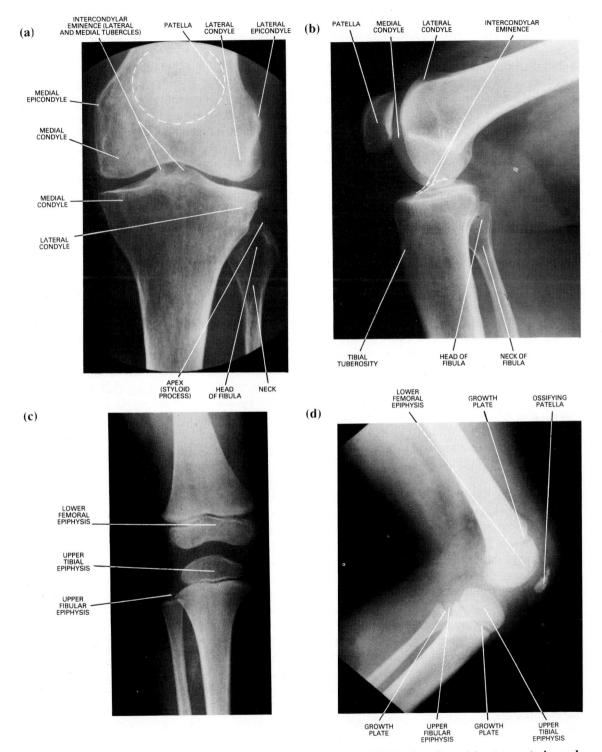

Figure 259   X-rays of the knee joint: (a) anteroposterior, (b) lateral with the knee bent, (c) anteroposterior and (d) lateral of a child aged about 4 years.

Because the pull of the quadriceps femoris is oblique the patella tends to be dislocated laterally. This is prevented by the greater forward projection of the lateral condyle as compared with that of the medial. In addition the muscle fibres of the vastus medialis extend more distally than those of the vastus lateralis and its lowest fibres are almost horizontal, so that in contraction of the quadriceps femoris the patella is pulled medially by the vastus medialis.

With the foot fixed on the ground the thigh can be flexed and extended on the leg. From the anatomical position, flexion of the thigh begins with some lateral rotation of the femur on the tibia probably due to the popliteus. As the femur slides on the tibia it also flexes due to the curvature of the femoral condyles. Flexion is more marked after the initiation of the movement. It should be emphasised that in most activities involving flexion of the thigh on the leg, the thigh is also flexed at the hip, and if the foot is fixed on the ground the leg is dorsiflexed on the foot. For example when sitting down or squatting these three movements (flexion at the hip, flexion at the knee and dorsiflexion at the ankle) take place at the same time, so that the tibia and femur are moving simultaneously on each other. When one limb is swinging during walking, flexion at the hip and knee takes place together. The final position of the thigh on the leg if the thigh is flexing at the knee is the same as that described in flexion of the leg on the thigh. When sitting down or squatting, the flexion at the knee is due to gravity and is controlled by the quadriceps femoris. The flexion which occurs when the foot is off the ground, together with flexion at the hip, as in walking, may be due to a passive swing or actively brought about by the hamstrings.

Extension of the thigh on the leg from the flexed position, as in standing up from the sitting or squatting position, is due to the quadriceps femoris. The femur slides backwards on the tibia and extends until the anterior end of the articular area on the lateral femoral condyle is reached. The femur now rotates medially about a longitudinal axis until the anterior end of the articular area of the medial femoral condyle meets the anterior part of the medial meniscus and the close-packed position is reached. This is the same as the final

position of extension of the leg on the thigh.

When the leg is flexed to a right angle on the thigh, the leg can be *rotated laterally* and *medially* for about 20° in each direction. This is due to a slackening of the fibular and tibial collateral ligaments. Lateral rotation is due to the biceps femoris and medial rotation to the semimembranosus, semitendinosus and popliteus. *Position one in ballet*, in which the feet are turned outwards through 180° (90° for each foot), is largely due to lateral rotation at the hip joints. It is difficult to attain the 180° so desired by the ballet dancer, but if the knees are bent, an additional 20° of lateral rotation at each knee can be added to the rotation at the hips. The limbs are then straightened at the knees and an apparent 180° are reached. When doing this, one is very conscious of the inner border of the foot being pressed against the floor to prevent the leg being rotated medially at the knee.

Active *abduction* and *adduction* and *backward* and *forward sliding* of the leg on the thigh are impossible. With the leg bent to a right angle at the knee a small amount of passive sliding is possible. The knee joint, in spite of the shallow socket provided by the flat tibial condyles for the curved femoral condyles, is remarkably stable because of its ligaments and muscles. (The menisci deepen to only a slight extent the tibial articular surfaces.) In a clinical examination of the knees all possible movements are investigated. The range of flexion and extension is measured. If the cruciate ligaments are torn passive gliding of the tibia on the femur is greatly increased — backward if the anterior ligament is torn and forward if it is the posterior which has ruptured. A torn tibial collateral ligament allows passive abduction of the leg on the thigh and a torn fibular collateral ligament allows passive adduction. Rotatory movements are also increased.

It is often stated that the stability of the knee joint depends only on a properly functioning quadriceps femoris. This is true in so far as in many activities the weight of the body falls behind the transverse axis of the knee joint or joints (sitting down, standing up, walking up or down a slope or stairs). A weak quadriceps femoris results in the knee giving way, in many situations. It should be emphasised that equally the ligaments make the knee joint stable. For example, a torn tibial collateral ligament results in an unstable knee unless the tear is repaired.

The Surface Anatomy of the Region of the Knee

Anteriorly the patella *with the tendon of the* quadriceps femoris *above and the* patellar ligament *below can be seen and felt, especially if the muscle is contracted so that the patella is pulled upwards. This movement also confirms that the muscle fibres of the* vastus medialis *extend almost to the patella as compared with those of the* vastus lateralis *which end 5 cm more proximally. The* characteristic hollows *at the sides of the patella and its ligament are lost if there is fluid in the knee joint.*

Laterally the head *of the* fibula, *situated more posteriorly than is expected, can be felt and also the* tendon *of the* biceps femoris *above it, especially if made more prominent by flexing the leg against resistance. Immediately in front of this tendon the lower end of the* iliotibial tract *can usually be seen and invariably palpated as it passes to the upper end of the tibia. The* common peroneal nerve *winding round the upper end of the fibula, 4 cm below its apex, is subcutaneous and can be rolled under one's finger.*

On the medial side posteriorly the bowed out tendon *of the* semitendinosus *superficial to the* tendon *of the* semimembranosus *can be seen and felt, especially if the leg is flexed at the knee. The* tendon *of the* gracilis *may be palpated more medially. If the fingers are pushed inwards towards the femur posterior to the lower end of the vastus medialis and anterior to these tendons, the* tendon *of the* adductor magnus *is felt as it passes to the* adductor tubercle.

Posteriorly the hollow of the popliteal fossa *is bounded above by the diverging hamstring muscles and below by the converging heads of the* gastrocnemius muscle. *Standing on the toes makes the two bellies of this muscle visible. With the knee bent the pulsations of the* popliteal artery *can be felt.*

With the leg at a right angle to the thigh the line *of the* knee joint *below the bulging* femoral condyles *and above the* tibial condyles *can be felt. This is important because the site of tenderness along this line helps to indicate which structure may be injured. Tenderness at the sides of the patellar ligament indicates that the infrapatellar folds have been nipped. More posteriorly, on either side, damaged cartilages are more likely to produce tenderness and further back torn ligaments are usually the cause.*

37

The Leg and Foot

The Skeleton of the Foot (figure 260)

The bones of the foot are the tarsal and metatarsal bones and the phalanges. The seven tarsal bones are comparable with the carpal bones but are much larger and their arrangement is different. The *talus* is the only bone to articulate with the tibia and fibula at the ankle joint (*talus = ankle*, Latin). It lies on the calcaneus and projects forwards on the medial side to articulate with the *navicular bone*. The *calcaneus* projects backwards and forms the prominence of the heel (*calx = heel*, Latin). Anteriorly it projects on the lateral side to articulate with the *cuboid bone*. The navicular articulates with the three *cuneiform bones* – *medial, intermediate* and *lateral*. Each cuneiform articulates with a *metatarsal bone* and the cuboid articulates with the two lateral metatarsals. The big toe has two *phalanges* and each of the remaining four toes has three.

The Talus. This is the second largest of the tarsal bones and has six surfaces. Most of the *superior trochlear surface* articulates with the distal surface of the tibia. This articular area is convex from front to back and concave from side to side and is wider anteriorly (figure 260(a)). In front of the articular area the talus narrows to form the *neck* and then widens to form the *head*, which is directed medially as well as forwards. The *inferior surface* has a large posterior concave articular facet and a smaller anterior flatter facet. Both articulate with the upper surface of the calcaneus (figure 272).

These facets are separated by a deep groove, the *sulcus tali*. The facets and sulcus are directed forwards and laterally. The anterior facet is often divided by a ridge and is continuous distally with the articular area of the head.

The *lateral surface* of the talus has a triangular articular area for the lateral malleolus and the lateral end of the sulcus tali lies in front of this area. On the *medial surface* of the talus there is a much smaller articular area for the medial malleolus. *Posteriorly*, behind the trochlear surface, the posterior process consists of *lateral* and *medial tubercles* which are separated by a groove. The lateral tubercle may form a separate bone, the *os trigonum*. *Anteriorly* the head has a convex, articular area for the navicular. This area is continuous with the anterior articular area for the calcaneus on the inferior surface of the head. Medially between these two facets a triangular articular area can be distinguished.

The Calcaneus. This is the largest of the tarsal bones and can be regarded as having six surfaces. The *superior (dorsal) surface* has about its middle a large convex articular area for the posterior concave area of the talus (figure 272). Anteriorly this area is separated by the *sulcus calcanei* from an articular area for the inferior part of the head of the talus. Frequently this anterior area is divided into two, the posterior of which is on the *sustentaculum tali*, a projection of bone overhanging the medial surface of the calcaneus. The *sinus tarsi* is formed by the sulcus tali and the sulcus calcanei

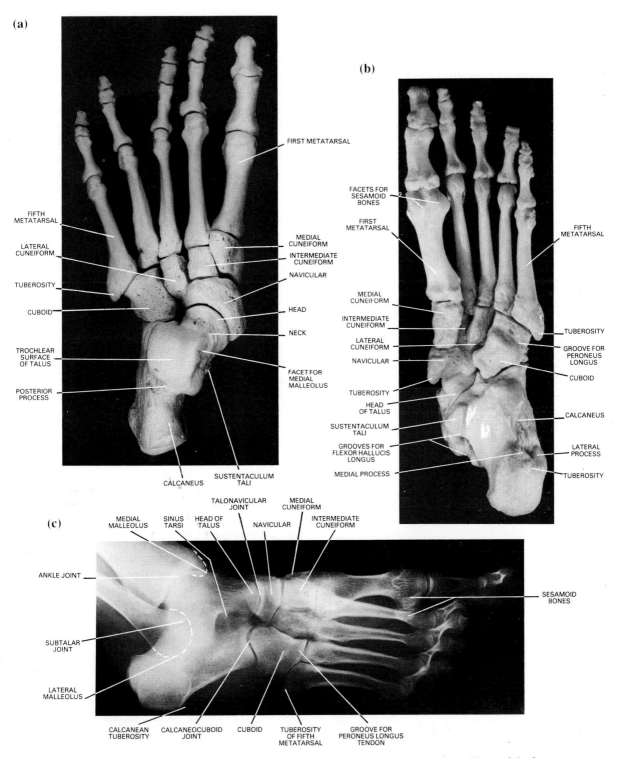

(a)

FIRST METATARSAL

FIFTH
METATARSAL

LATERAL
CUNEIFORM

TUBEROSITY

CUBOID

TROCHLEAR
SURFACE
OF TALUS

POSTERIOR
PROCESS

MEDIAL
CUNEIFORM

INTERMEDIATE
CUNEIFORM

NAVICULAR

HEAD

NECK

FACET FOR
MEDIAL
MALLEOLUS

CALCANEUS

SUSTENTACULUM
TALI

(b)

FACETS FOR
SESAMOID
BONES

FIRST
METATARSAL

MEDIAL
CUNEIFORM

INTERMEDIATE
CUNEIFORM

LATERAL
CUNEIFORM

NAVICULAR

TUBEROSITY

HEAD
OF TALUS

SUSTENTACULUM
TALI

GROOVES FOR
FLEXOR HALLUCIS
LONGUS

MEDIAL PROCESS

FIFTH
METATARSAL

TUBEROSITY

GROOVE FOR
PERONEUS
LONGUS

CUBOID

CALCANEUS

LATERAL
PROCESS

TUBEROSITY

(c)

MEDIAL
MALLEOLUS

SINUS
TARSI

HEAD OF
TALUS

TALONAVICULAR
JOINT

NAVICULAR

MEDIAL
CUNEIFORM

INTERMEDIATE
CUNEIFORM

ANKLE JOINT

SUBTALAR
JOINT

LATERAL
MALLEOLUS

SESAMOID
BONES

CALCANEAN
TUBEROSITY

CALCANEOCUBOID
JOINT

CUBOID

TUBEROSITY
OF FIFTH
METATARSAL

GROOVE FOR
PERONEUS LONGUS
TENDON

Figure 260   The bones of the foot: (a) dorsal view; (b) plantar view; (c) an oblique X-ray of the foot.

when the two bones articulate with each other. Behind the posterior articular area the upper surface of the calcaneus projects backwards behind the talus.

The *calcanean tuberosity*, divided by a groove into medial and lateral processes, is on the posterior part of the *inferior surface* (figure 260(b)). The inferior surface of the sustentaculum tali is deeply grooved. The posterior surface of the calcaneus has a transverse ridge which indicates the attachment of the tendo calcaneus. This ridge often has spicules of bone projecting upwards. The area above the ridge is smooth and the area below merges with the most posterior part of the inferior surface.

The *anterior surface* has a concavoconvex articular area for the posterior surface of the cuboid. The *lateral surface* has the *peroneal trochlea*, a small projection of bone about 2 cm inferior to the tip of the lateral malleolus. The main feature of the medial surface is the sustentaculum tali, which is about 2 cm inferior to the tip of the medial malleolus.

The Remaining Tarsal Bones. The boat-shaped *navicular bone* has on its proximal surface a concave articular area for the head of the talus. On its distal surface there are two vertical ridges producing three facets for the cuneiform bones. Medially the navicular projects downwards as a *tuberosity* which is palpable 2.5 cm in front of the sustentaculum tali. There may be a facet on the lateral surface for articulation with the cuboid.

The *cuboid bone* articulates proximally with the anterior end of the calcaneus and distally has two articular areas, a lateral which is triangular with a lateral apex for the base of the fifth metatarsal, and a medial which is rectangular for the base of the fourth metatarsal. The plantar surface has a *peroneal groove* which is directed medially and slightly forwards. Medially the cuboid articulates with the lateral cuneiform bone and sometimes with the navicular.

The three *cuneiform bones*, as their name suggests, are wedge-shaped. On the *medial cuneiform* the edge of the wedge is dorsal and on the *intermediate* and *lateral* the edge is plantar. Proximally the three cuneiforms articulate with the distal surface of the navicular. Distally the *medial cunei-*

form articulates with the base of the first metatarsal bone by a large kidney-shaped facet. Laterally the medial cuneiform articulates with the intermediate cuneiform and also the side of the base of the second metatarsal. The *intermediate cuneiform* articulates proximally with the middle facet on the distal surface of the navicular and distally with the base of the second metatarsal bone. The intermediate cuneiform is the smallest of the cuneiform bones. Proximally it is level with the other two but distally it is recessed between them, with the base of the second metatarsal in the recess. The lateral and medial surfaces of the intermediate cuneiform have articular and ligamentous areas for the lateral and medial cuneiforms respectively. The *lateral cuneiform* articulates proximally with the navicular, distally with the third metatarsal, laterally with the cuboid and medially with the intermediate cuneiform and lateral side of the base of the second metatarsal.

The Metatarsal Bones. Each of the five metatarsal bones has a proximal *base*, a distal *head* and an intervening *shaft*. The proximal surface of the base articulates with the tarsus (cuboid and cuneiforms) at the tarsometatarsal joints. The base in section is larger than the shaft which tapers as it passes distally and the head is larger in section than the shaft. The shaft of the lateral four metatarsals is curved with a dorsal convexity. The adjacent surfaces of the bases of the second, third, fourth and fifth metatarsal bones articulate with each other at the intermetatarsal joints. The bases of the second, third and fourth metatarsal bones are wedge-shaped with the base of the wedge on the dorsal surface and the base of the second metatarsal also articulates on its lateral and medial sides with the medial and lateral cuneiform bones. The articular area on the head for the base of the proximal phalanx extends further on to the plantar surface than on to the dorsal surface.

The *first metatarsal bone* is markedly different from the others, being shorter and much thicker, and its base as a rule does not articulate with the base of the second metatarsal. Its inferior and lateral surfaces are flat. The articular area on the plantar surface of the head has a median longitudinal ridge marking off an area on each side for articulation with a sesamoid bone.

The base of the fifth metatarsal is flattened in a dorsiplantar direction and laterally projects as the *tuberosity* (*styloid process*) of the fifth metatarsal.

The Phalanges. The *proximal phalanges* have a *base* with a proximal concave facet for the head of a metatarsal bone, a *shaft* which is compressed from side to side and a head which has a distal articular surface with two condyles. The *middle phalanges* of the lateral four toes are shorter and somewhat broader than the proximal and have a *base*, *shaft* and *head*. The articular area on the base has two concave areas for the condyles of the head of the proximal phalanx and the head has two small condyles. The *distal phalanges* are small and flattened. Distally they expand and have a prominence on the plantar aspect (the *tuberosity*). Occasionally the middle and distal phalanges of the little toe are fused.

The Ossification of the Bones of the Foot. The *tarsal bones* ossify in cartilage, each bone having a single centre. The *calcaneus* and *talus* begin to ossify during the third month of intra-uterine life and the *cuboid* just before birth. The *lateral cuneiform* ossifies in the first year after birth, the *medial cuneiform* in the second year and the *intermediate cuneiform* and *navicular* in the third year. The calcaneus usually has on its posterior surface a scale-like epiphysis which begins to ossify at about 7 years and fuses with the main part of the calcaneus at about 15 years. The lateral tubercle on the back of the talus may have its own centre of ossification and remain a separate bone (the *os trigonum*).

The *metatarsal bones* ossify in cartilage and have a primary centre for the shaft which appears about the eighth week of intra-uterine life. The lateral four metatarsals have a secondary centre for the head and the first a secondary centre for the base. These secondary centres begin to ossify about the third year and fuse with the shaft at about 18 years. There may also be a secondary centre for the head of the first metatarsal.

The *phalanges* ossify from a primary centre for the shaft which appears at about the 10th to 15th weeks of intra-uterine life, the distal phalanges ossifying before the proximal which ossify before the middle. The phalanges have an epiphysis for the base which ossifies between the second and eighth years and fuses with the shaft at about 18 years.

The Surface Features of the Leg and Foot

The bony prominences and tendons in the region of the knee joint are described on p. 457. The tibial tuberosity *at the proximal end of the front of the tibia can be easily felt. The* tibial anterior border *and* medial surface *are subcutaneous and can be followed downwards from the tuberosity to the* medial malleolus *which is also subcutaneous. Anterior to the medial malleolus the* great saphenous vein *is visible as it passes upwards on the medial side of the leg and behind the medial condyles of the tibia and femur.*

Only the upper and lower ends of the fibula, that is the head *and the* lateral malleolus, *are palpable. The intervening part of the bone is covered by muscles. The* small saphenous vein *lies behind the lateral malleolus and continues upwards towards the back of the knee.*

The individual bones of the tarsus are not distinguishable except for the head of the talus *in front of the malleoli, but the* sustentaculum tali *can be felt about 2 cm inferior to the medial malleolus. The* peroneal trochlea *on the lateral surface of the calcaneus is about 2.5 cm distal to the lateral malleolus. The* tuberosity of the navicular *is palpable on the medial border of the foot about 2.5 cm distal to the sustentaculum tali. The* tuberosity (styloid process) of the base of the fifth metatarsal *forms a prominence about halfway along the lateral border. On the dorsum of the foot the subcutaneous* plexus of veins *and sometimes some of the* subcutaneous nerves *to the digits can be seen. The* intermetatarsal spaces *between the shafts are palpable. The big toe is usually the longest, although a foot in which the second toe is longer than the first is not uncommon and is referred to as the* classical foot *because the sculptors of the ancient Greeks invariably carved a foot showing this characteristic.*

The Skin of the Leg and Foot (figure 275)

The skin of the lateral and adjacent anterior and posterior aspects of the leg are supplied by the *sural nerve* (L5, S1, 2) which is a branch of the tibial nerve. It is joined by the *communicating sural nerve* (L4, 5, S1) from the common peroneal nerve. The *lateral cutaneous nerve of the calf* (L4, 5, S1) from the common peroneal nerve is distributed to the upper lateral part of the leg. On the medial and adjacent anterior and posterior aspects of the leg the skin is supplied by the *saphenous nerve*, the continuation of the femoral nerve (L3, 4). The *posterior femoral cutaneous nerve* (S1, 2, 3) extends downwards to the middle of the calf.

The dorsum of the foot and the sides of the toes are supplied by the *superficial peroneal nerve* (L4, 5, S1) except for the adjacent sides of the big and second toes which are supplied by the *deep peroneal nerve* (L5, S1, 2). The *medial plantar nerve* (L4, 5) supplies the medial part of the skin of the sole and the medial three and a half toes. The *lateral plantar nerve* (S1, 2) supplies the lateral side of the sole and the lateral one and a half toes. These plantar nerves are the terminal branches of the tibial nerve.

The *dermatomes* are arranged as follows (figure 275). The fourth lumbar nerve supplies the skin of the medial side of the leg and foot as far as the ball of the big toe. The fifth lumbar nerve supplies the skin of the remainder of the big toe, the medial part of the dorsum of the foot and the lateral side of the leg. The first sacral nerve supplies the skin of the lateral side of the foot and the back of the heel.

The skin of the leg shows no special features. There is considerable variation in the thickness of the skin over different parts of the sole. The skin of weight-bearing areas, especially under the back of the heel and the heads of the metatarsal bones, is thick and the skin of the lateral side of the sole is thinner than that of the non-weight-bearing medial side. There are flexure lines on the sole and also papillary ridges on the plantar surface of the toes.

The Anterior and Lateral Regions of the Leg and the Dorsum of the Foot

A study of a transverse section through the middle of the leg is the best way to appreciate the arrangement of the structures in the different compartments formed by the bones and the septa of the deep fascia. A layer of *deep fascia* surrounds the structures and is continuous with the periosteum of the anteromedial surface of the tibia. The interosseous borders of the tibia and fibula are joined by an interosseous membrane. Septa pass inwards to the anterior and posterior borders of the fibula with the formation of *anterior (extensor)* and *lateral (peroneal)* compartments. The posterior region is separated into superficial and deep compartments by a transverse layer of fascia attached to the medial margin and the medial crest of the fibula. The proximal attachments of most of the muscles and their nerve supply are also indicated in the section.

The superficial and deep fasciae

The *superficial fascia* contains the cutaneous nerves referred to above — the sural and sural communicating nerves and lateral cutaneous nerve of the calf on the lateral side, the saphenous nerve on the medial side and the terminal branches of the posterior femoral cutaneous nerve on the upper part of the back of the calf. On the medial side of the leg the great saphenous vein and on the lateral side, the small saphenous vein pass upwards towards the knee.

The *deep fascia* of the leg, as already described, consists of an investing layer, intermuscular septa to the anterior and posterior borders of the fibula, and a transverse layer in the back of the leg. It is attached superiorly to the patella, patellar ligament, the head of the fibula and the condyles of the tibia, in the leg itself to the subcutaneous surface of the tibia, and inferiorly to the malleoli. In the region of the ankle on the dorsum and sides of the foot the fascia forms *retinacula* (retaining bands) for the tendons (p. 470).

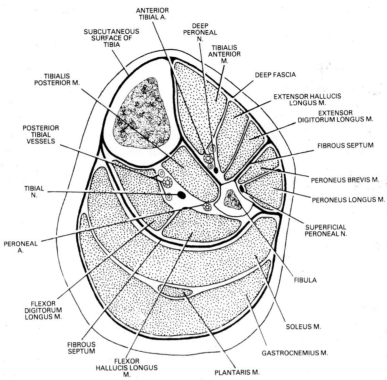

Figure 261 **A cross-section through the middle of the leg to show the arrangement of the fascia, muscles, arteries and nerves.**

The anterior (extensor) region (figure 262)

The structures in this compartment of fascia comprise the extensor digitorum longus, peroneus tertius, extensor hallucis longus and tibialis anterior muscles, the deep peroneal nerve and the anterior tibial vessels.

The Extensor Digitorum Longus, Peroneus Tertius and Extensor Hallucis Longus. These three muscles are attached to the fibula between its anterior and interosseous borders and to adjacent fascial structures such as the interosseous membrane, the intermuscular septum and the deep fascia of the leg. The extensor hallucis longus is medial and the peroneus tertius inferior to the extensor digitorum longus. All three muscles pass downwards deep to the extensor retinacula into the dorsum of the foot. The *extensor digitorum longus* divides into four tendons which go to the lateral four toes. Each tendon forms part of a dorsal digital expan-

sion to which contributions are made from the extensor digitorum brevis (except the little toe) and the lumbrical and interossei muscles. The expansion divides into three slips the middle of which is attached to the dorsal surface of the base of the middle phalanx and the outer two to the corresponding surface of the distal phalanx.

The *peroneus tertius* is regarded as a muscle split off from the extensor digitorum longus. It is attached to the dorsal surface of the base and shaft of the fifth metatarsal bone. The *extensor hallucis longus* ends in a tendon which is attached to the dorsal surface of the distal phalanx of the big toe.

All three muscles are supplied by the deep peroneal nerve (L5, S1). The long extensors extend the toes and dorsiflex the foot at the ankle. The peroneus tertius assists in dorsiflexing and everting the foot (turning the foot so that the sole faces outwards and upwards). This muscle is not always present. The development of an additional evertor in man is associated with the plantigrade position of the human foot in standing and walking.

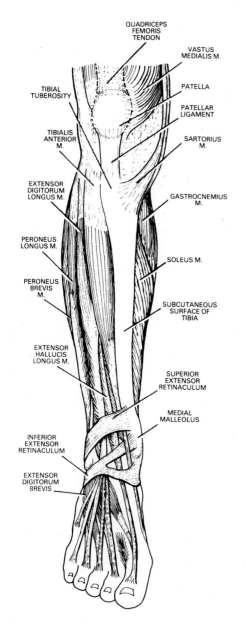

Figure 262   The anterior muscles of the leg and foot.

The Tibialis Anterior. This muscle is attached to the lateral surface of the tibia and adjacent part of the interosseous membrane. The muscle descends and forms a tendon which runs deep to the extensor retinacula and is attached to the medial side of the medial cuneiform and base of the first metatarsal. It is supplied by the deep peroneal nerve (L4, 5). Its actions are dorsiflexion and inversion

of the foot and maintenance of the medial longitudinal arch.

The tendons of all these muscles can be seen on the dorsum of the foot if the foot and toes are dorsiflexed (turned upwards). The most medial tendon going to the medial border of the foot is that of the tibialis anterior. *The tendon of the* extensor hallucis longus *is especially marked as it passes over the metatarsophalangeal joint of the big toe. The four tendons of the* extensor digitorum longus *are also easily identified.*

The Extensor Digitorum Brevis. This muscle is attached proximally to the anterosuperior surface of the calcaneus in front of the lateral malleolus. The muscle passes distally as four tendons which are attached to the medial four toes. The most medial tendon, which crosses the dorsalis pedis artery, is usually called the *extensor hallucis brevis*, which is attached to the dorsal surface of the base of the proximal phalanx of the big toe. The other three tendons are attached to the lateral side of the corresponding long extensor tendon of the second, third and fourth toes. The muscle, supplied by the deep peroneal nerve (S1, 2), dorsiflexes the toes. *On contraction the circular muscle belly can be seen in front of the lateral malleolus on the lateral side of the dorsum of the foot.* The extensor digitorum brevis is the only muscle of the digits of the hand and foot which gives off a tendon to the first digit (the big toe). This is taken to indicate the greater functional importance of the medial side of the foot.

The Anterior Tibial Vessels. The *anterior tibial artery* is one of the two terminal divisions of the popliteal artery. It begins posteriorly at the lower border of the popliteus, passes forwards through an opening on the upper part of the interosseous membrane and runs downwards on the membrane between the extensor hallucis longus, which is lateral, and the tibialis anterior, which is medial. The deep peroneal nerve is lateral to the artery. In the lower part of the leg the artery lies in front of the tibia and ankle joint, passes deep to the retinacula and is crossed from the lateral to the medial side by the tendon of the extensor hallucis longus. *The artery lies midway between the malleoli, where it can be felt pulsating lateral to the tendon of the extensor hallucis longus.* It continues on the dorsum of the foot as the *dorsalis pedis artery* which passes distally to the first intermetatarsal space. At the proximal end of the space the artery passes into the sole of the foot. In the dorsum of the foot the dorsalis pedis artery is superficial and lies medial to the extensor digitorum longus and lateral to the extensor hallucis longus. *The pulsation of the* anterior tibial *and* dorsalis pedis arteries *can be felt, the former midway between the malleoli and the latter as it passes through the proximal end of the first intermetatarsal space.* Checking the presence of pulsations in these arteries is a routine procedure in patients with diabetes mellitus and in old people. In both cases the peripheral arteries undergo degenerative changes.

The anterior tibial artery gives off branches to the anastomotic network round the knee joint, to the muscles, and to the anastomoses round the lateral and medial malleoli.

The dorsalis pedis artery gives off branches to the lateral and medial sides of the foot. Before passing to the plantar aspect of the foot the dorsalis pedis gives off the *arcuate artery*, which passes laterally over the bases of the metatarsal bones to the lateral border of the foot. The arcuate artery gives off three *metatarsal branches* which run forwards and divide to supply the sides of the lateral four digits. The sides of the first digital cleft and medial side of the big toe are supplied by a separate branch of the dorsalis pedis artery. The metatarsal arteries give off communicating branches to corresponding arteries in the sole of the foot.

The *anterior tibial veins* begin as upward continuations of veins associated with the dorsalis pedis artery. They pass backwards through the upper part of the interosseous membrane and join the posterior tibial veins to form the popliteal vein.

The Deep Peroneal (Anterior Tibial) Nerve (figure 263). This is one of the two terminal branches of the common peroneal nerve which divides in the peroneus longus muscle. The deep peroneal nerve passes anteriorly deep to the extensor digitorum longus to the front of the interosseous membrane and then downwards lateral to the anterior tibial artery between the extensor hallucis longus and

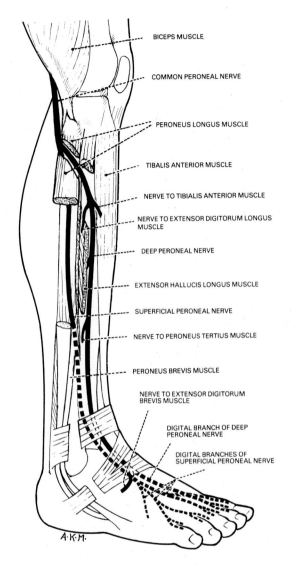

Figure 263   The distribution of the common peroneal nerve (reproduced from *Hamilton's Textbook of Human Anatomy* by courtesy of the Editors and The Macmillan Press).

tibialis anterior muscles. It supplies the extensor digitorum longus, peroneus tertius, extensor hallucis longus and tibialis anterior. At the level of the ankle joint the nerve divides into lateral and medial branches. The lateral supplies the extensor digitorum brevis and the joints of the lateral side of the foot. The medial branch is also articular but in addition supplies the skin of the adjacent sides of the first digital cleft.

The lateral (peroneal) region (figure 263)

This compartment of the leg is bounded by inter-muscular septa passing inwards to the anterior and posterior borders of the fibula. Superiorly the compartment is lateral, but due to what is often described as a lateral twist of the lower end of the fibula, the muscles inferiorly lie behind the lateral malleolus.

The Peroneus Longus and Brevis. The *longus* is attached to the head and the upper two-thirds of the lateral surface of the fibula and the neighbouring fascia. The *brevis* is attached to the lower two-thirds of the lateral surface of the fibula anterior to the longus. Both muscles form long tendons which run in a groove behind the lateral malleolus, where they are retained by a retinaculum. The tendons pass on to the lateral side of the calcaneus. The peroneus longus tendon lies below the peroneal trochlea (tubercle) and enters the sole of the foot to lie in a tunnel formed by the groove on the inferior surface of the cuboid and the long plantar ligament. The tendon passes obliquely forwards and medially and is attached to the lateral side of the medial cuneiform and base of the first metatarsal. The tendon of the peroneus brevis passes forwards above the peroneal trochlea, where both tendons are kept in position by a retinaculum, and is attached to the tubercle of the fifth metatarsal bone.

Both muscles are supplied by the superficial peroneal nerve (L5, S1, 2). They evert the foot and *can be identified as they pass above and below the peroneal trochlea if the foot is everted (turned outwards).* They are not important muscles in the movements of dorsiflexion and plantar flexion. The brevis, by pulling the lateral border of the foot upwards, may assist in maintaining the lateral longitudinal arch. The longus, since it passes below the lateral longitudinal arch, may act as a sling and support the arch. By pulling the lateral and medial ends of the transverse arch together the peroneus longus helps to maintain this arch. When standing on one lower limb, for example the right, the body sways from side to side. The peronei are active in this situation when the body is falling to the left.

The Superficial Peroneal Nerve (figure 263). The common peroneal nerve, as it lies in the peroneus longus, divides into the superficial and deep peroneal nerves. The superficial nerve runs downwards deep to the peroneus longus and then between that muscle and the extensor digitorum longus. The nerve supplies the two peronei muscles and becomes superficial in the distal third of the leg. It divides into a medial branch which supplies the skin on the medial side of the big toe and the adjacent sides of the second and third toes, and a lateral branch which supplies the skin on the adjacent sides of the third and fourth and fourth and fifth toes.

Lesions of the Common Peroneal Nerve. Because this nerve is subcutaneous as it winds round the fibula about 3–4 cm distal to the apex, it may be directly damaged by injury or involved in a fracture of this part of the fibula or pressed on by a badly applied external splint. If completely severed the movements of dorsiflexion of the foot and of the toes and eversion of the foot are lost. As a result the foot falls downwards if the leg is raised from the ground (the condition is called *foot-drop*). This is a considerable disability during walking since the toe is scraped along the ground unless the lower limb is markedly flexed at the hip and knee in the swing phase in each step. This increase in flexion at these joints produces a characteristic gait. The sensory loss due to the interruption of the common peroneal nerve is limited to the skin of the middle of the dorsum of the foot and a small part of the dorsal aspect of the digits.

The Posterior Region of the Leg (figure 264)

In this part of the leg, there is a group of superficial muscles, the gastrocnemius, soleus and plantaris, and a group of deep muscles, the flexor hallucis longus, flexor digitorum longus and tibialis posterior which, with the main vessels and nerve, pass downwards towards the medial malleolus before entering the sole of the foot.

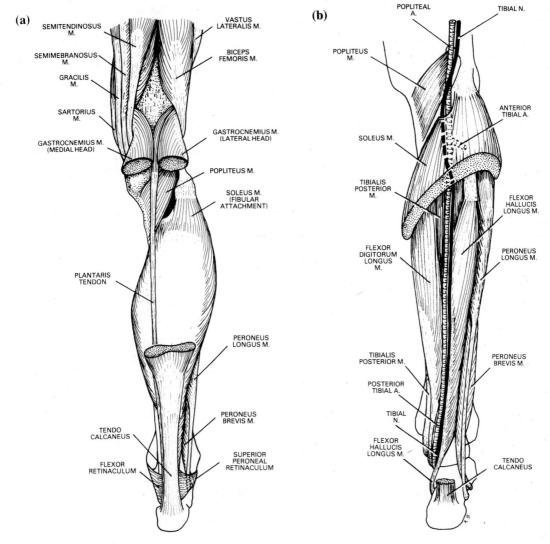

Figure 264   The posterior muscles of the leg: (a) superficial; (b) deep.

The superficial muscles

The Gastrocnemius. The upper attachment of this muscle by two heads to the lateral and medial femoral condyles is described on p. 477. The muscle fibres of the two heads are attached to the anterior surface of a broad tendon which narrows and joins the tendon of the soleus to form the *tendo calcaneus (Achillis).*

The Soleus. This muscle is deep to the gastrocnemius. It is attached superiorly to the upper quarter of the posterior surface of the fibula, to the soleal line on the back of the tibia, to the middle part of the medial border of the tibia and to a fibrous arch between the tibia and fibula over the popliteal vessels and tibial nerve where they pass downwards from the popliteal fossa into the leg. The muscle fibres are attached to the deep surface of its tendon which joins that of the gastrocnemius to form the tendo calcaneus. The adjacent surfaces of the soleus and gastrocnemius are aponeurotic. This may facilitate their sliding on each other when one muscle contracts independently of the other. The muscle fibres of the soleus extend much more distally than those of the gastrocnemius and bulge on each side of the upper part of the tendon of the gastrocnemius.

The Plantaris. The upper attachment of this muscle to the back of the femur above the lateral condyle is described on p. 447. The muscular part is about 8 cm long and ends in a long tendon which passes downwards and medially between the gastrocnemius and soleus to be attached to the medial side of the tendo calcaneus.

The Tendo Calcaneus. This tendon is about 15 cm long and is formed by the union of the tendons of the gastrocnemius, soleus and plantaris. It is attached to the middle of the posterior surface of the calcaneus and is separated from the upper half of this surface by a bursa.

The Nerve Supply and Actions of the Superficial Muscles. The three muscles are supplied by the tibial nerve (S1, 2). The branches leave the nerve in the lower part of the popliteal fossa between the two heads of the gastrocnemius.

The three muscles plantar flex the foot at the ankle. The gastrocnemius can also flex the leg on the thigh. These powerful muscles are involved in pulling the leg backwards on the fixed foot as in walking up stairs or standing up. By their controlled relaxation they are important in sitting down and walking down stairs. They are usually described as giving the body a thrust before the supporting limb leaves the ground at the end of the stance phase in walking. They certainly do this in running and jumping. In walking, however, it has been suggested that the calf muscles control the falling forwards of the body rather than propel it forwards.

The gastrocnemius can be used to demonstrate *active muscular insufficiency* which is due to the attachments of a muscle being so approximated that its contraction cannot produce any movement. If one lies on one's back with the thigh flexed at the hip and the leg flexed at the knee, the gastrocnemius remains slack in strong plantar flexion of the foot. This is most easily tested when lying on one's back in a bath.

When standing in the upright position (p. 489) the calf muscles are continuously but variably contracted because the body is falling forwards at the ankle joints.

The deep muscles and related structures (figures 264(b), 265)

Between the superficial and deep muscles there is a sheet of fascia attached to the medial crest of the fibula and the medial margin of the tibia. It is continuous superiorly with the fascia over the popliteus.

The Flexor Hallucis Longus. Proximally this muscle is attached to the posterior surface of the fibula between the peroneus longus and tibialis posterior muscles. It passes distally and ends in a long tendon which lies on the back of the lower end of the tibia, and then in the groove on the back of the talus. It passes deep to the flexor retinaculum, then below the sustentaculum tali and enters the sole of the foot deep to the superficial (first layer of) muscles. In the sole its tendon is crossed superficially by the tendon of the flexor digitorum longus, to which it may be attached, and runs forwards to become attached to the plantar surface of the base of the distal phalanx. As it approaches the phalanx the tendon lies in a groove between the two sesamoid bones in the two parts of the tendon of the flexor hallucis brevis.

The flexor hallucis longus is supplied by the tibial nerve (S2, 3) in the back of the calf. The muscle flexes the big toe at the interphalangeal and metacarpophalangeal joints and may assist in plantar flexion of the foot and the maintenance of the medial longitudinal arch. It has been suggested that it is an important muscle in controlling the forward movement of the body on the distal phalanx of the big toe at the terminal stage of the stance phase just before what is described as the toe-off stage of a step (p. 491).

The Flexor Digitorum Longus. This muscle is attached to the medial half of the posterior surface of the tibia below the level of the soleal line. Distally its tendon crosses superficial to the tendon of

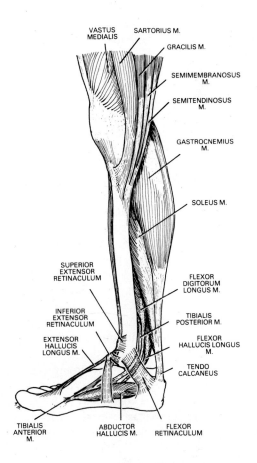

VASTUS MEDIALIS
SARTORIUS M.
GRACILIS M.
SEMIMEMBRANOSUS M.
SEMITENDINOSUS M.
GASTROCNEMIUS M.
SOLEUS M.
SUPERIOR EXTENSOR RETINACULUM
FLEXOR DIGITORUM LONGUS M.
INFERIOR EXTENSOR RETINACULUM
TIBIALIS POSTERIOR M.
EXTENSOR HALLUCIS LONGUS M.
FLEXOR HALLUCIS LONGUS M.
TENDO CALCANEUS
TIBIALIS ANTERIOR M.
ABDUCTOR HALLUCIS M.
FLEXOR RETINACULUM

Figure 265   The medial side of the leg and foot.

the tibialis posterior to reach its lateral side and lies medial to the tendon of the flexor hallucis longus as the three tendons wind round the medial malleolus deep to the flexor retinaculum. They enter the sole of the foot deep to the first layer of muscles. In the sole the tendon crosses superficial to the tendon of the flexor hallucis longus to which it is frequently attached (figure 267(b)). The tendon then divides into four to go to the lateral four toes. Each digital tendon passes through the digital tendon of the flexor digitorum brevis and is attached to the plantar surface of the distal phalanx.

The flexor digitorum longus is supplied by the tibial nerve (S2, 3). Its action is to flex the phalanges of the lateral four toes, a movement which may be important in gripping the ground in the late stance phase when walking on unshod feet.

In the sole the flexor accessorius is attached to the lateral border of the flexor digitorum longus and the lumbrical muscles are attached to the tendons. These muscles are described on p. 474 in chapter 38.

The Tibialis Posterior. Its proximal attachment is to the lateral half of the posterior surface of the tibia, the posterior surface of the fibula and the interosseous membrane between the two bones. It is overlapped by the flexor hallucis longus laterally and the flexor digitorum longus medially. Its tendon passes downwards and after being crossed superficially by the tendon of the flexor digitorum longus lies in a groove on the back of the tibia and then behind the medial malleolus deep to the flexor retinaculum. The tendon is medial to the deltoid (medial) ligament of the ankle joint before entering the sole. Its main attachment is to the tuberosity of the navicular but it sends slips to all the cuneiform bones, the bases of the middle three metatarsals and the cuboid (figure 267). There is also a tendinous slip passing backwards to the sustentaculum tali of the calcaneus.

The tibialis posterior is supplied by the tibial nerve (L4, 5). It is an invertor of the foot and may be involved in plantar flexion. It is also regarded as a support of the medial longitudinal arch. When standing on one lower limb, for example the right, the right tibialis posterior, together with the tibialis anterior, prevents the body falling laterally as it sways to the right.

The Posterior Tibial Vessels. The posterior tibial artery is a terminal branch of the popliteal artery which divides at the lower border of the popliteus. The artery continues downwards deep to the arch formed by the soleus and lies on the tibialis posterior with the flexor digitorum longus medially and the flexor hallucis longus laterally. The artery is at first deep to the soleus and the fascia between it and the deep muscles of the calf. Lower down, the artery is more superficial as it lies medial to the tendo calcaneus. It passes deep to the flexor retinaculum and abductor hallucis where it divides into its terminal branches, the *lateral* and *medial plantar arteries*. The tibial nerve crosses from the medial to the lateral side of the artery. *The artery can be felt pulsating midway between the medial malleolus and the prominence of the heel.*

The posterior tibial artery gives off muscular branches and a branch which winds round the neck of the fibula and takes part in the anastomoses round the knee joint. The *peroneal artery* is a large branch which arises near the upper end of the fibula and passes downwards on that bone towards the ankle, where it takes part in the anastomoses on the lateral side of the ankle. The peroneal artery supplies the muscles on the posterior and lateral side of the leg and gives off the nutrient artery to the fibula. The posterior tibial artery gives off the nutrient artery to the tibia and branches to the ankle anastomoses.

There are usually two *posterior tibial veins* which are formed by the union of the lateral and medial plantar veins. The veins receive communicating veins from the superficial veins of the leg and the calf muscles especially the soleus. The posterior tibial veins join the anterior tibial veins to form the popliteal vein.

The Tibial Nerve. The sciatic nerve divides into the tibial and common peroneal nerves about the middle of the back of the thigh. The tibial nerve (L4, 5, S1, 2, 3) continues downwards through the popliteal fossa and accompanies the posterior tibial artery at first on its medial side and lower down on its lateral side. The nerve has the same relations as the artery and divides deep to the abductor hallucis into the *lateral* and *medial plantar nerves*.

The branches of the tibial nerve in the popliteal fossa are described on p. 440. In the back of the leg the nerve supplies the tibialis posterior and the long flexor muscles.

In the upper part of the leg the tibial nerve gives off a cutaneous branch, the *sural nerve*, which becomes superficial about the middle of the calf where it is joined by the communicating sural branch of the common peroneal nerve. The sural nerve (L5, S1, 2) continues downwards lateral to the tendo calcaneus, below the lateral malleolus and along the lateral border of the foot. It supplies the skin on the lateral and posterior surfaces of the lower third of the leg and the lateral side of the foot. The tibial nerve also gives off medial calcaneal branches which supply the skin on the back and medial side of the heel.

The Retinacula and Synovial Sheaths of the Ankle (figure 266)

Several references have been made to thickenings of fascia lying over the tendons of the muscles of the leg as they pass into the foot. There are two *peroneal retinacula*. The *superior* is attached proximally to the back of the lateral malleolus and distally to the calcaneus posteriorly and holds the peroneal tendons in position behind the lateral malleolus. The *inferior* is attached to the side of the calcaneus where the peroneal tendons pass above and below the peroneal trochlea, and is continuous with the inferior extensor retinaculum. A continuous synovial sheath surrounds each of the peroneal tendons as they pass deep to the retinacula.

The *flexor retinaculum* is attached to the medial malleolus and passes backwards and downwards into the sole over the tendons of the tibialis anterior and flexor digitorum longus, the posterior tibial vessels, the tibial nerve and the tendon of the flexor hallucis longus which are arranged in that order from the medial to the lateral side. In the sole the retinaculum is continuous with the posterior part of the plantar aponeurosis and is attached to the medial part of the calcaneal tubercle. Each of the tendons deep to the retinaculum is enclosed in a synovial sheath, extending from above the medial malleolus to approximately the navicular bone.

The *superior extensor retinaculum* is attached to the anterior borders of the tibia and fibula and lies in front of the tendons of the tibialis anterior, long extensor muscles and peroneus tertius as they pass in front of the ankle into the dorsum of the foot. The anterior tibial vessels and deep peroneal nerve also pass deep to the retinaculum.

The *inferior extensor retinaculum* has a lateral attachment to the superior surface of the calcaneus. As it passes medially it divides into two limbs. The upper is attached to the medial malleolus and the lower passes into the sole to become attached to the plantar aponeurosis. The lateral part of the retinaculum forms a loop round the peroneus tertius and extensor digitorum longus, both of which are enclosed in a single synovial sheath as they lie in the loop. The upper limb of the retinaculum forms a loop round the extensor hallucis

(a)

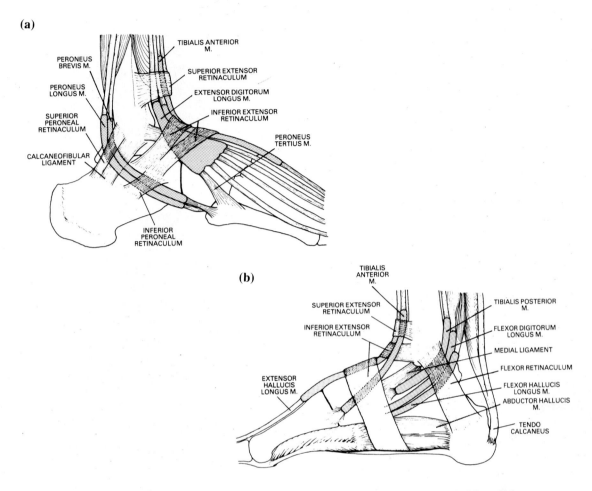

(b)

Figure 266 **The retinacula and synovial sheaths of the ankle: (a) lateral; (b) medial.**

longus but not round the tibialis anterior. The lower limb passes anterior to the two tendons, the dorsalis pedis artery and the deep peroneal nerve. The synovial sheath round the extensor hallucis longus extends from the inferior retinaculum to the base of the first metatarsal bone and that of the tibialis anterior lies deep to the superior retinaculum and the upper limb of the inferior.

The synovial sheaths allow the tendons to glide deep to the retinacula when the muscles contract. The retinacula prevent the tendons from bowing outwards under the skin. This improves the action of the muscles. Subjects who can dorsiflex the big toe at the metatarsophalangeal joint to about 90° demonstrate this bowing to a marked extent because there is no retinaculum over the tendon in

this part of its course. The retinacula were regarded by Paley as evidence of the divine construction of the human body. ('The effect of the ligament as a bandage can be made evident to the senses; for if it be cut, the tendon starts up. The simplicity, yet the cleverness of this contrivance, its exact resemblance to established resources of art, place it amongst the most indubitable manifestations of design with which we are acquainted.' From *Natural Theology; or Evidences of the Existence and Attributes of The Deity. Collected from the Appearances of Nature by William Paley, DD. Illustrated by a Series of Plates and Explanatory Notes by James Paxton, MRCS*, Vol. 1, 3rd edn, Oxford Univeristy Press, London, 1836.)

38

The Sole of the Foot

The innervation and gross structural features of the skin of the sole are described on p. 462. The general arrangement of the structures in the sole is similar to that in the palm. Some of the differences between the hand and foot have already been mentioned, particularly the large tarsal bones, the non-prehensile big toe and the shortness of the remaining toes. The arched form of the foot is a special feature.

The Plantar Aponeurosis

The central part of the aponeurosis is particularly strong and is attached proximally to the calcanean tuberosity. Distally it divides near the heads of the metatarsal bones into five slips which are attached superficially to the skin in the groove between the anterior part of the sole and the toes. The deeper part of each slip passes into the toes where it fuses with the fibrous sheath of the flexor tendons. The digital vessels and nerves enter the toes between the slips. The outer parts of the aponeurosis are much thinner and extend laterally and medially deep to the abductor digiti minimi and abductor hallucis respectively. Lateral and medial septa, passing deeply, separate the muscles of the sole into lateral, intermediate and medial groups.

In a manner similar to the palmar aponeurosis, the plantar aponeurosis is attached to the overlying skin by fibrous septa so that the skin does not slide on the aponeurosis. The plantar aponeurosis holds the anterior and posterior bases of the longitudinal arches together.

The Four Layers of the Muscles of the Sole (figure 267)

The muscles of the sole can be conveniently separated into four layers with the vessels and nerves lying between the first and second layers and the third and fourth layers.

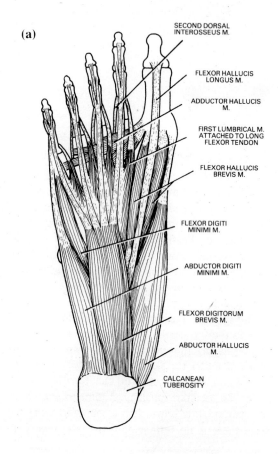

(a)

SECOND DORSAL INTEROSSEUS M.

FLEXOR HALLUCIS LONGUS M.

ADDUCTOR HALLUCIS M.

FIRST LUMBRICAL M. ATTACHED TO LONG FLEXOR TENDON

FLEXOR HALLUCIS BREVIS M.

FLEXOR DIGITI MINIMI M.

ABDUCTOR DIGITI MINIMI M.

FLEXOR DIGITORUM BREVIS M.

ABDUCTOR HALLUCIS M.

CALCANEAN TUBEROSITY

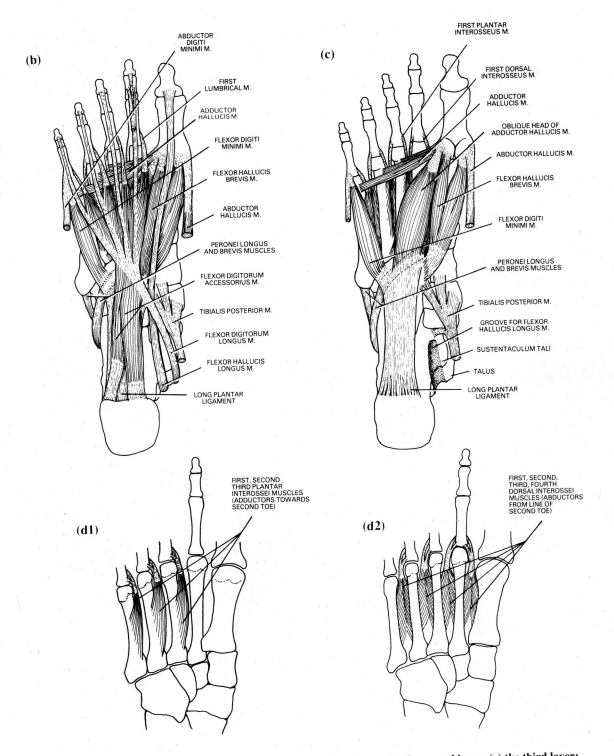

Figure 267 **The muscles of the sole of the foot: (a) the first layer; (b) the second layer; (c) the third layer; (d) the fourth layer.**

The first layer of muscles (figure 267(a))

This comprises three muscles, the lateral *abductor digiti minimi*, the medial *abductor hallucis* and the middle *flexor digitorum brevis*. All have a proximal attachment to the calcanean tuberosity and the deep surface of the plantar aponeurosis. Distally the abductor digiti minimi is attached to the lateral side of the base of the proximal phalanx of the little toe and the abductor hallucis to the medial side of the base of the proximal phalanx of the big toe. The flexor digitorum brevis divides into four tendons which go to the lateral four toes. Each tendon divides at the proximal phalanx into two slips, the inner parts of which cross deep to the tendon of the long flexor. The long flexor tendon passes forwards between the two slips and lies on the crossed part as it goes to the base of the distal phalanx. The short flexor tendon divides into two and is attached to the sides of the middle phalanx. The two tendons to each toe are enclosed in a fibro-osseous canal within which they are almost surrounded by a synovial sheath in a manner similar to the two tendons of the digits of the hand (p. 375).

The *lateral* and *medial plantar arteries* and *nerves* are the terminal branches of the posterior tibial artery and tibial nerve which divide deep to the flexor retinaculum. These vessels and nerves lie between the first and second layers of muscles. The medial plantar nerve supplies the abductor hallucis (S2, 3) and the flexor digitorum brevis (S2, 3) and then passes forwards towards the big toe. The lateral plantar nerve runs laterally and forwards deep to the flexor digitorum brevis and supplies the abductor digiti minimi (S2, 3).

The muscles of the first layer perform the movements which their names suggest and by their contraction assist in maintaining the longitudinal arches of the foot.

The second layer of muscles (figure 267(b))

It is simpler to regard this layer as being formed by the *tendons* of the *flexor hallucis longus* and *flexor digitorum longus*, together with the muscles associated with the tendons of the latter — the *flexor (digitorum) accessorius* and the *lumbricals*. The *flexor accessorius* is attached to the inferior surface of the calcaneus in front of the calcanean tuberosity and to its lateral surface. The muscle runs forwards and is attached to the lateral border of the tendon of the flexor digitorum longus. Its nerve supply is from the lateral plantar nerve (S2, 3). Its contraction straightens the oblique pull of the long tendons to the lateral four toes and it has been suggested that it maintains the action of the flexor digitorum longus when the muscle in the back of the calf relaxes.

There are four *lumbrical muscles*, numbered from the medial side. The first is attached to the medial side of the long flexor tendon to the second toe, and the remaining three to the adjacent sides of the four flexor tendons. The lumbricals pass forwards, wind round the medial side of the second to the fifth toes and each becomes attached to the dorsal digital expansion of its own toe.

The first lumbrical is supplied by the medial plantar nerve (S2, 3) and the second to the fourth by the lateral plantar nerve (S2, 3). The lumbrical muscles assist in plantar flexion at the metatarsophalangeal joints and dorsiflexion at the interphalangeal joints.

The third layer of muscles (figure 267(c))

These include the *flexor hallucis brevis*, *flexor digiti minimi brevis* and *adductor hallucis*. They are all in the forefoot, that is distal to the talus and calcaneus. The *flexor hallucis brevis* rather unexpectedly arises from the cuboid and lateral cuneiform bones and passing forwards divides into two parts which end in tendons. Each contains a sesamoid bone. One tendon is attached to the lateral side of the base of the proximal phalanx of the big toe with the adductor hallucis and the other to the medial side with the abductor hallucis. The muscle is supplied by the medial plantar nerve (S2, 3). Its action is to flex the proximal phalanx at the metatarsophalangeal joint of the big toe.

The *flexor digiti minimi brevis* is attached proximally to the base of the fifth metatarsal bone and distally to the lateral side of the base of the proximal phalanx with the abductor digiti minimi.

The muscle is supplied by the lateral plantar nerve (S2, 3) and acts as a flexor of the proximal phalanx at the metatarsophalangeal joint of the little toe.

The *adductor hallucis* has two heads, an *oblique* from the plantar surface of the bases of the middle three metatarsal bones, and a *transverse* head from the plantar ligaments of the metatarsophalangeal joints of the lateral three toes. The oblique head passes forwards and medially and the transverse head medially to join the lateral part of the flexor hallucis brevis and its sesamoid bone. The muscle is supplied by the lateral plantar nerve (S2, 3). In addition to pulling the big toe towards the second toe this muscle is regarded as an important structure in the maintenance of the transverse arch of the foot.

The fourth layer of muscles (figure 267(d))

In this plane of the sole of the foot the *tendon* of the *tibialis posterior* sends its several slips to the tarsal and metatarsal bones (p. 469) and the *tendon* of the *peroneus longus* lies in the groove on the plantar surface of the cuboid and passes medially to the medial cuneiform and first metatarsal bones (p. 466). Deep to these are the *plantar interossei*, of which there are three. The first is attached to the medial side of the shaft of the third metatarsal and passes to the medial side of the proximal phalanx of the third toe. The second and third plantar interossei have similar attachments to the fourth and fifth metatarsals and proximal phalanges of the fourth and fifth toes. There are four *dorsal interossei*. Each lies between adjacent metatarsals and is attached to the neighbouring shafts of these bones. The first dorsal interosseus is attached distally to the medial side of the proximal phalanx of the second toe. The second, third and fourth are attached to the lateral side of the proximal phalanx of the second, third and fourth toes respectively. All the interossei have extensions into the dorsal digital expansion of the toe with which each is associated.

The interossei are supplied by the lateral plantar nerve (S2, 3). The action of these muscles is related to the long axis of the second toe in a manner similar to the way in which the action of the interossei

of the hand are related to its middle digit. The plantar interossei of the sole adduct the third, fourth and fifth toes towards the second toe and the dorsal interossei abduct the second, third and fourth toes away from the long axis of the second toe.

The *lateral plantar artery* and *nerve* having reached the lateral side of the sole by passing between the first and second layers pass medially between the third and fourth layers.

The Nerves and Vessels of the Sole (figure 268)

These are the terminal branches of the tibial nerve and posterior tibial artery which divide deep to the flexor retinaculum and enter the sole deep to the abductor hallucis.

The Medial Plantar Nerve. This nerve runs forwards on the lateral side of the artery between the abductor hallucis and flexor digitorum brevis and supplies these two muscles, the flexor hallucis brevis and first lumbrical. The nerve also gives off digital branches to the medial side of the big toe and the adjacent sides of the first, second, third and fourth toes. These branches also innervate the nailbeds on the dorsal surface of the toes. The distribution of the medial plantar nerve, both muscular and cutaneous, has been compared with that of the median nerve in the hand (p. 396).

The Lateral Plantar Nerve. This nerve is lateral to the artery as they pass forwards and laterally between the flexor digitorum and flexor accessorius (between the first and second layers of muscles). It supplies the flexor accessorius and abductor digiti minimi and divides into superficial and deep branches. The deep branch passes medially deep to the adductor hallucis. The two branches supply the rest of the muscles of the sole — the remaining three lumbricals, all the interossei, the flexor digiti minimi brevis and adductor hallucis. The super-

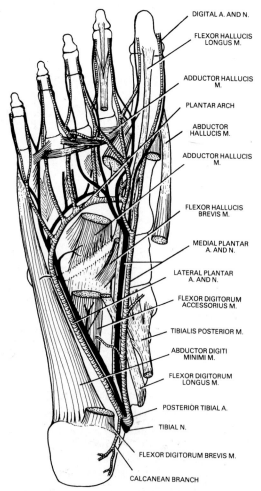

DIGITAL A. AND N.

FLEXOR HALLUCIS LONGUS M.

ADDUCTOR HALLUCIS M.

PLANTAR ARCH

ABDUCTOR HALLUCIS M.

ADDUCTOR HALLUCIS M.

FLEXOR HALLUCIS BREVIS M.

MEDIAL PLANTAR A. AND N.

LATERAL PLANTAR A. AND N.

FLEXOR DIGITORUM ACCESSORIUS M.

TIBIALIS POSTERIOR M.

ABDUCTOR DIGITI MINIMI M.

FLEXOR DIGITORUM LONGUS M.

POSTERIOR TIBIAL A.

TIBIAL N.

FLEXOR DIGITORUM BREVIS M.

CALCANEAN BRANCH

Figure 268   The arteries and nerves of the sole of the foot.

ficial branch gives off digital branches to the lateral side of the little toe and the adjacent sides of the fourth and fifth toes. The distribution of the lateral plantar nerve has been compared with that of the ulnar nerve in the hand (p. 396).

The Medial and Lateral Plantar Arteries. The *medial plantar artery* accompanies the medial plantar nerve which lies lateral to it. The artery gives off digital branches which run with the digital branches of the medial plantar nerve. The *lateral plantar artery* runs laterally and distally with the lateral plantar nerve on its lateral side and from the lateral border of the foot passes medially with the deep branch of that nerve forming the *plantar arterial arch* which is completed by the terminal part of the dorsalis pedis artery from the dorsal aspect of the foot. The plantar arch gives off metatarsal branches which divide and form digital branches. The metatarsal arteries give off proximal and distal perforating branches which pass dorsally in the metatarsal spaces to anastomose with the dorsal metatarsal arteries.

The Plantar Veins. The veins of the sole correspond with the arteries, digital veins forming metatarsal veins which form a plantar venous arch. The medial and lateral plantar veins drain this arch and unite deep to the flexor retinaculum to form the posterior tibial veins.

39

The Tibiofibular and Ankle Joints and the Joints of the Foot. The Arches of the Foot

The Tibiofibular Joints (figures 259(a), 269(a))

Unlike the radius and ulna, the fibula and tibia articulate with each other in such a way that no active movement between the two bones is possible. The *superior tibiofibular joint* is between the head of the fibula and the inferior surface of the lateral condyle of the tibia. It is a synovial joint of the plane type and has no special features except a thickening of the fibrous capsule anteriorly and posteriorly.

The shafts of the tibia and fibula are joined by an *interosseous membrane* which is attached to the

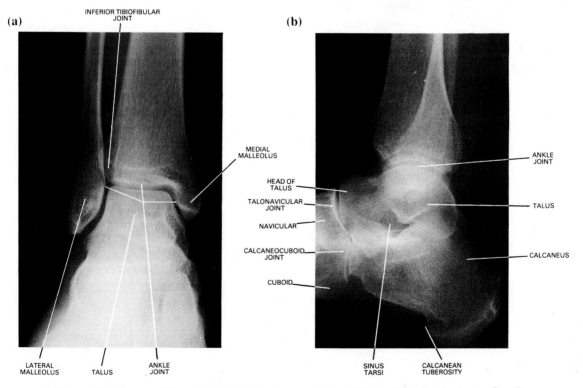

(a)

INFERIOR TIBIOFIBULAR JOINT

MEDIAL MALLEOLUS

LATERAL MALLEOLUS   TALUS   ANKLE JOINT

(b)

ANKLE JOINT

HEAD OF TALUS

TALONAVICULAR JOINT

NAVICULAR

TALUS

CALCANEOCUBOID JOINT

CALCANEUS

CUBOID

SINUS TARSI   CALCANEAN TUBEROSITY

Figure 269 X-rays of the ankle joint: (a) anteroposterior; (b) lateral (the foot is plantar flexed).

interosseous borders of the two bones. The fibres of the membrane pass downwards and laterally from the tibia to the fibula. The anterior tibial vessels pass through an opening in the upper part of the membrane and inferiorly the membrane is continuous with the interosseous ligament of the inferior tibiofibular joint. Several of the anterior and posterior muscles of the leg are attached to the surfaces of the membrane.

The *inferior tibiofibular joint* (figure 269(a)) is between the rough triangular area above the articular facet on the medial side of the lower end of the fibula and the concave fibular notch on the lateral side of the lower end of the tibia. It is a fibrous joint and the adjacent articulating surfaces of the tibia and fibula are joined by an *interosseous ligament*. The superficial parts of the two bones are united posteriorly by the *posterior tibiofibular ligament*, the lowest and deepest part of which forms the *inferior transverse tibiofibular ligament* (figure 270(c)). This ligament is attached laterally to the malleolar fossa of the fibula and medially to the posterior border of the articular area of the lower end of the tibia. The deep surface of the ligament forms part of the articulating socket for the talus at the ankle joint. The inferior tibiofibular joint provides a strong union between the lower ends of the two bones and contributes to the rigid mortice in which the talus moves at the ankle joint.

The Ankle (Talocrural) Joint (figures 269, 270)

This is a synovial joint of the hinge type. The distal surface of the tibia, the lateral surface of its malleolus and the medial surface of the fibular malleolus form an articular surface for the superior, medial and lateral surfaces of the talus. The superior articular surface of the talus, wider in front than behind, is convex anteroposteriorly and concave from side to side. The lateral articular area for the fibula is triangular and extends further distally than the medial articular area for the tibia. *The transverse line of the joint is about 1 cm above the tip of the medial malleolus, which lies about 1 cm*

above the tip of the lateral malleolus. The *fibrous capsule* is attached proximally to the edge of the articular area formed by the tibia and fibula and distally to the edges of the corresponding articular areas of the talus, except anteriorly where the capsule is attached to the neck of the talus in front of the articular edge. The *synovial membrane* lines the capsule and is reflected anteriorly on to the neck of the talus as far as the articular cartilage. The synovial membrane may extend a short distance upwards between the tibia and fibula.

The fibrous capsule is thin in front and behind, and posteriorly fuses with the inferior transverse tibiofibular ligament which forms part of the superior articular surface. On the medial side the *deltoid* or *medial ligament* is attached above to the medial malleolus (figure 270(b)). It has superficial fibres which are attached inferiorly to the sustentaculum tali, the plantar calcaneonavicular ligament and the tuberosity of the navicular. Its deep fibres are attached to the medial surface of the talus in front of and behind its medial articular area. The *lateral ligament*, a term which has been apparently abandoned, has three parts which are separate structures (figure 270(a), (c)). The *anterior talofibular ligament* passes downwards and forwards from the lateral malleolus to the lateral part of the neck of the talus. The *calcaneofibular ligament* passes downwards and backwards from the lateral malleolus to the lateral surface of the calcaneus. The *posterior talofibular ligament* is posterior to the joint and is attached to the malleolar fossa and the lateral tubercle of the talus.

The *structures related* to the front of the ankle joint are the tendons of the long extensors and the tibialis anterior, the anterior tibial vessels and the deep peroneal nerve as they pass from the leg to the foot (figure 270(d)). Posteriorly and medially the tendons of the long flexors and tibialis posterior, the posterior tibial vessels and tibial nerve pass deep to the flexor retinaculum into the sole. The peronei are posterolateral behind the fibular malleolus.

The *arteries* to the joint come from the malleolar branches of the anterior tibial and peroneal arteries and the *nerves* are branches of both the deep peroneal and the tibial nerves.

The terminology for the *movements* at the ankle

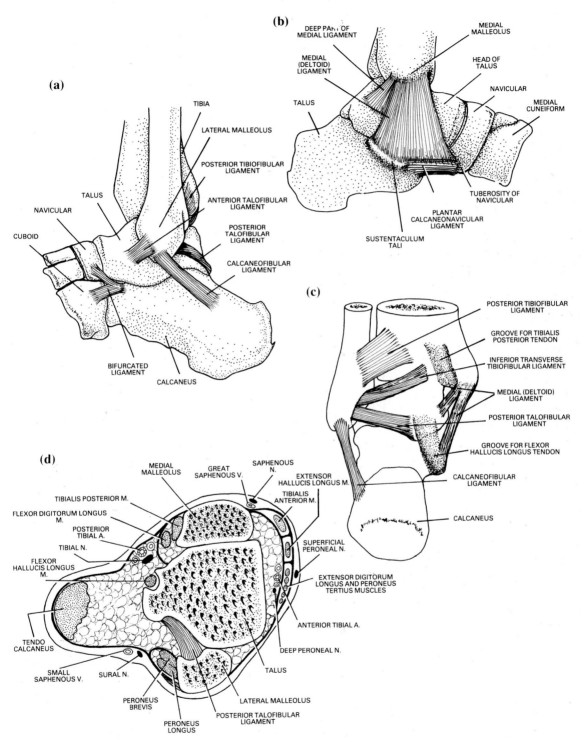

Figure 270 **The ankle joint: (a) the lateral ligaments; (b) the medial ligament; (c) the posterior ligaments; (d) the structures related to the joint.**

joint is difficult and the least confusing terms are *plantar flexion* for downward movement of the foot and *dorsiflexion* for upward movement. According to the names of the muscles downward movement is *flexion* and upward movement is *extension* but unfortunately these terms have had their meanings reversed and they should be avoided. (Physiologists in describing the movements of the lower limb in the spinal animal refer to flexion at the hip, knee and ankle, and flexion at the ankle refers to the upward movement of the foot. This is one of the reasons for the confusion.) Dorsiflexion from the neutral position, in which the foot is more or less at right angles to the leg, is less than plantar flexion and the total range of movement is about 90°. The wider part of the talus is wedged between the malleoli in dorsiflexion and causes the fibula to rotate laterally about a longitudinal axis through about 5°. Dorsiflexion is produced by the tibialis anterior, extensor hallucis longus, extensor digitorum longus and peroneus tertius supplied by the deep peroneal nerve (L4, 5). Plantar flexion is due mainly to the gastrocnemius and soleus supplied by the tibial nerve (S1, 2). The deep muscles of the calf may assist in plantar flexing of the foot. Dorsiflexion is limited by the tension of the calf muscles, the posterior fibres of the deltoid ligament and the calcaneofibular ligament, and the wedging of the talus between the malleoli. Plantar flexion is limited by tension in the anterior muscles, the anterior part of the deltoid ligament and the anterior talofibular ligament.

Injuries in the region of the ankle joint are common, although dislocation is rare. If the foot is turned excessively inwards or outwards it is not uncommon for the lateral or medial ligaments to be torn, resulting in a sprained ankle. The same movements can also cause a fracture of the malleoli. If the body falls to the right with the weight on the right foot which is fixed on the ground, the lateral malleolus may be fractured about 5 cm above its tip and the medial deltoid ligament torn. However, this ligament is very strong and more commonly the ligament remains intact and the tip of the medial malleolus is torn off the tibia. This fracture is named after Sir Percivall Pott and is usually referred to as an *abduction–eversion fracture* (Sir Percivall Pott, 1714–88, English

surgeon). The opposite movement of the body results in an *adduction–inversion fracture* (a *reverse Pott's fracture*). If the interosseous ligament is also torn, the whole ankle joint is disrupted and a fracture-dislocation occurs.

The Joints of the Foot (figure 260)

There are numerous synovial joints in the foot between the tarsal bones (*intertarsal joints*), the tarsal bones and the bases of the metatarsals (*tarsometatarsal joints*) and between the bases of the metatarsals (*intermetatarsal joints*), but only a few of them require a detailed description. Many of the joints are of the plane, synovial variety without any special features — the bones are held together by a fibrous capsule lined by synovial membrane and the cartilage-covered joint surfaces are more or less flat, so that there is little movement between the bones. Because weight is transmitted downwards and the foot is arched, the capsule is thickened on the plantar aspect of the joints and, if there are interosseous ligaments, they are nearer the concavity of the sole. There is one strong ligament on the dorsum of the foot, the *bifurcate ligament*, which is attached proximally to the dorsal surface of the calcaneus anterolateral to the head of the talus, and distally, after bifurcating, to the dorsal surfaces of the cuboid and the navicular (figure 270(a)).

In the sole there are three strong ligaments, two lateral and one medial (figure 271). On the lateral side the *long plantar ligament* is attached to the inferior surface of the calcaneus in front of the tuberosity and passes forwards over the groove in the cuboid for the tendon of the peroneus longus to become attached to the bases of the lateral metatarsal bones. The deep fibres of the ligament are attached to the edges of the groove and convert it into a tunnel for the tendon. The second ligament is the *plantar calcaneocuboid* (*short plantar*) *ligament*, which is attached to the plantar surface of the calcaneus in front of the attachment of the long plantar ligament and passes forwards to the cuboid behind the groove for the tendon. On the medial side of the sole the *plantar calcaneonavicular* (*spring*) *ligament* is attached posteriorly to the

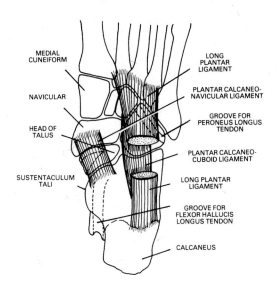

Figure 271   The main plantar ligaments of the foot.

sustentaculum tali and anteriorly to the plantar surface of the navicular. This ligament supports the head of the talus and its dorsal surface articulates directly with the head. The deltoid ligament is attached to its medial border. The tendons of the tibialis anterior and the long flexors lie on the plantar surface of the ligament as they pass into the foot. All three ligaments support the arches of the foot.

The joints associated with inversion and eversion (figure 272)

Inversion is a movement of the foot on the talus so that the sole is turned inwards and the medial border of the foot moves medially as well as upwards. *Eversion* is the opposite movement in which the sole is turned outwards and the lateral border moves laterally as well as upwards. Rotation of the foot about a longitudinal axis cannot occur without some adduction, as in inversion, or abduction, as in eversion, because of the arrangement of the joints involved. The movement takes place about an oblique axis through the superomedial part of the neck of the talus, the sinus tarsi and the inferolateral aspect of the calcaneus.

The joints involved are the *posterior talocalcanean (subtalar)* and the *talocalcaneonavicular.* The *subtalar joint* is behind the sinus tarsi and is formed by the concave facet on the inferior surface of the talus and the convex posterior facet on the back of the upper surface of the calcaneus. The fibrous capsule is attached to the edges of the joint and is thickened laterally and medially. The *interosseous ligament*, in the sinus tarsi, attached above to the sulcus tali and below to the sulcus calcanei, is an important ligament holding the two bones together and acting as the fulcrum round which the movements between the bones occur.

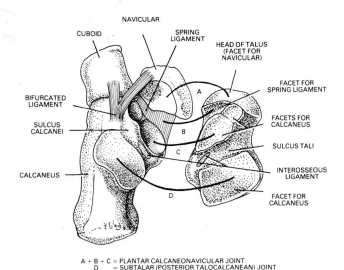

A + B + C = PLANTAR CALCANEONAVICULAR JOINT
D   = SUBTALAR (POSTERIOR TALOCALCANEAN) JOINT

Figure 272   The main joints involved in inversion and eversion.

The *talocalcaneonavicular joint* is between the head of the talus and the socket formed by the middle and anterior facets on the upper surface of the calcaneus, the superior surface of the spring ligament and the proximal surface of the navicular. As compared with the rest of the intertarsal joints, the reciprocal surfaces of the talocalcaneonavicular and subtalar joints are markedly curved. This accounts for the considerable range of movement between the foot and the talus. The muscles producing inversion are the tibialis anterior supplied by the deep peroneal nerve (L4, 5) and the tibialis posterior supplied by the tibial nerve (L4, 5). The evertors are the peroneus longus and peroneus brevis, supplied by the superficial peroneal nerve (L5, S1) and the peroneus tertius, supplied by the deep peroneal nerve (L4, 5).

Inversion is maximal with the foot plantar flexed. This is due to the disposition of the ligaments of the ankle, especially the calcaneofibular, which is slack in plantar flexion. The deltoid ligament is slackened if the foot is inverted. Eversion is maximal with the foot dorsiflexed because the deltoid ligament is slack and the movement relaxes the calcaneofibular ligament. It is suggested that inversion is increased when the foot is plantar flexed because the narrow part of the talus lies between the malleoli and allows the talus to move. This would equally apply to eversion but eversion is almost impossible if the foot is fully plantar flexed.

The *transverse tarsal joint* is the name given to the combined *talonavicular* and *calcaneocuboid joints* (figure 260). Movements of the foot distal to these joints, that is movements on the talus and calcaneus, can occur. This may add to the range of inversion and eversion but the contribution is limited. The bifurcated ligament prevents this to some extent. Evidence that inversion and eversion do not occur at the transverse tarsal joint was obtained following operative fusion of the talus and calcaneus for the treatment of fractures of the calcaneus involving its articular facets for the talus. (These fractures occur as a result of landing on one's heels when falling from a height.) It was found that the movements of inversion and eversion were very severely limited following the operation. Plantar flexion and dorsiflexion also take place at the transverse tarsal joint, normally to a very limited extent, but plantar flexion can be marked in the feet of female ballet dancers when they dance on points.

The terms *supination* and *pronation* of the foot are used as synonyms for inversion and eversion but it has been suggested that these terms should refer to the movements of the forefoot on the talus and calcaneus when the foot is on the ground. Supination occurs when the lateral border of the anterior part of the foot moves downwards and pronation when the medial border of the forefoot is brought downwards towards the ground.

The metatarsophalangeal and interphalangeal joints

The *metatarsophalangeal joints* are ellipsoid synovial joints between the convex heads of the metatarsals and the concave bases of the proximal phalanges. The articular area on the head extends on to its plantar surface. In the lateral four toes the fibrous capsule is thickened on the plantar surface where it is grooved for the flexor tendons. In the big toe the plantar surface of the metatarsal head has a ridge. On either side of the ridge there is a groove for the sesamoid bone embedded in the capsule which is fused with the two parts of the flexor hallucis brevis. The plantar parts of the capsules are joined on each side to the *deep transverse metatarsal ligaments* which separate the interossei from the lumbrical muscles and digital vessels and nerves. There are also *collateral ligaments* passing from the sides of the metatarsal heads to the sides of the bases of the phalanges in a plantar direction.

The main movements at these joints are plantar flexion and dorsiflexion. Dorsiflexion is much more extensive than plantar flexion, as can be seen when moving the toes with the foot off the ground. Dorsiflexion is important in the end of the stance phase of walking before the toes leave the ground. In this movement of the body on to the toes, the weight of the body produces the movement. Active dorsiflexion at the metatarsophalangeal joints is due to the long extensor muscles and the extensor digitorum brevis supplied by the deep peroneal nerve (L4, 5). Active plantar flexion is brought about by the long flexor muscles in the calf and the short flexor muscles in the sole supplied by the tibial nerve or its terminal branches (S2, 3).

To a limited extent the toes can be moved away from and towards a longitudinal line represented by the second toe. Movement of the toes away from the second toe is called *abduction* and the opposite movement, *adduction*. The big toe is abducted by the abductor hallucis and adducted by the adductor hallucis. The third and fourth toes are abducted by the third and fourth dorsal interosseus respectively and the little toe by the abductor digiti minimi. The second toe is abducted to either side by the first and second dorsal interossei. Each of the lateral three toes is adducted by a plantar interosseus. All the muscles are supplied by S2, 3 through the lateral plantar nerve except the abductor hallucis which is supplied by the medial plantar nerve.

The structure of the *interphalangeal joints*, proximal and distal in the lateral four toes, is similar to that of the interphalangeal joints of the digits of the hand. The heads of the proximal and middle phalanges have two small condyles which articulate with the reciprocally curved bases of the middle and distal phalanges. The interphalangeal joint of the big toe has similar articular areas. Dorsiflexion and plantar flexion occur at these joints but plantar flexion is much more extensive than dorsiflexion. The muscles involved in these movements are the same as those producing the movements at the metatarsophalangeal joints. The long flexors act at both interphalangeal joints, and the short flexors at only the proximal joints.

The amount of dorsiflexion at the interphalangeal joint of the big toe is in inverse proportion to dorsiflexion at the metatarsophalangeal joint. Although the total dorsiflexion at both joints is normally more than adequate for the purposes of walking, a condition called *hallux rigidus* occurs in which there is limited dorsiflexion at the metatarsophalangeal joint. Walking is painful and treatment without surgery is difficult.

The limited plantar flexion at the metatarsophalangeal joint and limited dorsiflexion at the interphalangeal joint of the big toe are utilised by female ballet dancers who, when on points, put their big toes in this position so that the joints lock

and the ligaments carry the weight of the body. The form of the ballet shoe assists the dancer to maintain this position and she is discouraged from going on to points without wearing a shoe.

The Arches of the Foot (figures 273, 274)

Examination of the normal foot or a footprint or an X-ray of the foot confirms that the sole is arched anteroposteriorly and transversely and is best described as forming half a dome. The anteroposterior curve is most marked on the medial side, is called the *medial longitudinal arch* and consists of the calcaneus behind, the talus at the summit and the navicular, cuneiforms and medial three metatarsals in front. The heads of the metatarsals are regarded as the anterior end of the arch. The *lateral longitudinal arch*, much flatter than the medial, lies along the lateral border of the foot and is almost non-existent. It is formed posteriorly by the calcaneus and anteriorly by the cuboid and the

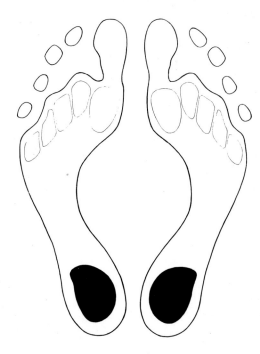

Figure 273   A footprint (reproduced from *Hamilton's Textbook of Human Anatomy* **by courtesy of the Editors and The Macmillan Press).**

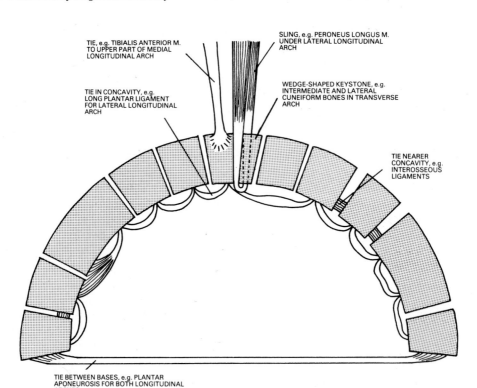

TIE, e.g. TIBIALIS ANTERIOR M.
TO UPPER PART OF MEDIAL
LONGITUDINAL ARCH

SLING, e.g. PERONEUS LONGUS M.
UNDER LATERAL LONGITUDINAL
ARCH

TIE IN CONCAVITY, e.g.
LONG PLANTAR LIGAMENT
FOR LATERAL LONGITUDINAL
ARCH

WEDGE-SHAPED KEYSTONE, e.g.
INTERMEDIATE AND LATERAL
CUNEIFORM BONES IN TRANSVERSE
ARCH

TIE NEARER
CONCAVITY, e.g.
INTEROSSEOUS
LIGAMENTS

TIE BETWEEN BASES, e.g. PLANTAR
APONEUROSIS FOR BOTH LONGITUDINAL
ARCHES

Figure 274   Structures which can maintain a segmented arch.

lateral two metatarsals, the heads of which form the anterior base of the arch. The *transverse arch*, really half an arch, is most marked in the region of the cuneiforms and the bases of the metatarsals.

An arch can be maintained in a number of ways, as is indicated in figure 274. Some of these are present in the arches of the human foot but the importance of each is difficult to determine. In the medial and lateral longitudinal arches the bases are tied by the plantar aponeurosis and the short superficial muscles (the abductor hallucis, flexor digitorum brevis and abductor hallucis). The bones forming the arches are held together by the plantar ligaments, especially the spring ligament on the medial side and the long plantar and plantar calcaneocuboid ligaments on the lateral side. The interosseous ligaments being nearer the concavity of the arch also prevent its collapse. The muscles which pull the medial border of the foot upwards (the tibialis anterior and tibialis posterior) assist in maintaining the arch and the long flexor muscles whose tendons pass into the foot under the medial

longitudinal arch act like a sling. The peroneus brevis and tertius pull upwards on the lateral longitudinal arch and the peroneus longus acts like a sling in support of this arch. The shape of the bones does not contribute to the maintenance of either of the longitudinal arches. On the contrary the weight of the body drives the head of the talus downwards between the calcaneus and navicular and this is resisted by the spring ligament.

In the case of the transverse arch the wedge-shape of the intermediate and lateral cuneiforms and the adjacent bases of the second, third and fourth metatarsals helps to maintain the arch. The tendon of the peroneus longus, the oblique head of the adductor hallucis and the flexor hallucis brevis assist in holding the bases of the arch together. In the region of the heads of the metatarsals the transverse metatarsal ligaments prevent spreading of the bones and the transverse head of the adductor hallucis can pull the ends of the arch together. The mobility of this part of the foot can be easily demonstrated by pressing the heads of the first and fifth metatarsals together and producing a transverse arch.

An arched foot has the advantage of being resilient in response to the varying forces to which it is subjected. Segmentation of the arch permits movements, for example the movements of inversion and eversion and to some extent the movement of the forefoot (the part anterior to the transverse tarsal joint), on the remainder of the foot, but segmentation produces instability. Several mechanisms, as outlined above, are involved in coping with this and of these the muscles are regarded as being the most important. There is considerable evidence, however, that, when standing, the muscles related to the arches are inactive and that the ligaments maintain the arched form of the foot. In activities, such as walking and running, the muscles to some extent play a part in supporting the arches.

Weakness of the muscles causes a condition called *falling arches* and this suggests that the ligaments alone cannot support the arches over a long period of time. The usual treatment for falling arches, which is a painful condition, consists of exercising the muscles. The problem is that the treatment is not always successful and the patient, against the doctor's advice, buys an arched metal support which is placed in the shoe. This support relieves the pain but does not restore the muscle function. Falling arches may be progressive and fully developed *fallen arches* are painless. This is accompanied by changes in the shape of the bones and stretched ligaments. The foot, however, does not function well when walking long distances or running.

One must be aware of the apparent flat foot in young children in whom the normal concavity of the medial side of the foot is reduced or absent because of underlying fat. A very mobile foot, seen in ballet dancers and certain individuals with a more than normal range of movement between the bones of the foot, often appears flat when standing but becomes arched when not weight-bearing.

40

The Venous and Lymphatic Drainage and Segmental Innervation

Most of these topics have been described in the various regions of the limb and will therefore be dealt with briefly.

The Venous Drainage of the Lower Limb

The main veins of the lower limb are *superficial* and *deep*. The important *superficial veins* are the *great* (*long*) and *small* (*short*) *saphenous veins* (p. 426 and p. 439). They both begin in the region of the ankle by draining the *dorsal venous plexus* and for most of their course are subcutaneous. The dorsal venous plexus receives *dorsal digital* and *metatarsal veins*. The great saphenous vein is on the medial side and passes upwards in front of the medial malleolus on the medial side of the leg behind the saphenous nerve. The vein curves behind the medial condyles of the tibia and femur, continues upwards in the thigh and passes through the saphenous opening in the deep fascia to end in the femoral vein.

The great saphenous vein receives a number of tributaries in the leg and thigh, and also before it passes through the saphenous opening, but the communications with the deep veins, particularly in the leg, are the most important. The great saphenous vein has a number of valves. There are also valves in the communicating veins and these are arranged so that blood passes from the superficial to the deep veins. If these valves become incompetent, muscle contraction pushes blood from the deep veins into the superficial which become vari-

cose. The valves in the great saphenous vein also become incompetent. The venous return from the lower limb is due largely to the contraction of the muscles, especially the soleus, whose function in this respect is referred to as the *soleal pump*.

The *small saphenous vein* passes behind the lateral malleolus, runs upwards in the back of the leg medial to the sural nerve and pierces the deep fascia to join the popliteal vein. It has tributaries from the lateral side of the leg and communicates superficially with the great saphenous vein and also with the deep veins of the leg.

The *deep veins* of the limb begin as *digital* and *metatarsal veins* in the sole and form *lateral* and *medial plantar veins*. These form the *posterior tibial veins* (p. 470). The *anterior tibial veins* are described on p. 465. These pass through the upper part of the interosseous membrane and join the posterior tibial veins to form the *popliteal vein*. The popliteal vein (p. 440) passes upwards through the popliteal fossa and through the opening in the adductor magnus to form the *femoral vein* (p. 431). The femoral vein becomes the *external iliac vein* deep to the inguinal ligament. Its main tributary is the *deep femoral vein* (*vena profunda femoris*).

The Lymphatic Drainage of the Lower Limb

The tissues of the lower limb are drained by either *subcutaneous lymphatic vessels* or *deep vessels* related to the main blood vessels. Most of the superficial vessels accompany the great saphenous vein and end in the *superficial inguinal lymph nodes* (figure 100) which lie near the termination of that vein (p. 427). The vessels from the lateral side of the foot and leg follow the small saphenous vein and end in the *popliteal lymph nodes* (p. 440). The efferents from these nodes accompany the main vessels and drain into the *deep inguinal lymph nodes* which are near the femoral vein or in the femoral canal. The superficial vessels from the buttock drain into the lateral nodes of the *upper superficial inguinal nodes*.

The vessels from the deep tissues of the lower limb end in the deep inguinal nodes near the femoral vein. The deep tissues of the buttock drain into the *internal iliac nodes* in the pelvis.

The arrangement of the *inguinal lymph nodes* is described on p. 427. There are *superficial* nodes

arranged as an *upper* group inferior and parallel to the inguinal ligament and a *lower* group along the termination of the great saphenous vein. The medial nodes of the upper group receive lymphatic vessels from the external genitalia, the lower part of the vagina and anal canal and the anterior abdominal wall below the level of the umbilicus. The superficial nodes drain into the external iliac nodes and are also connected to the deep nodes whose efferent vessels pass to the external iliac nodes.

The Segmental Innervation of the Lower Limb

The segmental innervation of the skin of the lower limb and the nerves involved are summarised in

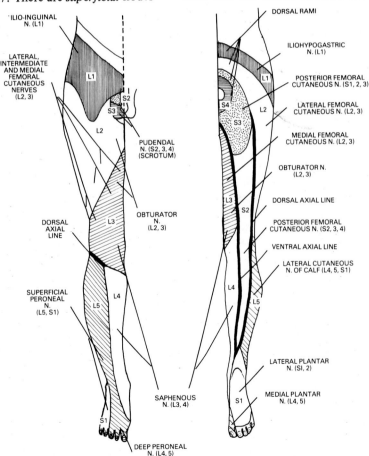

Figure 275   The segmental innervation of the skin of the lower limb.

figure 275 and have been described on pp. 426 and 462.

The *axial lines* indicating where adjacent areas of skin are not supplied by consecutive segments of the spinal cord are also shown. Again it must be emphasised that there is considerable overlap between consecutive segments so that division of a single spinal nerve does not result in complete anaesthesia of the segment of skin supplied by it. Lesions of the lumbar and sacral spinal nerves result in sensory disturbances such as pain or sensory loss along their distribution, depending on whether the nerve is pressed on or interrupted.

To some extent there is a segmental innervation related to the movements at the joints of the limb. *Flexion and adduction at the hip* are carried out by muscles supplied by the second, third and fourth lumbar spinal nerves and *extension and abduction* by muscles supplied by the fifth lumbar and first sacral nerves. Probably the fourth lumbar and second sacral nerves are also involved. *Lateral rotation* involves the fifth lumbar and first sacral nerves. *Medial rotation* involves the same nerves (fifth lumbar and first sacral) if the main muscles used are the tensor fasciae latae and the gluteus minimus. The idea that the iliacus and psoas are medial rotators (L2, 3) dies hard. *Flexion at the knee* by the hamstring muscles involves the fifth lumbar and first and second sacral nerves and *extension* by the quadriceps the second, third and fourth lumbar nerves. *Dorsiflexion at the ankle* is produced by the anterior muscles of the leg, which are supplied by the fourth and fifth lumbar nerves. *Plantar flexion* involves the first and second sacral nerves. *Inversion* is related to the same spinal cord segments as those involved in dorsiflexion and *eversion* to the fifth lumbar and first sacral segments. Table 7 summarises the spinal cord segments related to the different movements.

Table 7

Joint	Movements	Segmental innervation
Hip	Flexion and adduction	L2, 3, 4
	Extension and abduction	L4, 5, S1, 2
	Lateral rotation	L(4) 5, S1 (2)
	Medial rotation	L5, S1, 2
Knee	Flexion	L5, S1
	Extension	L2, 3, 4
Ankle	Dorsiflexion	L4, 5
	Plantar flexion	S1, 2
Subtalar	Inversion	L4, 5
	Eversion	L5, S1

41

Human Posture and Walking

The way in which human beings stand and walk is unique in the animal kingdom. The unique features are the plantigrade position of the foot (the foot is everted so that the sole is on the ground), the foot is more or less at right angles to the leg, and the leg, thigh and trunk are vertically above each other. This bipedal gait is also unique among the primates, whose mode of progression involves the use of one or both of the forelimbs. The exception is the orang-utan which occasionally straightens the trunk on the thigh and the thigh on the leg and shuffles forward for a few paces before returning to its normal flexed position. Birds are bipedal but their knees and thighs are markedly flexed and a large part of their trunk projects backwards behind the pelvis. The attainment of the upright posture and bipedal locomotion is regarded as of great evolutionary significance because it freed the fore-limbs and enabled them to be used for new and more skilled activities (with the consequent de-velopment of the forebrain). Although in this chapter only what may be called the peripheral mechanisms are considered, it must be stressed that the characteristic posture and locomotion of human beings require the coordinating mechanisms organised by the nervous system.

Posture

Although posture is not static and there is an in-finite number of postures, it is accepted that what is called the standing-at-ease position can be used as a basic posture for description and study. In this position the weight is born evenly on both feet, which are about 25 cm apart and slightly turned out, the upper limbs are at the sides of the trunk or behind the back with the hands held lightly together, and the subject stands comfortably and looks straight ahead. In this position it has been shown that the centre of gravity of the body is situated about 55 per cent of the individual's height above the ground (this is about the level of the second sacral vertebra). A vertical line through this centre of gravity is about 3 cm in front of this vertebra and bisects the base on which we stand, namely the heel and the heads of the metatarsals. The relation of this line to the foot can be deter-mined by the method illustrated in figure 276. This line (*the line of gravity* or *weight*) always falls in front of the ankle joints (figure 276), usually slightly in front of the transverse axes of the knee joints and behind the transverse axes of the hip joints. When standing in this position there is a backward and forward swaying movement and although the swaying is not visible to the naked eye it is easily demonstrated by placing a light on the top of the head and watching the light moving on the ceiling. There is a slight side to side swaying more difficult to demonstrate. The anteroposterior swaying is not sufficient to bring the line of weight behind the ankle joints. The maintenance of the upright position in relation to the ankle joints requires continuous but variable contraction of the calf muscles, especially the soleus. The anterior muscles of the leg show no activity in the standing-at-ease position.

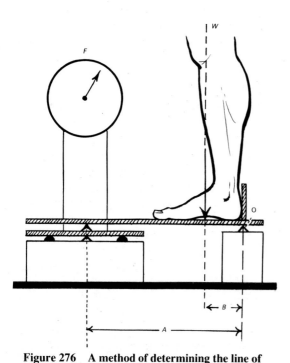

Figure 276   A method of determining the line of gravity (or weight) in relation to the heel and heads of the metatarsals. W (weight of body) $\times B = F$ (weight recorded) $\times A$ (these are equal moments about O).
Therefore $B = (F/W) \times A$ (where B and A are measured in centimetres and F and W in kilograms body weight) (reproduced from *Hamilton's Textbook of Human Anatomy* by courtesy of the Editors and The Macmillan Press).

The vertical line through the centre of gravity of that part of the body above the knee joints passes in front of the transverse axis through these joints. Maintenance of the erect posture at the knees in most people does not require any muscle activity because the ligaments at the back of the knee joints can resist the forward bending of the body at these joints without contraction of the posterior muscles, mainly the hamstrings. Exaggerated backward swaying immediately results in contraction of the quadriceps femoris muscle and forward swaying in contraction of the hamstrings, although the latter muscles may be acting primarily at the hip joints. The posterior ligaments of the knee joint can resist a force of more than 700 kg (the average weight of an adult is 70–75 kg).

The line of gravity of that part of the body above the hip joints passes behind their transverse axis so that the body is falling backwards. This is prevented by the powerful ligaments anterior to the hip joints. In most subjects there is no evidence of contraction of either the anterior or posterior muscles of the hip joints. If, however, the centre of gravity is moved forwards either by swaying forwards or by raising the upper limbs at the shoulder joints the hamstrings become active. Their contraction in this situation prevents further extension at the knee joints as well as flexion at the hip joints.

In relation to the vertebral column the situation is more complex because the column does not act as a single entity. It appears that, as seen from the back, the part of the body above the lumbar concavity is falling backwards and the part above the lower part of the thoracic convexity is falling forwards. The head is falling forwards on the cervical vertebrae. Consequently there is usually no activity of the back muscles in the lumbar concavity, marked activity in those of the lower part of the thoracic convexity and slight activity in the muscles of the back of the neck. The last observation is unexpected, but an examination of the position and plane of the joints between the articular processes of the cervical vertebrae and their posterior ligaments, especially the ligamentum nuchae, indicates a built-in mechanical stability which resists the flexion force of the weight of the head.

That the upright posture is maintained with very little muscle activity is borne out by the observation that there is only a small increase in oxygen consumption in the upright position as compared with that observed when lying down. It appears that ligaments bear weight without the assistance of muscles, but normally they do so for only short periods of time. Most people (about two-thirds), when standing without the opportunity to lean or sit on some stable structure, shift their weight from one limb to the other. In this posture the same muscle groups in the supporting limb are active as when standing with the weight on both limbs.

Certain muscles are labelled *postural muscles* — the erector spinae of the vertebral column, the gluteus maximus, the quadriceps femoris and the soleus. Not all of them, however, are active in the upright posture, but all of them are required to attain this posture if not to maintain it. They are used, for example, when standing up from the sitting position or maintaining a flexed position of the trunk, thigh and leg.

The terms *good* and *bad posture* are often used with the implication that the way in which one stands can have a considerable influence on causing certain ailments not only of the locomotor system, for example backache, but also of the internal organs. The evidence for this is non-existent, although one cannot deny that a certain mode of standing (or sitting) is aesthetically more pleasing than another. The terms *good* and *bad* and even *upright* in relation to posture seem to take on a moral connotation, an aspect of the subject which need not be discussed here.

Locomotion

The lower limbs are used in different ways to move the body from one place to another, as in walking, running and jumping. An analysis of each of these activities would be too lengthy as well as too difficult, but some of the basic features of what is involved in walking on a flat surface are given. If asked to walk at their own rate healthy adults have a step frequency of about 50–55 per minute. This number refers to the complete cycle which one limb undergoes and is often doubled to correspond with the number of times each limb is in contact with the ground in 1 min. It is accepted that one step should be regarded as beginning when the heel strikes the ground and ending when it strikes the ground again (*heel strike to heel strike*) and it is assumed that the other limb goes through the same cycle (figure 277). The foot is on the ground for about three-fifths of the cycle (*stance phase*) and off the ground for about two-fifths (*swing phase*). Both feet are on the ground twice in each step for about one-fifth of the cycle (*double stance phase*). The stance phase may be subdivided into early, middle and late stages to distinguish the period during which the heel, whole foot and toes are on the ground. *Toe off* refers to the end of the stance phase as the foot leaves the ground. These different phases can be determined by means of cinephotography, which can also be used to analyse in a fairly crude way the movements taking place at the hip, knee and ankle joints. It is not possible to determine which muscles are active during the various stages of a step because many of the movements are due to the passive swing of the whole limb or its segments. Electromyography, the recording of the electrical changes in a muscle when it contracts, has been used to determine which muscles are active during walking.

From heel strike to heel strike the limb moves from flexion to extension at the hip (stance phase, figure 277, 0–14) and then into flexion again (swing phase, figure 277, 15–0). The gluteus maximus and hamstrings are active during the early part of the stance phase until the body is vertically over the supporting limb. They then relax and the remainder of the extension movement is due to the forward momentum of the body. During the whole of the stance phase the gluteus medius on the supporting side contracts to prevent the body falling on to the unsupported side. Since extension at the hip is limited, the length of the step is increased by rotating the pelvis about a vertical axis at the hip by means of the gluteus medius and minimus. This is often called a medial rotation of the pelvis because the movement of the body on the lower limb at the hip is similar to medial rotation of the free lower limb at the hip joint. During the swing phase, the flexor muscles of the thigh at the hip are active in the first half of the movement but the rest of the movement is due to the forward momentum of the limb. During this phase there is some lateral rotation at the hip joint and the outer part of the heel strikes the ground first, an observation which can be confirmed by examining the wear on the heel of any pair of shoes.

At the knee, there is extension during the whole of the stance phase (figure 277, 0–14), except for the very early stages when the knee is slightly flexed. The quadriceps femoris is therefore contracted during the early stage of the stance phase. Before the end of the stance phase and during the first half of the swing phase the leg is flexed at the knee (figure 277, 12–16) and in the second part of this phase the leg is extended (figure 277, 17–0). In about 50 per cent of individuals the flexion is not accompanied by contraction of the hamstrings and the movement is due to the leg swinging backwards without muscle contraction. Similarly, ex-

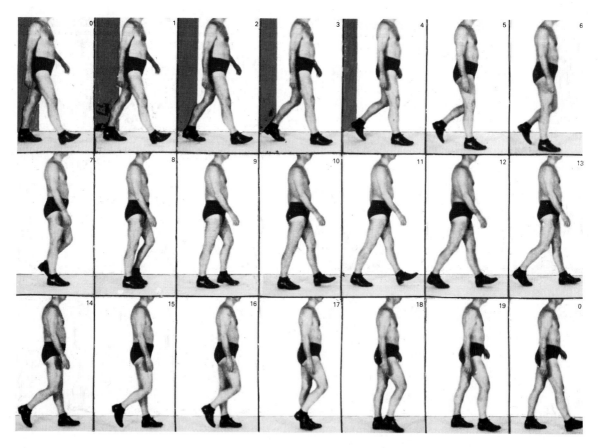

Figure 277   The stages of one step (reproduced from *Hamilton's Textbook of Human Anatomy* **by courtesy of the Editors and The Macmillan Press).**

tension is not due to the action of the quadriceps femoris, which contracts only at the end of the swing phase. The hamstrings contract at the end of the swing phase probably to control the forward swing of the leg due to its own momentum.

At the ankle the foot is dorsiflexed at heel strike (figure 277, 0) and is then plantar flexed (figure 277, 1–3). When the foot is flat on the ground the body moves over the foot, the equivalent of dorsiflexion at the ankle (figure 277, 4–12). As the foot moves on to the toes at the end of the stance phase it becomes plantar flexed (figure 277, 13–14). During the swing phase (figure 277, 15–0) the foot is dorsiflexed to assist the limb to clear the ground (flexion at the hip and knee are the other means whereby this is achieved). There is considerable variation in the way in which the

tibialis anterior contracts just before, during and at the end of the swing phase. In the majority of individuals it contracts twice, just before heel strike and at the beginning of the swing phase. In these people during the swing phase the muscle relaxes. This is contrary to the accepted idea that the tibialis anterior contracts during the whole of the swing phase so that the foot does not drop. In some people the contraction of the tibialis anterior is reduced and in others maintained throughout the swing phase. The contraction of the tibialis anterior persists into the early part of the stance phase when the foot is inverted. The soleus and gastrocnemius are active during most of the stance phase (figure 277, 5–12) and it has always been maintained that this is essential for the propulsive movement imparted to the body as it rises on to the toes. There is no doubt that the calf muscles provide this propulsive movement in running and a powerful lifting movement in walking up stairs but in normal walking on flat ground these muscles may control the falling forwards of the body after the centre of gravity moves in front of the supporting foot.

The erector spinae on both sides contract twice in each step corresponding with the alternate heel strike of the right and left limbs. This contraction prevents the flexion of the trunk which would occur due to its forward momentum as the body decelerates on heel strike.

In order to minimise the amount of energy used in walking, the body utilises the vertical movements of its centre of gravity during the stance phase. The velocity of the centre of gravity also changes as the body decelerates and accelerates. One may regard the lower limb during the single part of the stance phase (figure 277, 4–10) as a lever with the fulcrum at the ankle. The centre of gravity is at its lowest at heel strike and is then raised during extension at the hip by the kinetic energy of the body assisted by the gluteus maximus and hamstrings.

During the swing phase (figure 277, 14–0) the lower limb may be regarded as a pendulum swinging forwards at the hip from extension to flexion. Similarly the flexion and extension at the knee are pendulum-like movements of the leg on the thigh.

The nailing or pinning of fractures of the neck of the femur and more recently the replacement of the hip joint by a prosthesis have made it necessary to know the forces acting on the bones forming the hip joint, so that the materials which are used do not break. It has been estimated that the head and neck of the femur are subjected at heel strike to a force five or six times the body weight. In addition there are also the problems of the reaction of the materials used to the milieu in which they are placed and also their effects on the surrounding tissues.

Index